Practical Geriatric Oncology

The risk of cancer increases with age, and the number of older adults seeking treatment is increasing dramatically in line with the aging population. The care of older patients differs from that of younger adults because of differences in the biology of the tumor, age-related differences in host physiology, comorbidity burden, and psychosocial issues that might have an effect on the efficacy and side effects of cancer therapy. *Practical Geriatric Oncology* is comprehensive and evidence based. It synthesizes the growing literature in this field and provides practical guidelines on the care of older adults with cancer.

The book covers patient assessment, management of solid tumors and hematologic malignancies, the impact of age on the pharmacology of cancer therapy, surgical oncology and radiation oncology in the older adult, symptom management, and supportive care.

In addition to serving as core reading for oncologists and hematologists, the book will be useful for other health care professionals who provide oncology care, including surgeons, radiation oncologists, palliative care doctors, primary care providers, geriatricians, and nurses.

Arti Hurria, MD, is a geriatrician and oncologist who focuses on the care of older patients with cancer. She completed a geriatric fellowship in the Harvard Geriatric Fellowship Program, followed by a hematology-oncology fellowship at Memorial Sloan-Kettering Cancer Center (MSKCC). She subsequently joined the faculty at MSKCC, where she served as coprincipal investigator on the institutional NIH P20 grant "Development of an Aging and Cancer Center at MSKCC." In fall 2006, Dr. Hurria joined the City of Hope as director of the Cancer and Aging Research Program. Dr. Hurria is a cadre member of the Cancer and Leukemia Group B, Cancer in the Elderly Committee, and is a recipient of the Paul Beeson Career Development Award in Aging Research and the American Society of Clinical Oncology–Association of Specialty Professors Junior Development Award in Geriatric Oncology. She serves on the editorial board of the *Journal of the National Cancer Institute, Journal of Clinical Oncology*, and *Oncologist*.

Harvey Jay Cohen, MD, is a geriatrician and oncologist who serves in several professional roles at Duke University Medical Center, including as Walter Kempner Professor and chair for the Department of Medicine, director of the Center for the Study of Aging and Human Development, and principal investigator of the Duke Claude Pepper Older Americans Independence Center. In addition, he chairs the Cancer in the Elderly Committee for Cancer and Leukemia Group B and cochairs the Task Force on Cancer and Aging for the American Association for Cancer Research. He is a member of the International Association of Gerontology Governing Board and a past president of the American Geriatrics Society, the Gerontological Society of America, and the International Society of Geriatric Oncology. Dr. Cohen is on the editorial board of the *Journal of Gerontology: Medical Sciences*, the international editorial board of *Geriatrics and Gerontology International*, and the editorial advisory board of both the *American Journal of Geriatric Pharmacotherapy* and *Research News*. He has received the Joseph T. Freeman Award and the Kent Award from the Gerontological Society of America, the Jahnigen Memorial Award from the American Geriatrics Society, the Paul Calabresi Award from the International Society of Geriatric Oncology, and the Clinically Based Research Mentoring Award from Duke University.

Practical Geriatric Oncology

Edited by

Arti Hurria
City of Hope

Harvey Jay Cohen
Duke University Medical Center

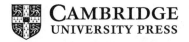

CAMBRIDGE UNIVERSITY PRESS
Cambridge, New York, Melbourne, Madrid, Cape Town, Singapore,
São Paulo, Delhi, Dubai, Tokyo, Mexico City

Cambridge University Press
32 Avenue of the Americas, New York, NY 10013-2473, USA

www.cambridge.org
Information on this title: www.cambridge.org/9780521513197

First published 2010

Printed in the United States of America

*A catalog record for this publication is available from the
British Library.*

Library of Congress Cataloging in Publication Data

Practical geriatric oncology / edited by Arti Hurria,
Harvey Jay Cohen.
   p. ; cm.
Includes bibliographical references and index.
ISBN 978-0-521-51319-7 (hardback)
1. Geriatric oncology. I. Hurria, Arti. II. Cohen, Harvey Jay.
III. Title.
[DNLM: 1. Neoplasms–therapy. 2. Aged. QZ 266]
RC281.A34P73 2010
618.97′6994–dc22
                                                    2010028275

ISBN 978-0-521-51319-7 Hardback

Contents

v

Contributors

Matti S. Aapro, MD
Institut Multidisciplinaire d'Oncologie
Clinique de Genolier
Genolier, Switzerland

Amy P. Abernethy, MD
Division of Medical Oncology
Duke University Medical Center
Durham, NC, USA

Andrew S. Artz, MD, MS
Section of Hematology/Oncology
University of Chicago Medical Center
Chicago, IL, USA

Riccardo A. Audisio, MD, FRCS
Division of Surgery and Oncology
University of Liverpool, St. Helens Hospital
St. Helens, UK

Dean F. Bajorin, MD
Genitourinary Oncology Service
Memorial Sloan-Kettering Cancer Center
New York, NY, USA

Chandra P. Belani, MD
Penn State Cancer Institute
Hershey Medical Center
Hershey, PA, USA

Stephen A. Bernard, MD
Division of Hematology and Oncology
University of North Carolina School of Medicine
Chapel Hill, NC, USA

Anne H. Blaes, MD
Division of Hematology/Oncology/Transplant
University of Minnesota
Minneapolis, MN, USA

Tami Borneman, RN, MSN, CNS
Division of Nursing Research and Education
Department of Population Sciences
City of Hope National Medical Center
Duarte, CA, USA

Leslie J. Bryan, MD
Center for Palliative Care
Department of Medicine
Duke University Medical Center
Durham, NC, USA

Thomas A. Buchholz, MD
Department of Radiation Oncology
University of Texas M. D. Anderson
  Cancer Center
Houston, TX, USA

Gurkamal Chatta, MD
Division of Hematology/Oncology
University of Pittsburgh
VA Pittsburgh Healthcare System
Pittsburgh, PA, USA

Harvey Jay Cohen, MD
Department of Medicine and Center for the
  Study of Aging
Duke University Medical Center
Durham, NC, USA

Jeffrey Crawford, MD
Division of Medical Oncology
Duke University Medical Center
Durham, NC, USA

David C. Currow, BMed, MPH, FRACP
Department of Palliative and Supportive Services
Division of Medicine, Flinders University
Bedford Park, Australia

Leona Downey, MD
Division of Hematology/Oncology
University of Arizona
Tucson, AZ, USA

Katja Elbert-Avila, MD
Center for Palliative Care
Department of Medicine
Duke University Medical Center
Durham, NC, USA

William B. Ershler, MD
Clinical Research Branch
National Institute on Aging
Baltimore, MD, USA

Betty Ferrell, RN, PhD, FAAN
Division of Nursing Research and Education
Department of Population Sciences
City of Hope National Medical Center
Duarte, CA, USA

Anthony Nicholas Galanos, MD
Center for Palliative Care
Department of Medicine
Duke University Medical Center
Durham, NC, USA

Suzanne Gaskell, MBChB
Department of Medicine
Southport and Formby Hospital NHS Trust
Southport, UK

Richard M. Goldberg, MD
Division of Hematology and Oncology
University of North Carolina School of Medicine
Chapel Hill, NC, USA

Vivian von Gruenigen, MD
Division of Gynecologic Oncology
University Hospitals Case Medical Center
Cleveland, OH, USA

Mark T. Hegel, PhD
Department of Psychiatry
Norris Cotton Cancer Center
Dartmouth-Hitchcock Medical Center
Lebanon, NH, USA

Arti Hurria, MD
Cancer and Aging Research Program
City of Hope National Medical Center
Duarte, CA, USA

Jimmy Hwang, MD
Division of Hematology/Oncology
Lombardi Comprehensive Cancer Center
Washington, DC, USA

Harman P. Kaur, MD
James Wilmot Cancer Center
University of Rochester
Rochester, NY, USA

Gretchen Kimmick, MD
Division of Hematology/Oncology
Duke University Medical Center
Durham, NC, USA

Julie A. Kish, MD, FACP
Division of Head and Neck Oncology
H. Lee Moffitt Cancer Center and
    Research Institute
Tampa, FL, USA

Heidi D. Klepin, MD, MS
Section of Hematology and Oncology
Wake Forest University School of Medicine
Winston-Salem, NC, USA

Alice B. Kornblith, PhD
Psycho-oncology Research Program
Division of Women's Cancers
Dana-Farber Cancer Institute
Boston, MA, USA

Amrita Y. Krishnan, MD, FACP
Division of Hematology and
    Hematopoietic Cell Transplantation
City of Hope National Medical Center
Duarte, CA, USA

Siri R. Kristjansson, MD
Department of Geriatric Medicine
Ullevaal University Hospital
Oslo, Norway

Nicole M. Kuderer, MD
Health Services, Effectiveness and Outcomes
    Research Program, Division of Medical
    Oncology
Duke University School of Medicine and Duke
    Comprehensive Cancer Center
Durham, NC, USA

Stuart M. Lichtman, MD
Clinical Geriatrics Program
Memorial Sloan-Kettering Cancer Center
Commack and New York, NY, USA

Andrew Liman, MD
Division of Hematology/Oncology
University of Pittsburgh
VA Pittsburgh Healthcare System
Pittsburgh, PA, USA

Gijsberta van Londen, MS, MD
University of Pittsburgh School of Medicine
Pittsburgh, PA, USA

Gary H. Lyman, MD, MPH, FRCPEd
Health Services, Effectiveness and Outcomes
    Research Program, Division of Medical
    Oncology
Duke University School of Medicine and Duke
    Comprehensive Cancer Center
Durham, NC, USA

Matthew S. McKinney, MD
Department of Internal Medicine
Duke University Medical Center
Durham, NC, USA

Matthew I. Milowsky, MD
Genitourinary Oncology Service
Memorial Sloan-Kettering Cancer Center
New York, NY, USA

Supriya Gupta Mohile, MD, MS
James Wilmot Cancer Center
University of Rochester
Rochester, NY, USA

Joseph O. Moore, MD
Divisions of Medical Oncology and Geriatrics
Duke University Medical Center
Durham, NC, USA

Vicki A. Morrison, MD
Sections of Hematology/Oncology and Infectious
    Disease
VA Medical Center
Minneapolis, MN, USA

Christian J. Nelson, PhD
Department of Psychiatry and
    Behavioral Sciences
Memorial Sloan-Kettering Cancer Center
New York, NY, USA

Bayard L. Powell, MD
Section of Hematology and Oncology
Wake Forest University School of Medicine
Winston-Salem, NC, USA

Laura Raftery, MD
Division of Hematology and Oncology
University of North Carolina School of Medicine
Chapel Hill, NC, USA

Suresh S. Ramalingam, MD
Winship Cancer Institute
Emory University
Atlanta, GA, USA

Arati V. Rao, MD
Division of Medical Oncology and Cell Therapy
Durham VA Medical Center
Durham, NC, USA

Andrew J. Roth, MD
Department of Psychiatry and
    Behavioral Sciences
Memorial Sloan-Kettering Cancer Center
New York, NY, USA

Michelle Shayne, MD
Division of Hematology/Oncology
University of Rochester School of Medicine
    and Dentistry
Rochester, NY, USA

Shahzad Siddique, MD
Division of Hematology/Oncology
Lombardi Comprehensive Cancer Center
Washington, DC, USA

Benjamin D. Smith, MD
Radiation Oncology Flight USAF Medical Corps
Lackland, TX
Department of Radiation Oncology
The University of Texas M. D. Anderson Cancer
    Center
Houston, TX, USA

Richard Maury Stone, MD
Adult Acute Leukemia Program
Dana-Farber Cancer Institute
Boston, MA, USA

Stephanie Studenski, MD, MPH
Department of Medicine (Geriatrics)
University of Pittsburgh School of Medicine
Pittsburgh, PA, USA

Virginia Sun, RN, MSN, ANP
Division of Nursing Research and Education
Department of Population Sciences
City of Hope National Medical Center
Duarte, CA, USA

William P. Tew, MD
Gynecologic Medical Oncology Service
Department of Medicine
Memorial Sloan-Kettering Cancer Center
New York, NY, USA

Tiffany A. Traina, MD
Breast Cancer Medicine Service
Memorial Sloan-Kettering Cancer Center
New York, NY, USA

Martha Wadleigh, MD
Dana-Farber Cancer Institute
Boston, MA, USA

Mark I. Weinberger, PhD
Department of Psychiatry
Weill Cornell Medical College
White Plains, NY, USA

Jane L. Wheeler, MSPH
Division of Medical Oncology
Duke University Medical Center
Durham, NC, USA

Hans Wildiers, MD, PhD
Department of General Medical Oncology
University Hospital Gasthuisberg
Leuven, Belgium

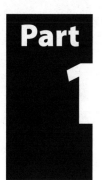

Part 1

Key principles in geriatric oncology

Geriatric assessment for the older adult with cancer

Arti Hurria and Harvey Jay Cohen

A. The aging population in the United States and worldwide

Cancer is a disease associated with aging. Approximately 60 percent of cancer incidence and 70 percent of cancer mortality occur in adults over 65 years of age.[1] Thus the principles of geriatrics are particularly relevant in today's field of oncology and will become even more relevant as the United States and world populations age.

Over the past century, the population of individuals aged 65 years and older grew 10-fold, increasing from 3.1 million in the year 1900 to 35 million in the year 2000.[2] This number is expected to double from 2000 to 2030 as baby boomers (born 1946–1964) start to reach age 65 in 2011 (Figure 1.1). By 2030, the population aged 65 years and older is projected to account for almost 20 percent (about one in five) of the population.[2] Along with the increase in the absolute number of older adults, life expectancy is also increasing. From 1900 to 2000, average life expectancy in the United States increased from 47.3 to 76.9 years.[2] After 2030, the population considered to be the oldest old (aged 85 years and older) is projected to increase rapidly as baby boomers reach and surpass age 85.

Similar growth in the older population is projected to take place across the world. In the year 2000, 420 million people worldwide were aged 65 years and older, representing 7 percent of the world's population. By 2030, this number is projected to double to 974 million, with 70 percent of older adults living in developing countries.[2] Projecting into the future, from 2100 to 2300, centenarians (those individuals aged 100 years and older) will be the fastest-growing segment of the world population, with an anticipated ninefold increase in the proportion of the population (from 0.2% to 1.8%).[3]

B. The association between cancer and aging

There is a clear association between cancer and aging. The median age of diagnosis for cancer at all sites is 67 years, and the median age of death from cancer is 73.[1] The aging of the U.S. population is expected to contribute to an increase in the total yearly cancer incidence. From 2010 to 2030, the total projected cancer incidence will increase 45 percent, from 1.6 million in 2010 to 2.3 million in 2030. This increase in cancer incidence is largely driven by an increase in cancer in older adults, with a 67 percent increase in cancer incidence anticipated in older adults compared with an 11 percent increase in younger adults.[4] The most common tumor types are those that commonly afflict older adults, that is, prostate, lung, and colon cancer in men and breast, lung, and colorectal cancer in women.[a]

C. Assessment of older adults with cancer: Integrating geriatric principles in oncology care

Along with increasing age comes a decrease in physiologic reserve; however, the aging process is heterogeneous and occurs at variable rates among different individuals. It is not uncommon to hear doctors use the phrase "a young 80-year-old" or "an old 80-year-old," implying that factors other than age affect an older adult's life expectancy. Understanding or objectively quantifying an older adult's physiologic reserve is an important part of cancer treatment planning; however, there is no standard tool in oncology practice with which to assess an older adult's physiologic reserve, to help weigh the risks and benefits of cancer treatment in the older adult, or to guide treatment decisions.

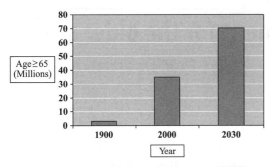

Figure 1.1 Projected aging of the U.S. population.[147,148]

Geriatricians utilize a geriatric assessment in daily practice as a means of quantifying this physiologic reserve and understanding other factors that may influence overall survival, treatment tolerance, quality of life, or the ability to follow a particular treatment regimen. This assessment consists of an evaluation of functional status, comorbid medical conditions, cognitive function, psychological state, and social support. The patient's medication list is also reviewed to assess for drug interactions, duplicative or unnecessary medications, or drugs that may carry a high risk of side effects, with consideration for discontinuing or substituting medications, as appropriate. Consideration is also given to the potential costs of therapy and the ability of the patient to absorb these costs.

One could argue that a geriatric assessment should be performed for patients of all ages, particularly those with cancer who are facing a possibly life-threatening diagnosis that may require intensive treatment. However, this assessment is especially valuable in the older adult, in whom competing causes of morbidity and mortality (often a consequence of the aging process) need to be considered to weigh the potential risks and benefits of cancer therapy. In this chapter, we review the domains of a geriatric assessment with a particular focus on emerging literature that demonstrates how an understanding of these factors can support the care of an older adult with cancer. In addition, we summarize the evolving literature that demonstrates the potential for incorporating physiologic and biologic markers as part of the assessment.

C.1. The role of functional status

The Karnofsky Performance Status (KPS) Scale[5] or the Eastern Cooperative Oncology Group (ECOG) Performance Status Scale is commonly used to assess functional status in oncology practice.[6] These scales predict morbidity and mortality among all patients with cancer. They require the clinician to choose a number that best describes the patient's overall level of daily activity and need for assistance with activities. A decline in function is presumed to be secondary to the cancer and cancer-associated symptoms. This assessment does not provide a detailed evaluation of the patient's baseline level of functioning (regardless of cancer), which is an independent predictor of morbidity and mortality in the geriatric population.

A geriatrician's evaluation of functional status includes an assessment of the patient's ability to complete activities of daily living (ADLs) and instrumental activities of daily living (IADLs). ADLs are basic self-care skills required to maintain independence in the home such as the ability to bathe, dress, toilet, transfer, maintain continence, and feed oneself.[7] IADLs are skills required to maintain independence in the community such as the ability to take transportation, prepare meals, use the telephone, manage money, take medications, shop, travel, and do laundry.[8] Requiring assistance with ADLs or IADLs is associated with an increased risk of further functional decline,[9] hospitalization,[9] nursing home placement,[9] cognitive dysfunction,[10] and mortality.[9,11–14] In a study of community-dwelling older adults, patients who required assistance in one or more ADLs had 9.8-fold (95% confidence interval [CI] 6.8–14.0) increased odds of being institutionalized and 8.6-fold (95% CI 6.6–11.0) increased odds of mortality within 6 years. Patients who required assistance with one or more IADLs had 6.7-fold (95% CI 4.6–9.6) increased odds of being institutionalized and 6.6-fold (95% CI 5.1–8.6) increased odds of mortality within 6 years (Figure 1.2).[9]

Measuring functional status at only one time point provides just part of the picture. Emerging reports demonstrate the importance of functional transitions and the impact of transient versus permanent declines in physical function. Declines in physical function that persist over time are associated with poorer overall survival and increased risk of subsequent hospitalization compared with declines in physical function that are transient.[9,15] These data suggest that measuring functional status at several points along the trajectory of illness provides valuable prognostic information.

From a practical standpoint, assessing an older adult's functional status should be an integral part of determining whether the patient can comply

Figure 1.2 Association of baseline functional status with risk of institutionalization and mortality 6 years later.[9] Abbreviations are as follows: CI, confidence interval; IADL, instrumental activities of daily living; ADL, activities of daily living.

Baseline: Functional Status (1984)	Follow-up (1990)	
	Risk of Institutionalization Odds Ratio (95% CI)	Risk of Mortality Odds Ratio (95% CI)
IADL Assistance	6.7 (4.6, 9.6)	6.6 (5.1, 8.6)
ADL Assistance (Moderate)	9.8 (6.8, 14.0)	8.6 (6.6, 11.0)
ADL Assistance (Severe)	17.0 (9.1, 32.0)	30.0 (18.0, 15.0)

with an oncology treatment plan. For example, when planning a daily radiation schedule, the physician needs to know whether the patient can drive to the appointment or whether he or she has other means of transportation. This is particularly important for the oncology population because a diagnosis of cancer is associated with an increased need for assistance with ADLs and IADLs, and this increased need for assistance continues among cancer survivors (Figure 1.3).[16,17] In studies of older adults with cancer, requiring assistance in ADLs and IADLs is particularly common. For example, in a study of 363 older patients with cancer, 9 percent required assistance with ADLs and 38 percent required assistance with IADLs,[18] despite that all patients had an ECOG performance score of less than 2. In another study of older adults with metastatic breast cancer, 26 percent of patients required assistance with ADLs and 73 percent required assistance with IADLs.[19] The need for assistance with ADLs is even greater among patients who are hospitalized.

For example, in a study of older adults with cancer who were admitted to an acute care for elders unit, 45 percent of patients required assistance with ADLs.[20]

A survey of oncologists and primary care providers demonstrated that health status (functional status plus comorbid conditions) plays a significant role in adjuvant treatment decisions for older adults with breast cancer.[21] Although functional impairment influences treatment decisions and is common among the oncology population, there is no standard tool used in daily practice to determine how functional status affects the risks and benefits of cancer therapy with an older adult and how this unique health status should be integrated into treatment decisions. Emerging data do suggest that the ability to complete IADLs is associated with cancer prognosis and risk of toxicity to chemotherapy. Among older adults with advanced lung cancer, for example, requiring assistance with IADLs and pretreatment quality of life were reported as independent

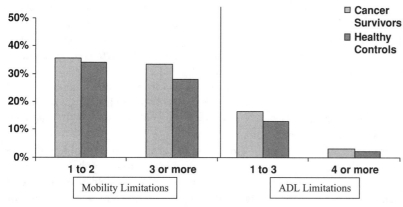

Figure 1.3 More mobility limitations and ADL limitations of cancer survivors.[17]

predictors of median survival.[22] In another study of 63 patients with acute myelogenous leukemia across all ages (range 19–85, median 61), requiring assistance with IADLs, KPS score, and the presence of unfavorable cytogenetics were independent predictors of overall survival.[23]

C.2. Comorbidity

With increasing age, there is an increase in the number of comorbid medical conditions that may have an impact on a patient's risk of morbidity, mortality, and tolerance to cancer therapy. Therefore an integral part of oncology decisions is to decide whether the patient's life expectancy is more likely to be limited by the cancer or another comorbid medical condition, whether a comorbid medical condition will affect treatment tolerance, and what the interactions of the comorbid medical conditions with the patient's cancer will be. Studies in the cancer literature suggest a low correlation between measures of comorbidity and functional status,[24] with each being an independent prognostic factor for overall survival.[25]

Among patients with cancer, comorbid medical conditions influence overall survival. This was illustrated in an observational prospective cohort study of 17,712 patients with a variety of cancers, in which the severity of comorbidity was significantly associated with survival, independent of cancer stage.[26] In another study of patients with early-stage breast cancer, patients with three or more comorbid conditions (out of seven selected comorbid medical conditions) were 20 times more likely to die of a cause other than breast cancer.[27] A similar impact of comorbidity on overall survival was demonstrated in another study of older adults with stage I breast cancer who received tamoxifen and were randomized to postlumpectomy radiation versus no radiation.[28] Whereas radiation decreased the risk of local recurrence, radiation had no impact on overall survival, with most patients dying of another cause. In a study of patients with advanced lung cancer, increased comorbidity (as assessed by the Charlson Comorbidity Index[29]) was associated with poorer overall survival (Figure 1.4).[30]

On the other hand, the risk from cancer might outweigh the risk of dying from another comorbid illness, underscoring the importance of treating an older adult with a cancer that carries a poorer prognosis. This was demonstrated in a study of patients aged 65 years and older with breast cancer (the majority with node-positive dis-

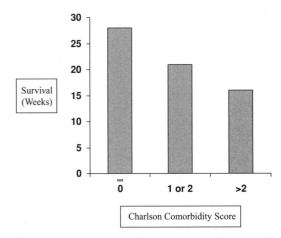

Figure 1.4 Increased comorbidity associated with decreased survival in advanced lung cancer.[30]

ease) who were randomized to a standard adjuvant polychemotherapy regimen versus an experimental arm of oral monochemotherapy to decrease the risk of relapse. With 2.4 years of follow-up, patients who received standard chemotherapy had a statistically significant improvement in overall and disease-free survival. Therefore treatment affected breast cancer–specific mortality within a relatively short period of follow-up, and within this follow-up period, only 2 percent of patients enrolled in the study died of a cause not related to breast cancer or treatment.[31]

Common treatments in the oncology population may exacerbate or unmask comorbid illnesses. For example, steroids are often prescribed as chemotherapy premedications to prevent nausea or an allergic reaction. They may also be included as a part of the cancer treatment regimen such as in the cyclophosphamide, doxorubicin, vincristine, and prednisone (CHOP) regimen for lymphoma. These steroids could exacerbate diabetes or unmask glucose intolerance. In addition, comorbid conditions place the patient at risk for treatment-associated side effects. Taxanes or other neurotoxic drugs can exacerbate underlying neuropathy. A diagnosis of hypertension (present in almost half of all adults aged 70 years or older[32]) is a known risk factor for trastuzumab-associated cardiomyopathy.[33,34] In addition, hypertension is a risk factor for anthracycline-associated cardiomyopathy.

Comorbid medical conditions could influence whether a patient is able to complete a prescribed chemotherapy course. In a study of patients with advanced lung cancer randomized to poly- or single-agent chemotherapy, comorbidity (defined as a Charlson score greater than 2, compared to 2 or less) was associated with increased likelihood of discontinuing treatment.[30] In a study of patients with breast cancer, comorbidity was a better predictor of the toxicity risk from adjuvant chemotherapy than age alone.[35] Comorbid medical conditions also influence cancer prognosis. In a large randomized study of adjuvant chemotherapy for colon cancer, patients with diabetes experienced a significantly higher rate of disease recurrence and overall mortality, independent of predictors for colon cancer recurrence.[36]

Several tools are available to assess the prognostic impact of comorbidity among older adults in general; however, few tools have been developed specifically for older adults with cancer. Piccirillo and colleagues evaluated the prognostic importance of comorbidity among patients with cancer (46.3% aged 65 years or older) using the Adult Comorbidity Evaluation–27, which yields an overall comorbidity level (none, mild, moderate, or severe).[26] This comorbidity level is used to estimate the hazard ratio for overall survival within a variety of tumor types. Other tools evaluate the risk of mortality among all older adults and have included a diagnosis of cancer as one variable in the model. For example, Walter and colleagues developed and validated a prognostic index for 1-year mortality among older adults who have been hospitalized. A diagnosis of cancer (solitary vs. metastatic) was among the six risk factors (male sex, ADL dependency, congestive heart failure, cancer, creatinine value, and albumin level) considered for 1-year mortality.[37] In another index developed by Lee and colleagues, a diagnosis of cancer was 1 of 12 variables (including age, sex, comorbid medical conditions, and functional status) that predicted a 4-year risk of mortality.[38] The Charlson Comorbidity Index ranks and compares comorbid medical conditions that increase the 1-year risk of mortality; it also includes a diagnosis of cancer among the comorbid illnesses included in the index.[39] A Charlson Comorbidity Index that takes into account the impact of age in addition to comorbid conditions is also available.[40]

C.3. Cognition

In the geriatric population, the prevalence of cognitive impairment increases with age and is associated with an increased risk for functional decline and an increased risk of mortality.[41-43] In a study of older adults with chronic medical illnesses (including cancer), the effects on mortality of cognitive impairment and chronic medical illnesses are additive.[44] Patients with cancer may be predisposed to cognitive problems for a variety of reasons, including symptoms, fatigue, pain, and depression.[45] Cognitive problems often go unrecognized. In a study of older adults with cancer admitted to an acute care for elders unit, 27 percent of patients scored above the abnormal range on the short "Blessed Test," while 36 percent of patients did not have delirium or dementia documented in their charts.[20]

Cognitive impairment may lead to a delay in cancer diagnosis and variations in cancer treatment patterns. In a study utilizing the Surveillance, Epidemiology, and End Result (SEER)-Medicare database, patients with colon cancer and dementia were twice as likely to have colon cancer reported after death (on an autopsy or death certificate). Of those who were diagnosed while they were alive, patients with dementia were less likely to obtain a pathologic diagnosis, undergo surgical resection, or receive adjuvant chemotherapy.[46] Cognitive impairment is associated with a lower likelihood of receiving cancer therapy. In a study of older adults with cancer, advanced age and decreased mental status were associated with a decreased likelihood of surgery.[47]

Cancer therapy may be associated with cognitive side effects, which have been described in the breast cancer literature[48-58]; however, few studies have specifically focused on older adults or on patients with baseline cognitive problems.[56,59] Nevertheless, among older adults, the impact of therapy on cognitive or functional status significantly influences the patients' preferences for life-sustaining therapy. This was demonstrated in a study of patients aged 60 years and older who had a limited life expectancy because of cancer or other chronic illness (congestive heart failure or chronic obstructive pulmonary disease). In this survey, patients responded that they would forego a life-sustaining therapy if the outcome was survival but severe cognitive (88.8%) or functional (74.4%) impairment.[60]

Studies of the impact of cancer and/or cancer therapy on cognitive function of cancer survivors have reported conflicting results.[17,61,62] A population-based sample of patients aged 55 years and older demonstrated no difference in self-reported cognitive function in cancer survivors (survived cancer 4 or more years) versus controls.[17] Neuropsychological and radiology studies demonstrate a different result. In a study of twins aged 65 years and older, of which one was a cancer survivor and the other had no history of cancer, the cancer survivor twin was more likely to have cognitive dysfunction than the unaffected twin.[62] Another study of survivors of breast cancer and lymphoma demonstrated that survivors treated with systemic chemotherapy scored lower on neuropsychological tests than survivors who had not received chemotherapy.[61] Furthermore, positron emission tomography scans of the brain in breast cancer survivors 5–10 years after chemotherapy demonstrated altered activity in the frontocortical, cerebellar, and basal ganglia compared with subjects who had not received chemotherapy.[63] Another study of breast cancer survivors demonstrated that those who had received chemotherapy had differences in information processing on electrophysiologic tests.[64]

From a practical standpoint, an assessment of cognitive function is necessary prior to prescription of cancer therapy to ensure that the patient can provide informed consent and understand the risks, benefits, and alternatives of the therapy. The health care team needs to be sure that the patient understands the side effects of therapy and the indications of when to seek help. In addition, with the increase in oral cancer therapies, an assessment of cognitive function is necessary to be sure that the patient will comply with the schedule. Taking too few pills could be ineffective, and in some cases, taking too many pills could be lethal. Enlisting the patient's social support for assistance can be critical to ensuring success of the cancer treatment and minimizing the risk of toxicity.

C.4. Nutritional status

Among community-dwelling older adults, a low body mass index (BMI), weight loss, and weight cycling (loss and subsequent gain or vice versa) increase the risk of mortality.[65,66] In a study of 4,317 nonsmoking men and women aged 65–100 years, there was an inverse relationship between BMI and mortality. Women with a BMI less than 20 were at highest risk for 5-year mortality.[67] A study of 4,714 older adults demonstrated that weight loss of 5 percent or more was associated with an increased risk of mortality.[68] In another study of 247 patients aged 65 years and older, weight loss of more than 4 percent of body weight was an independent predictor of mortality.[66,67]

Weight loss and malnutrition are common among patients with cancer. A study of 3,047 patients enrolled in ECOG protocols demonstrated that weight loss prior to initiation of

chemotherapy varied from 31 percent in patients with favorable non-Hodgkin's lymphoma to 87 percent in patients with gastric cancer. Weight loss was associated with decreased performance status, lower chemotherapy response rates, and decreased median survival.[69] Weight loss prior to diagnosis or treatment has been associated with poor outcomes in multiple tumor types, including an association between weight loss and poorer quality of life.[70,71] Patients with mild cognitive impairment or dementia are at increased risk for malnutrition.[72] As part of a nutritional evaluation, it is important to distinguish whether reversible factors associated with weight loss are present, including difficulty chewing because of poorly fitting dentures or mucositis, inability to shop or cook, or medication side effects. Nutritional intervention should be tailored to the individual patient, depending on the cancer treatment and the patient's clinical condition and nutritional status. The intervention can range from evaluating and treating reversible causes to diet counseling, oral supplementation, or enteral or total parenteral nutrition.[73]

C.5. Psychological state and social support

Depression in older adults is associated with functional decline, increased need for informal caregiving, and increased utilization of health care resources.[74-78] The number of comorbid conditions is associated with an increased risk of depression and anxiety among older adults.[79] Patients with cancer may be at particular risk, secondary to the potentially life-threatening nature of the diagnosis, associated symptomatology, or need for aggressive therapy. A study of 2,924 outpatients with cancer demonstrated that 7.8 percent reported thinking in the past 2 weeks that they would be better off dead or had thoughts of hurting themselves, with risk factors including clinically significant emotional distress ($p < .001$), substantial pain ($p < .001$), and older age ($p = .029$).[80] A case-control study of adults aged 65 years and older with a variety of medical illnesses demonstrated that the only medical illness associated with an increased risk of suicide was cancer (odds ratio 2.3, 95% CI 1.1–4.8). Older adults with concomitant psychiatric disorders, including affective disorder, anxiety/personality disorder, treatment with antidepressants, and treatment with opioid analgesics, were also at an increased risk for suicide.[81]

The psychological impact of cancer may be further heightened by social isolation. Social isolation and loneliness are associated with increased morbidity and mortality in older adults.[82–86] Shifts in the configuration and structure of family networks (such as dissolution of a joint-family living arrangement and geographic dispersion of families) may have an impact on an older adult's available social support during cancer treatment. The presence of social support may play a role in the type of cancer treatment received and the cancer prognosis. A study utilizing the SEER-Medicare database of women aged 65 years and older demonstrated that unmarried women were more likely to be diagnosed with a higher stage of breast cancer, were less likely to receive definitive therapy, and were at an increased risk of death from breast cancer after controlling for cancer stage and size at diagnosis.[87] In addition, a lack of social support can influence a patient's psychological state, as described previously, as can the patient's adherence to medication.[88]

C.6. Performing a geriatric assessment in oncology practice

There are several potential approaches to performing a geriatric assessment in an oncology practice. The approach depends on the goal of the assessment (clinical care vs. research tool) as well as on the time and resources available to perform this assessment and to act on the results. The National Comprehensive Cancer Network practice guideline in *Senior Adult Oncology* outlines a brief approach to a geriatric assessment, including a description of several screening tools for each geriatric assessment domain and potential action based on a "positive" screen.[89] Others have utilized a mailed geriatric assessment that can be completed prior to the office visit and subsequently reviewed by the clinical team.[90,91] A primarily self-administered geriatric assessment for inclusion in cooperative group clinical trials is being evaluated within the Cancer and Leukemia Group B (CALGB).[92]

D. Age-related changes in physiology

Physiologic and biologic predictors of aging and vulnerability among the general geriatric population may be particularly applicable to the oncology population. Either cancer or cancer treatment can be considered a physiological stressor, and age-related diminution in physiologic reserve may affect tolerance to cancer treatment. Furthermore, patients may be affected by physiologic derangements that are distinct from clinically diagnosed conditions. Recognizing that everyone experiences a spectrum of health across multiple domains, the National Institute on Aging Comorbidity Task Force proposed that comorbidity be considered as the total burden of biologic dysfunction, including subclinical dysfunction and physiologic changes as well as clinically diagnosed chronic conditions.[61]

D.1. Age and organ function

Aging is associated with a decline in organ function that occurs at a unique pace in each individual. With increasing age, there is a decrease in cerebral blood flow, loss of neurons, and a decrease in brain weight.[93–95] Age-related neurological changes include a slowing of reaction time and a decrease in the ability to learn or acquire new material; however, delayed recall is preserved.[96–98] Normal age-related neurological changes do not affect usual daily functioning. Aging is also associated with a decrease in both vision and hearing, with the formation of cataracts, presbyopia (impaired ability to focus on near objects), decreased contrast sensitivity, impaired dark vision, and loss of high-frequency hearing.[99] Practical suggestions to compensate for these age-related changes include speaking slowly and clearly, turning toward the patient when speaking, using adequate lighting, and writing instructions in large letters using black ink on white paper to maximize contrast. In addition, removal of cataracts and utilizing glasses or a hearing aid can help with eyesight and hearing.

Cardiovascular changes with aging include arterial stiffening and an increase in systolic blood pressure. While resting heart rate does not change, there is a decrease in the maximum heart rate in response to stress.[100] Similarly, the ejection fraction response to stress is blunted.[101] Aging is associated with changes in pulmonary physiology, including a decrease in FEV1 (forced expiratory volume in 1 second), vital capacity, and diffusing capacity.[102] With increasing age, a change in body composition accompanies a loss of muscle and bone mass.[103] Renal and hepatic mass and blood flow decrease with age. Biopsies of the liver demonstrate a decrease in cytochrome P450 with age[104]; however, aging is not associated with a change in liver function tests. Similarly,

9

age-related decreases in renal function are not evident when checking a serum creatinine alone—measurement of the glomerular filtration rate provides a more accurate estimate of renal function.[105,106] The age-related decrease in glomerular filtration rate is estimated at 0.75 mL/minute/year; however, approximately one-third of all patients will have no change in glomerular filtration rate with aging.[107]

D.2. Age and bone marrow

There is a decrease in bone marrow reserve and an increase in bone marrow fat with age. Although the aged marrow has less proliferative capacity,[108] under steady state conditions, peripheral blood counts remain within normal limits. In the geriatric population, the presence of anemia is associated with an increased risk of morbidity and mortality. For example, in a study of community-dwelling people aged 85 years and older, anemia was an independent predictor of mortality (mortality risk 1.60 [95% CI 1.24–2.06] for women and 2.29 [95% CI 1.60–3.26] for men).[109] In another study of residents in a skilled nursing facility, the presence of anemia was associated with increased risk of hospitalization.[110]

Among older adults with cancer, the age-related decrease in bone marrow reserve is associated with an increased risk of myelosuppression and myelosuppressive-associated complications from chemotherapy.[111,112] In patients receiving adjuvant chemotherapy for breast cancer, Silber and colleagues found that the first-cycle nadir neutrophil count predicted subsequent neutropenia, treatment delays, or dose reduction.[113] Dees and colleagues performed a prospective pharmacologic evaluation of patients receiving adjuvant AC (doxorubicin 60 mg/m^2 IV and cyclophosphamide 600 mg/m^2 IV every 21 days) and demonstrated an age-related decrease in nadir absolute neutrophil count. After four cycles of AC, the mean nadir absolute neutrophil count was significantly lower for patients aged 65 years and older than for those aged less than 65 years ($p = .01$).[114]

For patients with cancer, the presence of anemia is associated with an increased susceptibility to myelosuppression with certain antineoplastic drugs. For example, the epipodophllotoxins, anthracyclines, and camptothecins are heavily bound to red blood cells. With a progressive decrease in hemoglobin, the distribution volume of these drugs increases.[115] In a cohort of older adults receiving adjuvant chemotherapy for breast

cancer, a greater decrease in white blood cell count, absolute neutrophil count, or hemoglobin level from cycle 1 to cycle 2 was associated with increased risks of grade 3 or 4 toxicity, including febrile neutropenia and hospitalization.[116]

D.3. Inflammation, coagulation, and physiologic dysregulation in older adults

It has been hypothesized that aging is associated with a dysregulation in inflammation and coagulation. There is an age-associated increase in levels of pro-inflammatory cytokines such as interleukin-6 (IL-6) and C-reactive protein (CRP).[117–119] Physiologic dysregulation in the domains of inflammation and coagulation has been associated with functional decline and mortality.[120–127] Among 1,723 older persons in the Duke Established Populations for Epidemiologic Studies of the Elderly, those with higher levels of D-dimer and IL-6 at baseline were significantly more likely to subsequently experience functional decline or death.[128] In a prospective longitudinal study of healthy nondisabled older adults, higher circulating levels of IL-6 and CRP were associated with an increased risk of mortality. The joint elevation of both values was associated with a 2.6 times greater mortality compared with lower values of both.[120]

Serum levels of inflammation and coagulation have been associated with poorer physical function and clinical frailty. Serum measures of inflammation (CRP) and coagulation (factor VIII, D-dimer) were associated with clinical frailty among 4,735 community-dwelling adults aged 65 years and older participating in the Cardiovascular Health Study.[126] In a different analysis derived from the same study population, the authors found an inverse relation between inflammation and physical activity.[129] In another study of 880 highly functional older men and women who participated in the MacArthur Studies of Successful Aging, a higher IL-6 and CRP level was associated with poor walking speed and grip strength; however, there was no correlation between these measures and subsequent functional decline over a 7-year period in those who were able to participate in the follow-up physical function testing. Of note, those who died or were unable to undergo testing had higher baseline IL-6 and CRP levels and slower walking speeds.[123] Serum markers of inflammation, especially IL-6 and CRP, are prospectively associated with cognitive decline in well-functioning older adults.[130] Inflammatory markers have also been associated with coronary artery disease,[131] insulin resistance,[117] risk for type 2 diabetes,[132] changes in bone density,[133] and renal insufficiency.[134]

D.4. Inflammation, coagulation, and physiologic dysregulation in patients with cancer

The importance of elevated levels of CRP, IL-6, and D-dimer has also been demonstrated in the oncology literature. Chronic inflammation may produce reactive oxygen species that result in DNA damage, activation of growth factors, and inhibition of apoptosis.[135–137] Increased levels of IL-6 may be associated with a worse prognosis for patients with breast cancer as well as a higher likelihood of metastasis by up-regulating the expression of adhesion molecules on endothelial cells as well as increasing the production of vascular endothelial growth factor (VEGF.)[138] In a study of patients with prostate cancer, elevated levels of IL-6 were seen in patients with clinically evident hormone refractory disease compared with patients who were normal controls or who had prostatitis, benign prostatic hypertrophy, or localized and recurrent disease.[139] Higher IL-6 levels in patients with advanced non-small-cell lung cancer were associated with poorer survival and poorer performance status.[140] Higher preoperative levels of CRP were associated with poorer overall survival in a study of patients with localized renal cancer.[141] In a study of patients with metastatic renal cell cancer, an "inflammation-based prognostic score" consisting of CRP and albumin level demonstrated that an elevated CRP level and low albumin were associated with cancer-specific survival.[142]

Baseline D-dimer levels were a stronger predictor of overall survival and disease progression than CEA levels among patients with metastatic colon cancer.[143] Among patients with operable breast cancer, elevated plasma D-dimer levels were markers of lymphovascular invasion, clinical stage, and lymph node involvement.[144] Some studies have suggested that CRP is associated with cancer risk, although higher levels of CRP were not associated with breast cancer among the 27,000 plus women in the Women's Health Study.[145,146]

In summary, markers of inflammation and coagulation have been associated with an increased risk of mortality and functional decline in the aging population. Emerging data are demonstrating the applicability of these biomarkers in older adults with cancer.

E. Conclusion

The fields of geriatrics and oncology unite through the care of older adults with cancer. Chronological age tells relatively little about an older adult's physiological age. The factors covered in a geriatric assessment measure independent clinical predictors of morbidity and mortality in older adults and hence provide a more comprehensive understanding of an older adult's health status. Understanding age-related changes in physiology and biomarkers of aging also provides insight into the functional age of an older adult. Incorporating this geriatric knowledge into oncology care would facilitate decision making regarding the risks and benefits of cancer therapy, help identify vulnerable older adults at risk for chemotherapy toxicity, and guide rational interventions to decrease risk. The ultimate goal of applying geriatric principles to an aging oncology population is to preserve the function and well-being of older adults with cancer.

Endnote

a. Excludes squamous and basal cell skin cancers and in situ carcinomas except urinary bladder.

References

1. SEER cancer statistics review, 1975–2005. National Cancer Institute Web site. Available at: http://seer.cancer.gov/csr/1975_2005/.

2. He W, Sengupta M, Velkoff V, et al. *U.S. Census Bureau, current population reports, P23-209, 65+ in the United States: 2005*. Washington, DC: U.S. Government Printing Office; 2005.

3. Department of Economic and Social Affairs/Population Division. World population to 2300. United Nations Web site. Available at: http://secint24.un.org/esa/population/publications/longrange2/WorldPop2300final.pdf.

4. Smith BD, Smith GL, Hurria A, et al. Future of cancer incidence in the United States: burdens upon an aging, changing nation. *J Clin Oncol.* 2009;27(17):2758–2765.

5. Karnofsky D, Burchenal J. The clinical evaluation of chemotherapeutic agents in cancer. In: Macleod CM, ed. *Evaluation of Chemotherapeutic Agents*. New York: Columbia University Press; 1948: 191–205.

6. Zubrod C, Schneiderman M, Frei E. Appraisal of methods for the study of chemotherapy of cancer in man: comparative therapeutic trial of nitrogen mustard and triethylene thiophosphoramide. *J Chron Dis.* 1960;11:7–33.

7. Katz S, Ford AB, Moskowitz RW, et al. Studies of illness in the aged. The index of ADL: a standardized measure of biological and psychosocial function. *J Am Med Assoc.* 1963;185:914–919.

8. Lawton MP, Brody EM. Assessment of older people: self-maintaining and instrumental activities of daily living. *Gerontologist.* 1969;9(3):179–186.

9. Mor V, Wilcox V, Rakowski W, et al. Functional transitions among the elderly: patterns, predictors, and related hospital use. *Am J Public Health* 1994;84:1274–1280.

10. Barberger-Gateau P, Fabrigoule C, Helmer C, et al. Functional impairment in instrumental activities of daily living: an early clinical sign of dementia? *J Am Geriatr Soc.* 1999;47(6)(4): 456–462.

11. Reuben DB, Rubenstein LV, Hirsch SH, et al. Value of functional status as a predictor of mortality: results of a prospective study. *Am J Med.* 1992;93:663–669.

12. Ponzetto M, Maero B, Maina P, et al. Risk factors for early and late mortality in hospitalized older patients: the continuing importance of functional status. *J Gerontol A Biol Sci Med Sci.* Series A. 2003;58 (11):1049–1054.

13. Inouye SK, Peduzzi PN, Robison JT, et al. Importance of functional measures in predicting mortality among older hospitalized patients. *J Am Med Assoc.* 1998;279(15):1187–1193.

14. Sleiman I, Rozzini R, Barbisoni P, et al. Functional trajectories during hospitalization: a prognostic sign for elderly patients. *J Gerontol A Biol Sci Med Sci.* Series A. 2009;64(6):659–663.

15. Sleiman I, Rozzini R, Barbisoni P, et al. Functional trajectories during hospitalization: a prognostic sign for elderly patients. *J Gerontol A Biol Sci Med Sci.* Series A. 2009;64(6):659–663.

16. Stafford RS, Cyr PL. The impact of cancer on the physical function of the elderly and their utilization of health care. *Cancer.* 1997;80(10): 1973–1980.

17. Keating NL, Norredam M, Landrum MB, et al. Physical and mental health status of older long-term cancer survivors. *J Am Geriatr Soc.* 2005;53(12):2145–2152.

18. Repetto L, Fratino L, Audisio RA, et al. Comprehensive geriatric assessment adds information to Eastern Cooperative Oncology Group performance status in elderly cancer patients: an Italian Group for Geriatric Oncology Study. *J Clin Oncol.* 2002;20(2):494–502.

19. Del Mastro L, Perrone F, Repetto L, et al. Weekly paclitaxel as first-line chemotherapy in elderly advanced breast cancer patients: a phase II study of the Gruppo Italiano di Oncologia Geriatrica (GIOGer). *Ann Oncol.* 2005;16(2):253–258.

20. Flood KL, Carroll MB, Le CV, et al. Geriatric syndromes in elderly patients admitted to an oncology-acute care for elders unit. *J Clin Oncol.* 2006;24(15):2298–2303.

21. Hurria A, Wong FL, Villaluna D, et al. The role of age and health in treatment recommendations for older adults with breast cancer: the perspective of oncologists and primary care providers. *J Clin Oncol.* 2008;26(33):5386–5392.

22. Maione P, Perrone F, Gallo C, et al. Pretreatment quality of life and functional status assessment significantly predict survival of elderly patients with advanced non-small-cell lung cancer receiving chemotherapy: a prognostic analysis of the multicenter Italian lung cancer in the elderly study. *J Clin Oncol.* 2005;23(28):6865–6872.

23. Wedding U, Rohrig B, Klippstein A, et al. Impairment in functional status and survival in patients with acute myeloid leukaemia. *J Cancer Res Clin Oncol.* 2006;132(10):665–671.

24. Extermann M, Overcash J, Lyman GH, et al. Comorbidity and functional status are independent in older cancer patients. *J Clin Oncol.* 1998;16(4):1582–1587.

25. Firat S, Bousamra M, Gore E, et al. Comorbidity and KPS are independent prognostic factors in stage I non-small-cell lung cancer. *Int J Radiat Oncol Biol Phys.* 2002;52:1047–1057.

26. Piccirillo JF, Tierney RM, Costas I, et al. Prognostic importance of comorbidity in a hospital-based cancer registry. *J Am Med Assoc.* 2004;291(20):2441–2447.

27. Satariano WA, Ragland DR. The effect of comorbidity on 3-year survival of women with primary breast cancer. *Ann Intern Med.* 1994;120:104–110.

28. Hughes KS, Schnaper LA, Berry D, et al. Lumpectomy plus breast cancer. *N Engl J Med.* 2004;351(10):971–977.

29. Charlson ME, Pompei P, Ales KL, et al. A new method of classifying prognostic comorbidity in longitudinal studies: development and validation. *J Chron Dis.* 1987;40(5):373–383.

30. Frasci G, Lorusso V, Panza N, et al. Gemcitabine plus vinorelbine versus vinorelbine alone in elderly patients with advanced non-small-cell lung cancer. *J Clin Oncol.* 2000;18(13):2529–2536.

31. Muss HB, Berry DA, Cirrincione CT, et al. Adjuvant chemotherapy in older women with early-stage breast cancer. *N Engl J Med.* 2009;360(20):2055–2065.

32. Covinsky KE, Hilton J, Lindquist K, et al. Development and validation of an index to predict activity of daily living dependence in community-dwelling elders. *Med Care.* 2006;44(2):149–157.

33. Suter TM, Procter M, van Veldhuisen DJ, et al. Trastuzumab-associated cardiac adverse effects in the herceptin adjuvant trial. *J Clin Oncol.* 2007;25(25):3859–3865.

34. Perez EA, Suman VJ, Davidson NE, et al. Cardiac safety analysis of doxorubicin and cyclophosphamide followed by paclitaxel with or without trastuzumab in the North Central Cancer Treatment Group N9831 adjuvant breast cancer trial. *J Clin Oncol.* 2008;26(8):1231–1238.

35. Zauderer M, Patil S, Hurria A. Feasibility and toxicity of dose-dense adjuvant chemotherapy in older women with breast cancer. *Breast Cancer Res Treat.* 2008;117(1):205–210.

36. Meyerhardt JA, Catalano PJ, Haller DG, et al. Impact of diabetes mellitus on outcomes in patients with colon cancer. *J Clin Oncol.* 2003;21(3):433–440.

37. Walter LC, Brand RJ, Counsell SR, et al. Development and validation of a prognostic index for 1-year mortality in older adults after hospitalization. *J Am Med Assoc.* 2001;285(23):2987–2994.

38. Lee SJ, Lindquist K, Segal MR, et al. Development and validation of a prognostic index for 4-year mortality in older adults. *J Am Med Assoc.* 2006;295(7):801–808.

39. Charlson ME, Pompei P, Ales KL, et al. A new method of classifying prognostic comorbidity in longitudinal studies: development and validation. *J Chron Dis.* 1987;40(5):373–383.

40. Charlson M, Szatrowski TP, Peterson J, et al. Validation of a combined comorbidity index. *J Clin Epidemiol.* 1994;47(11):1245–1251.

41. Eagles JM, Beattie JA, Restall DB, et al. Relation between cognitive impairment and early death in the elderly. *Br Med J.* 1990;300(6719):239–240.

42. Wolfson C, Wolfson DB, Asgharian M, et al. A reevaluation of the duration of survival after the onset of dementia. *N Engl J Med.* 2001;344(15):1111–1116.

43. Landi F, Onder G, Cattel C, et al. Functional status and clinical correlates in cognitively impaired community-living older people. *J Geriatr Psychiatry Neurol.* 2001;14(1):21–27.

44. Feil D, Marmon T, Unutzer J. Cognitive impairment, chronic medical illness, and risk of mortality in an elderly cohort. *Am J Geriatr Psychiatry.* 2003;11(5):551–560.

45. Rogers LQ, Courneya KS, Robbins KT, et al. Factors associated with fatigue, sleep, and cognitive function among patients with head and neck cancer. *Head Neck.* 2008;30(10):1310–1317.

46. Gupta SK, Lamont EB. Patterns of presentation, diagnosis, and treatment in older patients with colon cancer and comorbid dementia. *J Am Geriatr Soc.* 2004;52(10):1681–1687.

47. Goodwin JS, Hunt WC, Samet JM. Determinants of cancer therapy in elderly patients. *Cancer.* 1993;72(2):594–601.

48. Weineke M, Dienst E. Neuropsychological assessment of cognitive functioning following chemotherapy for breast cancer. *Psychooncology.* 1995;4:61–66.

49. van Dam FS, Schagen SB, Muller MJ, et al. Impairment of cognitive function in women receiving adjuvant treatment for high-risk breast cancer: high-dose versus standard-dose chemotherapy. *J Natl Cancer Inst.* 1998;90(3):210–218.

50. Schagen SB, van Dam FS, Muller MJ, et al. Cognitive deficits after postoperative adjuvant chemotherapy for breast carcinoma. *Cancer.* 1999;85(3):640–650.

51. Schagen SB, Muller MJ, Boogerd W, et al. Cognitive dysfunction and chemotherapy: neuropsychological findings in perspective. *Clin Breast Cancer.* 2002;3(suppl 3):S100–108.

52. Brezden CB, Phillips KA, Abdolell M, et al. Cognitive function in breast cancer patients receiving adjuvant chemotherapy. *J Clin Oncol.* 2000;18(14):2695–2701.

53. Tchen N, Juffs HG, Downie FP, et al. Cognitive function, fatigue, and menopausal symptoms in

women receiving adjuvant chemotherapy for breast cancer. *J Clin Oncol*. 2003;21(22): 4175–4183.

54. Castellon SA, Ganz PA, Bower JE, et al. Neurocognitive performance in breast cancer survivors exposed to adjuvant chemotherapy and tamoxifen. *J Clin Exp Neuropsychol*. 2004;26(7): 955–969.

55. Wefel JS, Lenzi R, Theriault RL, et al. The cognitive sequelae of standard-dose adjuvant chemotherapy in women with breast carcinoma: results of a prospective, randomized, longitudinal trial. *Cancer*. 2004;100(11):2292–2299.

56. Hurria A, Rosen C, Hudis C, et al. Cognitive function of older patients receiving adjuvant chemotherapy for breast cancer: a pilot prospective longitudinal study. *J Am Geriatr Soc*. 2006;54(6):925–931.

57. Ernst T, Chang L, Cooray D, et al. The effects of tamoxifen and estrogen on brain metabolism in elderly women. *J Natl Cancer Inst*. 2002;94(8): 592–597.

58. Shilling V, Jenkins V, Morris R, et al. The effects of adjuvant chemotherapy on cognition in women with breast cancer: preliminary results of an observational longitudinal study. *Breast*. 2005; 14(2):142–150.

59. Hurria A, Somlo G, Ahles T. Renaming "chemobrain." *Cancer Invest*. 2007;25(6): 373–377.

60. Fried TR, Bradley EH, Towle VR, et al. Understanding the treatment preferences of seriously ill patients. *N Engl J Med*. 2002;346(14): 1061–1066.

61. Ahles TA, Saykin AJ, Furstenberg CT, et al. Neuropsychologic impact of standard-dose systemic chemotherapy in long-term survivors of breast cancer and lymphoma. *J Clin Oncol*. 2002;20(2):485–493.

62. Heflin LH, Meyerowitz BE, Hall P, et al. Cancer as a risk factor for long-term cognitive deficits and dementia. *J Natl Cancer Inst*. 2005;97(11): 854–856.

63. Silverman DH, Dy CJ, Castellon SA, et al. Altered frontocortical, cerebellar, and basal ganglia activity in adjuvant-treated breast cancer survivors 5–10 years after chemotherapy. *Breast Cancer Res Treat*. 2006;103(3):303–311.

64. Kreukels BP, Schagen SB, Ridderinkhof KR, et al. Electrophysiological correlates of information processing in breast-cancer patients treated with adjuvant chemotherapy. *Breast Cancer Res Treat*. 2005;94(1):53–61.

65. Reynolds MW, Fredman L, Langenberg P, et al. Weight, weight change, mortality in a random sample of older community-dwelling women. *J Am Geriatr Soc*. 1999;47(12):1409–1414.

66. Wallace JI, Schwartz RS, LaCroix AZ, et al. Involuntary weight loss in older outpatients: incidence and clinical significance. *J Am Geriatr Soc*. 1995;43(4):329–337.

67. Diehr P, Bild DE, Harris TB, et al. Body mass index and mortality in nonsmoking older adults: the Cardiovascular Health Study. *Am J Public Health*. 1998;88(4):623–629.

68. Newman AB, Yanez D, Harris T, et al. Weight change in old age and its association with mortality. *J Am Geriatr Soc*. 2001;49(10): 1309–1318.

69. Dewys WD, Begg C, Lavin PT, Band PR, et al. Prognostic effect of weight loss prior to chemotherapy in cancer patients. Eastern Cooperative Oncology Group. *Am J Med*. 1980;69(4):491–497.

70. Andreyev HJ, Norman, AR, Oates J, Cunningham D. Why do patients with weight loss have a worse outcome when undergoing chemotherapy for gastrointestinal malignancies? *Eur J Cancer*. 1998;34(4):503–509.

71. Buccheri G, Ferrigno D. Importance of weight loss definition in the prognostic evaluation of non-small-cell lung cancer. *Lung Cancer*. 2001;34(3):433–440.

72. Orsitto G, Cascavilla L, Franceschi M, et al. Influence of cognitive impairment and comorbidity on disability in hospitalized elderly patients. *J Nutr Health Aging*. 2005;9(3): 194–198.

73. Nourissat A, Vasson MP, Merrouche Y, et al. Relationship between nutritional status and quality of life in patients with cancer. *Eur J Cancer*. 2008;44(9):1238–1242.

74. Penninx BW, Guralnik JM, Ferrucci L, et al. Depressive symptoms and physical decline in community-dwelling older persons. *J Am Med Assoc*. 1998;279(21):1720–1726.

75. Langa KM, Valenstein MA, Fendrick AM, et al. Extent and cost of informal caregiving for older Americans with symptoms of depression. *Am J Psychiatry*. 2004;161(5):857–863.

76. Kua J. The prevalence of psychological and psychiatric sequelae of cancer in the elderly – how much do we know? *Ann Acad Med Singapore*. 2005;34(3):250–256.

77. Dalle Carbonare L, Maggi S, Noale M, et al. Physical disability and depressive symptomatology in an elderly population: a complex relationship. The Italian Longitudinal Study on Aging (ILSA). *Am J Geriatr Psychiatry*. 2009;17(2):144–154.

78. Bruce ML, Seeman TE, Merrill SS, et al. The impact of depressive symptomatology on physical disability: MacArthur Studies of Successful Aging. *Am J Public Health*. 1994;84(11):1796–1799.

79. Penninx BW, Beekman AT, Ormel J, et al. Psychological status among elderly people with chronic diseases: does type of disease play a part? *J Psychosom Res.* 1996;40(5):521–534.

80. Walker J, Waters RA, Murray G, et al. Better off dead: suicidal thoughts in cancer patients. *J Clin Oncol.* 2008;26(29):4725–4730.

81. Miller M, Mogun H, Azrael D, et al. Cancer and the risk of suicide in older Americans. *J Clin Oncol.* 2008;26(29):4720–4724.

82. Seeman TE, Kaplan GA, Knudsen L, et al. Social network ties and mortality among the elderly in the Alameda County Study. *Am J Epidemiol.* 1987;126(4):714–723.

83. Tomaka J, Thompson S, Palacios R. The relation of social isolation, loneliness, and social support to disease outcomes among the elderly. *J Aging Health.* 2006;18(3):359–384.

84. House JS, Landis KR, Umberson D. Social relationships and health. *Science.* 1988;241(4865):540–545.

85. Golden J, Conroy RM, Bruce I, et al. Loneliness, social support networks, mood and wellbeing in community-dwelling elderly. *Int J Geriatr Psychiatry.* 2009;24(7):694–700.

86. Iwasaki M, Otani T, Sunaga R, et al. Social networks and mortality based on the Komo-Ise cohort study in Japan. *Int J Epidemiol.* 2002;31(6): 1208–1218.

87. Osborne C, Ostir GV, Du X, et al. The influence of marital status on the stage at diagnosis, treatment, and survival of older women with breast cancer. *Breast Cancer Res Treat.* 2005;93(1):41–77.

88. DiMatteo MR. Social support and patient adherence to medical treatment: a meta-analysis. *Health Psychol.* 2004;23(2):207–218.

89. NCCN practice guidelines in oncology: senior adult oncology. National Comprehensive Cancer Network Web site. Available at: http://www.nccn.org/professionals/physician_gls/PDF/senior.pdf.

90. Ingram SS, Seo PH, Martell RE, et al. Comprehensive assessment of the elderly cancer patient: the feasibility of self-report methodology. *J Clin Oncol.* 2002;20(3):770–775.

91. Hurria A, Lichtman SM, Gardes J, et al. Identifying vulnerable older adults with cancer: integrating geriatric assessment into oncology practice. *J Am Geriatr Soc.* 2007;55(10): 1604–1608.

92. Hurria A, Gupta S, Zauderer M, et al. Developing a cancer-specific geriatric assessment: a feasibility study. *Cancer.* 2005;104(9):1998–2005.

93. Larsson A, Skoog I, Aevarsson AA, et al. Regional cerebral blood flow in normal individuals aged 40, 75 and 88 years studied by 99Tc(m)-d,l-HMPAO SPET. *Nucl Med Commun.* 2001;22(7):741–746.

94. Ito H, Kanno I, Ibaraki M, et al. Effect of aging on cerebral vascular response to Paco2 changes in humans as measured by positron emission tomography. *J Cereb Blood Flow Metab.* 2002;22(8):997–1003.

95. Meier-Ruge W, Ulrich J, Bruhlmann M, et al. Age-related white matter atrophy in the human brain. *Ann N Y Acad Sci.* 1992;673:260–269.

96. Fozard JL, Vercryssen M, Reynolds SL, et al. Age differences and changes in reaction time: the Baltimore Longitudinal Study of Aging. *J Gerontol.* 1994;49(4):P179–189.

97. Petersen RC, Smith G, Kokmen E, et al. Memory function in normal aging. *Neurology.* 1992;42(2):396–401.

98. Small SA, Stern Y, Tang M, et al. Selective decline in memory function among healthy elderly. *Neurology.* 1999;52(7):1392–1396.

99. Helzner EP, Cauley JA, Pratt SR, et al. Race and sex differences in age-related hearing loss: the Health, Aging and Body Composition Study. *J Am Geriatr Soc.* 2005;53(12):2119–2127.

100. Tanaka H, Monahan KD, Seals DR. Age-predicted maximal heart rate revisited. *J Am Coll Cardiol.* 2001;37(1):153–156.

101. Ferrari AU, Radaelli A, Centola M. Invited review: aging and the cardiovascular system. *J Appl Physiol.* 2003;95(6):2591–2597.

102. Sawhney R, Sehl M, Naeim A. Physiologic aspects of aging: impact on cancer management and decision making, part I. *Cancer J.* 2005;11(6): 449–460.

103. Short KR, Nair KS. Mechanisms of sarcopenia of aging. *J Endocrinol Invest.* 1999;22(suppl 5): 95–105.

104. Sotaniemi EA, Arranto AJ, Pelkonen O, et al. Age and cytochrome P450-linked drug metabolism in humans: an analysis of 226 subjects with equal histopathologic conditions. *Clin Pharmacol Ther.* 1997;61(3):331–339.

105. Fehrman-Ekholm I, Skeppholm L. Renal function in the elderly (>70 years old) measured by means of iohexol clearance, serum creatinine, serum urea and estimated clearance. *Scand J Urol Nephrol.* 2004;38(1):73–77.

106. Rimon E, Kagansky N, Cojocaru L, et al. Can creatinine clearance be accurately predicted by formulae in octogenarian in-patients? *Q J Med.* 2004;97(5):281–287.

107. Lindeman RD, Tobin J, Shock NW. Longitudinal studies on the rate of decline in renal function with age. *J Am Geriatr Soc.* 1985;33(4):278–285.

108. Tsuboi I, Morimoto K, Horie T, et al. Age-related changes in various hemopoietic progenitor cells in senescence-accelerated (SAM-P) mice. *Exp Hematol.* 1991;19(9):874–877.

15

109. Izaks GJ, Westendorp RG, Knook DL. The definition of anemia in older persons. *J Am Med Assoc.* 1999;281(18):1714–1717.

110. Artz AS, Fergusson D, Drinka PJ, et al. Prevalence of anemia in skilled-nursing home residents. *Arch Gerontol Geriatr.* 2004;39(3):201–206.

111. Gomez H, Hidalgo M, Casanova L, et al. Risk factors for treatment-related death in elderly patients with aggressive non-Hodgkin's lymphoma: results of a multivariate analysis. *J Clin Oncol.* 1998;16(6):2065–2069.

112. Balducci L, Cohen HJ, Engstrom PF, et al. Senior adult oncology clinical practice guidelines in oncology. *J Natl Compr Canc Netw.* 2005;3(4):572–590.

113. Silber JH, Fridman M, DiPaola RS, et al. First-cycle blood counts and subsequent neutropenia, dose reduction, or delay in early-stage breast cancer therapy. *J Clin Oncol.* 1998;16(7):2392–2400.

114. Dees EC, O'Reilly S, Goodman SN, et al. A prospective pharmacologic evaluation of age-related toxicity of adjuvant chemotherapy in women with breast cancer. *Cancer Invest.* 2000;18(6):521–529.

115. Repetto L, Carreca I, Maraninchi D, et al. Use of growth factors in the elderly patient with cancer: a report from the Second International Society for Geriatric Oncology (SIOG) 2001 meeting. *Crit Rev Oncol Hematol.* 2003;45(2):123–128.

116. Hurria A, Brogan K, Panageas KS, et al. Change in cycle 1 to cycle 2 haematological counts predicts toxicity in older patients with breast cancer receiving adjuvant chemotherapy. *Drugs Aging.* 2005;22(8):709–715.

117. Abbatecola AM, Ferrucci L, Grella R, et al. Diverse effect of inflammatory markers on insulin resistance and insulin-resistance syndrome in the elderly. *J Am Geriatr Soc.* 2004;52(3):399–404.

118. Roubenoff R, Harris TB, Abad LW, et al. Monocyte cytokine production in an elderly population: effect of age and inflammation. *J Gerontol.* 1998;53(1):M20–26.

119. Fagiolo U, Cossarizza A, Scala E, et al. Increased cytokine production in mononuclear cells of healthy elderly people. *Eur J Immunol.* 1993;23(9):2375–2378.

120. Harris TB, Ferrucci L, Tracy RP, et al. Associations of elevated interleukin-6 and C-reactive protein levels with mortality in the elderly. *Am J Med.* 1999;106(5):506–512.

121. Reuben DB, Ferrucci L, Wallace R, et al. The prognostic value of serum albumin in healthy older persons with low and high serum interleukin-6 (IL-6) levels. *J Am Geriatr Soc.* 2000;48(11):1404–1407.

122. Reuben DB, Cheh AI, Harris TB, et al. Peripheral blood markers of inflammation predict mortality and functional decline in high-functioning community-dwelling older persons. *J Am Geriatr Soc.* 2002;50(4):638–644.

123. Taaffe DR, Harris TB, Ferrucci L, et al. Cross-sectional and prospective relationships of interleukin-6 and C-reactive protein with physical performance in elderly persons: MacArthur studies of successful aging. *J Gerontol.* 2000;55(12):M709–715.

124. Leng S, Chaves P, Koenig K, et al. Serum interleukin-6 and hemoglobin as physiological correlates in the geriatric syndrome of frailty: a pilot study. *J Am Geriatr Soc.* 2002;50(7):1268–1271.

125. Leng SX, Xue QL, Tian J, et al. Inflammation and frailty in older women. *J Am Geriatr Soc.* 2007;55(6):864–871.

126. Walston J, McBurnie MA, Newman A, et al. Frailty and activation of the inflammation and coagulation systems with and without clinical comorbidities: results from the Cardiovascular Health Study. *Arch Intern Med.* 2002;162(20):2333–2341.

127. Cesari M, Penninx BW, Pahor M, et al. Inflammatory markers and physical performance in older persons: the InCHIANTI study. *J Gerontol.* 2004;59(3):242–248.

128. Cohen HJ, Harris T, Pieper CF. Coagulation and activation of inflammatory pathways in the development of functional decline and mortality in the elderly. *Am J Med.* 2003;114(3):180–187.

129. Geffken DF, Cushman M, Burke GL, et al. Association between physical activity and markers of inflammation in a healthy elderly population. *Am J Epidemiol.* 2001;153(3):242–250.

130. Yaffe K, Lindquist K, Penninx BW, et al. Inflammatory markers and cognition in well-functioning African-American and white elders. *Neurology.* 2003;61(1):76–80.

131. Pai JK, Pischon T, Ma J, et al. Inflammatory markers and the risk of coronary heart disease in men and women. *N Engl J Med.* 2004;351(25):2599–2610.

132. Spranger J, Kroke A, Mohlig M, et al. Inflammatory cytokines and the risk to develop type 2 diabetes: results of the prospective population-based European Prospective Investigation into Cancer and Nutrition (EPIC)-Potsdam Study. *Diabetes.* 2003;52(3):812–817.

133. Ding C, Parameswaran V, Udayan R, et al. Circulating levels of inflammatory markers predict change in bone mineral density and resorption in older adults: a longitudinal study. *J Clin Endocrinol Metab.* 2008;93(5):1952–1958.

134. Shlipak MG, Fried LF, Crump C, et al. Elevations of inflammatory and procoagulant biomarkers in elderly persons with renal insufficiency. *Circulation.* 2003;107(1):87–92.

135. Coussens LM, Werb Z. Inflammation and cancer. *Nature.* 2002;420(6917):860–867.

136. Ames BN, Gold LS. The causes and prevention of cancer: the role of environment. *Biotherapy.* 1998;11:205–220.

137. Christensen S, Hagen TM, Shigenaga MK, et al. Chronic inflammation, mutation, and cancer. In: Parsonnet J, ed. *Microbes and Malignancy: Infection as a Cause of Human Cancers.* New York: Oxford University Press; 1999:35–88.

138. Caruso C, Lio D, Cavallone L, et al. Aging, longevity, inflammation, and cancer. *Ann N Y Acad Sci.* 2004;1028:1–13.

139. Drachenberg DE, Elgamal AA, Rowbotham R, et al. Circulating levels of interleukin-6 in patients with hormone refractory prostate cancer. *Prostate.* 1999;41(2):127–133.

140. Songur N, Kuru B, Kalkan F, et al. Serum interleukin-6 levels correlate with malnutrition and survival in patients with advanced non-small cell lung cancer. *Tumori.* 2004;90(2):196–200.

141. Lamb GW, McArdle PA, Ramsey S, et al. The relationship between the local and systemic inflammatory responses and survival in patients undergoing resection for localized renal cancer. *BJU Int.* 2008;102(6):756–761.

142. Ramsey S, Lamb GW, Aitchison M, et al. Evaluation of an inflammation-based prognostic score in patients with metastatic renal cancer. *Cancer.* 2007;109(2):205–212.

143. Blackwell K, Hurwitz H, Lieberman G, et al. Circulating D-dimer levels are better predictors of overall survival and disease progression than carcinoembryonic antigen levels in patients with metastatic colorectal carcinoma. *Cancer.* 2004;101(1):77–82.

144. Blackwell K, Haroon Z, Broadwater G, et al. Plasma D-dimer levels in operable breast cancer patients correlate with clinical stage and axillary lymph node status. *J Clin Oncol.* 2000;18(3):600–608.

145. Zhang SM, Lin J, Cook NR, et al. C-reactive protein and risk of breast cancer. *J Natl Cancer Inst.* 2007;99(11):890–894.

146. Siemes C, Visser LE, Coebergh JW, et al. C-reactive protein levels, variation in the C-reactive protein gene, and cancer risk: the Rotterdam Study. *J Clin Oncol.* 2006;24(33):5216–5222.

147. Yancik R. Cancer burden in the aged: an epidemiologic and demographic overview. *Cancer.* 1997;80(7):1273–1283.

148. Profile of general demographic characteristics 2000. 2000 Census of Population and Housing United States. Available at: http://www.census.gov/prod/cen2000/dp1/2kh00.pdf.

2 Pharmacology and unique side effects of chemotherapy in older adults

Hans Wildiers and Matti S. Aapro

A. Introduction

Physiology and bodily functions are known to modify with increasing age. These changes can have a considerable impact on the pharmacokinetic (PK) processes of absorption, distribution, metabolism, and excretion of administered drugs. For many drugs, these changes are not clinically relevant, but for drugs with low therapeutic index, such as chemotherapy, this can have dramatic consequences. Increased drug levels can lead to increased side effects in elderly who already have diminished reserve capacities to deal with these toxicities.

This chapter will discuss two important issues related to specific chemotherapeutic agents in older patients: first, we will discuss specific aspects of the pharmacology of different chemotherapeutic drugs in older adults, focusing on clinical implications; second, we will discuss side effects of chemotherapy for specific agents and general side effects as well. Practical recommendations and future perspectives will be discussed.

B. General pharmacological issues related to chemotherapy in elderly cancer patients

Age can have an effect on most pharmacokinetic parameters, including absorption, volume of distribution, hepatic drug metabolism, and excretion[1] (see Table 2.1). Diminished *absorption* can occur because of atrophic gastritis, decreased gastric motility and secretions, or decreased intraluminal surface area, possibly resulting in reduced effectiveness. However, it is still controversial whether decreased absorption actually occurs with age.[2] Polypharmacy with multiple concomitant medications can alter absorption by binding drugs in the gastrointestinal tract, by changing absorption or pH, and by competition for carrier sites.[3]

The *volume of distribution* (Vd) is a function of body composition, serum protein profile, and blood cells. A progressive increase in body fat and a decline in body water generally occur with increasing age. These changes tend to reduce the Vd of water-soluble drugs, such as anthracyclines, and increase those of fat-soluble compounds, such as carmustine. Plasma albumin levels can decrease because of the aging process and/or because of concomitant pathophysiological processes that will clearly influence the concentration of the unbound or free fraction of drug in the plasma, especially those that are highly protein bound.[4,5]

Hepatic function is also modified by aging: decreases in liver size (by 18%–44%), blood flow, albumin production, and cytochrome P450 function have all been reported.[6] Also, drug interactions at the level of hepatic metabolization (or to a lesser extent at other levels such as drug binding or renal elimination) are an important issue in elderly because drug intake increases with increasing age.[4,7]

The decreasing *renal excretion* of drugs is the most predictable and easily measurable pharmacokinetic change, as the glomerular filtration rate (GFR) declines on average with age by about 1 mL/min per year from the age of 40 years.[8] For drugs that are predominantly renally excreted, the dose usually needs to be reduced when the creatinine clearance (CrCl) is below 60 mL/min.

Despite previous knowledge, great uncertainty exists regarding the optimal dose of chemotherapy for older patients. By the way, this is not so much different from younger patients in whom identical drugs can also have dramatic differences in pharmacology with subsequent over- or underdosing in some patients. It is hoped that pharmacogenomics in the near future will allow for better titration of the doses of chemotherapy in individuals. Because interindividual heterogeneity, related to differences in aging processes and development of comorbid diseases, increases with age, dose individualization is of utmost importance in older patients. At present, we can use available data on pharmacology to titrate the doses, and this can

Table 2.1 Pharmacokinetic parameters that might change with aging.

Parameter changes	Clinical consequences
Absorption: decreased	Oral chemotherapy (e.g., capecitabine) might be less effective in elderly
Volume of distribution: decreased	Serum concentrations and toxicity of several chemotherapeutics might increase (e.g., cisplatin, taxanes, etoposide, irinotecan)
Hepatic metabolism: decreased	Not well known, may affect serum concentrations of chemotherapeutics eliminated by hepatic metabolism (e.g., taxanes, cyclophosphamide, anthracyclines)
Renal excretion: decreased	Dosing should be adapted to present recommendations to avoid excessive serum concentrations and toxicity from renally excreted chemotherapeutics (e.g., carboplatin, topotecan, methotrexate)

Note. From Wildiers,[15] with permission.

already eliminate partial differences in drug exposure. Dose adaptation in elderly is a double-edged sword (see Table 2.2). On one hand, overdosing can lead to important toxicity. Elderly individuals also have much less capability to deal with toxicity related to diminished functional reserve capacities. Dehydration can lead more quickly to renal insufficiency, and neutropenic infection can lead to more dramatic infections and treatment related/induced death.[9] On the other hand, great care is warranted when making dose reductions because the antitumor effect may also decrease. For instance, a 50 percent initial dose reduction of cyclophosphamide, doxorubicin, vincristine, and prednisone (CHOP) in patients aged 65 years and older is inferior to the full dose in patients with non-Hodgkin's lymphomas (NHL).[10] Also, less intensive chemotherapy, such as etoposide, mitoxantrone, and prednimustine (VMP), is less effective than standard CHOP chemotherapy in NHL in the elderly (over 69 years of age).[11] However, the VMP schedule is still effective with an objective response rate of 50 percent, less toxicity, and fewer toxic deaths. Hematological growth factors could help in maintaining dose intensity while decreasing hematological toxicity but do not alleviate nonhematological toxicities. A lot depends on the clinical situation and goals of therapy (see Table 2.3). In a curative setting, such as lymphomas, dose intensity is critical and should be maintained if possible to optimize chances of cure. In an adjuvant setting, several studies suggest that low-dose or soft chemotherapy is associated with decreased efficacy. For breast cancer, for instance, cyclophosphamide, methotrexate, and fluorouracil (CMF) chemotherapy was not as effective if a dose intensity of 85 percent could not be reached.[12] A recent study showed that classical chemotherapy with doxorubicin and cyclophosphamide (AC) or CMF is superior to capecitabine, the latter being an oral drug incorrectly thought to be more easily manageable in elderly patients. In a metastatic setting, however, there is no hard proof that dose intensity is crucial. The main goals of treatment are palliative, that is, controlling disease as long as possible while causing as little toxicity as possible.

C. Pharmacology and side effects of specific anticancer drugs in elderly individuals

An overview of age-related specific pharmacological data on frequently used chemotherapeutic agents is shown in Table 2.4. More details on these drugs, and information on other less frequently used chemotherapeutic agents, can be found in several recent reviews.[13–15]

Table 2.2 Systematic dose adaptation of chemotherapy in elderly cancer patients is a double-edged sword.

	Advantages	Disadvantages
	Debilitating toxicity can probably be avoided in many cases	Underdosing might lead to severe undertreatment
	The dose can be up-titrated in case of good tolerance	Progression can occur not related to intrinsic chemoresistance but to insufficient dosing

Table 2.3 Purpose of treatment in elderly patients with cancer and consequences.

	Curative setting	Adjuvant setting	Palliative setting
Setting	Curative intent in advanced disease	Curative intent in (possibly) micrometastatic disease	Palliative intent in advanced disease
Examples	Lymphomas, germ cell tumors	Adjuvant setting in breast cancer, colon cancer	Advanced disease in cancer of the breast, colon, lung, etc.
Attitude	Some toxicity is acceptable if it is well managed	Always weigh advantages (usually rather small) vs. disadvantages (toxicity, morbidity of treatment)	Quality of life is paramount; significant toxicity is generally not acceptable
	Aim to maintain dose intensity to optimize chances of cure	Take age of patient into account when aiming for increased survival in an often far future	Omitting chemotherapy can be the best option in some patients
	Remember pharmacological principles and alternations in the elderly	Dose intensity can be very important to have any gain at all	Definitely consider dose modifications based on pharmacological parameters and alternations in elderly

Note. From Wildiers et al.,[15] with permission.

C.1. Alkylating agents

Cyclophosphamide (CPA) can be given orally and is very well absorbed, with a true bioavailability close to 100 percent. CPA by itself is inactive and is transformed in the liver into active metabolites, which are ultimately eliminated by hepatic metabolism and in 20–25 percent by renal excretion. One study of 44 women with breast cancer, aged 35–79 years and treated with CPA and doxorubicin, showed no age-related differences in the clearance of CPA.[16] An accumulation of toxic alkylating metabolites is expected in renal insufficiency, justifying a dose reduction of 20–30 percent, depending on the degree of the renal insufficiency.[17] At the pharmacodynamic level, it has been shown that circulating monocytes in the elderly (over 72 years vs. less than 25 years in age) are less able to recuperate from CPA-induced DNA damage,[18] which can explain the increased risk of myelosuppression, the predominant toxicity of CPA, in the elderly.

C.2. Platinum compounds

Cisplatin is an important drug in several tumor types, but the metabolism of cisplatin is not fully understood. It is partly excreted renally (20–70%), and dose adjustment recommendations have been made: 75 percent of the regular dose for a CrCl less than or equal to 60 mL/min and 50 percent for a CrCl less than or equal to 45 mL/min; no data are available for a CrCl less than or equal to 30 mL/min.[19] However, the nonreversible plasma protein binding of cisplatin also should be considered as an important elimination process as only the unbound plasma cisplatin concentrations represent the active fraction. Plasma protein binding of cisplatin is greater than the plasma protein binding of other platinum compounds (e.g., carboplatin). In addition to renal function, age is an independent and significant predictor of the area under the curve (AUC) of the free ultrafilterable platinum fraction (U-Pt) and total plasma platinum, with a higher AUC with increasing age.[20] The maximum concentration (Cmax) of U-Pt has been shown to correlate significantly with nephrotoxicity,[21] and it may be appropriate to reduce the rate of infusion in the elderly.[22] Renal function should be considered as a major pharmacodynamic parameter for cisplatin as renal insufficiency represents the major toxicity, together with magnesium wasting, nausea and vomiting, peripheral neuropathy, auditory impairment (which can be problematic since age-related hearing loss is already frequent), and myelosuppression. Severe nausea and vomiting have been markedly reduced by the use of adequate antiemetic treatment regimens. Intravenous hydration has reduced acute nephrotoxicity to less than 5 percent. In conclusion, increased AUC and toxicity in elderly patients prohibit the use of high-dose cisplatin. Cisplatin could be used at the lower range of dosage (e.g., 60 mg/m^2) and at a reduced infusion rate (e.g., over 24 hours) to

Table 2.4 Age-related effects on pharmacokinetics of frequently used chemotherapeutics and consequences.

Alkylating agents
- **Cyclophosphamide:**
  - PK not different, some increased toxicity on PD level
  - Important liver metabolism, effect of age-related decrease in hepatic function is unknown
  - Adapt to renal function
  - No arguments for a priori dose reduction in elderly
- **Cisplatin**
  - Increased AUC and toxicity in elderly
  - Adapt to renal function
  - Consider the lower range of dosage (e.g., 60 mg/m^2) and preferably at a reduced infusion rate (e.g., over 24 hours)
- **Carboplatin**
  - Adapt to renal function (Calvert formula)
- **Oxaliplatin**
  - No arguments for a priori dose reduction in elderly

Taxanes
- **Paclitaxel**
  - Conflicting PK data on paclitaxel clearance in elderly
  - Several trials show feasibility of both 3-weekly and weekly paclitaxel in elderly patients
  - No arguments for a priori dose reduction in elderly
- **Docetaxel**
  - Docetaxel PK is at most only minimally influenced by age
  - Elderly patients are somewhat more vulnerable to side effects, but like for PK, interpatient variability is larger than age-related variability
  - In principle, standard regimens of docetaxel can be used (dose and schedule depend on clinical setting), but high dose needs to be given with caution

Topoisomerase inhibitors
- **Etoposide (topo II)**
  - High variability in oral absorption
  - Increased AUC and toxicity in elderly
  - Dose adaptation according to albumin, bilirubin, renal function should be considered
- **Irinotecan (topo I)**
  - Increased AUC and diarrhea in elderly
  - A lower dose (e.g., 300 mg/m^2 q3w instead of 350 mg/m^2 q3w) could be considered for age ≥70
- **Topotecan (topo I)**
  - Adapt to renal function
  - Consider weekly regimens (less myelosuppression)

Table 2.4 (*cont.*)

Antimetabolites
- **Methotrexate**
  - AUC possibly increased
  - Adapt to renal function
- **Fluorouracil**
  - PK and toxicity not majorly influenced
- **Capecitabine**
  - Lower dose such as 1,000 mg/m^2 twice daily instead of 1,250 mg/m^2 seems equally effective with fewer side effects
  - Adapt to renal function
- **Gemcitabine**
  - Unpredictable PK
  - Generally good tolerance in elderly

Antitumor antibiotics
- **Doxorubicin**
  - Increased peak plasma concentrations
  - Increased myelosuppression and cardiotoxicity
  - At full dose (cyclophosphamide, doxorubicin, vincristine, and prednisone; doxorubicin and cyclophosphamide), relatively toxic
  - Possible solutions:
    - Dose reduction if being given in palliative setting
    - Alternative administration regimens, e.g., weekly
    - Liposomal forms
    - Removal of doxorubicin in lymphoma regimens
    - Growth factors

Note. Based on Lichtman et al.[14] and Wildiers et al.[100] Reprinted from Wildiers,[15] with permission from Elsevier. PK = pharmacokinetics; AUC = area under the curve; PD = pharmacodynamics.

avoid excessive toxicity in elderly. Hydration must be monitored carefully to prevent fluid overload. The concomitant use of other potentially nephrotoxic drugs should be avoided.

Carboplatin, in contrast to cisplatin, has very limited protein binding. It is completely eliminated through the kidneys and has a unique method of dosing based on the GFR and the targeted AUC that has permitted the individualization of the carboplatin dose for maximum effect with tolerable side effects. The Calvert formula provides an accurate and safe dose[23]:

$$\text{Dose (mg)} = \text{target AUC} \times (\text{GFR} + 25),$$

where AUC = AUC of free carboplatin

$(\text{mg/mL} \times \text{min}).$

There is some controversy over the optimal way of determining GFR.[24] Several methods are available, the most popular being determination of creatinine clearance, which involves 24-hour urine collections, or from the Cockcroft-Gault equation using serum creatinine. Because of the low incidence of nonhematologic toxicity and the quite similar efficacy, carboplatin can replace cisplatin in the palliative setting or in case adverse effects of cisplatin are problematic.

Oxaliplatin, like cisplatin, is strongly protein bound. The kidneys eliminate approximately 30–50 percent of the drug, and the AUC of the free fraction correlates with CrCl. However, in patients with normal or moderately impaired renal function (CrCl range 27–57 mL/min), no increased toxicity was observed, suggesting that it can be safely administered without dose adjustment or hydration in moderate renal dysfunction.[25] Patients with a severe decrease in GFR should have a dose reduction. In the meta-analysis from Goldberg and colleagues that involved patients receiving FOLFOX 4 for colorectal cancer,[26] there was no difference in toxicity or efficacy between younger and (selected) older patients. Also the combination of oxaliplatin and capecitabine was feasible and effective in older patients, and there was no relationship between response and patient age, Eastern Cooperative Oncology Group performance status, or the ability to perform activities of daily living (ADLs) or instrumental ADLs.[27,28] The rate of neurotoxicity secondary to oxaliplatin-based chemotherapy has not been shown to be any greater in the elderly than in younger patients. There are no data to support dose reduction based on age alone.

C.3. Taxanes

Paclitaxel and docetaxel are extensively metabolized in the liver. The majority of paclitaxel and docetaxel is protein bound (97% and 94%, respectively). Only a small amount is excreted renally, and, in principle, these drugs can be employed at full doses even if renal function is impaired. Both drugs are extensively metabolized in the liver by the cytochrome P450 system and are excreted in bile, resulting in increased toxicity when administered to patients with impaired liver function.[29] The repetitive administration of corticosteroids should be monitored carefully because these can also cause significant toxicity in the elderly. Neuropathy can be troublesome and debilitating, especially for elderly patients with unsteady balance. An extensive review on the use of taxanes in elderly breast cancer patients pro-

vides more details,[30] but the most important issues are summarized in the following paragraphs.

Paclitaxel was developed as a 3-weekly schedule but is currently often used as a weekly regimen because toxicity is diminished while efficacy is at least as good (in breast cancer, it is even better) as in 3-weekly regimens.[31] A Cancer and Leukemia Group B trial showed a modest but significant decrease in clearance of total paclitaxel with increasing age and also an increase in white blood cell nadir, although this did not result in increased fever and neutropenia.[32] This decreased clearance seems partly induced by decreased clearance of the formulation vehicle Cremophor EL. Moreover, unbound paclitaxel might be a better predictor of clinically relevant exposure than total paclitaxel.[33] So there is still some controversy on the effect of age on paclitaxel pharmacology. However, several trials indicate the feasibility of both 3-weekly and weekly paclitaxel in elderly patients. There is no basis for a dose reduction based on age alone for classical standard dose or schedule.

Docetaxel undergoes extensive metabolization by cytochrome CYP3A4, which is by far the strongest predictor of docetaxel clearance and, together with albumin/α1-acid glycoprotein (AAG), accounts for 72 percent of the interpatient variation in clearance.[34] Attempts have been made to predict docetaxel PK by measurement of CYP3A4 activity by the erythromycin breath test or by plasma AAG concentration or urinary cortisol ratio, but this is unvalidated and difficult to implement in routine clinical care. Population PK studies suggest that docetaxel clearance decreases with age and hypoalbuminemia, but only by 7 and 8 percent, respectively.[35] Small, specific phase I trials in elderly cancer patients treated with docetaxel every 3 weeks have been performed with contradictory results.[36,37] As with paclitaxel, weekly-dose docetaxel regimens have been investigated, and they seem to decrease toxicity without loss of efficacy,[38] except perhaps in prostate cancer, where a 3-weekly regimen was slightly more effective than weekly docetaxel.[39] Neutropenia was limited with weekly regimens, but fatigue and lacrimation were often incapacitating. Various dosages (e.g., 20–35 mg/m^2 weekly or 60–100 mg/m^2 every 3 weeks) and regimens (rest weeks at various time points) have been used. There are no significant data to support dose modification of docetaxel based on age alone. Docetaxel pharmacokinetics are at most only minimally influenced by age. Any age-related changes are minimal compared to interpatient variability in metabolism. However, elderly patients are somewhat more vulnerable to adverse effects, but here as well, interpatient variability is larger than age-related variability. In principle, standard regimens of docetaxel can be used (e.g., 30–36 mg/m^2 weekly with a rest week at regular time points or 75 mg/m^2 every 3-week regimen). The choice between weekly and 3-weekly regimens can depend on the setting (e.g., in prostate cancer, 75 mg/m^2 every 3 weeks is the standard) and on potential adverse effects (if neutropenia should be avoided, weekly regimens are preferred). Nanoparticle-bound paclitaxel is a promising taxane formulation with low risk of allergy not requiring corticosteroids, but no studies have yet been done specifically in the elderly.

C.4. Topoisomerase interactive agents

The pharmacokinetics of *etoposide* are quite unpredictable and vary considerably between individuals; even more variability is to be expected in the elderly. The oral formulation poses even more problems than the intravenous formulation because intestinal absorption can also vary significantly.[40] Impaired renal function leads to a decrease in drug clearance rates, and dose modification has been proposed.[14] Increased age was a significant predictor of decreased etoposide clearance, increased AUC, and increased hematological toxicity, and in elderly patients with normal organ function, a small dose reduction and/or careful monitoring is advised.[41,42]

Irinotecan (CPT-11) is converted by decarboxylation in the liver into the active metabolite SN-38, which is 1,000 times more cytotoxic than the parent compound. Only a small amount is excreted in the urine, indicating that dose adjustment is not needed in patients with renal dysfunction. It can be given as a weekly or 3-weekly dose. The weekly and 3-weekly regimens showed similar efficacy and quality of life but differences in toxicity.[43] Therapy with CPT-11 is feasible in older patients, but some studies indicate somewhat higher toxicity, mainly delayed diarrhea,[44,45] which can be problematic in elderly individuals who have less capability of dealing with dehydration. A pharmacokinetic study demonstrated clearly that age is a significant independent predictor of the AUC of CPT-11.[46] It has been suggested that patients older than 70 years, patients with prior pelvic irradiation, or patients with poor performance status start at reduced doses. However, there are no good data to support a specific dose modification. A more recent retrospective but large study[47] demonstrated no difference in toxicity and efficacy in older patients and recommended standard dosing. Further studies are necessary to demonstrate whether a reduced initial dose is preferable in elderly cancer patients.

Topotecan is about 40 percent renally excreted, but there is also a substantial concentration in bile.[48] Dose adjustments are required in extensively pretreated patients and in those with moderate but not mild renal impairment because of the risk of increased toxicity. A specific dose modification has been proposed, based on CrCl, for the standard intravenous dose of 1.5 mg/m^2/d for 5 days every 3 weeks.[49] Weekly regimens seem to be effective with decreased risk of hematological toxicity.[50]

C.5. Antimetabolites

Methotrexate (MTX) is mainly excreted by the renal route and is inhibited by nonsteroidal anti-inflammatory drugs, cephalosporins, and several other drugs. The dose of MTX should be adjusted according to renal function, and recommendations have been proposed.[51] Increased toxicity has been observed in elderly patients receiving low-dose, long-term methotrexate. The methotrexate half-life and clearance have been shown to be significantly prolonged in older patients.[52] The dose of MTX should thus carefully be adjusted in the elderly population, based on renal function.

5-Fluorouracil (5-FU) pharmacokinetics are only marginally influenced by age.[53,54] At most, 15–20 percent of the drug is excreted renally; some authors suggest a dose reduction to 80 percent in severe renal failure, but this is not really evidence based.[55] At the level of toxicity, there is also controversy. Some studies have suggested increased toxicity in elderly,[56,57] while a pooled analysis of adjuvant chemotherapy for resected colon cancer in 3,351 elderly patients[58] showed no significant interactions between age, efficacy, and toxicity (except for leukopenia in one of the seven trials studied). It seems that otherwise healthy older patients with colorectal cancer obtain benefits from adjuvant chemotherapy that are not much different from those experienced by younger patients, while the benefits might be much lower in elderly patients with comorbidities and impaired functional status.[59] The data suggest no reason to reduce the dose for intravenous fluoropyrimidines, unless there is severe renal dysfunction or comorbidity. There are some data to suggest that women may be at higher risk of toxicity than men because of a decrease in the enzyme used to metabolize 5-FU in women compared to men.[54]

Capecitabine is an oral prodrug of 5-FU that is extensively metabolized in the liver to 5-FU, and over 70 percent of the dose is recovered in the urine. This necessitates dose reduction in case of renal dysfunction,[60] which is quite common in the elderly. The pharmacokinetics of capecitabine are not affected by age in patients with normal renal function.[61] Studies in elderly breast cancer patients showed that the dose of capecitabine might be reduced from 1,250 to 1,000 mg/m^2 with equal efficacy but reduced toxicity.[62]

Gemcitabine seems to require dose adaptation in patients with hepatic and renal dysfunction on the basis of clinical pharmacokinetic data.[63] However, there is a lack of correlation between pharmacokinetic parameters and toxicity that has made it impossible to provide any specific dose recommendations. Nevertheless, caution is required in patients with renal or hepatic impairment. The total clearance and half-life of gemcitabine are influenced by age and sex, with a longer half-life with increasing age and in men.[64] However, gemcitabine as a single agent causes minimal toxicity in elderly patients, and the side effect profile does not seem to be affected by patient age, leading to dose recommendations in the elderly that are no different than for the general population.[65–67]

C.6. Antitumor antibiotics

Doxorubicin is probably the most commonly used anthracycline drug. It is metabolized and excreted primarily through the hepatobiliary route, while renal excretion is very low, not necessitating dose adjustment in case of renal failure. Increased peak plasma levels have been observed in older patients.[13,68] Some studies suggest that the drug's peak concentration correlates with efficacy, whereas toxicity is most likely a function of both peak and exposure.[69] Anthracyclines can cause cardiac dysfunction, and older patients are at higher risk. This increased incidence of anthracycline-related cardiomyopathy over the age of 70 is most likely due to a combination of factors, including a higher prevalence of preexisting conditions restricting the functional reserve of the myocardium. Certainly in a situation like adjuvant therapy for early breast cancer, where a large proportion of patients are cured, treatment-induced cardiac toxicity can be troublesome. A large study used the Surveillance, Epidemiology, and End Results Medicare database and included women with no history of chronic heart failure (CHF) who were aged 66–80 years and diagnosed with stage I–III breast cancer from 1992 to 2002.[70] A total of 43,338 women were included. Anthracycline-treated women were younger, with fewer comorbidities and more advanced disease than women who received nonanthracycline or no chemotherapy ($p < .001$ for each). The adjusted hazard ratio for CHF was 1.26 (95% confidence interval 1.12–1.42) for women aged 66–70 years treated with anthracycline compared with other chemotherapy. It can thus be concluded that women aged 66–70 years who received adjuvant anthracyclines had significantly higher rates of CHF. The difference in rates of CHF continued to increase through more than 10 years of follow-up. The benefit of adjuvant chemotherapy in breast cancer can be rather small and might be counterbalanced by treatment-induced toxicity. The expected advantages and disadvantages should always be balanced when making treatment decisions. Also, in NHL, doxorubicin in elderly patients has been extensively studied. Large prospective studies of elderly patients (older than 60 years) with NHL receiving doxorubicin (50 mg/m^2) in the CHOP regimen have shown that this regimen can be used in the elderly but is associated with a higher degree of toxicity and a toxic death rate of 7.6–15 percent.[71,72]

Several attempts have been made to deal with increased toxicity in elderly, including dose reduction, alternative administration regimens, removal of doxorubicin from the multidrug regimen, and the use of hematological growth factors. Great care is warranted when doxorubicin is combined with new therapies such as trastuzumab, a recombinant monoclonal antibody against HER2, where a clear additive cardiotoxic effect occurs.[73] When doxorubicin is administered by continuous infusion or in small daily doses, the incidence of drug-related cardiotoxicity seems to be reduced significantly.[69] Weekly low-dose doxorubicin has also been studied in elderly patients with the potential benefit of inducing less neutropenia and lower peak plasma levels, which might be related to cardiac toxicity. Dexrazoxane can also reduce cardiac toxicity, but this needs to be confirmed and investigated specifically in the elderly population.[74] In addition, it is unclear whether the addition of dexrazoxane may impact antitumor efficacy. Liposomal formulations of doxorubicin have been shown to prevent cardiotoxicity while providing comparable antitumor activity.[75] They may be very beneficial in elderly patients with anthracycline-sensitive disease, but the experience in the elderly is limited.

There are no strict guidelines for the dose adjustment of doxorubicin on the basis of age, but great care is recommended in the elderly given the observed increased toxicity, and doses higher than 50–60 mg/m^2 should be avoided. It has been suggested that in patients over the age of 70 years, regardless of coexisting heart disease, a cumulative doxorubicin dose of 450 mg/m^2 should not be exceeded, whereas in younger patients, a 550 mg/m^2 threshold is used.[76] Several other strategies (slower infusion rate, low-dose weekly regimens, liposomal forms, etc.) have been proposed in an effort to reduce the toxicity.

D. General side effects of chemotherapy in older adults with cancer

Several drug-specific side effects that increase in older patients have been mentioned in the previous section. Elderly patients have a decreased tolerability to chemotherapy in general, with increased incidence of various toxicities. Myelosuppression and mucositis are less drug-specific and will be briefly discussed in this chapter. The greater incidence and severity of toxicity in the elderly mean that they require more supportive care. The aggressive and effective management of toxicity associated with chemotherapy is, therefore, crucial in this population.

D.1. Myelosuppression

Myelosuppression is the major dose-limiting toxicity of many modern chemotherapeutic drugs. Retrospective analyses of data from clinical trials in patients with solid tumors show no correlation between age and myelosuppression.[77–80] These retrospective studies show that age itself should not be a contraindication for cancer therapy. Severe selection bias was present in these studies, however, limiting the generalizability of these conclusions to the general geriatric population. Elderly are clearly underrepresented in clinical studies – certainly patients above the age of 80 years. Moreover, conventional enrollment criteria ensured that the older patients had disproportionately few comorbidities and good performance status.

In contrast, age was found to be a definite independent risk factor for neutropenia in patients older than 60 years with lymphoma in a number of prospective clinical trials of CHOP or reg-

imens with equivalent toxicity.[81–87] The conclusion is that age is clearly associated with a greater risk of grade 4 neutropenia, neutropenia-related infection, and mortality. Not only the incidence but also the severity of myelosuppression increases in elderly receiving chemotherapy, resulting in longer hospital stays and higher inpatient mortality.[88] The risk of neutropenia and its complications, including death, is highest in the early cycles of chemotherapy.[81,89,90] Because of this risk and the potential for better outcomes, prophylaxis with a colony-stimulating factor beginning in the first cycle should be considered in elderly patients.[91]

Age-related data on anemia and trombopenia are less available but are probably also relevant.

D.2. Mucositis

Chemotherapeutic drugs such as Irinotecan and fluorouracil are well known to induce intestinal mucositis, and liposomal anthracyclines cause more oral mucositis than classic anthracyclines; however, many other chemotherapeutic drugs also can induce mucositis to various degrees. Older persons seem to be more susceptible to mucosal toxicities, such as cystitis, gastritis, and stomatitis, and intestinal mucositis, which can lead to diarrhea.[92–94] In studies of 5-FU-containing regimens for colorectal cancer or CMF for breast cancer, advanced age predicted more frequent and more severe diarrhea and stomatitis.[93–95] Mucositis can lead to dehydration and can become life threatening, and elderly individuals are more prone to this.[93,94]

E. Practical recommendations

Specific recommendations can be made when chemotherapy is considered in elderly cancer patients[15]:

1. *Treatment individualization* is important in oncology but is even more important in the elderly because interindividual heterogeneity dramatically increases with increasing age.
2. Perform some form of geriatric assessment at 70 years or more of age.[96]
3. *Supportive or protective* agents, such as hematological growth factors or antiemetics, should be considered and can play a key role in diminishing toxicity in the elderly.[97]
4. *Beware of the risk of drug interactions.* Because many elderly patients are on multiple medications, there can be a great influence on the pharmacokinetics of anticancer drugs.[98]

5. *Compliance needs to be monitored.* For intravenous drugs, this is not an issue, but for oral drugs like capecitabine or temozolomide, or for supportive drugs like antiemetics and growth factors, this is important.

6. *The possibility of less toxic therapy.* Older cancer patients (over 70 years) undergoing classical chemotherapy have a higher risk of experiencing toxicity. Several studies show that chemotherapy is generally well tolerated with a limited impact on independence, comorbidity, and quality of life, but selection bias might be present. Targeted therapies do not induce classic side effects of chemotherapy in general (hair loss, deep neutropenia, nausea and vomiting) and are certainly promising for elderly individuals, but care is warranted because specific side effects might also occur. Angiogenesis inhibitors, for instance, can cause thrombosis and hypertension, and age is an important risk factor.

7. *Maintain adequate hydration.* Elderly patients have a tendency to drink less, especially when feeling ill, and are more intolerant of dehydration. Poor hydration can lead to decreased clearance and increased toxicity, especially for drugs subject to renal excretion.

8. *Define the aim of chemotherapy* (see Table 2.3).

9. *Check renal function in elderly cancer patients.* The International Society of Geriatric Oncology has made specific guidelines on the determination of renal function in elderly[24] as well as on dose adaptation of specific chemotherapeutic agents in renal dysfunction.[99] Prior to drug therapy in elderly patients with cancer, assessment and optimization of hydration status and evaluation of renal function to establish any need for dose adjustment are required. Serum creatinine alone is insufficient as a means of evaluating renal function. More accurate tools, including creatinine clearance methods such as the Cockcroft-Gault method (CG), are available and are generally good indices of renal function status of the patient. However, in elderly patients, the CG and other similar formulas are not as accurate as in the younger population. More recently developed tools, such as the Modification of Diet in Renal Disease (MDRD) equation may be the estimation of choice in elderly patients, whereas the CG estimate can be used in subjects younger than 65 years. However, the

aMDRD (abbreviated MDRD) has generally not been validated for dose calculation of chemotherapy, and the CG may be more practical. Moreover, in extremes of obesity and cachexia and at very high and low creatinine values, no single tool is really accurate. The best estimate of GFR is provided by direct methods such as ^{51}Cr-EDTA or inulin measurement. Within each drug class, preference may be given to agents less likely to be influenced by renal clearance. Within each drug class, preference may be given to agents less likely to be toxic to the kidneys or for which appropriate methods of prevention for renal toxicity exist. Coadministration of known nephrotoxic drugs, such as nonsteroidal anti-inflammatory drugs (NSAIDs), should be avoided or minimized.

10. *Be aware of clinical data for specific chemotherapy drugs.* This is summarized in Table 2.4, based on two recent reviews.[13,14] As mentioned, many clinical and pharmacological data on pharmacokinetics of chemotherapy are available. However, it should be stated that dose adaptation based on age-related pharmacological changes is an unvalidated approach because clinical trials prospectively testing the efficacy and toxicity of age-related dose adaptation versus standard dosing are lacking.

F. Future perspectives

The management of the elderly patient with cancer represents an increasingly common challenge. Physicians and oncologists should be familiar with the age-related changes in physiology that affect the disposition and response to drugs in older patients. The impact of these changes on the availability, efficacy, and toxicity of most classical anticancer drugs is not always well documented. In general, and for most drugs, age itself is not a contraindication to full-dose chemotherapy. Cancer chemotherapy in the elderly may best be considered as an example of the need for dose optimization in individual patients. By considering the basic principles of the pharmacokinetics and pharmacodynamics of these agents, therapy can be optimized. For most agents, it is not possible to provide clear level I guidelines for dose modification on the basis of age. However, one should consider the statement that "if it was not due to the extreme variability, medicine would be a science and not an art." The geriatric population is preeminently a heterogeneous population at all levels, and therefore it will be very difficult to provide simple guidelines. Despite these difficulties, if the important physiological changes in elderly patients are kept in mind, severe toxicity or toxic deaths can be avoided. The fine balance between increased efficacy plus higher toxicity and potentially lesser efficacy, but better tolerability, can frequently swing to the latter because it is just this severe toxicity that is often unacceptable to elderly patients. The decision to modify the dose of an anticancer agent still lies with the bedside clinician, who must integrate knowledge of pharmacology with the type of cancer and condition of the elderly patient. It is evident that more pharmacological studies of anticancer agents in the elderly are required. It is reassuring that there is more and more interest and focus on the elderly population such as the increasing development of clinical trials specifically directed to elderly individuals.

References

1. Vestal RE. Aging and pharmacology. *Cancer* 1997;80:1302–1310.

2. Johnson SL, Mayersohn M, Conrad KA. Gastrointestinal absorption as a function of age: xylose absorption in healthy adults. *Clin Pharmacol Ther.* 1985;38:331–335.

3. Skirvin JA, Lichtman SM. Pharmacokinetic considerations of oral chemotherapy in elderly patients with cancer. *Drugs Aging.* 2002;19:25–42.

4. Wallace SM, Verbeeck RK. Plasma protein binding of drugs in the elderly. *Clin Pharmacokinet.* 1987;12:41–72.

5. Yuen GJ. Altered pharmacokinetics in the elderly. *Clin Geriatr Med.* 1990;6:257–267.

6. Egorin MJ. Cancer pharmacology in the elderly. *Semin Oncol.* 1993;20:43–49.

7. Balis FM. Pharmacokinetic drug interactions of commonly used anticancer drugs. *Clin Pharmacokinet.* 1986;11:223–235.

8. Brenner BM, Meyer TW, Hostetter TH. Dietary protein intake and the progressive nature of kidney disease: the role of hemodynamically mediated glomerular injury in the pathogenesis of progressive glomerular sclerosis in aging, renal ablation, and intrinsic renal disease. *N Engl J Med.* 1982;307:652–659.

9. Muss HB, Woolf S, Berry D, et al. Adjuvant chemotherapy in older and younger women with lymph node-positive breast cancer. *J Am Med Assoc.* 2005;293:1073–1081.

10. Dixon DO, Neilan B, Jones SE, et al. Effect of age on therapeutic outcome in advanced diffuse histiocytic lymphoma: the Southwest Oncology Group experience. *J Clin Oncol.* 1986;4:295–305.

11. Tirelli U, Errante D, Van Glabbeke M, et al. CHOP is the standard regimen in patients > or = 70 years of age with intermediate-grade and high-grade non-Hodgkin's lymphoma: results of a randomized study of the European Organization for Research and Treatment of Cancer Lymphoma Cooperative Study Group. *J Clin Oncol.* 1998;16:27–34.

12. Bonadonna G, Valagussa P. Dose-response effect of adjuvant chemotherapy in breast cancer. *N Engl J Med.* 1981;304:10–15.

13. Wildiers H, Highley MS, de Bruijn EA, et al. Pharmacology of anticancer drugs in the elderly population. *Clin Pharmacokinet.* 2003;42: 1213–1242.

14. Lichtman SM, Wildiers H, Chatelut E, et al. International Society of Geriatric Oncology chemotherapy taskforce: evaluation of chemotherapy in older patients – an analysis of the medical literature. *J Clin Oncol.* 2007;25:1832–1843.

15. Wildiers H. Mastering chemotherapy dose reduction in elderly cancer patients. *Eur J Cancer.* 2007;43:2235–2241.

16. Dees EC, O'Reilly S, Goodman SN, et al. A prospective pharmacologic evaluation of age-related toxicity of adjuvant chemotherapy in women with breast cancer. *Cancer Invest.* 2000;18:521–529.

17. Moore MJ. Clinical pharmacokinetics of cyclophosphamide. *Clin Pharmacokinet.* 1991;20: 194–208.

18. Rudd GN, Hartley JA, Souhami RL. Persistence of cisplatin-induced DNA interstrand crosslinking in peripheral blood mononuclear cells from elderly and young individuals. *Cancer Chemother Pharmacol.* 1995;35:323–326.

19. Kintzel PE, Dorr RT. Anticancer drug renal toxicity and elimination: dosing guidelines for altered renal function. *Cancer Treat Rev.* 1995;21:33–64.

20. Yamamoto N, Tamura T, Maeda M, et al. The influence of ageing on cisplatin pharmacokinetics in lung cancer patients with normal organ function. *Cancer Chemother Pharmacol.* 1995;36:102–106.

21. Reece PA, Stafford I, Russell J, et al. Creatinine clearance as a predictor of ultrafilterable platinum disposition in cancer patients treated with cisplatin: relationship between peak ultrafilterable platinum plasma levels and nephrotoxicity. *J Clin Oncol.* 1987;5:304–309.

22. Baker SD, Grochow LB. Pharmacology of cancer chemotherapy in the older person. *Clin Geriatr Med.* 1997;13:169–183.

23. Calvert AH, Newell DR, Gumbrell LA, et al. Carboplatin dosage: prospective evaluation of a simple formula based on renal function. *J Clin Oncol.* 1989;7:1748–1756.

24. Launay-Vacher V, Chatelut E, Lichtman SM, et al. Renal insufficiency in elderly cancer patients: International Society of Geriatric Oncology clinical practice recommendations. *Ann Oncol.* 2007;18:1314–1321.

25. Massari C, Brienza S, Rotarski M, et al. Pharmacokinetics of oxaliplatin in patients with normal versus impaired renal function. *Cancer Chemother Pharmacol.* 2000;45:157–164.

26. Goldberg RM, Tabah-Fisch I, Bleiberg H, et al. Pooled analysis of safety and efficacy of oxaliplatin plus fluorouracil/leucovorin administered bimonthly in elderly patients with colorectal cancer. *J Clin Oncol.* 2006;24:4085–4091.

27. Feliu J, Salud A, Escudero P, et al. XELOX (capecitabine plus oxaliplatin) as first-line treatment for elderly patients over 70 years of age with advanced colorectal cancer. *Br J Cancer.* 2006;94:969–975.

28. Comella P, Natale D, Farris A, et al. Capecitabine plus oxaliplatin for the first-line treatment of elderly patients with metastatic colorectal carcinoma: final results of the Southern Italy Cooperative Oncology Group Trial 0108. *Cancer*. 2005;104:282–289.

29. Venook AP, Egorin MJ, Rosner GL, et al. Phase I and pharmacokinetic trial of paclitaxel in patients with hepatic dysfunction: Cancer and Leukemia Group B 9264. *J Clin Oncol*. 1998;16:1811–1819.

30. Wildiers H, Paridaens R. Taxanes in elderly breast cancer patients. *Cancer Treat Rev*. 2004;30:333–342.

31. Seidman AD, Berry D, Cirrincione C, et al. Randomized phase III trial of weekly compared with every-3-weeks paclitaxel for metastatic breast cancer, with trastuzumab for all HER-2 overexpressors and random assignment to trastuzumab or not in HER-2 nonoverexpressors: final results of Cancer and Leukemia Group B protocol 9840. *J Clin Oncol*. 2008;26:1642–1649.

32. Lichtman SM, Hollis D, Miller AA, et al. Prospective evaluation of the relationship of patient age and paclitaxel clinical pharmacology: Cancer and Leukemia Group B (CALGB 9762). *J Clin Oncol*. 2006;24:1846–1851.

33. Smorenburg CH, ten Tije AJ, Verweij J, et al. Altered clearance of unbound paclitaxel in elderly patients with metastatic breast cancer. *Eur J Cancer*. 2003;39:196–202.

34. Hirth J, Watkins PB, Strawderman M, et al. The effect of an individual's cytochrome CYP3A4 activity on docetaxel clearance. *Clin Cancer Res*. 2000;6:1255–1258.

35. Bruno R, Vivier N, Veyrat-Follet C, et al. Population pharmacokinetics and pharmacokinetic-pharmacodynamic relationships for docetaxel. *Invest New Drugs*. 2001;19:163–169.

36. Girre V, Beuzeboc P, Livartowski A, et al. Docetaxel in elderly patients: phase I and pharmacokinetic study [abstract number 2113]. *Proc Am Soc Clin Oncol*. 2005. JOURNAL OF CLINICAL ONCOLOGY Volume: 23 Issue: 16 Pages: 162S-162S Part: Part 1 Suppl. S Supplement: Part 1 Suppl. S Published: JUN 1 2005

37. Zanetta S, Albrand G, Bachelot T, et al. A phase I trial of docetaxel every 21 days in elderly patients with metastatic breast cancer [abstract]. *Ann Oncol*. 2000;11:XX. ANNALS OF ONCOLOGY Volume: 11 Pages: 73-73 Supplement: Suppl. 4 Meeting Abstract: 322PD Published: 2000

38. Hainsworth JD, Burris III HA, Litchy S, et al. Weekly docetaxel in the treatment of elderly patients with advanced nonsmall cell lung carcinoma: a Minnie Pearl Cancer Research Network phase II trial. *Cancer*. 2000;89:328–333.

39. Tannock IF, de WR, Berry WR, et al. Docetaxel plus prednisone or mitoxantrone plus prednisone for advanced prostate cancer. *N Engl J Med*. 2004;351:1502–1512.

40. Souhami RL, Spiro SG, Rudd RM, et al. Five-day oral etoposide treatment for advanced small-cell lung cancer: randomized comparison with intravenous chemotherapy. *J Natl Cancer Inst*. 1997;89:577–580.

41. Joel SP, Shah R, Slevin ML. Etoposide dosage and pharmacodynamics. *Cancer Chemother Pharmacol*. 1994;34(suppl):69–75.

42. Miller AA, Rosner GL, Ratain MJ, et al. Pharmacology of 21-day oral etoposide given in combination with I.V. cisplatin in patients with extensive-stage small cell lung cancer: a Cancer and Leukemia Group B study (CALGB 9062). *Clin Cancer Res*. 1997;3:719–725.

43. Fuchs CS, Moore MR, Harker G, et al. Phase III comparison of two irinotecan dosing regimens in second-line therapy of metastatic colorectal cancer. *J Clin Oncol*. 2003;21:807–814.

44. Aparicio T, Desrame J, Lecomte T, et al. Oxaliplatin- or irinotecan-based chemotherapy for metastatic colorectal cancer in the elderly. *Br J Cancer*. 2003;89:1439–1444.

45. Sastre J, Marcuello E, Masutti B, et al. Irinotecan in combination with fluorouracil in a 48-hour continuous infusion as first-line chemotherapy for elderly patients with metastatic colorectal cancer: a Spanish cooperative group for the treatment of digestive tumors study. *J Clin Oncol*. 2005;23:3545–3551.

46. Miya T, Goya T, Fujii H, et al. Factors affecting the pharmacokinetics of CPT-11: the body mass index, age and sex are independent predictors of pharmacokinetic parameters of CPT-11. *Invest New Drugs*. 2001;19:61–67.

47. Chau I, Norman AR, Cunningham D, et al. Elderly patients with fluoropyrimidine and thymidylate synthase inhibitor-resistant advanced colorectal cancer derive similar benefit without excessive toxicity when treated with irinotecan monotherapy. *Br J Cancer*. 2004;91:1453–1458.

48. Herben VM, Bokkel Huinink WW, Beijnen JH. Clinical pharmacokinetics of topotecan. *Clin Pharmacokinet*. 1996;31:85–102.

49. O'Reilly S, Armstrong DK, Grochow LB. Life-threatening myelosuppression in patients with occult renal impairment receiving topotecan. *Gynecol Oncol*. 1997;67:329–330.

50. Armstrong DK. Topotecan dosing guidelines in ovarian cancer: reduction and management of hematologic toxicity. *Oncologist*. 2004;9:33–42.

51. Gelman RS, Taylor SG. Cyclophosphamide, methotrexate, and 5-fluorouracil chemotherapy in women more than 65 years old with advanced breast cancer: the elimination of age trends in toxicity by using doses based on creatinine clearance. *J Clin Oncol*. 1984;2:1404–1413.

52. Kristensen LO, Weismann K, Hutters L. Renal function and the rate of disappearance of methotrexate from serum. *Eur J Clin Pharmacol.* 1975;8:439–444.

53. Port RE, Daniel B, Ding RW, et al. Relative importance of dose, body surface area, sex, and age for 5-fluorouracil clearance. *Oncology.* 1991;48:277–281.

54. Milano G, Etienne MC, Cassuto-Viguier E, et al. Influence of sex and age on fluorouracil clearance. *J Clin Oncol.* 1992;10:1171–1175.

55. Young AM, Daryanani S, Kerr DJ. Can pharmacokinetic monitoring improve clinical use of fluorouracil? *Clin Pharmacokinet.* 1999;36:391–398.

56. Stein BN, Petrelli NJ, Douglass HO, et al. Age and sex are independent predictors of 5-fluorouracil toxicity – analysis of a large-scale phase-III trial. *Cancer.* 1995;75:11–17.

57. Weinerman B, Rayner H, Venne A, et al. Increased incidence and severity of stomatitis in women treated with 5-fluorouracil and leucovorin [abstract No 1176]. *Proc Am Soc Clin Oncol.* 1998.

58. Sargent DJ, Goldberg RM, Jacobson SD, et al. A pooled analysis of adjuvant chemotherapy for resected colon cancer in elderly patients. *N Engl J Med.* 2001;345:1091–1097.

59. Balducci L. The geriatric cancer patient: equal benefit from equal treatment. *Cancer Control.* 2001;8:1–25.

60. Poole C, Gardiner J, Twelves C, et al. Effect of renal impairment on the pharmacokinetics and tolerability of capecitabine (Xeloda) in cancer patients. *Cancer Chemother Pharmacol.* 2002;49:225–234.

61. Cassidy J, Twelves C, Cameron D, et al. Bioequivalence of two tablet formulations of capecitabine and exploration of age, gender, body surface area, and creatinine clearance as factors influencing systemic exposure in cancer patients. *Cancer Chemother Pharmacol.* 1999;44:453–460.

62. Bajetta E, Procopio G, Celio L, et al. Safety and efficacy of two different doses of capecitabine in the treatment of advanced breast cancer in older women. *J Clin Oncol.* 2005;23:2155–2161.

63. Venook AP, Egorin MJ, Rosner GL, et al. Phase I and pharmacokinetic trial of gemcitabine in patients with hepatic or renal dysfunction: Cancer and Leukemia Group B 9565. *J Clin Oncol.* 2000;18:2780–2787.

64. Lichtman SM, Skirvin JA. Pharmacology of antineoplastic agents in older cancer patients. *Oncology.* 2000;14:1743–1755.

65. Shepherd FA, Abratt RP, Anderson H, et al. Gemcitabine in the treatment of elderly patients with advanced non-small cell lung cancer. *Semin Oncol.* 1997;24:S7-50–S7-55.

66. Martin C, Ardizzoni A, Rosso R. Gemcitabine: safety profile and efficacy in non-small cell lung cancer unaffected by age. *Aging.* 1997;9:297–303.

67. Martoni A, Di Fabio F, Guaraldi M, et al. Prospective phase II study of single-agent gemcitabine in untreated elderly patients with stage IIIB/IV non-small-cell lung cancer. *Am J Clin Oncol.* 2001;24:614–617.

68. Robert J, Hoerni B. Age dependence of the early-phase pharmacokinetics of doxorubicin. *Cancer Res.* 1983;43:4467–4469.

69. Legha SS, Benjamin RS, Mackay B, et al. Reduction of doxorubicin cardiotoxicity by prolonged continuous intravenous infusion. *Ann Intern Med.* 1982;96:133–139.

70. Pinder MC, Duan Z, Goodwin JS, et al. Congestive heart failure in older women treated with adjuvant anthracycline chemotherapy for breast cancer. *J Clin Oncol.* 2007;25:3808–3815.

71. Sonneveld P, Deridder M, Vanderlelie H, et al. Comparison of doxorubicin and mitoxantrone in the treatment of elderly patients with advanced diffuse non-Hodgkins-lymphoma using CHOP versus CNOP chemotherapy. *J Clin Oncol.* 1995;13:2530–2539.

72. Coiffier B, Lepage E, Briere J, et al. CHOP chemotherapy plus rituximab compared with CHOP alone in elderly patients with diffuse large-B-cell lymphoma. *N Engl J Med.* 2002;346:235–242.

73. Slamon DJ, Leyland-Jones B, Shak S, et al. Use of chemotherapy plus a monoclonal antibody against HER2 for metastatic breast cancer that overexpresses HER2. *N Engl J Med.* 2001; 344:783–792.

74. Swain SM, Whaley FS, Gerber MC, et al. Cardioprotection with dexrazoxane for doxorubicin-containing therapy in advanced breast cancer. *J Clin Oncol.* 1997;15:1318–1332.

75. Harris L, Batist G, Belt R, et al. Liposome-encapsulated doxorubicin compared with conventional doxorubicin in a randomized multicenter trial as first-line therapy of metastatic breast carcinoma. *Cancer.* 2002;94:25–36.

76. Buzdar AU, Marcus C, Smith TL, et al. Early and delayed clinical cardiotoxicity of doxorubicin. *Cancer.* 1985;55:2761–2765.

77. Gelman RS, Taylor SG. Cyclophosphamide, methotrexate, and 5-fluorouracil chemotherapy in women more than 65 years old with advanced breast cancer: the elimination of age trends in toxicity by using doses based on creatinine clearance. *J Clin Oncol.* 1984;2:1404–1413.

78. Ibrahim NK, Frye DK, Buzdar AU, et al. Doxorubicin-based chemotherapy in elderly patients with metastatic breast cancer: tolerance and outcome. *Arch Intern Med.* 1996;156:882–888.

79. Begg CB, Carbone PP. Clinical trials and drug toxicity in the elderly: the experience of the Eastern Cooperative Oncology Group. *Cancer.* 1983;52:1986–1992.

80. Giovanazzi-Bannon S, Rademaker A, Lai G, et al. Treatment tolerance of elderly cancer patients entered onto phase II clinical trials: an Illinois Cancer Center study. *J Clin Oncol.* 1994;12:2447–2452.

81. Bastion Y, Blay JY, Divine M, et al. Elderly patients with aggressive non-Hodgkin's lymphoma: disease presentation, response to treatment, and survival – a Groupe d'Etude des Lymphomes de l'Adulte study on 453 patients older than 69 years. *J Clin Oncol.* 1997;15:2945–2953.

82. Bertini M, Freilone R, Vitolo U, et al. P-VEBEC: a new 8-weekly schedule with or without rG-CSF for elderly patients with aggressive non-Hodgkin's lymphoma (NHL). *Ann Oncol.* 1994;5:895–900.

83. Gomez H, Mas L, Casanova L, et al. Elderly patients with aggressive non-Hodgkin's lymphoma treated with CHOP chemotherapy plus granulocyte-macrophage colony-stimulating factor: identification of two age subgroups with differing hematologic toxicity. *J Clin Oncol.* 1998;16:2352–2358.

84. O'Reilly SE, Connors JM, Howdle S, et al. In search of an optimal regimen for elderly patients with advanced-stage diffuse large-cell lymphoma: results of a phase II study of P/DOCE chemotherapy. *J Clin Oncol.* 1993;11:2250–2257.

85. Sonneveld P, Deridder M, Vanderlelie H, et al. Comparison of doxorubicin and mitoxantrone in the treatment of elderly patients with advanced diffuse non-Hodgkins-lymphoma using CHOP versus CNOP chemotherapy. *J Clin Oncol.* 1995;13:2530–2539.

86. Tirelli U, Zagonel V, Serraino D, et al. Non-Hodgkins lymphomas in 137 patients aged 70 years or older – a retrospective European Organization for Research and Treatment of Cancer lymphoma group-study. *J Clin Oncol.* 1988;6:1708–1713.

87. Zinzani PL, Storti S, Zaccaria A, et al. Elderly aggressive-histology non-Hodgkin's lymphoma: first-line VNCOP-B regimen experience on 350 patients. *Blood.* 1999;94:33–38.

88. Morrison VA, Picozzi V, Scott S, et al. The impact of age on delivered dose intensity and hospitalizations for febrile neutropenia in patients with intermediate-grade non-Hodgkin's lymphoma receiving initial CHOP chemotherapy: a risk factor analysis. *Clin Lymphoma.* 2001;2:47–56.

89. Gomez H, Hidalgo M, Casanova L, et al. Risk factors for treatment-related death in elderly patients with aggressive non-Hodgkin's lymphoma: results of a multivariate analysis. *J Clin Oncol.* 1998;16:2065–2069.

90. Zinzani PL, Pavone E, Storti S, et al. Randomized trial with or without granulocyte colony-stimulating factor as adjunct to induction VNCOP-B treatment of elderly high-grade non-Hodgkin's lymphoma. *Blood.* 1997;89:3974–3979.

91. Balducci L, Repetto L. Increased risk of myelotoxicity in elderly patients with non-Hodgkin lymphoma – the case for routine prophylaxis with colony-stimulating factor beginning in the first cycle of chemotherapy. *Cancer.* 2004;100:6–11.

92. Balducci L, Corcoran MB. Antineoplastic chemotherapy of the older cancer patient. *Hematol Oncol Clin N Am.* 2000;14:193–212

93. Crivellari D, Bonetti M, Castiglione-Gertsch M, et al. Burdens and benefits of adjuvant cyclophosphamide, methotrexate, and fluorouracil and tamoxifen for elderly patients with breast cancer: the International Breast Cancer Study Group trial VII. *J Clin Oncol.* 2000;18:1412–1422.

94. Stein BN, Petrelli NJ, Douglass HO, et al. Age and sex are independent predictors of 5-fluorouracil toxicity – analysis of a large-scale phase-III trial. *Cancer.* 1995;75:11–17.

95. Popescu RA, Norman A, Ross PJ, et al. Adjuvant or palliative chemotherapy for colorectal cancer in patients 70 years or older. *J Clin Oncol.* 1999;17:2412–2418.

96. Extermann M, Aapro M, Bernabei RB, et al. Use of comprehensive geriatric assessment in older cancer patients: recommendations from the task force on CGA of the International Society of Geriatric Oncology (SIOG). *Crit Rev Oncol Hematol.* 2005;55:241–252.

97. Aapro MS, Cameron DA, Pettengell R, et al. EORTC guidelines for the use of granulocyte-colony stimulating factor to reduce the incidence of chemotherapy-induced febrile neutropenia in adult patients with lymphomas and solid tumours. *Eur J Cancer.* 2006;42:2433–2453.

98. Loadman PM, Bibby MC. Pharmacokinetic drug interactions with anticancer drugs. *Clin Pharmacokinet.* 1994;26:486–500.

99. Lichtman SM, Wildiers H, Launay-Vacher V, et al. International Society of Geriatric Oncology (SIOG) recommendations for the adjustment of dosing in elderly cancer patients with renal insufficiency. *Eur J Cancer.* 2007;43:14–34.

100. Wildiers H, Highley MS, de Bruijn EA, et al. Pharmacology of anticancer drugs in the elderly population. *Clin Pharmacokinet.* 2003;42:1213–1242.

Pharmacology and unique side effects of hormonal therapy in older adults

Leona Downey

As a majority of breast cancers in elderly women are hormone receptor positive and therefore driven by estrogen-related growth, hormonal therapies, such as the selective estrogen receptor modulators (SERMs) or the aromatase inhibitors (AIs), play a primary role in the treatment of these women. These medications function through different mechanisms to prevent estrogen's stimulation of breast cancer cell growth. The drugs' different mechanisms of action result in unique side effects for each class. Though these side effects can occur in women of any age, normal physiologic changes of aging, polypharmacy, and age-associated comorbidities can make the use of hormonal therapy more complex in older patients. Because elderly women have been underrepresented in breast cancer clinical trials, there are few published data on the differential side effect profiles of hormonal therapies in old versus young women. However, increasing awareness of the need for geriatric oncology studies should result in improved evidence-based recommendations for this population.

A. Tamoxifen

A.1. Pharmacology and metabolism

Tamoxifen, an oral nonsteroidal antiestrogen, or selective estrogen receptor modulator, functions by binding to the estrogen receptor, competitively inhibiting estrogen binding. Tamoxifen was first used in the treatment of metastatic breast cancer in the 1970s and has since been used in the treatment of women with all stages of breast cancer as well as in women at high risk of breast cancer. Tamoxifen is dosed daily and has a terminal elimination half-life of 5–7 days. Tamoxifen is converted to its more active metabolite, endoxifen, by the hepatic cytochrome P450 enzyme 2D6 (CYP2D6). Variation in CYP2D6 activity has been shown to affect tamoxifen metabolism to endoxifen and can therefore limit the drug's ability to function as an antiestrogen. CYP2D6 activity may

be altered by inherited variation in 2D6 genotype or by concurrent medications that decrease 2D6 activity.[1,2] For example, patients who are homozygous for a variant 2D6 allele, resulting in impaired tamoxifen metabolism, have decreased endoxifen concentrations, and this has been correlated with poor breast cancer–specific outcomes.[3] Similarly, patients taking tamoxifen concurrently with a drug that is a potent 2D6 inhibitor have also been found to have poorer outcomes.[4] The 2D6 inhibitors vary in their degree of inhibition, with the potent inhibitors having the greatest effect. Neither inherited CYP2D6 genotypes nor drug interactions are specifically more likely in elderly patients. However, many elderly are on multiple medications, making the likelihood of a concurrent 2D6 inhibitor more probable. See Table 3.1 for common inhibitors of CYP2D6. The degree of 2D6 inhibition reported varies by source for many of the drugs, but clearly paroxetine and fluoxetine are the most potent inhibitors. Venlafaxine appears to have no clinically significant effect on 2D6 activity and tamoxifen metabolism.[1] Therefore, if an antidepressant is needed for a patient on tamoxifen, venlafaxine is preferred. Care should be taken to avoid any inhibitor of 2D6 in combination with tamoxifen.

The effects on tamoxifen metabolism of impaired liver function, as in cirrhosis, are not known, and no formal recommendations exist for tamoxifen dose adjustments in hepatic insufficiency. Though the liver parenchymal volume does decline as a normal function of aging, variation in metabolic function of the liver with aging is quite variable, and there is no evidence that tamoxifen metabolism is less vigorous in normal older individuals. In addition, the available data on the efficacy of tamoxifen by age suggest that it is as effective in reducing breast cancer risk in older versus younger patients, supporting the theory that aging alone does not significantly affect hepatic metabolism of tamoxifen. However, this could be more clearly demonstrated if studied specifically in a cohort of elderly patients.

Table 3.1 CYP2D6 inhibitors.

Degree of CYP2D6 inhibition	Drugs
Potent inhibitors	Fluoxetine (Prozac), paroxetine (Paxil)
Moderate inhibitors	Duloxetine (Cymbalta), sertraline (Zoloft), buproprion[a] (Wellbutrin), cimetidine, amiodarone, doxepin, haloperidol
Weak inhibitors	Mirtazapin (Remeron), celecoxib
No inhibition	Venlafaxine (Effexor)
Unclear	Citalopram (Celexa), escitalopram (Lexapro)

[a]Buproprion is listed as a potent or moderate inhibitor in various sources.[1–5]

B. Tamoxifen side effects

Tamoxifen is referred to as a selective estrogen receptor modulator because the drug's effect on the estrogen receptor varies, or is "selective" in different tissues. Tamoxifen's anti–breast cancer properties result from having an estrogen-antagonist effect on the estrogen receptor in the breast, meaning that tamoxifen binding results in inhibition of this estrogen receptor (ER) and its downstream signaling. On the contrary, tamoxifen has an estrogen-agonist effect in other tissues, including the uterus, the bone, and the vascular system. Tamoxifen derives its side effect profile from the variable effects of ER binding in these different tissues.

B.1. Thromboembolic disease

One of the most life-threatening adverse effects associated with tamoxifen is venous thromboembolic disease. In a meta-analysis of 32 randomized controlled trials of tamoxifen for adjuvant treatment or risk reduction, the relative risk (RR) of pulmonary embolus was 1.88 for tamoxifen versus control.[6] Similarly, tamoxifen was associated with a statistically significant increased risk of stroke, with an RR of 1.49. The risks of both stroke and pulmonary embolism were even greater when trials of only postmenopausal women were considered, with RR of 1.68 and 2.46, respectively. However, these authors did not perform multivariate analysis to evaluate the contribution of age or other risk factors for thromboembolic disease such as hyperlipidemia, hypertension, or prior thrombophlebitis. One study that calculated age-adjusted mortality rates for tamoxifen-treated patients for specific causes of death demonstrated that the risk of death by thromboembolic episode was significantly associated with age. In this study, tamoxifen treatment was associated with an increase in thromboembolic deaths per 1,000 women of +1.3, +3.3, +7.5, and +15.0 for women aged 50, 60, 70, and 80 years, respectively.[7] Again, multivariate analysis was not possible, but the increase in risk of thromboembolic disease with age is likely due to an increased likelihood of underlying risk factors for the complication in that patient population.

There does not appear to be an increase in coronary artery thrombosis or ischemic heart disease with tamoxifen treatment. Some studies have suggested that tamoxifen may actually decrease the risk of myocardial infarction or myocardial infarction death,[6] while others have shown no effect on this outcome. Tamoxifen has been clearly associated with a beneficial effect on the lipid profile, with a decrease in total cholesterol and LDL cholesterol and an increase or neutral effect on HDL cholesterol. This may translate to improved cardiovascular risk.

B.2. Endometrial carcinoma

Tamoxifen has partial estrogen-agonist activity when binding to the ER in the uterus, resulting in stimulation of this receptor. Therefore tamoxifen, like unopposed estrogen, results in stimulation of the endometrial lining, which may be manifested by endometrial thickening, endometrial hyperplasia, and rarely endometrial carcinoma. In the meta-analysis of tamoxifen trials, tamoxifen treatment was associated with a relative risk of endometrial cancer of 2.7 compared to control treated groups.[6] When trials evaluating only postmenopausal women were considered, the risk was even greater, with an RR of 3.18, suggesting that the risk is more significant in older women. In another study, the 10-year risk of mortality from endometrial carcinoma was significantly associated with increased age. The use of tamoxifen was associated with an excess risk of death from endometrial carcinoma per 1,000 women of +1.0, +3.8, +8.1, and +8.0 for women aged 50, 60, 70, and 80 years, respectively.[7]

The aromatase inhibitors do not increase the risk of endometrial carcinoma and may actually be able to reverse some of the increased risk associated with tamoxifen when used in sequence. For example, the incidence of endometrial carcinoma

Table 3.2 Endometrial carcinoma incidence in adjuvant hormonal therapy trials.[8–10]

	Endometrial cancer incidence		
	ATAC	IES	ABCSG/ARNO
Tamoxifen alone	0.8%	0.46%	0.43%
AI alone	0.2%		
Tamoxifen followed by AI		0.21%	0.06%
Median follow-up (months)	100	56	28

ATAC: Arimidex, Tamoxifen, Alone, or in Combination
IES: Intergroup Exemestane Study
ABCSG: Austrian Breast & Colorectal Cancer Study Group
ARNO: Arimidex-Nolvadex
AI: Aromatase inhibitor

in the Arimidex, Tamoxifen, Alone or in Combination (ATAC) trial, which compared 5 years of adjuvant tamoxifen to 5 years of adjuvant anastrozole, was 0.8 percent for tamoxifen and 0.2 percent for anastrozole.[8] In contrast, studies of sequential therapy including tamoxifen followed by an AI versus tamoxifen alone suggest that the risk of endometrial cancer in the sequential arms is significantly lower than that seen in the tamoxifen-alone arms. For example, in the Intergroup Exemestane Study, comparing 5 years of tamoxifen versus 2 years of tamoxifen followed by 3 years of exemestane, the incidence of endometrial carcinoma was 0.46 percent versus 0.21 percent, respectively.[9] Similarly, Austrian Breast and Colorectal Cancer Study Group/Arimidex-Nolvadex 95, which compared tamoxifen to tamoxifen followed by anastrozole, revealed that the endometrial carcinoma incidence was 0.43 percent versus 0.06 percent.[10] Therefore it appears in cross-study comparisons that the incidence of endometrial carcinoma with tamoxifen may be reduced when an aromatase inhibitor is used in sequence as well (Table 3.2). Of course, cross-trial comparisons must be interpreted with caution. However, a prospective study of transvaginal ultrasound to assess endometrial thickness in women receiving AI therapy following long-term tamoxifen therapy supported the theory that AI therapy can reverse the effects of tamoxifen on the endometrium. In this study, postmenopausal breast cancer patients who had received tamoxifen for at least 2.5 years and were being switched to an AI were followed with serial transvaginal ultrasound.[11] Fifty-five

percent of those patients had a decline in endometrial thickness, and an additional 38 percent had stable endometrial thickness. Longer duration of AI therapy was associated with a higher likelihood of endometrial thinning. No comment was made on the association of age with this effect.

B.3. Cognitive function

Estrogens were historically thought to have a beneficial effect on brain metabolism, and potentially with a lower risk of dementia. However, there are conflicting data on this topic, and it remains controversial. For example, in the Heart and Estrogen/Progestin Replacement Study, over 1,000 women randomized to hormone replacement versus placebo were evaluated for cognitive effects. This study showed no significant difference between the two arms in cognitive function as measured by six different standardized tests.[12] On the other hand, the Women's Health Initiative Memory Study evaluated cognitive change in elderly women randomized to estrogen replacement versus placebo or estrogen and progestin replacement versus placebo. In this study, the hormone replacement study appeared to be associated with a higher incidence of dementia and mild cognitive impairment compared to placebo.[13]

This raises concerns that there may be a relationship between breast cancer hormonal therapies and cognitive function or dementia. A study of magnetic resonance spectroscopy to assess biochemical markers of brain injury and metabolism suggests that tamoxifen results in activity in the brain similar to that seen with estrogen.[14] Therefore tamoxifen may have estrogen agonist effects in the brain, as it does in some other tissues. Raloxifene (another SERM) was shown to result in a reduced risk of cognitive decline in non–breast cancer patients receiving raloxifene for osteoporosis.[15] Interestingly, this was seen only in the 120 mg/d dose but not in the 60 mg/d dose. A small pilot study compared patients treated on ATAC with a control group of healthy patients and evaluated for cognitive decline.[16] This study was not powered to compare differences in patients treated with tamoxifen versus an AI but did demonstrate that patients receiving hormonal therapy on ATAC had decreased verbal memory performance compared to the controls. Another study evaluated patients with breast cancer who were treated with either tamoxifen or anastrozole in a nonrandomized fashion and found that anastrozole was associated with poorer verbal and visual learning and memory compared to women receiving tamoxifen.[17] In this small study, the anastrozole patients were older than the tamoxifen-treated patients, but the difference in cognitive function remained when data were controlled for age, education, and depression. This raises concerns that the additional estrogen deprivation that results from aromatase inhibitor therapy may worsen cognitive decline. However, in a cognitive function substudy of the International Breast Cancer Intervention Study (IBIS) II trial, a trial of anastrozole versus placebo as chemoprevention in women at high risk of breast cancer, there was no difference in cognitive performance in AI- versus placebo-treated patients.[18] Therefore there is no clear pattern of cognitive effects related to breast cancer hormonal therapy, and many studies present conflicting results. Cognitive function must be assessed in further hormonal therapy studies to better elucidate the risk of cognitive decline as this could significantly affect the risk-benefit ratio of the use of hormonal therapy in older women with breast cancer.

B.4. Other

Other common effects of tamoxifen treatment include hot flashes and vaginal discharge. Hot flashes clearly do occur in elderly women treated with tamoxifen more frequently than placebo.[19] However, it is unclear from the literature if hot flashes are more or less common in older versus younger tamoxifen-treated patients. In anecdotal experience, tamoxifen-induced hot flashes are more severe in younger or perimenopausal women compared to elderly women. Many nonestrogen medications are available for the treatment of hot flashes in breast cancer patients. As described earlier, caution should be taken when prescribing antidepressants as treatment for hot flashes. Venlafaxine (Effexor) and gabapentin (Neurontin) are two safe options for the treatment of hot flashes in women on tamoxifen. Neither is approved by the U.S. Food and Drug Association for this indication, but both have been studied and demonstrated efficacy in the treatment of hot flashes in breast cancer patients.[20,21] The vaginal discharge seen with tamoxifen therapy is generally clear and mucoid and can actually provide wanted improvement in the vaginal dryness often seen in elderly women. Finally, tamoxifen is known to result in improved bone mineral density in postmenopausal women because of its estrogen-agonist effect in the bone.

C. Aromatase inhibitors

C.1. Pharmacology and metabolism

The current aromatase inhibitors in clinical use include anastrozole (Arimidex), letrozole (Femara), and exemestane (Aromasin). These medications decrease circulating estrogen levels by inhibiting peripheral conversion of other steroid hormones to estrogen. Because they function only to prevent peripheral estrogen production and have no effect on ovarian estrogen production, they are effective only in postmenopausal women. Anastrozole and letrozole are nonsteroidal aromatase inhibitors that bind reversibly to the enzyme aromatase. Exemestane, on the other hand, is a steroidal aromatase inhibitor that binds irreversibly. Head-to-head studies are ongoing to compare the efficacy and toxicity of these different AIs, but results of these studies are pending. Individual studies evaluating each of the three AIs suggest that their toxicity profiles are similar. All the AIs are dosed orally daily, and terminal elimination half-lives are approximately 2 days for anastrozole and letrozole and approximately 24 hours for exemestane. The AIs are metabolized primarily by the liver and are excreted in urine and feces. No dose adjustments are suggested for any of the AIs for age, renal insufficiency, or hepatic insufficiency with anastrozole or exemestane. For letrozole, in patients with severe hepatic insufficiency, a dose reduction is recommended. Unlike tamoxifen, these drugs do not appear to require activation or conversion to a more active metabolite, suggesting that there should be no major inhibitory drug interaction.

D. Aromatase inhibitor side effects

Older women generally appear to tolerate AI therapy well. In an efficacy and tolerability study of elderly women being treated in the National Cancer Institute of Canada MA.17 trial, evaluating extended adjuvant AI therapy versus placebo, there was no significant difference in toxicity or quality of life in AI- versus placebo-treated women over the age of 70 years.[22] However, there are a few AI-specific adverse events that must be considered in elderly women being evaluated for AI therapy.

D.1. Bone loss

The most significant and concerning adverse effect associated with the AIs is loss of bone density, which occurs because of the loss of circulating estrogen. In all the studies comparing adjuvant AI therapy to tamoxifen, the AI has been associated with a statistically significant increase in bone loss and fracture.[16–18] These studies suggest that the annual bone loss with aromatase inhibitor therapy is 1.6–2.6 percent per year, compared to an average annual loss of 1 percent in healthy postmenopausal women.[23] Therefore the baseline bone density prior to initiating AI therapy is key to assessing the risk of subsequent bone loss. In ATAC, no patient with normal bone density or mild osteopenia (T score greater than –1.5) at baseline developed osteoporosis over 5 years of treatment.[24] In this study, the rate of bone loss was greatest in those women who were within 4 years of menopause compared to women who were more than 4 years from menopause. This might suggest that the effect is less abrupt in older women.

The bone mineral density loss in AI-treated patients does not appear to be independently associated with age.[24,25] In an analysis of Breast International Group (BIG) 1-98 study (letrozole vs. tamoxifen) by age, the risk of fracture was higher in letrozole-treated patients, but this was generally consistent across age groups for those over age 54 years,[26] meaning that the increase in fracture risk was similar for all age groups. However, the rate of bone loss and the risk of fracture are associated with other risk factors, including lower baseline bone density and lower baseline estradiol levels.[24] These risk factors may be more prevalent in older women. Other risk factors for osteoporosis in non–breast cancer patients include prior osteoporosis-related fracture, lower body mass index, smoking, and steroid medication use. These factors have not been clearly demonstrated in AI-induced bone loss but may also contribute to the risk. Some of these risk factors may be also higher in older versus younger patients.

Interestingly, in the 100-month follow-up of ATAC, the increased fracture rate associated with anastrozole was seen only during active treatment and appeared to normalize after completion of therapy.[27] Therefore it is not likely a permanent side effect.

D.2. Treatment options for bone loss

A number of studies have been performed to evaluate the efficacy of bisphosphonate therapy in reducing the risk of breast cancer treatment–associated bone loss. The use of intravenous zole-dronic acid, given as 4 mg intravenously every 6 months, in patients receiving adjuvant letrozole was studied to determine whether upfront use of zoledronic acid was superior to delayed use, in which zoledronic acid was initiated once a decline in bone mineral density (to a T score of –2.0 or worse) was demonstrated or a fracture occurred.[28] In this study, upfront zoledronic acid resulted in increased bone mineral density over baseline, while the delayed group demonstrated decreased BMD over baseline. Upfront-treated patients also demonstrated a decrease in markers of bone turnover. No significant difference was seen in the incidence of fracture, but the overall incidence of fracture was low in both groups. Interestingly, this study also demonstrated a decrease in risk of breast cancer recurrence associated with upfront zoledronic acid. Novel inhibitors of bone loss have also been studied in preventing AI-associated loss of bone density. Denosumab is a monoclonal antibody targeting RANK ligand and results in increased bone density by inhibiting osteoclast-mediated bone resorption. A randomized trial of subcutaneous denosumab versus placebo given every 6 months in AI-treated patients revealed an increase of 4.8 percent in lumbar spine BMD with denosumab compared to a decrease of 0.7 percent with placebo.[29] Denosumab is also being studied for the treatment of bone metastasis.

As demonstrated in the study of zoledronic acid for BMD in AI-treated patients,[28] the use of intravenous bisphosphonates has been thought to be associated with a potential to also decrease breast cancer recurrence. Another study of zolendronic acid as adjuvant treatment of breast cancer in premenopausal women also confirmed an absolute benefit in breast cancer recurrence with zoledronic acid given every 6 months versus placebo.[30] Additional studies, such as SWOG 0307, are ongoing to define the optimal schedule of zoledronic acid administration and to define whether oral bisphosphonates might have similar breast cancer benefits. None of these studies have demonstrated variable effects by age.

D.3. Joint pain and stiffness

The most common symptomatic adverse effect of the aromatase inhibitors is joint pain and stiffness. This symptom has been seen in non–breast cancer patients with low estrogen levels. The exact cause of this pain syndrome is not well understood but likely relates to a loss of estrogen's beneficial effect on the joint or on the nervous system. In the adjuvant clinical trials of AI therapy, the incidence of joint pain or musculoskeletal symptoms is quite variable but has been shown to be as high as 47 percent.[31] Some patients have joint pain severe enough to limit their activities, and this significant a pain syndrome can result in discontinuation of the medication. In a retrospective exploratory analysis of ATAC, a number of risk factors for AI-associated arthralgias were defined.[32] Age was not associated with this symptom. However, body mass index over 30, prior use of hormone replacement therapy, and prior chemotherapy were all associated with the development of AI-associated joint pain. These may all be related to the rate or degree of change in circulating estrogen levels with treatment. For example, obese women would have higher baseline estrogen levels because of estrogen production in adipose tissue, so the decline with AI therapy in these women could be greater than that seen in thin women.

Studies have evaluated joint imaging as a means to better understand AI-associated joint symptoms. One such study prospectively performed joint magnetic resonance imaging (MRI), rheumatologic exam, and pain questionnaires in a small group of 17 women receiving tamoxifen or an aromatase inhibitor.[33] This study demonstrated that patients on AI therapy, but not patients on tamoxifen, had a significant decline in grip strength and a significant increase in tenosynovial changes by MRI. No effect of age was described in this study.

D.4. Lipid profile and cardiovascular risk

There remains controversy about the effect of aromatase inhibitor therapy on the lipid profile and risk of cardiovascular disease. Initial adjuvant trials comparing the aromatase inhibitors with tamoxifen suggested a detrimental effect of the AI on the lipids and potentially an increase in cardiovascular events. For example, in BIG 1-98, comparing upfront letrozole to tamoxifen in early-stage breast cancer, letrozole was associated with a significantly higher incidence of hyperlipidemia (43% vs. 19%) and a nonsignificant trend toward cardiovascular events.[34] Similarly, in the first report of the ATAC trial, anastrozole was associated with a nonsignificant trend toward higher ischemic cardiovascular disease.[35] However, the reporting of these events has been variable, and

it is unclear whether the AIs truly have a detrimental effect or whether the difference is because of a lack of the beneficial effects of tamoxifen. In fact, when AIs are compared to placebo, there appears to be no significant change in lipid profile or cardiovascular events. For example, in MA.17, comparing letrozole to placebo after completion of tamoxifen, the risk of cardiovascular event was 5.8 percent versus 5.6 percent, $p = .76$. One overall review of the available literature suggests that the AIs are not associated with a significant increase in risk of cardiovascular events.[36] Another meta-analysis demonstrated that the AIs are associated with a significant increase in grade 3–4 cardiovascular adverse events compared to tamoxifen.[37] However, the absolute difference was small and the number needed to harm was 180 patients.

These data have not been well described with respect to age or other underlying risk factors for cardiovascular disease such as hypertension, diabetes, hyperlipidemia, or smoking. In BIG 1-98, the overall incidence of cardiac events and ischemic cardiac events was similar between letrozole- and tamoxifen-treated patients.[26] However, after adjusting for risk factors, a significant difference was seen in time to first grade 3–5 ischemic cardiac events favoring tamoxifen in the women aged 65–74. This difference was not seen in women under 65 or over 74. Underlying cardiac risk factors (hypertension, prior cardiac event) were highest in the women over 74 but were fairly well balanced in the two treatment arms for all age groups. The fact that the cardiac event difference was not seen in the oldest subgroup makes it difficult to make a clear statement that AI-related cardiac toxicity is real or age related. Another study evaluating the relationship of baseline factors (age, cardiovascular disease, osteoporosis, and others) with competing causes of death in patients treated on MA.17 has been published.[38] In this study, age *was* associated with an increased mortality from non–breast cancer causes. Underlying cardiovascular disease was also associated with an increased risk of non–cancer related death. Treatment with letrozole was associated with a higher risk of death from noncancer causes compared to placebo in patients with underlying cardiovascular disease. Interestingly, in patients without underlying cardiovascular disease, letrozole was associated with a lower risk of death from noncancer causes. Clearly these data need to be confirmed in other studies.

As older patients undoubtedly have a higher incidence of some of the underlying cardiovascular risk factors, it is possible that there may be a subset of patients who do have an increase in cardiac risk, but this has not been clearly demonstrated. Given the serious nature of cardiovascular events, this should be better evaluated in existing databases and future prospective studies.

D.5. Atrophic vaginitis

A common symptom of estrogen loss with menopause is atrophic vaginitis. This may cause pain, frequent urinary tract infections, bleeding, and dyspareunia. The decline in circulating estrogen resulting from the AIs can produce worsening atrophy of vaginal epithelium and increase these symptoms.[39] Lubricants and moisturizers are first-line treatments for these symptoms but are insufficient for some patients. Few studies have evaluated the use of topical estrogens for this symptom in patients on AI therapy, but there is concern about the degree of systemic absorption and the possibility that this may increase breast cancer recurrence risk. Some formulations of vaginal estrogen (Vagifem and Estring) are felt to have minimal enduring systemic absorption and therefore may not result in clinically significant increase in breast cancer risk. This has been poorly studied to date. However, one small study of six patients receiving adjuvant AI therapy followed serum estradiol levels over 12 weeks of Vagifem therapy.[40] Serum estradiol levels rose consistently at 2 weeks of therapy, but in the majority of patients (4/6), the levels then declined again by week 4. These authors concluded that vaginal estrogen should not be used in this group. However, their data raise the question of whether the systemic absorption occurs only early in treatment, when the vaginal mucosa is thin and fragile, but then may not be persistently absorbed. Controversy remains about this issue, and the clinical relevance of a transient elevation in serum estradiol is not known. Investigators are evaluating alternatives, such as vaginal vitamin E or vaginal testosterone, for this symptom.

D.6. Cognitive function

The studies regarding AIs and cognitive function are described earlier in Section B.3.

Table 3.3 Common effects associated with hormonal therapy for breast cancer.

Tamoxifen	Aromatase inhibitors
Venous thromboembolism	Bone loss
Endometrial carcinoma	Arthralgia/stiffness
Hot flashes	Atrophic vaginitis
Vaginal discharge	? Lipid effect
Improved lipids	? Cardiovascular risk
Improved bone density	? Cognitive function

Note. See text for further description.

E. Conclusions and future directions

The hormonal therapies used in breast cancer can result in a variety of side effects in women of any age (see Table 3.3). As described elsewhere in this text, elderly patients are clearly underrepresented in cancer clinical trials. This results in a dearth of controlled data on treatment-related side effects in this population. As elderly patients are quite variable and often have complicated comorbidities, controlled data are absolutely necessary to clarify the differential contribution of age, treatment, and underlying risk factors to any toxicity. Existing data do suggest that elderly women are at an increased risk of venous thromboembolic disease and endometrial cancer with tamoxifen use compared to younger women. The effect of age on AI side effects is unclear, and the interaction of age and comorbidity with AI-induced bone loss and the potential for adverse cardiac risk and dementia must be better elucidated. Though the efficacy of the aromatase inhibitors is clear and appears to be independent of age, the potential risk of serious side effects must be taken into account when planning treatment.

Further studies are clearly needed to better define these toxicity profiles associated with breast cancer hormonal therapies in older patients. These studies should focus on the effects of polypharmacy, comorbidity, physiologic changes of aging, and geriatric syndromes on drug effect. Similarly, these studies must address the drug's effect on those same conditions. The currently available literature does not allow us to adequately address these issues, and it is imperative that future studies do.

References

1. Jin Y, Desta Z, Stearns V, et al. CYP2D6 genotype, anti-depressant use, and tamoxifen metabolism during adjuvant breast cancer treatment. *J Natl Cancer Inst*. 2005;97(1):30–39.

2. Hemeryck A, Belpaire FM. Selective serotonin reuptake inhibitors and cytochrome P-450 mediated drug interactions: an update. *Curr Drug Metab*. 2002;3(1):13–37.

3. Schroth W, Antoniadou L, Fritz P, et al. Breast cancer treatment outcome with adjuvant tamoxifen relative to patient CYP2D6 and CYP2C19 genotypes. *J Clinical Oncology* 2007;25(33):5187–5193.

4. Goetz MP, Knox SK, Suman VJ, et al. The impact of cytochrome P450 2D6 metabolism in women receiving adjuvant tamoxifen. *Breast Cancer Res Treat*. 2007;101(1):113–121.

5. Defining genetic influences on pharmocologic responses. Indiana University School of Medicine Web site. Available at: http://www.drug-interactions.com.

6. Braithwaite RS, Chlebowski RT, Lau J, et al. Meta-analysis of vascular and neoplastic events associated with tamoxifen. *J Gen Intern Med*. 2003;18:937–947.

7. Ragaz J, Coldman A. Survival impact of adjuvant tamoxifen on competing causes of mortality in breast cancer survivors, with analysis of mortality from contralateral breast cancer, cardiovascular events, endometrial cancer, and thromboembolic episodes. *J Clin Oncol*. 1998;16(6):2018–2024.

8. Howell A, Cuzick J, Baum M, et al. Results of the ATAC (arimidex, tamoxifen alone or in combination) trial after completion of 5 years' adjuvant treatment for breast cancer. *Lancet*. 2005;365:60–62.

9. Coombes RC, Hall E, Gibson LJ, et al. A randomized trial of exemestane after two to three years of tamoxifen therapy in post-menopausal women with primary breast cancer. *N Engl J Med*. 2004;350:1081–1092.

10. Jakesz R, Jonat W, Gnant M, et al. Switching of post-menopausal women with endocrine-responsive early breast cancer to anastrozole after 2 years' adjuvant tamoxifen: combined results of the ABCSG trial 8 and ARNO 95 trial. *Lancet*. 2005;366:455–462.

11. Markovitch O, Tepper R, Fishman A, et al. Aromatase inhibitors reverse tamoxifen induced endometrial ultrasonographic changes in post-menopausal breast cancer patients. *Breast Cancer Res Treat*. 2007;101(2):185–190.

12. Grady D, Yaffe K, Kristof M, et al. Effect of post-menopausal hormone therapy on cognitive function: the Heart and Estrogen/Progestin Replacement Study. *Am J Med*. 2002;113(7):543–548.

13. Shumaker SA, Legault C, Kuller L, et al. Conjugated equine estrogens and incidence of probable dementia and mild cognitive impairment in postmenopausal women: Women's Health Initiative Memory Study. *J Am Med Assoc*. 2004;291(24):2947–2958.

14. Ernst T, Chang L, Cooray D, et al. The effects of tamoxifen and estrogen on brain metabolism in elderly women. *J Natl Cancer Inst*. 2002;94(8):592–597.

15. Yaffe K, Krueger K, Cummings SR, et al. Effect of raloxifene on prevention of dementia and cognitive impairment in older women: the Multiple Outcomes of Raloxifene Evaluation (MORE) randomized trial. *Am J Psychiatry*. 2005;162(4):683–690.

16. Jenkins VA, Shilling V, Fallowfield L, et al. Does hormone therapy for the treatment of breast cancer have a detrimental effect on memory and cognition? A pilot study. *Psychooncology*. 2004;13:61–66.

17. Bender CM, Sereika SM, Brufsky AM, et al. Memory impairments with adjuvant anastrozole versus tamoxifen in women with early-stage breast cancer. *Menopause*. 2007;14(6):995–998.

18. Jenkins VA, Ambroisine LM, Atkins L, et al. Effects of anastrozole on cognitive performance in postmenopausal women: a randomized, double blind chemoprevention trial (IBIS II). *Lancet Oncol*. 2008;9:953–961.

19. Cummings FJ, Gray R, Davis TE, et al. Tamoxifen versus placebo: double blind adjuvant trial in elderly women with stage II breast cancer. *NCI Monogr*. 1986;1:119–123.

20. Toulis KA, Tzellos T, Kouvelas D, et al. Gabapentin for the treatment of hot flushes in women with natural or tamoxifen induced menopause: a systematic review and meta-analysis. *Clin Therap*. 2009;31(2):221–235.

21. Buijs C, Mom CH, Willemse PH, et al. Venlafaxine versus clonidine for the treatment of hot flashes in breast cancer patients: a double-blind, randomized cross-over study. *Breast Cancer Res Treat*. 2009;115(3):573–580.

22. Muss H, Tu D, Ingle JN, et al. Efficacy, toxicity, and quality of life in older women with early-stage breast cancer treated with letrozole or placebo after 5 years of tamoxifen: NCIC CTC Intergroup Trial MA.17. *J Clin Oncol*. 2008;26(12):1956–1964.

23. Consensus Development Statement. Who are candidates for prevention and treatment of osteoporosis? *Osteoporos Int*. 1997;7:1–6.

24. Eastell R, Adams JE, Coleman RE, et al. Effect of anastrozole on bone mineral density: 5-year result from the anastrozole, tamoxifen, alone or in

combination trial 18233230. *J Clin Oncol*. 2008; 26(7):1051–1057.

25. Coleman RE, Banks LM, Girgis SI, et al. Skeletal effects of exemestane on bone-mineral density, bone biomarkers, and fracture incidence in post-menopausal women with early breast cancer participating in the Intergroup Exemestane Study (IES): a randomized controlled trial. *Lancet Oncol*. 2007;8:119–127.

26. Crivellari D, Sun Z, Coates AS, et al. Letrozole versus tamoxifen for elderly patients with endocrine responsive early breast cancer: the BIG 1-98 trial. *J Clin Oncol* 2008;28(12):1972–1979.

27. ATAC Trialists' group effect of anastrozole and tamoxifen as adjuvant treatment for early stage breast cancer: 100 month analysis of the ATAC trial. *Lancet Oncol*. 2007;9:45–53.

28. Brufsky A, Bundred N, Coleman R, et al. Integrated analysis of zoledronic acid for prevention of aromatase inhibitor associated bone loss in post-menopausal women with early breast cancer receiving adjuvant letrozole. *Oncologist*. 2008;13:503–514.

29. Ellis GK, Bone HG, Chlebowski R, et al. Randomized trial of denosumab in patients receiving adjuvant aromatase inhibitors for nonmetastatic breast cancer. *J Clin Oncol*. 2008;26(30):4875–4882

30. Gnant, M, Mlineritsch, B, Schippinger, W, et al. Endocrine therapy plus zoledronic acid in pre-menopausal breast cancer. *New Engl J Med*. 2009; 360: 679–691.

31. Crew KD, Greenlee H, Capodice J, et al. Prevalence of joint symptoms in post-menopausal women taking aromatase inhibitors for early stage breast cancer. *J Clin Oncol*. 2007;25(25):3877–3883.

32. Sestak I, Cuzick J, Sapunar F, et al. Risk factors for joint symptoms in patients enrolled in the ATAC trial: a retrospective, exploratory analysis. *Lancet Oncol*. 2008;9:866–872.

33. Morales L, Pans S, Verschueren K, et al. Prospective study to assess short-term intra-articular and tenosynovial changes in the aromatase inhibitor-associated arthralgia syndrome. *J Clin Oncol* 2008;26(19):3147–3152.

34. Thurlimann B, Keshaviah A, Coates AS, (BIG 1-98 Collaborative Group). A comparison of letrozole and tamoxifen in postmenopausal women with early breast cancer. *N Engl J Med*. 2005;353(26): 2747–2757.

35. ATAC Trialists Group. Anastrozole alone or in combination with tamoxifen for adjuvant treatment of postmenopausal women with early breast cancer: first results of the ATAC trial. *Lancet*. 2002;359:2131–2139.

36. Filippatos TD, Liberopoulos, EN, Pavlidis N, et al. Effect of hormonal treatment on lipids in patients with cancer. *Cancer Treat Rev*. 2009;35,2: 175–184.

37. Cuppone F, Bria E, Verma S, et al. Do adjuvant aromatase inhibitors increase the cardiovascular risk in post-menopausal women with early breast cancer: a meta-analysis of published trials. *Cancer*. 2008;112(2):260–267.

38. Chapman JW, Meng D, Shepherd L, et al. Competing causes of death from a randomized trial of extended adjuvant endocrine therapy for breast cancer. *J Natl Cancer Inst*. 2008;100(4): 252–260.

39. Derzko C, Elliott S, Lam W. Management of sexual dysfunction in postmenopausal breast cancer patients taking adjuvant aromatase inhibitor therapy. *Curr Oncol*. 2007;14(suppl 1):20–40.

40. Kendall A, Dowsett M, Folkerd E, et al. Caution: vaginal estradiol appears to be contraindicated in postmenopausal women on adjuvant aromatase inhibitors. *Ann Oncol*. 2006;17(4):584–587.

4

Drug utilization, adherence, and unique side effects of targeted therapy in older adults

Tiffany A. Traina and Stuart M. Lichtman

A. Introduction

Cancer is a disease of older adults. Approximately 60 percent of cancer diagnoses and 70 percent of cancer mortality occur in individuals aged 65 years and older.[1] As the general population ages and life expectancy increases, the number of older adults with cancer is growing. Several unique challenges arise in caring for older adults with cancer. In particular, the physiologic changes associated with aging can have an impact on the pharmacokinetics and pharmacodynamics of cancer therapies. The effects of these age-related changes on drug dosing and tolerance have been understudied as clinical trials that set the standards for oncology care and drug approval have typically focused on a younger patient population.[2,3] In this chapter, we will review the physiologic changes associated with aging and how they may impact the safety, tolerability, and efficacy of and adherence to cancer treatment. We will also review the limited data of novel targeted oncology drugs in the elderly.

B. Physiologic changes with aging

Aging is a heterogenous process; however, some characteristic changes in physiology and organ function can have an impact on the pharmacology and toxicity of anticancer therapy. For example, age-related changes in the gastrointestinal tract may affect drug absorption. These changes include a decrease in splanchnic blood flow, gastrointestinal motility, secretion of digestive enzymes, and mucosal atrophy.[4,5] With increasing age, hepatic mass decreases, and there is a decrease in the cytochrome P450 content in liver biopsies, although the impact of these declines on hepatic function remains controversial.[6-8] There is a decrease in renal mass and renal blood flow with aging.[9] These age-related changes in renal function could affect the pharmacology of anticancer drugs. A serum creatinine is often used to approximate renal function in younger adults; however, it is a poor indicator of renal function in older adults because of a decrease in muscle mass with age.[10] On average, the glomerular filtration rate decreases by approximately 0.75 mL/min/yr after age 40; however, this decrease is not universal, and approximately one-third of all patients will have no change in creatinine clearance with age.[11] Various equations have been used to estimate glomerular filtration rate, including the Cockcroft-Gault, Jeliffe, Wright, and modification of diet in renal disease (MDRD) formulas. The Cockcroft-Gault and Jeliffe formulas have primarily been validated in younger patients without renal disease.[12,13] The Wright formula is more accurate than the Cockcroft-Gault formula in elderly patients with a glomerular filtration rate of more than 50 mL/min.[14] The MDRD formula is more accurate than other formulas in patients with chronic renal disease. This formula takes into account age, sex, ethnicity, serum creatinine, blood urea nitrogen, and albumin.[15,16] With increasing age, body composition changes, body fat increases, and total body water decreases. This in turn increases the volume distribution of drugs that are lipid soluble and decreases the volume distribution of drugs that are water soluble. Hypoalbuminemia and anemia can lead to an increase in the volume distribution of drugs that are bound to albumin or hemoglobin, respectively. There is also an increase in bone marrow fat and a decrease in bone marrow reserve with age. This decrease in bone marrow reserve places older adults at increased risk for myelosuppressive complications from chemotherapy.[9] Each of these physiologic changes that accompany aging could affect the pharmacokinetics and pharmacodynamics of anticancer therapies. There are a number of reviews that discuss the pharmacology of chemotherapy in older patients.[17-20]

Targeted therapy has been less well studied. Many of the targeted drugs are oral, which makes issues of polypharmacy, compliance, and adherence particularly important. Polypharmacy can affect the metabolism of drugs, particularly drugs that utilize the cytochrome P450 system, making them vulnerable to drug interactions.

B.1. Polypharmacy

Persons over the age of 65 years represent approximately 15 percent of the population but account for more than one-third of all prescription drugs taken and an even higher percentage of nonprescription drugs.[21] Polypharmacy and nonadherence to medications are well documented problems among elderly patients. The simultaneous use of many drugs in a given patient can produce noxious effects. The term *polypharmacy* means "many drugs" and is used to indicate the use of more medications than are clinically indicated or warranted. The elderly cancer patient often needs additional medications prescribed to treat possible side effects of other drugs.[22]

Polypharmacy is a complex issue that can often lead to nonadherence; adverse drug reactions; drug-drug interactions; and increased emergency room visits, hospitalizations, and nursing home admissions.[23] Elderly patients often visit several specialists along with their oncologist and general practitioner. This may result in multiple prescriptions.

B.2. Nonadherence

The World Health Organization describes adherence as the extent to which a person's behavior corresponds with agreed recommendations from a health care provider. The terms *adherence* and *nonadherence* introduce an element of equality in the clinician-patient relationship and reinforce the fact that patients may choose not to follow the clinician's advice. Adherence issues are not well understood, and the specific process of medication adherence is difficult to measure with any degree of accuracy. Clinicians generally assume that patients are taking medications as prescribed and believe their patients when they say they are doing so.[24] However, numerous studies have shown poor adherence with beneficial medications.

A patient's adherence to a medication regimen is primarily determined by his or her assessment of risks and benefits.[24] Some factors that come into play are economics of filling or refilling a prescription, dosing frequency, and side effects. Patients tend to be more adherent when starting a drug regimen (approximately 20% of new prescriptions and 85% of refills are never filled).

There has been the development of oral anticancer drugs. Some of the advantages to oral therapy are that it can be taken at home and that it eliminates the need for intravenous access. One major disadvantage is that it shifts many of the responsibilities of managing the regimen and monitoring for doses and toxicity from the oncologist to the patient.

Adherence has been found to be variable, ranging from 20 to 100 percent, even though adherence was measured in the context of clinical trials, which is the optimal situation of highly motivated and supervised patients.[24] Partridge and colleagues concluded that nonadherence may have a substantial impact on the therapeutic success or failure of oral regimens for the prevention or treatment of malignancies.

In a study of patients receiving imatinib, the overall adherence rate was 75 percent, and only 50 percent of the patients were 100 percent compliant.[25] A study of adherence to anastrozole therapy in early-stage breast cancer reported that approximately one in four women with early-stage breast cancer may not be optimally adherent.[26]

Strategies to improve appropriate prescribing and adherence in the oncology setting are needed. Adherence behavior is not stable and may change over time, necessitating the regular use of detection methods (e.g., self-report, pill count, or therapeutic outcome). Some of the major risk factors of poor adherence include cognitive impairment, treatment of asymptomatic disease, adverse effects of medications, patient's lack of belief in the benefit of treatment, a poor provider-patient relationship, and inadequate follow-up.[27]

One of the most effective steps to ensure appropriate prescribing is to review all the medications the patient is on at every visit. This process is now called medication reconciliation. It is used to help avoid duplication of therapy, drug-drug interactions, and drug-disease interactions. At Memorial Sloan-Kettering Cancer Center, we are conducting a pilot program using the so-called brown-bag approach. A medication management clinic for older adults is conducted where all the medications are brought to the pharmacist and reviewed directly. Dates of refills are assessed, and adherence is determined by the number of pills remaining in the bottles. An assessment is conducted to determine the current use of all medications and to determine the patient's knowledge about his or her medications.

Patient education is a cornerstone in achieving medication adherence and preventing polypharmacy. Many factors influence the effectiveness of educational efforts. Decisions must be made as to what information should be provided to patients about their illnesses and drug therapy. It is important for the clinician to recognize when the information provided is too comprehensive or detailed (e.g., a discussion of all adverse effects of a medication that alarms the patient) as this may discourage the patient from taking the medication. The goal of patient education is to provide information that the patient can understand and use. The anticipated benefits of therapy should be explained. Clinicians should confirm the patient's understanding about the information he or she received by asking the patient to repeat dosing instructions and discussing the patient's expectations for treatment. Involving the patient in the decision-making process about treatment may also increase patient motivation and enhance adherence. Because extended family and primary caregivers can influence a patient's adherence significantly, in some cases, involving them in the educational process may facilitate adherence.[28] Because of the complexity of chemotherapy, educating additional caregivers is beneficial even when the patient is capable of following the treatment regimen without any assistance.

Several types of medication containers have been developed to help patients organize their medications and to monitor self-administration of the drugs. Recommending the patient buy a pillbox organizer may be helpful. Also, providing a calendar with the patient's oral chemotherapy schedule can help ensure accuracy in adhering to the correct dose and schedule.[28]

Polypharmacy has been associated with increased rates of potentially inappropriate medication use and harmful drug interactions. Beers and colleagues developed criteria to identify inappropriate use of medications in seniors residing in nursing homes based on a risk-benefit definition of appropriateness. The criteria, known as the Beers criteria, include two aspects of medication use: (1) drugs that should be avoided in seniors and (2) dosages, frequencies, or durations that should not be exceeded. The Beers criteria were updated in 1997 and again in 2003.[29,30] The updated Beers criteria grouped these drugs into two categories: (1) drugs that should be avoided in seniors and (2) drugs that should be avoided in patients who have a certain condition or diagnosis. The Beers criteria for screening potentially inappropriate medication use in older adults have been widely used as a guide in analyzing prescribing trends in the elderly and have been applied to general hospital and long-term care facility settings.[31,32] A drug evaluation reported that three medications accounted for one-third of emergency department visits for adverse drug events in older adults: warfarin (17.3%), insulin (13.0%), and digoxin (3.2%).[33]

C. Specific targeted therapies

C.1. Endocrine therapy

Endocrine therapy is perhaps the oldest example of so-called targeted therapy as oophorectomy was first proposed as a treatment for advanced breast cancer in 1889.[34] Since that time, drugs that inhibit the estrogen receptor (ER) (i.e., selective estrogen receptor modulators [SERMs]) or the production of estrogen (i.e., aromatase inhibitors [AIs]) have become the most commonly used systemic treatments in older patients with hormone receptor–positive breast cancer in both the adjuvant and metastatic settings.

C.2. Tamoxifen

Tamoxifen is a SERM that competes with estrogen for binding at the ER. Its antagonism of ER has had a significant role in reducing the risk of breast cancer recurrence and death in women aged 70 years and older with early-stage, ER-positive breast cancer when used for 5 years.[35] However, the use of this SERM is associated with side effects of particular importance to older breast cancer patients. Tamoxifen demonstrates partial estrogen-agonist effects, leading to an increased risk of thromboembolism, ischemic cerebrovascular events, endometrial hyperplasia, endometrial cancer, and risk of cataract development.[36] The risk of endometrial cancer, albeit small, is almost exclusively seen in patients older than 50 years of age.[37] These potential risks may significantly impact the safety and tolerability of tamoxifen in older patients with breast cancer with underlying comorbid conditions. Though tamoxifen remains the mainstay of treatment for premenopausal women with ER-positive breast cancer, newer targeted therapies directed at estrogen production have offered postmenopausal women a potentially safer alternative.

C.3. Aromatase inhibitors

AIs suppress estrogen levels in postmenopausal women by blocking aromatase, the enzyme responsible for the peripheral conversion of androgenic substrates into estrogen. Several randomized trials have shown superior disease-free survival associated with AIs compared to tamoxifen for the adjuvant treatment of postmenopausal women with hormone receptor–positive, early-stage breast cancer.[38-41] AIs have been associated with an increased incidence of musculoskeletal symptoms, osteoporosis, and rate of fractures rather than the endometrial toxicity and hypercoagulability seen with tamoxifen. However, one large randomized trial of letrozole versus observation following 5 years of tamoxifen enrolled more than 1,300 women over the age of 70 years and found no significant difference in toxicities between the letrozole and placebo groups.[42] Unrelated to treatment, women 70 years of age and older had significantly higher incidences of fracture, new osteoporosis, and cardiac disease, but there were no significant differences between the two treatment groups in fractures (6% letrozole vs. 8% placebo), the development of osteoporosis (10% letrozole vs. 8% placebo), or cardiac disease (10% letrozole vs. 11% placebo). A meta-analysis of several randomized AI studies has suggested an increased risk for grade 3–4 cardiovascular complications (relative risk 1.31, $p = .007$) compared with tamoxifen.[43] The impact of these clinically relevant side effects and the high cost of nongeneric AIs on adherence to therapy remains unclear. These data also suggest that toxicities may vary within subgroups of the older oncology patient.

D. Monoclonal antibodies

D.1. Bevacizumab

Age-related toxicity is seen with bevacizumab, the humanized monoclonal antibody that inhibits vascular endothelial growth factor (VEGF). Incorporation of this monoclonal antibody in first-line therapy in advanced colorectal cancer has shown improvement in progression-free and overall survival.[44-46] A retrospective pooled analysis of five randomized studies in 1,745 patients demonstrated that patients aged 65 years and older who were treated with chemotherapy and bevacizumab had an increased risk of arterial thromboembolic events compared with those aged under 65 years (7.1% vs. 2.5%). Risk factors for development of an arterial thromboembolic event included age over 65 years and a history of a prior arterial thromboembolic event.[47] In a prospective observational cohort, there was a higher rate of arterial thrombotic events. The other observed toxicities did not differ by age. The authors concluded that the results indicate that age alone should not be a barrier to using bevacizumab-containing regimens in older patients. But caution still needs to be observed for patients at higher risk of arterial thrombotic events.[48]

A phase III study (E4599) of patients with advanced non-small-cell lung cancer (NSCLC) who received paclitaxel (P) and carboplatin (C) were randomized to receive bevacizumab (B) or placebo. A retrospective outcome analysis was performed on patients 70 years of age and older.[49] Among the older patients, there was a trend toward higher response rate (29% vs. 17%, $p = .067$) and progression-free survival (5.9 vs. 4.9 months, $p = .063$) with the bevacizumab, although overall survival (PCB = 11.3 months, PC = 12.1 months, $p = 0.4$) was similar. Grade 3–5 toxicities occurred in 87 percent of elderly patients with PCB versus 61 percent with PC ($p < .001$), with seven treatment-related deaths in the bevacizumab arm compared to patients treated with chemotherapy alone. Elderly patients had higher incidence of grade 3–5 neutropenia, bleeding, and proteinuria with bevacizumab. The study concluded that in elderly patients with NSCLC, the addition of bevacizumab was associated with a higher degree of toxicity but no obvious improvement in survival.

Bevacizumab is also approved for the first-line treatment of metastatic breast cancer in combination with paclitaxel.[50] A small retrospective study of patients older than 65 years of age receiving bevacizumab with chemotherapy for advanced breast cancer found an increased incidence of thrombosis, bleeding, gastrointestinal perforation, and neutropenic fever than previously reported.[51] Twenty-five percent of patients in this small population discontinued use of bevacizumab due to an adverse event. These data suggest that disease-specific studies of novel targeted agents may need to be conducted in the older cancer patient to determine whether the benefits and risks associated with these agents are similar to those seen in younger patients.

D.2. Trastuzumab

Trastuzumab is a humanized monoclonal antibody that targets the HER2-neu receptor. Its use in combination with chemotherapy for the treatment of women with advanced and early-stage, HER2-amplified or overexpressed breast cancer has improved overall survival.[52] However, cardiac toxicity has been associated with its use, particularly in patients who received concomitant anthracycline-based chemotherapy. For patients over the age of 60 years, the response and overall survival advantage to trastuzumab-based therapy was maintained; however, the risk of cardiac dysfunction was higher (11% in those aged under 60 years vs. 21% in those aged over 60 years).[53]

Patients with cardiac comorbidities were excluded from most of the adjuvant trastuzumab studies, thereby eliminating many older patients with HER2-positive breast cancer. For example, only 16 percent of patients in the Herceptin Adjuvant (HERA) trial were aged 60 years or older.[54] Unplanned subset analyses and small retrospective studies have examined the risks and benefits of trastuzumab in older HER2-positive patients.[55] With the limited data available, the benefit of adjuvant trastuzumab for women aged over 60 years seems to outweigh the risks at this time. However, the cardiac risks associated with trastuzumab must be carefully considered in the context of comorbid conditions for the older HER2-positive patient, and a dialogue between the oncologist and patient should review the individual risk-benefit ratio.

D.3. Cetuximab

Cetuximab is a chimeric monoclonal antibody directed to the exo-domain of the epidermal growth factor receptor (EGFR) that has been shown to be active against metastatic colorectal cancer after failure of standard therapies.[56–58] Furthermore, despite documented resistance to irinotecan, its use in combination with irinotecan is more active than single-agent therapy, suggesting some extent of drug resistance reversal.[56] Data pertaining to cetuximab in elderly patients are very scarce, and there are no data suggesting an influence of age on cetuximab clearance.[59] In a review of older patients, diarrhea occurred in 45 patients (80%) and was grade 3 or 4 in 10 and 1 patients, respectively (20%, grades 3–4). This degree of toxicity may be very significant for an older and possibly frail patient population. It emphasizes the need for close monitoring and supportive care (i.e., hydration).[60] Panitumumab would be expected to have a similar toxicity profile.[61,62] Cetuximab is approved for treatment of head and neck cancer with radiotherapy.[63] It provides an alternative to patients who cannot tolerate or are ineligible for cisplatin therapy.

D.4. Rituximab

Rituximab is a chimeric murine/human monoclonal antibody directed against the CD20 antigen of B lymphocytes. It is approved by the U.S. Food and Drug Administration (FDA) for the treatment of patients with relapsed or refractory low-grade or follicular, CD20-positive, B-cell non-Hodgkin's lymphoma. Few studies have evaluated rituximab in the geriatric oncology population despite the large proportion of elderly patients of the total lymphoma population. However, the combination of rituximab with cyclophosphamide, adriamycin, vincristine, prednisone (CHOP), even in a dose-dense fashion, appears well tolerated and effective in patients over 60 years of age with aggressive non-Hodgkin's lymphoma.[64–66]

E. Signal transduction inhibitors

E.1. Imatinib

The development of imatinib mesylate has redefined the management of chronic myeloid leukemia (CML).[67] It is an orally administered tyrosine kinase inhibitor that is metabolized with the cytochrome P450 isoenzyme 3A4.[68] It is characterized by the presence of a balanced translocation between chromosomes 9 and 22, t(9;22)(q34;q11.2), which produces a chimeric gene, BCR-ABL. This in turn translates into a fusion protein product with increased tyrosine kinase activity that is pathophysiologically linked to CML. Thus it represented an ideal target for therapeutic intervention because inhibition of the BCR-ABL kinase activity could lead to the elimination of leukemic cells while sparing normal cells. Nearly all patients with CML in chronic phase treated with imatinib achieve a complete hematologic response, and 80–90 percent of those treated in the early chronic phase achieve a complete cytogenetic response. With the excitement of the success of this approach came the realization of additional complexities in the pathophysiology and clinical course of CML. One example is the development of resistance to imatinib through point mutations in the kinase domain of BCR-ABL. More than 30 different mutations have been reported that vary in their extent of preventing inhibition by imatinib and their proliferative potential. Mutations have been identified in 30–50 percent of patients who become resistant to imatinib. Several other mechanisms of resistance have been identified, but how often they occur is less clear. These include BCR-ABL-dependent (e.g., overexpression and amplification) and BCR-ABL-independent mechanisms (e.g., overexpression of Src-related kinases). Imatinib has been used in elderly patients with chronic-phase CML and

Philadelphia-positive ALL with similar efficacy as with younger patients.[69,70]

GI stromal tumors (GISTs) are malignant tumors that arise from precursor cells of the interstitial cells of Cajal in the GI tract. Eighty-six percent of GISTs harbor activating mutations of the KIT or PDGFR genes, leading to ligand-independent activation of these receptor tyrosine kinases and tumor growth in vitro. These mutations are likely to be very early events in the oncogenesis of these tumors. Although resistant to conventional chemotherapy, these tumors have been shown to be extremely sensitive to targeted therapy with imatinib, a tyrosine kinase inhibitor selectively blocking KIT and PDGFR. Eight-five to 90 percent of patients with GIST experience tumor control with imatinib, including objective tumor response and stable disease according to Response Evaluation Criteria in Solid Tumors, both being correlated with a similar prolonged overall survival. A strong correlation between the antitumor activity of imatinib and the site of KIT and PDGFR mutations has been reported.[71]

E.2. Erlotinib

Erlotinib targets the tyrosine kinase domain of the EGFR. The National Cancer Institute of Canada Clinical Trials Group BR.21 study randomly assigned patients who had experienced failure with first- or second-line chemotherapy to erlotinib or placebo in a two-to-one ratio. Treatment with erlotinib resulted in a significant survival benefit over placebo.[72] Because no randomized studies have been reported to document the efficacy and tolerance of elderly patients treated with EGFR inhibitors, a retrospective analysis of patients treated in the BR.21 study was performed.[73] Response rates were similar between age groups. Elderly patients, compared with young patients, had significantly more overall and severe (grade 3 and 4) toxicity (35% vs. 18%, $p < .001$) and were more likely to discontinue treatment as a result of treatment-related toxicity (12% vs. 3%, $p < .0001$) and had lower relative dose intensity (64% vs. 82% received more than 90% planned dose, $p < .001$). The elderly were more likely than the younger group to have grade 3 rash, fatigue, stomatitis, or dehydration as well as any grade of anorexia (26% vs. 16%, $p = .03$) and fatigue (22% vs. 14%, $p = .04$). Elderly patients treated with erlotinib gain similar survival and quality of life (QOL) benefits as younger patients. The issue of toxicity is significant in that erlotinib is often used as a single agent in the poor–performance status and frail patient.

A phase II study of erlotinib as first-line therapy for patients aged 70 years and older with advanced non-small-cell lung cancer demonstrated that 12 percent of patients on the study required discontinuation of therapy.[74]

Erlotinib has been studied in patients with end-organ dysfunction.[75] Patients with renal dysfunction tolerate 150 mg of erlotinib daily and seem to have an erlotinib clearance similar to patients without organ dysfunction. Patients with hepatic dysfunction should be treated at a reduced dose (i.e., 75 mg daily) consistent with their reduced clearance.

E.3. Sorafenib and sunitinib

Raf, which is an essential serine/threonine kinase constituent of the mitogen-activated protein kinase signaling pathway and a downstream effector of the central signal transduction mediator Ras, is activated in a wide range of human malignancies and is therefore recognized as a strategic target for therapeutic drug development. Sorafenib, an orally active multikinase inhibitor with effects on tumor cell proliferation and tumor angiogenesis, was initially identified as a Raf kinase inhibitor. It also inhibits vascular endothelial growth factor receptors 1, 2, and 3; platelet-derived growth factor receptor; FMS-like tyrosine kinase 3; c-Kit protein; and RET receptor tyrosine kinase. Sorafenib is approved by the FDA for the treatment of renal[76] and hepatocellular carcinomas[77] and has also demonstrated activity in a number of other malignancies.[78] As in the development of other new drugs, sorafenib was initially tested in patients with adequate hepatic and renal function, and the recommended continuous daily dose is 400 mg twice a day for such patients. The most common side effects include hand-foot skin reactions, diarrhea, fatigue, rash, and hypertension. Sorafenib is primarily metabolized in the liver (predominantly by CYP3A4). A study of patients with hepatic and renal dysfunction has been reported with dosing recommendations.[78]

Sunitinib malate is an oral, multitargeted tyrosine kinase inhibitor of VEGF receptors (VEGFR-1, -2, and -3) and platelet-derived growth factor receptors that has been shown to improve progression-free survival compared with interferon-alfa in previously untreated patients with clear-cell metastatic renal cell carcinoma.[79,80] It is also approved for imatinib-resistant GIST tumors.[81]

The toxicity of sorafenib and sunitinib of most concern in the elderly is cardiac.[82] In one observational evaluation of 86 patients treated with either sunitinib or sorafenib at a single institution, 74 patients were available for cardiovascular monitoring. Thirty-three percent of evaluable patients experienced a cardiac event, 40.5 percent had electrocardiogram changes, and 18 percent were symptomatic. Seven patients (9.4%) were seriously compromised and required intermediate care and/or intensive care admission. All patients recovered after cardiovascular management (i.e., medication, coronary angiography, pacemaker implantation, heart surgery) and were considered eligible for tyrosine kinase inhibitor continuation. Statistically, there was no significant survival difference between patients who experienced a cardiac event and those who did not experience a cardiac event. The authors concluded that cardiac damage from these medications is a largely underestimated phenomenon but is manageable if patients have careful cardiovascular monitoring and cardiac treatment at the first signs of myocardial damage.

E.4. Lapatinib

Lapatinib is a dual HER1- and HER2-tyrosine kinase inhibitor. It is FDA approved, in combination with capecitabine, for the treatment of advanced HER2-positive breast cancer that has progressed following treatment with trastuzumab-based chemotherapy.[83] The effects of age on the pharmacokinetics of lapatinib have not been published. Thus far, no overall differences in safety or effectiveness of the combination of lapatinib and capecitabine were observed between patients aged older than 65 years and younger subjects; however, only 17 percent of patients in the early lapatinib trials were over 65 years of age.

Of significant concern is the cardiac toxicity associated with this HER2-targeted therapy. In a meta-analysis examining the cardiac safety data of over 3,500 patients enrolled on 43 lapatinib clinical trials, approximately 1.6 percent of patients experienced a decline in left ventricular ejection fraction (LVEF), and 0.2 percent developed symptoms of congestive heart failure.[84] The incidence of cardiac events did not seem to vary significantly based on prior anthracycline or trastuzumab exposure, both agents with known cardiac toxicity. For the 31 patients with available follow-up data who had a decline in LVEF, all recovered LVEF function. Therefore investigators conclude that lapatinib produces low levels of severe congestive heart failure, which appears to be mostly reversible. Nevertheless, predictors of HER2-targeted cardiac toxicity have been described and include patients over 50 years of age with baseline cardiac dysfunction, and use of hypertensive medications.[83] Careful cardiac monitoring of left ventricular ejection fraction in the older patient with HER2-positive breast cancer is imperative.

F. Conclusions

The oncology community includes a large proportion of patients 70 years of age and older. The most common cancers in the United States (i.e., breast, lung, and colorectal cancers) have an age-related incidence suggesting that the concerns of geriatric oncology are widely applicable to the general oncologist.

The development of novel, targeted therapies has helped to improve survival for patients with cancer (i.e., trastuzumab in breast cancer and bevacizumab in colon cancer). Rituximab has significantly altered the natural history of B-cell non-Hodgkin's lymphoma. And agents such as imatinib, sorafenib, sunitinib, and erlotinib have improved the outcomes of patients with renal cell cancer, pancreatic tumors, and GIST. It seems that the older cancer patient may benefit from these biologic therapies; however, special attention must be paid to the unique toxicities of these agents. Targeted therapies are not entirely benign, as evidenced by the cardiac toxicity associated with trastuzumab and lapatinib or the arterial thrombotic events associated with bevacizumab. Clinical trials that characterize the treatment needs and goals of therapy in elderly cancer patients are ongoing. Additional trials are necessary to clarify the risk-benefit ratio of newer targeted agents in the elderly cancer patient as differences in physiology, organ function reserves, social and financial resources, and decreased resilience to toxicity may all influence outcomes for this special patient population.

References

1. Yancik R, Ries LA. Aging and cancer in America: demographic and epidemiologic perspectives. *Hematol Oncol Clin North Am.* 2000;14:17–23.

2. Hutchins LF, Unger JM, Crowley JJ, et al. Underrepresentation of patients 65 years of age or older in cancer-treatment trials. *N Engl J Med.* 1999;341:2061–2067.

3. Talarico L, Chen G, Pazdur R. Enrollment of elderly patients in clinical trials for cancer drug registration: a 7-year experience by the US Food and Drug Administration. *J Clin Oncol.* 2004;22:4626–4631.

4. Yuen GJ. Altered pharmacokinetics in the elderly. *Clin Geriatr Med.* 1990;6:257–267.

5. Baker SD, Grochow LB. Pharmacology of cancer chemotherapy in the older person. *Clin Geriatr Med.* 1997;13:169–183.

6. Sotaniemi EA, Arranto AJ, Pelkonen O, et al. Age and cytochrome P450-linked drug metabolism in humans: an analysis of 226 subjects with equal histopathologic conditions. *Clin Pharmacol Ther.* 1997;61:331–339.

7. Sawhney R, Sehl M, Naeim A. Physiologic aspects of aging: impact on cancer management and decision making, part I. *Cancer J.* 2005;11:449–460.

8. Shah RR. Drug development and use in the elderly: search for the right dose and dosing regimen (parts I and II). *Br J Clin Pharmacol.* 2004;58:452–469.

9. Vestal RE. Aging and pharmacology. *Cancer.* 1997;80:1302–1310.

10. Fehrman-Ekholm I, Skeppholm L. Renal function in the elderly (>70 years old) measured by means of iohexol clearance, serum creatinine, serum urea and estimated clearance. *Scand J Urol Nephrol.* 2004;38:73–77.

11. Lindeman RD, Tobin J, Shock NW. Longitudinal studies on the rate of decline in renal function with age. *J Am Geriatr Soc.* 1985;33:278–285.

12. Burkhardt H, Bojarsky G, Gretz N, Gladisch R. Creatinine clearance, Cockcroft-Gault formula and cystatin C: estimators of true glomerular filtration rate in the elderly? *Gerontology.* 2002;48:140–146.

13. Rimon E, Kagansky N, Cojocaru L, et al. Can creatinine clearance be accurately predicted by formulae in octogenarian in-patients? *Q J Med.* 2004;97:281–287.

14. Marx GM, Blake GM, Galani E, et al. Evaluation of the Cockroft-Gault, Jelliffe and Wright formulae in estimating renal function in elderly cancer patients. *Ann Oncol.* 2004;15:291–295.

15. Levey AS, Bosch JP, Lewis JB, et al. A more accurate method to estimate glomerular filtration rate from serum creatinine: a new prediction equation. Modification of Diet in Renal Disease Study Group. *Ann Intern Med.* 1999;130:461–470.

16. Lichtman SM, Wildiers H, Launay-Vacher V, et al. International Society of Geriatric Oncology (SIOG) recommendations for the adjustment of dosing in elderly cancer patients with renal insufficiency. *Eur J Cancer.* 2007;43:14–34.

17. Hurria A, Lichtman SM. Clinical pharmacology of cancer therapies in older adults. *Br J Cancer.* 2008;98:517–522.

18. Lichtman SM. Older patients and the shifting focus of cancer care. *Oncology.* 2009;23:86, 88.

19. Lichtman SM, Wildiers H, Chatelut E, et al. International Society of Geriatric Oncology Chemotherapy Taskforce: evaluation of chemotherapy in older patients – an analysis of the medical literature. *J Clin Oncol.* 2007;25:1832–1843.

20. Lichtman SM. Therapy insight: therapeutic challenges in the treatment of elderly cancer patients. *Natl Clin Pract Oncol.* 2006;3:86–93.

21. Fulton MM, Allen ER. Polypharmacy in the elderly: a literature review. *J Am Acad Nurse Pract.* 2005;17:123–132.

22. Lichtman SM, Boparai MK. Anticancer drug therapy in the older cancer patient: pharmacology and polypharmacy. *Curr Treat Options Oncol.* 2008;9:191–203.

23. Bergman-Evans B. AIDES to improving medication adherence in older adults. *Geriatr Nurs.* 2006;27:174–182; quiz 83.

24. Partridge AH, Avorn J, Wang PS, et al. Adherence to therapy with oral antineoplastic agents. *J Natl Cancer Inst.* 2002;94:652–661.

25. Tsang J, Rudychev I, Pescatore SL. Prescription compliance and persistency in chronic myelogenous leukemia (CML) and gastrointestinal stromal tumor (GIST) patients (pts) on imatinib (IM). *J Clin Oncol Meet Abstr.* 2006;24:6119.

26. Partridge AH, LaFountain A, Mayer E, et al. Adherence to initial adjuvant anastrozole therapy among women with early-stage breast cancer. *J Clin Oncol.* 2008;26:556–562.

27. Osterberg L, Blaschke T. Adherence to medication. *N Engl J Med.* 2005;353:487–497.

28. Hartigan K. Patient education: the cornerstone of successful oral chemotherapy treatment. *Clin J Oncol Nurs.* 2003;7:21–24.

29. Fick DM, Cooper JW, Wade WE, et al. Updating the Beers criteria for potentially inappropriate medication use in older adults: results of a US consensus panel of experts. *Arch Intern Med.* 2003;163:2716–2724.

30. Beers MH. Explicit criteria for determining potentially inappropriate medication use by the elderly: an update. *Arch Intern Med.* 1997;157:1531–1536.

31. Barry PJ, O'Keefe N, O'Connor KA, et al. Inappropriate prescribing in the elderly: a comparison of the Beers criteria and the improved prescribing in the elderly tool (IPET) in acutely ill elderly hospitalized patients. *J Clin Pharm Ther.* 2006;31:617–626.

32. Cannon KT, Choi MM, Zuniga MA. Potentially inappropriate medication use in elderly patients receiving home health care: a retrospective data analysis. *Am J Geriatr Pharmacother.* 2006;4:134–143.

33. Budnitz DS, Shehab N, Kegler SR, et al. Medication use leading to emergency department visits for adverse drug events in older adults. *Ann Intern Med.* 2007;147:755–765.

34. Love RR, Philips J. Oophorectomy for breast cancer: history revisited. *J Natl Cancer Inst.* 2002;94:1433–1434.

35. Early Breast Cancer Trialists' Collaborative Group. Effects of chemotherapy and hormonal therapy for early breast cancer on recurrence and a 15-year survival: an overview of the randomised trials. *Lancet.* 2005;365:1687–1717.

36. Osborne CK. Tamoxifen in the treatment of breast cancer. *N Engl J Med.* 1998;339:1609–1618.

37. Braithwaite RS, Chlebowski RT, Lau J, et al. Meta-analysis of vascular and neoplastic events associated with tamoxifen. *J Gen Intern Med.* 2003;18:937–947.

38. Baum M, Budzar AU, Cuzick J, et al. Anastrozole alone or in combination with tamoxifen versus tamoxifen alone for adjuvant treatment of postmenopausal women with early breast cancer: first results of the ATAC randomised trial. *Lancet.* 2002;359:2131–2139.

39. Goss PE, Ingle JN, Martino S, et al. Randomized trial of letrozole following tamoxifen as extended adjuvant therapy in receptor-positive breast cancer: updated findings from NCIC CTG MA.17. *J Natl Cancer Inst.* 2005;97:1262–1271.

40. Coombes RC, Hall E, Gibson LJ, et al. A randomized trial of exemestane after two to three years of tamoxifen therapy in postmenopausal women with primary breast cancer. *N Engl J Med.* 2004;350:1081–1092.

41. Thurlimann BJ, Keshaviah A, Mouridsen H, et al. BIG 1–98: randomized double-blind phase III study to evaluate letrozole (L) vs. tamoxifen (T) as adjuvant endocrine therapy for postmenopausal women with receptor-positive breast cancer. *Proc Am Soc Clin Oncol.* 2005;23(suppl 16):511.

42. Muss HB, Tu D, Ingle JN, et al. Efficacy, toxicity, and quality of life in older women with early-stage breast cancer treated with letrozole or placebo after 5 years of tamoxifen: NCIC CTG intergroup trial MA.17. *J Clin Oncol.* 2008;26:1956–1964.

43. Cuppone F, Bria E, Verma S, et al. Do adjuvant aromatase inhibitors increase the cardiovascular risk in postmenopausal women with early breast cancer? Meta-analysis of randomized trials. *Cancer.* 2008;112:260–267.

44. Saltz L, Clarke S, Díaz-Rubio E, et al. Bevacizumab in combination with oxaliplatin-based chemotherapy as first-line therapy in metastatic colorectal cancer: a randomized phase III study. *J Clin Oncol.* 2008;26:2013–2019.

45. Hurwitz H, Fehrenbacher L, Novotny W, et al. Bevacizumab plus irinotecan, fluorouracil, and leucovorin for metastatic colorectal cancer. *N Engl J Med.* 2004;350:2335–2342.

46. Kabbinavar FF, Schulz J, McCleod M, et al. Addition of bevacizumab to bolus fluorouracil and leucovorin in first-line metastatic colorectal cancer: results of a randomized phase II trial. *J Clin Oncol.* 2005;23:3697–3705.

47. Scappaticci FA, Skillings JR, Holden SN, et al. Arterial thromboembolic events in patients with metastatic carcinoma treated with chemotherapy and bevacizumab. *J Natl Cancer Inst.* 2007;99:1232–1239.

48. Kozloff MF, Sugrue MM, Purdie DM, et al. Safety and effectiveness of bevacizumab (BV) and chemotherapy (CT) in elderly patients (pts) with metastatic colorectal cancer (mCRC): results from the BRiTE observational cohort study. *Proc Am Soc Clin Oncol.* 2008;26:4026.

49. Ramalingam SS, Dahlberg SE, Langer CJ, et al. Outcomes for elderly, advanced-stage non small-cell lung cancer patients treated with bevacizumab in combination with carboplatin and paclitaxel: analysis of Eastern Cooperative Oncology Group Trial 4599. *J Clin Oncol.* 2008;26:60–65.

50. FDA approval for bevacizumab. National Cancer Institute Web site. Available at: http://www.cancer.gov/cancertopics/druginfo/fda-bevacizumab.

51. Richardson S, Dickler M, Dang C, et al. Tolerance of bevacizumab in an older patient population: The Memorial Sloan-Kettering Cancer Center (MSKCC) experience. *Proc Am Soc Clin Oncol.* 2008;26(suppl 15):9569.

52. Slamon DJ, Leyland-Jones B, Shak S, et al. Use of chemotherapy plus a monoclonal antibody against HER2 for metastatic breast cancer that overexpresses HER2. *N Engl J Med.* 2001;344:783–792.

53. Fyfe GA, Mass R, Murphy M. Survival benefit of traztuzumab (Herceptin) and chemotherapy in older (age > 60) patients. *Proc Am Soc Clin Oncol.* 2001;20:189.

54. Piccart-Gebhart MJ, Procter M, Leyland-Jones B, et al. Trastuzumab after adjuvant chemotherapy in HER2-positive breast cancer. *N Engl J Med.* 2005;353:1659–1672.

55. Gupta A, Mekan S, Eckman M. Trastuzumab for all? A decision analysis examining tradeoffs between efficacy and cardiac toxicity of adjuvant therapy in HER2-positive breast cancer. *Proc Am Soc Clin Oncol.* 2006;24(suppl 18): 6022.

56. Cunningham D, Humblet Y, Siena S, et al. Cetuximab monotherapy and cetuximab plus irinotecan in irinotecan-refractory metastatic colorectal cancer. *N Engl J Med.* 2004;351:337–345.

57. Lenz HJ, Van Cutsem E, Khambata-Ford S, et al. Multicenter phase II and translational study of cetuximab in metastatic colorectal carcinoma refractory to irinotecan, oxaliplatin, and fluoropyrimidines. *J Clin Oncol.* 2006;24:4914–4921.

58. Gebbia V, Del Prete S, Borsellino N, et al. Efficacy and safety of cetuximab/irinotecan in chemotherapy-refractory metastatic colorectal adenocarcinomas: a clinical practice setting, multicenter experience. *Clin Colorectal Cancer.* 2006;5:422–428.

59. Vincenzi B, Santini D, Rabitti C, et al. Cetuximab and irinotecan as third-line therapy in advanced colorectal cancer patients: a single centre phase II trial. *Br J Cancer.* 2006;94:792–797.

60. Bouchahda M, Macarulla T, Spano JP, et al. Cetuximab efficacy and safety in a retrospective cohort of elderly patients with heavily pretreated metastatic colorectal cancer. *Crit Rev Oncol Hematol.* 2008;67:255–262.

61. Rocha-Lima CM, Soares HP, Raez LE, et al. EGFR targeting of solid tumors. *Cancer Control.* 2007;14:295–304.

62. Van Cutsem E, Peeters M, Siena S, et al. Open-label phase III trial of panitumumab plus best supportive care compared with best supportive care alone in patients with chemotherapy-refractory metastatic colorectal cancer. *J Clin Oncol.* 2007;25:1658–1664.

63. Bonner JA, Harari PM, Giralt J, et al. Radiotherapy plus cetuximab for squamous-cell carcinoma of the head and neck. *N Engl J Med.* 2006;354:567–578.

64. Coiffier B, Haioun C, Ketterer N, et al. Rituximab (anti-CD20 monoclonal antibody) for the treatment of patients with relapsing or refractory aggressive lymphoma: a multicenter phase II study. *Blood.* 1998;92:1927–1932.

65. Coiffier B, Lepage E, Briere J, et al. CHOP chemotherapy plus rituximab compared with CHOP alone in elderly patients with diffuse large-B-cell lymphoma. *N Engl J Med.* 2002;346:235–242.

66. Habermann TM, Weller EA, Morrison VA, et al. Rituximab-CHOP versus CHOP alone or with maintenance rituximab in older patients with diffuse large B-cell lymphoma. *J Clin Oncol.* 2006;24:3121–3127.

67. Cortes J, Kantarjian H. New targeted approaches in chronic myeloid leukemia. *J Clin Oncol.* 2005;23:6316–6324.

68. Peng B, Hayes M, Resta D, et al. Pharmacokinetics and pharmacodynamics of imatinib in a phase I trial with chronic myeloid leukemia patients. *J Clin Oncol.* 2004;22:935–942.

69. Brandwein JM, Gupta V, Wells RA, et al. Treatment of elderly patients with acute lymphoblastic leukemia – evidence for a benefit of imatinib in BCR-ABL positive patients. *Leuk Res.* 2005;29:1381–1386.

70. Latagliata R, Breccia M, Carmosino I, et al. Elderly patients with Ph+ chronic myelogenous leukemia (CML): results of imatinib mesylate treatment. *Leuk Res.* 2005;29:287–291.

71. Blay JY, Le Cesne A, Ray-Coquard I, et al. Prospective multicentric randomized phase III study of imatinib in patients with advanced gastrointestinal stromal tumors comparing interruption versus continuation of treatment beyond 1 year: the French Sarcoma Group. *J Clin Oncol.* 2007;25:1107–1113.

72. Shepherd FA, Rodrigues Pereira J, Ciuleanu T, et al. Erlotinib in previously treated non-small-cell lung cancer. *N Engl J Med.* 2005;353:123–132.

73. Wheatley-Price P, Ding K, Seymour L, et al. Erlotinib for advanced non-small-cell lung cancer in the elderly: an analysis of the National Cancer Institute of Canada Clinical Trials Group Study BR.21. *J Clin Oncol.* 2008;26:2350–2357.

74. Jackman DM, Yeap BY, Lindeman NI, et al. Phase II clinical trial of chemotherapy-naive patients > or = 70 years of age treated with erlotinib for advanced non-small-cell lung cancer. *J Clin Oncol.* 2007;25:760–766.

75. Miller AA, Murry DJ, Owzar K, et al. Phase I and pharmacokinetic study of erlotinib for solid tumors in patients with hepatic or renal dysfunction: CALGB 60101. *J Clin Oncol.* 2007;25:3055–3060.

76. Ratain MJ, Eisen T, Stadler WM, et al. Phase II placebo-controlled randomized discontinuation trial of sorafenib in patients with metastatic renal cell carcinoma. *J Clin Oncol.* 2006;24: 2505–2512.

77. Llovet JM, Ricci S, Mazzaferro V, et al. Sorafenib in advanced hepatocellular carcinoma. *N Engl J Med.* 2008;359:378–390.

78. Miller AA, Murry DJ, Owzar K, et al. Phase I and pharmacokinetic study of sorafenib in patients with hepatic or renal dysfunction: CALGB 60301. *J Clin Oncol.* 2009;27:1800–1805.

79. Rini BI, Michaelson MD, Rosenberg JE, et al. Antitumor activity and biomarker analysis of sunitinib in patients with bevacizumab-refractory metastatic renal cell carcinoma. *J Clin Oncol.* 2008;26:3743–3748.

80. Motzer RJ, Hutson TE, Tomczak P, et al. Sunitinib versus interferon alfa in metastatic renal-cell carcinoma. *N Engl J Med.* 2007;356:115–124.

81. Joensuu H. Sunitinib for imatinib-resistant GIST. *Lancet.* 2006;368:1303–1304.

82. Schmidinger M, Zielinski CC, Vogl UM, et al. Cardiac toxicity of sunitinib and sorafenib in patients with metastatic renal cell carcinoma. *J Clin Oncol.* 2008;26:5204–5212.

83. Geyer CE, Forster J, Lindquist D, et al. Lapatinib plus capecitabine for HER2-positive advanced breast cancer. *N Engl J Med.* 2006;355:2733–2743.

84. Perez EA. Cardiac toxicity of ErbB2-targeted therapies: what do we know? *Clin Breast Cancer.* 2008;8(suppl 3):114–120.

Key principles in geriatric oncology

5 Principles of surgical oncology in older adults

Suzanne Gaskell, Siri R. Kristjansson, and Riccardo A. Audisio

Despite the outstanding achievements of medicine in the knowledge and management of cancer, surgery remains the treatment of choice for most malignancies. Although some surgical procedures are not based on stringent evidence and were never tested within randomized controlled trials (RCTs), they are frequently accepted as the best standard of care. The majority of surgical patients do receive treatment based on satisfactory evidence (categories 1 and 2), with approximately 25 percent of patients receiving treatments based on data retrieved from RCTs. General surgery, especially surgical oncology, is evidence based, even if the proportion of surgical treatments supported by randomized controlled trial evidence is smaller than that found in general medicine.[1]

Regrettably, evidence surrounding the management of elderly patients with cancer from categories 1 and 2 is scanty. Although a handful of clinical trials in this area have been conducted, interestingly, their findings have not been universally adopted.

Surgical procedures are difficult to validate within clinical trials.[2,3] This explains the lack of robust evidence when the elderly age group is taken into account. Although they may share tumor characteristics with the younger age group, their expectations and treatment goals are deeply different. It is for this reason that the findings of any RCT cannot be extrapolated and transposed to the elderly group. Also, wider variations in fitness for surgery and thus operative risk need to be considered. Careful preoperative staging, skillful surgical technique, and optimal perioperative management with a multimodal approach are therefore mandatory. These issues are not discussed here as they are not specific to cancer patients alone.

The multidisciplinary approach is, as always, of great importance when treating elderly patients because of the need for close interactions between professionals throughout the course of disease. It has been shown that this approach can improve measurable outcomes and quality of life.[4-6]

A. Defining the targets

For elderly patients with cancer, the decision whether to undergo treatment may be a compromise between loss of function and/or independence as a consequence of treatment versus the extension of life. A higher prevalence of disability and limited physiological reserves means that elderly patients have a higher risk of developing protracted postoperative disability. Only a few studies have looked at this: in a study by Lawrence and colleagues that looked at 372 consecutive patients over the age of 60 years who underwent elective major abdominal surgery, 10–50 percent (depending on the measure) had prolonged disability and had not recovered to their preoperative statuses by 6 months.[7] Potentially modifiable factors predicting a slow postoperative recovery were the occurrence of serious postoperative complications and poor preoperative physical function. Amemiya and colleagues followed 223 patients aged 75 years and older who underwent elective surgery for gastric and colorectal cancer for 6 months. They found that only 3 percent of patients showed a decline in activities of daily living after 6 months, and quality of life was reported to be equal to or better than preoperative levels.[8] Considerations about postoperative functional status and quality of life are essential for decision making in the cohort of elderly patients with cancer undergoing surgery, and more data on these issues are warranted.

B. Breast cancer

Treatment guidelines and practice standards have been developed for the surgical management of elderly patients with breast cancer.[9] Overall, breast cancer surgery–related mortality in the elderly population is low, ranging from 0 to 0.3 percent.[10,11] Anesthesia with paravertebral nerve block or a local anesthetic with or without sedation should be taken into account before denying removal of the tumor.[12]

Assumptions that elderly patients have a reduced life expectancy and should therefore receive less aggressive forms of breast cancer treatment have meant that hormonal treatment *without* surgery has been considered a reasonable treatment option, particularly in very old and frail patients.[13] The impact of omitting surgery (and treating with primary endocrine therapy) on overall survival is not clear and differs between studies. Four of these studies compared tamoxifen monotherapy versus surgery alone.[14-17] The Group for Research on Endocrine Therapy in the Elderly trial used a more informative design where treatment with surgery and adjuvant tamoxifen[18] showed a nonsignificant benefit in overall survival in comparison to treatment with tamoxifen alone. Moreover, a significantly higher proportion of patients treated with tamoxifen alone experienced local relapse for which subsequent salvage breast cancer surgery would have been necessitated. Another study randomized 455 women aged 70 years or older with operable breast cancer into groups who received either treatment with surgery and tamoxifen or tamoxifen alone.[19] There was an increase in breast cancer–specific mortality and overall mortality in those who had no surgery (hazard ratio 1.68, 95% confidence interval [CI] 1.15–2.47 and 1.29, 1.04–1.59, respectively). A Cochrane meta-analysis has confirmed that hormonal treatment with tamoxifen alone is inferior to surgery (with or without hormonal treatment) for the local control and progression-free survival of breast cancer in medically fit older women.[20] However, surgery did not result in a significantly improved overall survival.

Neoadjuvant treatment with aromatase inhibitors in postmenopausal patients with breast cancer has shown better response rates than tamoxifen.[21-23] There are no specific data evaluating treatment with an aromatase inhibitor alone versus surgery combined with an aromatase inhibitor in this cohort. This approach warrants further investigation, preferably in older patients who have a limited life expectancy and in whom the omission of surgery is unlikely to affect breast cancer–specific mortality.

The extent of axillary dissection is also a matter of debate. Interesting results of an RCT were published by Martelli et al., who evaluated the utility of an axillary dissection for early-stage (T1N0 M0) breast cancer in the elderly.[24] After a follow-up of 60 months, no significant difference in overall mortality, breast cancer–specific mortality, and crude cumulative incidence of breast events (local recurrence or metachronous cancer) between the two groups (quadrantectomy ± axillary dissection) was found. Only 2 out of 110 patients in the arm that omitted axillary dissection developed overt axillary involvement (8 and 40 months after surgery). It was concluded that elderly patients with T1N0 breast cancer can be treated with conservative surgery and no axillary dissection without adversely affecting breast cancer–specific mortality or overall survival. These findings were recently confirmed in trial 10-93 of the International Breast Cancer Study Group.[25] However, on several occasions, breast surgeons have performed a delayed dissection for recurrent axillary disease several years after the primary tumor was removed and the axilla was left intact. The need for considering axillary evaluation at time of primary breast surgery is supported by findings from the European Institute of Oncology (EIO) study in Milan,[26] in which elderly postmenopausal women were found to be more likely to present with pathologically involved axillary nodes.

Sentinel-node biopsy is proven to be a feasible and useful procedure in elderly women with breast cancer measuring less than 3 cm in maximum diameter.[27] It allows appropriate staging with the benefits of reduced morbidity and can be performed under local anesthesia. However, it is questionable whether a frail, elderly woman should be exposed to the risks of undergoing an anesthetic twice in the case of positivity, rather than being offered an axillary dissection at the time of initial breast surgery.

Recommendations follow:

- Hormonal treatment alone for elderly patients with breast cancer is an inferior option to surgical excision and should be only considered in frail individuals who cannot tolerate the procedure.
- Surgical removal of the primary tumor results in improved mortality rates and should not be denied, particularly when one considers the low operative mortality.
- The need of axillary dissection is questionable and still under investigation.
- Sentinel-node biopsy is feasible in elderly patients.

C. Colorectal cancer

In the attempt to rationalize the approach toward elderly patients with colorectal cancer (CRC), a task force has been set up by the International

Society of Geriatric Oncology (SIOG). Their recommendations, including surgical recommendations, were recently published.[28] Surgery is indisputably the most successful treatment modality for colorectal tumors. The improvement in the survival of patients with CRC has largely been a result of the decrease in operative mortality and the increase in resection rates, possibly coupled with a more aggressive approach to the treatment of local or distant recurrences.[29]

A registry-based study of 6,457 patients with CRC, diagnosed between 1985 and 1992 in hospitals connected to the Rotterdam Cancer Registry, emphasizes the disparity in the treatment patterns between elderly and younger patients.[30] Overall, 87 percent of the patients underwent resection, but the resection rates were lower for patients over 89 years of age (67%) and for patients with rectal cancer (83%). The postoperative mortality rate was 1 percent for patients under 60 years of age and steadily increased with age. For patients over 80 years of age, the operative risk was 10 percent. According to a multivariate analysis, gender, age, subsite, and stage were defined as independent prognostic factors. Another study of patients in their eighth and ninth decades showed that postoperative mortality increased from 8 percent between 80 and 84 years to 13 percent between 85 and 89 years and to 20 percent for those in their nineties.[31]

A systematic review of 28 independent studies conducted by the Colorectal Cancer Collaborative Group[32] involving a total of 34,194 patients compared the outcomes after colorectal surgery for patients aged 65–74 years, 75–84 years, and 85 or more years with those for patients aged under 65 years. The findings showed that elderly patients had an increased number of comorbidities, were more likely to present with advanced disease, were more likely to undergo emergency surgery, and were less likely to have curative surgery than younger patients. In concordance with the Rotterdam study, the incidence of postoperative morbidity and mortality increased with advancing age. Overall survival was also reduced in elderly patients, but for cancer-specific survival, the age-related differences were far less striking. Thus the relationship between age and outcomes from CRC surgery is complex and may be confounded by differences in stage at presentation, tumor site, the type of treatment received, and preexisting comorbidities, for example, the presence of chronic obstructive pulmonary disease (COPD) and deep venous thrombosis, which lead to an increased risk of developing postoperative complications.[33]

However, there is little doubt that carefully selected elderly patients benefit from surgery since a large proportion survive for 2 or more years after surgery irrespective of age. A recommendation in support of this came from an analysis of the long-term outcomes after surgical intervention in 9,501 patients with rectal cancer aged over 80 years. It concluded that "age should not deter surgeons from offering optimal therapy to good-risk patients."[34]

It appears that in the case of elective surgery, long-term-cancer-related and short-term morbidity and mortality outcomes for elderly patients are similar to those of younger patients.[35] An analysis of selected series suggests that age is not a risk factor for local recurrence and that the rate of distant recurrence can be lower in elderly patients.[36] On the other hand, consistent data demonstrate how preexisting comorbidities strongly influenced the type of resection performed (elective vs. emergency) and as a consequence, the long-term outcome is influenced.[37] Elderly patients with comorbidities are being treated less aggressively and face a poorer survival than those with no concomitant disease.[38]

Furthermore, results from a cost analysis performed on a consecutive series of patients with CRC show that there are no differences in cost when treating when treating patients 65 years and older compared to younger patients.[39]

Although it has been suggested that the development of complications among patients undergoing surgery for CRC can be predicted by the presence of comorbidity,[40] it should be acknowledged that almost all patients with stage I–III colon cancer or rectal cancer usually undergo surgery regardless of age or comorbidity.[41] On the other hand, there is unanimous agreement that emergency colorectal surgery in elderly patients should be avoided whenever possible because of the profound operative mortality.[42] A recent study from Denmark investigating 2,000 acute patients with obstruction, perforation or bleeding demonstrated how such complications are more than tripled for patients in the seventh decade (24%), rising to 35 percent in the eighth decade and 48 percent thereafter. Interestingly, this study demonstrated how surgical complications (i.e., after-bleeds requiring surgery, wound dehiscence requiring surgery, anastomotic leak, intestinal obstruction requiring surgery, abdominal abscess, and stoma complications requiring surgery) may be responsible for 20 percent of postoperative deaths, while medical complications (i.e., apoplexy, myocardial infarction or heart failure, pneumonia, sepsis, need for dialysis, deep vein thrombosis, embolism, and respiratory failure) were responsible for 58 percent of postoperative mortality rates.[43]

For this reason, every effort should be taken to prevent such complications, particularly obstruction. The use of colorectal stents in treating obstruction as a bridge to surgery should be considered in elderly patients. This technique succeeds in decompressing the bowel in 88–94 percent of cases with a minimal mortality (0.4%–0.6%), as demonstrated by two systematic reviews.[44,45]

The available evidence suggests that long-term survival for fit, elderly patients with CRC undergoing surgery is similar to that of younger patients, although it is recognized that overall survival is poorer in elderly patients because of other factors.

Recommendations follow:

- Emergency colorectal surgery should be avoided where possible because of its high morbidity and mortality.
- The use of colorectal stents should be considered whenever appropriate to facilitate elective surgery 1–2 weeks after the patient has presented as an emergency.
- Elective surgery and careful treatment planning should be the pathways of choice.

D. Hepatic, pancreatic, and biliary surgery

Even with the recent advances in chemotherapy, 5-year survival in patients with colorectal cancer with liver metastases receiving only palliative chemotherapy is 0–4%, and none are cured.[46,47] The active treatment of elderly patients with metastatic colorectal cancer presents us with a dilemma when evaluating the benefits and risks of surgery. Most studies reporting outcomes after hepatic resection in the elderly deal with mixed tumor types, including a substantial number of patients with hepatocellular carcinoma and different types of resection, making informed conclusions difficult.

The largest single-center series of liver resections for colorectal liver metastases in patients aged over 70 years has recently been reported from Aintree University Hospital.[48] Interestingly, this is also the first single-center study that attempts to evaluate the impact of neoadjuvant chemotherapy in elderly patients undergoing liver resection. Postoperative morbidity and mortality rates (38.5% and 4.9%, respectively) are consistent with previous series in older and younger patients, confirming that there is no significantly increased operative risk among selected elderly patients.[49–51] There is clear evidence that patients with CRC who are aged over 70 years and undergo liver resection achieve clinically significant progression-free[51] and 5-year survivals.[52]

This is important in light of the recommendation that liver resection should be undertaken in patients with resectable hepatic metastases wherever possible.[53] Mortality is, however, higher in those over the age of 70 (4.5% vs. 1.5%).[48]

Liver failure is a worrying but rare complication after liver resection (3.9% in the Aintree series). A higher risk of developing liver failure is found in elderly patients, resulting in a more conservative surgical selection policy.[54,55]

Perioperative chemotherapy with FOLFOX 4 is routinely prescribed in most patients with liver metastases from primary colorectal cancer: it was proven to be compatible with major liver surgery and capable of increasing progression-free survival in eligible and resected patients.[56] Neoadjuvant chemotherapy is nevertheless seldom prescribed to elderly patients; there is concern that an age-related reduced hepatic functional reserve increases the risk for life-threatening hepatotoxicity (sinusoidal congestion and thrombosis) caused by Oxaliplatin. This was not confirmed in the Aintree series, in which only 1 out of the 34 patients receiving FOLFOX developed liver failure. Interestingly, there was no difference in postoperative complication rates when patients who did or did not receive neoadjuvant chemotherapy were compared.

An important factor influencing postoperative survival is primary tumor category. Surprisingly, patients with a T3 primary tumor showed inferior overall and disease-free survival compared to T4 tumors. This may suggest an increased tendency for early metastatic spread in T3 tumors compared with the more locally progressive T4 tumors.[57] Overall and disease-free survival are better for those patients who undergo resection of only one or two liver segments when compared to those undergoing major liver resection. Although no significant difference in postoperative complication rates is evident between the groups, postoperative mortality is increased after major hepatic resection, thus affecting long-term survival. Recurrence rates are generally lower after minor liver resections, and this could be explained by surgeons adopting a more favorable selection process. Furthermore, the improved long-term outcomes found in patients treated with a limited resection may be the result of their initial presentation being one of less aggressive liver involvement and not actually the difference in surgical approach. These findings indicate that extensive anatomic resections are no longer justified. When one excludes postoperative mortality, disease-free survival rates at 1, 3, and 5 years are similar in elderly and younger patients.[58]

Despite the scarce data surrounding resection of gallbladder and hilar bile duct cancers in the elderly, evidence from a large series concluded that advanced age per se is not a risk factor for poor outcomes.[59]

Comparable findings are also reported for pancreatic resection in elderly patients with either ampullary or pancreatic cancer. It is widely known that the survival benefit of pancreaticoduodenectomy is limited in all age groups. However, this operation is the sole curative option. Postoperative mortality and morbidity, length of hospital stay, and long-term survival after periampullary and pancreatic resection were reported to be similar in selected series of elderly patients compared to those in younger patient cohorts.[60]

The presence of comorbid conditions, particularly COPD, is associated with poor short-term outcomes[61,62] and the aforementioned prognostic factors should be carefully assessed when considering surgical options in the management of elderly patients with malignant hepatobiliary tumors. Alternatively, palliative symptom management and pain control should be considered[63] to optimize quality of life whenever cure is unlikely.

Recommendations follow:

- Patient selection should be based on the patient's level of fitness, comorbidities, extent of surgery, and life expectancy because HPB surgery is often associated with a high operative mortality.

E. Upper gastrointestinal surgery

Overall prevalence rates of gastric cancer are decreasing, but the increasing life expectancy has resulted in a large number of elderly patients with gastric cancer presenting on surgical wards. In fact, one-third of gastric cancers occur at age 70 and beyond.[64,65]

An overview from the last decade demonstrated that surgery can be safely performed and that the outcomes achieved by the elderly are similar to those of younger patients.[66] However, it is likely that only fit senior patients were considered for surgery in this study, thus introducing a significant selection bias. It would be interesting to investigate whether postoperative mortality and morbidity can be reduced by using preoperative risk assessment tools to select patients appropriately. This would allow the tailoring of care, with less aggressive treatments being offered to the frail cohort to minimize postoperative negative outcomes. Less extensive surgical strategies such as combined resections or extensive lymphadenectomies may result in acceptable survival rates, a better quality of life, and a reduced operative mortality.[67]

This hypothesis was investigated in a study from Berlin that compared different age groups undergoing surgery for gastric cancer.[68] The analysis showed that despite a less extensive lymph node dissection in the elderly group (aged over 75 years), the tumor-related survival rate was not reduced, implying that the prognostic power of D2 lymph node dissection may not be as influential in older patients. The authors observed a higher prevalence of comorbidity in the older group, resulting in significantly higher rates of non-tumor-related long-term mortality. This conforms with previous observations.[69,70] A small series from Cagliari has confirmed that an adequate quality of life can be achieved from utilizing this strategy of tailored surgery.[71] Overall, elderly patients who were offered extensive surgical procedures (i.e., total gastrectomy and extensive lymphadenectomy) appeared to have similar long-term outcomes as younger patients, and it was elegantly demonstrated how patients' age appears to be the only independent variable correlating with the occurrence of postoperative complications.[72,73]

Recommendations follow:

- Gastric cancer surgery is feasible and can be safely delivered to selected series of elderly patients.
- The value of extensive resections and lymphadenectomy is yet to be demonstrated.

F. Thoracic surgery

Although half of all lung cancer cases occur in patients aged 65 years or older,[74] fewer surgical options are offered to the elderly because of suspected frailty, higher risk for complications, and less active life expectancy.[75] This differential treatment between young and elderly patients is unjustified. Age alone should not be a contraindication to thoracic surgery, which is proven to be safe in selected groups of the elderly population.[76,77]

Together with an aging population, advances in neoadjuvant therapies and wide availability of minimally invasive techniques mean that an increasing number of elderly patients with lung cancer will be candidates for surgical management.[78]

Risk assessment is paramount in the identification of elderly patients who may be suitable for surgery and those with high-risk profiles that would need additional special care. The evaluation of pulmonary and cardiac function is of particular importance. A greater understanding of other potential prognostic factors is important to avoid instigating aggressive and unnecessary treatment in patients who will not benefit from it.[79,80]

Given the improvement in morbidity and mortality figures, minimally invasive surgical techniques may prove advantageous for the less fit elderly patient. Additional benefits may be gained from these new surgical techniques, such as a lesser degree of postoperative pain, a quicker return to the home environment, and a decreased incidence of postoperative cognitive dysfunction, as a result of less surgical and anesthetic stress.

In 1995, the Lung Cancer Study Group published the results of a prospective randomized trial[81] that compared lobectomies with limited resections (including segmentectomies). Patients who underwent limited resections had a higher incidence of local recurrence and a marginally significant worse survival when compared to those who had lobectomies. Another study reported higher local recurrence rates and shorter survival among patients who had wedge resections in comparison to those who had lobectomies.[82] Lobectomy is, therefore, still considered the standard of care for stage T1 lung cancer in patients with an adequate cardiorespiratory reserve. Less extensive resections constitute a reasonable alternative for patients with a limited respiratory reserve and thus unable to tolerate a lobectomy.[83]

The difference in recurrence and survival between patients who have undergone lobec-tomies and those who have undergone limited resections may not be as stark in the elderly as in younger patients. Elderly patients have a higher rate of perioperative complications,[84] a higher probability of presenting with early-stage disease,[85] a reduced respiratory reserve, and a shorter life expectancy than their younger counterparts, making limited resections with a curative intent a reasonable alternative. The reduction in morbidity and mortality provided by limited resections should benefit the elderly given their reduced cardiac and respiratory reserve, associated comorbidities, and higher propensity for surgical complications. Some studies[86,87] have demonstrated a similar survival rate in limited resections and lobectomies among elderly patients. This is providing that the resection includes all foci of the tumor and provides a margin microscopically free of disease. These findings were affirmed in an analysis of a large multi-institutional database that found that the difference in long-term survival between the two treatment modalities disappeared after 71 years of age.[88] Although earlier-stage tumors were found among the elderly, curative surgery was less frequently offered to this cohort; almost 30 percent of elderly patients were denied surgery or were offered only palliative surgery, compared to 8 percent among the younger group.

Recommendations follow:

- Individual outcomes and quality of life measures are to be prioritized when planning treatment and during patient counseling.
- Limited resections may provide similar survival rates to lobectomies among the elderly.
- Video-assisted thoracoscopic surgery is a promising technique particularly suitable for elderly patients.

G. Head and neck cancer surgery

Head and neck cancer represents the eighth leading cause of cancer mortality worldwide.[89] Surgery is practical for elderly patients with head and neck cancers because positive outcomes have been reported in selected series of thyroid, laryngeal, and mixed head and neck cancers.[90–93] Mortality rates as low as 3.5 percent have been reported (median 7%) with almost 50 percent postoperative deaths resulting from pulmonary complications.[94] Associated medical conditions are highly prevalent in this group of patients, alcohol abuse and heavy smoking typically being the most common, alongside others such as hypertension, arrhythmias, congestive heart failure, COPD, and diabetes.[95] Sanabria and colleagues also noted that age is an independent negative prognostic indicator.

Piccirillo modified the Kaplan-Feinstein comorbidity index and developed the Adult Comorbidity Evaluation–27, which is widely utilized in the assessment of elderly head and neck cancer patients.[96,97,98] No significant differences in quality of life have been found between elderly and younger patients when measured 3 months after treatment.

Recommendations follow:

- Head and neck cancer surgery is feasible and can be safely delivered to selected elderly patients.
- Surgery achieves good oncological and functional results that improve quality of life, no matter the patient's age.
- Patient selection is crucial; this can be achieved with the use of extensive preoperative evaluations.

H. Conclusions

A large amount of data regarding elderly cancer patients can be retrieved from the literature to demonstrate the feasibility of surgical procedures and, most frequently, positive short- and long-term outcomes. It is unfortunate that these series inevitably selected the small minority of fit elderly individuals, while the frail ones were not considered.[66] No final conclusion can be drawn on the surgical management of this age group until all patients undergo preoperative Comprehensive Geriatric Assessment (CGA).

Adverse postoperative outcomes are more common in older patients, particularly delirium, cardiac events and lung infection.[99] Postoperative complications affect quality of life, long-term outcomes, hospital stay and total costs.[100] It is important to note that most series reporting on postoperative complications after surgery have not included the occurrence of delirium.

The development of guidelines for the surgical management of elderly cancer patients should

be strongly considered such as SIOG breast[9] and SIOG colorectal cancer guidelines.[28] However, it is imperative that one personalizes care with the aim of tailoring treatment options to each individual patient. This should be based on life expectancy, patient preference and fitness to undergo surgery and anesthesia. To improve our understanding of patient fitness, CGA tools commonly utilized by geriatricians, have been put into practice. The use of the Pre-operative Assessment of Cancer in the Elderly (PACE) has identified the factors that impinge on outcome.[101] PACE is a composite of validated questionnaires, including the CGA and others such as the Eastern Cooperative Oncology Group Performance Status, American Society of Anesthesiologists classification, Physiological and Operative Severity Score for Enumeration of Mortality and Morbidity (POSSUM), and the Portsmouth variation of POSSUM including pathological data. It has been shown that the PACE questionnaire takes only 20 minutes to complete; is practical, inexpensive and acceptable; it can be clearly comprehended by elderly patients.[102] The use of PACE has demonstrated that disability, measured as dependency in instrumental activities of daily living (IADLs) is associated with a 50 percent increase in the relative risk of developing postoperative complications. Multivariate analysis identified moderate to severe fatigue and dependency in IADLs as the most important independent predictors of postoperative complications. Dependency in basic activities of daily living, IADLs or low performance status as associated with an extended hospital stay. Another study of elderly patients electively operated for colorectal cancer showed that patients who are categorized as frail, based on a preoperative CGA, experience a significantly higher rate of severe postoperative complications compared to patients classified as not frail (62% vs. 36%, $p = .005$).[103] These findings indicate that preoperative risk assessments of elderly patients should include elements of CGA. Accurate patient selection is crucial to avoid overtreating frail individuals while offering state-of-the-art management to all others. It is essential to address these issues when counseling elderly patients and consenting them for an operation.

References

1. Howes N, Chagla L, Thorpe M, et al. Surgical practice is evidence based. *Br J Surg.* 1997;84(9):1220–1223.

2. Glasziou P, Chalmers I, Rawlins M, et al. When are randomised trials unnecessary? Picking signal from noise. *Br Med J.* 2007;334(7589): 349–351.

3. McCulloch P. Surgical professionalism in the 21st century. *Lancet.* 2006;367(9505):177–181.

4. Ferguson MK, Reeder LB, Mick R. Optimizing selection of patients for major lung resection. *J Thorac Cardiovasc Surg.* 1995;109:275–281; discussion 281–283.

5. Reilly JJ Jr, Mentzer SJ, Sugarbaker DJ. Preoperative assessment of patients undergoing pulmonary resection. *Chest.* 1993;103(suppl): 342–345.

6. Cain HD, Stevens PM, Adaniya R. Preoperative pulmonary function and complications after cardiovascular surgery. *Chest.* 1979;76: 130–135.

7. Lawrence VA, Hazuda HP, Cornell JE, et al. Functional independence after major abdominal surgery in the elderly. *J Am Coll Surg.* 2004;199: 762–772.

8. Amemiya T, Oda K, Ando M, et al. Activities of daily living and quality of life of elderly patients after elective surgery for gastric and colorectal cancers. *Ann Surg.* 2007;246:222–228.

9. Wildiers H, Kunkler I, Biganzoli L, et al. Management of breast cancer in elderly individuals: recommendations of the International Society of Geriatric Oncology. *Lancet Oncol.* 2007;8(12):1101–1115.

10. Gennari R, Curigliano G, Rotmensz N, et al. Breast carcinoma in elderly women – features of disease presentation, choice of local and systemic treatments compared with younger postmenopausal patients. *Cancer.* 2004;101: 1302–1310.

11. Gennari R, Rotmensz N, Perego E, et al. Sentinel node biopsy in elderly breast cancer patients. *Surg Oncol.* 2004;13:193–196.

12. Naijarian MM, Johnson JM, Landercasper J, et al. Paravertebral block: an alternative to general anaesthesia in breast cancer surgery. *Ann Surg.* 2003;69:213–218.

13. Rai S, Stotter A. Management of elderly patients with breast cancer: the time for surgery. *Anz J Surg.* 2005;75:863–865.

14. Fentiman IS, Christiaens MR, Paridaens R, et al. Treatment of operable breast cancer in the elderly: a randomised clinical trial EORTC 10851 comparing tamoxifen alone with modified radical mastectomy. *Eur J Cancer.* 2003;39:309–316.

15. Robertson JFR, Todd JH, Ellis IO, et al. Comparison of mastectomy with tamoxifen for treating elderly patients with operable breast cancer. *Br Med J.* 1988;297:511–514.

16. Gazet JC, Ford HT, Coombes RC, et al. Prospective randomized trial of tamoxifen vs surgery in elderly patients with breast cancer. *Eur J Surg Oncol.* 1994;20:207–214.

17. van Dalsen AD, de Vries JE. Treatment of breast cancer in elderly patients. *J Surg Oncol.* 1995;60:80–82.

18. Mustacchi G, Ceccherini R, Milani S, et al. Tamoxifen alone versus adjuvant tamoxifen or operable breast cancer of the elderly: long-term results of the phase III randomized controlled multicenter GRETA trial. *Ann Oncol.* 2003;14: 414–420.

19. Fennessy M, Bates T, MacRae K, et al. Late follow-up of a randomized trial of surgery plus tamoxifen versus tamoxifen alone in women aged over 70 years with operable breast cancer. *Br J Surg.* 2004;91:699–704.

20. Hind D, Wyld L, Reed MW. Surgery, with or without tamoxifen, vs tamoxifen alone for older women with operable breast cancer: Cochrane review. *Br J Cancer.* 2007;96(7):1025–1029.

21. Smith IE, Dowsett M, Ebbs SR, et al. Neoadjuvant treatment of postmenopausal breast cancer with anastrozole, tamoxifen, or both in combination: the Immediate Preoperative Anastrozole, Tamoxifen, or Combined with Tamoxifen (IMPACT) multicenter double-blind randomized trial. *J Clin Oncol.* 2005;23:5108–5116.

22. Ellis MJ, Coop A, Singh B, et al. Letrozole is more effective neoadjuvant endocrine therapy than tamoxifen for ErbB-1- and/or ErbB-2-positive, estrogen receptor-positive primary breast cancer: evidence from a phase III randomized trial. *J Clin Oncol.* 2001;19(18):3808–3816.

23. Buzdar AU. "Arimidex" (anastrozole) versus tamoxifen as adjuvant therapy in postmenopausal women with early breast cancer-efficacy overview. *J Steroid Biochem Mol Biol.* 2003;86:399–403.

24. Martelli G, Boracchi P, De Palo M, et al. A randomized trial comparing axillary dissection to no axillary dissection in older patients with T1N0 breast cancer: results after 5 years of follow-up. *Ann Surg.* 2005;242(1):1–6.

25. Rudenstam CM, Zahrieh D, Forbes JF, et al. Randomized trial comparing axillary clearance versus no axillary clearance in older patients with breast cancer: first results of International Breast Cancer Study Group Trial 10-93. *J Clin Oncol.* 2006;24(3):337–344.

26. Gennari R, Curigliano G, Rotmensz N. Breast carcinoma in elderly women: features of disease presentation, choice of local and systemic

treatments compared with younger postmenopausal patients. *Cancer*. 2004;101(6): 1302–1310.

27. Gennari R, Rotmensz N, Perego E, et al. Sentinel node biopsy in elderly breast cancer patients. *Surg Oncol*. 2004;13(4):193–196.

28. Papamichael D, Audisio R, Horiot JC, et al. Treatment of the elderly colorectal cancer patient: SIOG expert recommendations. *Ann Oncol*. 2009;20(1):5–16.

29. Mitry E, Bouvier AM, Esteve J, et al. Improvement in colorectal cancer survival: a population-based study. *Eur J Cancer*. 2005;41:2297–2303.

30. Damhuis RA, Wereldsma JC, Wiggers T. The influence of age on resection rates and postoperative mortality in 6457 patients with colorectal cancer. *Int J Colorectal Dis*. 1996;11:45–48.

31. Damhuis RA, Meurs CJ, Meijer WS. Postoperative mortality after cancer surgery in octogenarians and nonagenarians: results from a series of 5,390 patients. *World J Surg Oncol*. 2005;3:71.

32. Colorectal Cancer Collaborative Group. Surgery for colorectal cancer in elderly patients: a systematic review. *Lancet*. 2000;356:968–974.

33. Lemmens VE, Janssen-Heijnen ML, Houterman S, et al. Which comorbid conditions predict complications after surgery for colorectal cancer? *World J Surg*. 2007;31(1):192–199.

34. Kiran RP, Pokala N, Dudrick SJ. Long-term outcome after operative intervention for rectal cancer in patients aged over 80 years: analysis of 9,501 patients. *Dis Colon Rectum*. 2007;50: 604–610.

35. Audisio RA, Veronesi P, Ferrario L, et al. Elective surgery for gastrointestinal tumours in the elderly. *Ann Oncol*. 1997;8:317–326.

36. Manfredi S, Bouvier AM, Lepage C, et al. Incidence and patterns of recurrence after resection for cure of colonic cancer in a well defined population. *Br J Surg*. 2006;93:1115–1122.

37. Fallahzadeh H, Mays ET. Preexisting disease as a predictor of the outcome of colectomy. *Am J Surg*. 1991;162:497–498.

38. Lemmens VE, Janssen-Heijnen ML, Verheij CD, et al. Co-morbidity leads to altered treatment and worse survival of elderly patients with colorectal cancer. *Br J Surg*. 2005;92(5):615–623.

39. Audisio RA, Cazzaniga M, Robertson C, et al. Elective surgery for colorectal cancer in the aged: a clinical-economical evaluation. *Br J Cancer*. 1997;76(3):382–384.

40. Lemmens VE, Janssen-Heijnen ML, Houterman S, et al. Which comorbid conditions predict complications after surgery for colorectal cancer? *World J Surg*. 2007;31(1):192–199.

41. Janssen-Heijnen ML, Maas HA, Houterman S, et al. Comorbidity in older surgical cancer patients: influence on patient care and outcome. *Eur J Cancer*. 2007;43(15):2179–2193.

42. Hessman O, Bergkvist L, Ström S. Colorectal cancer in patients over 75 years of age – determinants of outcome. *Eur J Surg Oncol*. 1997;23(1):13–19.

43. Iversen LH, Bülow S, Christensen IJ, et al. Postoperative medical complications are the main cause of early death after emergency surgery for colonic cancer. *Br J Surg*. 2008;95(8): 1012–1019.

44. Khot UP, Lang AW, Murali K, et al. Systematic review of the efficacy and safety of colorectal stents. *Br J Surg*. 2002;89(9):1096–1102.

45. Sebastian S, Johnston S, Geoghegan T, et al. Pooled analysis of the efficacy and safety of self-expanding metal stenting in malignant colorectal obstruction. *Am J Gastroenterol*. 2004;99(10):2051–2057.

46. Yun HR, Lee WY, Lee OS, et al. The prognostic factors of stage IV colorectal cancer and assessment of proper treatment according to the patient's status. *Int J Colorectal Dis*. 2007;22(11): 1301–1310.

47. Okuno K. Surgical treatment for digestive cancer: current issues – colon cancer. *Dig Surg*. 2007; 24(2):108–114.

48. de Liguori Carino N, van Leeuwen BL, Ghaneh P, et al. Liver resection for colorectal liver metastases in older patients. *Crit Rev Oncol Hematol*. 2008;67(3):273–278.

49. Fong Y, Blumgart LH, Fortner JG, et al. Pancreatic or liver resection for malignancy is safe and effective for the elderly. *Ann Surg*. 1995;222(4): 426–434.

50. Mazzoni G, Tocchi A, Miccini M, et al. Surgical treatment of liver metastases from colorectal cancer in elderly patients. *Int J Colorectal Dis*. 2007;22(1):77–83.

51. Menon KV, Al Mukhtar A, Aldouri A, et al. Outcomes after major hepatectomy in elderly patients. *J Am Coll Surg*. 2006;203(5):677–683.

52. Mazzoni G, Tocchi A, Miccini M, et al. Surgical treatment of liver metastases from colorectal cancer in elderly patients. *Int J Colorectal Dis*. 2007;22:77–83.

53. Van Cutsem E, Nordlinger B, Adam R, et al. Towards a pan-European consensus on the treatment of patients with colorectal liver metastases. *Eur J Cancer*. 2006;42:2212–2221.

54. Kimura F, Miyazaki M, Suwa T, et al. Reduction of hepatic acute phase response after partial hepatectomy in elderly patients. *Res Exp Med (Berl)* 1996;196(5):281–290.

55. Aalami OO, Fang TD, Song HM, et al. Physiological features of aging persons. *Arch Surg.* 2003;138(10):1068–1076.

56. Nordlinger B, Sorbye H, Glimelius B, et al. Perioperative chemotherapy with FOLFOX 4 and surgery versus surgery alone for resectable liver metastases from colorectal cancer (EORTC Intergroup trial 40983): a randomised controlled trial. *Lancet.* 2008;371(9617):1007–1016.

57. de Liguori Carino N, van Leeuwen BL, Ghaneh P, et al. Liver resection for colorectal liver metastases in older patients. *Crit Rev Oncol Hematol.* 2008;67(3):273–278.

58. Figueras J, Ramos E, López-Ben S, et al. Surgical treatment of liver metastases from colorectal carcinoma in elderly patients: when is it worthwhile? *Clin Transl Oncol.* 2007;9(6): 392–400.

59. Petrowsky H, Clavien PA. Should we deny surgery for malignant hepato-pancreatico-biliary tumors to elderly patients? *World J Surg.* 2005;29(9):1093–1100.

60. Casadei R, Zanini N, Morselli-Labate AM, et al. Prognostic factors in periampullary and pancreatic tumor resection in elderly patients. *World J Surg.* 2006;30(11):1992–2001.

61. Brozzetti S, Mazzoni G, Miccini M, et al. Surgical treatment of pancreatic head carcinoma in elderly patients. *Arch Surg.* 2006;141(2):137–142.

62. Petrowsky H, Clavien PA. Should we deny surgery for malignant hepato-pancreatico-biliary tumors to elderly patients? *World J Surg.* 2005;29(9):1093–1100.

63. Cruciani RA, Jain S. Pancreatic pain: a mini review. *Pancreatology.* 2008;8(3):230–235.

64. Levi F, Lucchini F, Negri E, et al. Changed trends of cancer mortality in the elderly. *Ann Oncol.* 2001;12(10):1467–1477.

65. Takeda J, Tanaka T, Koufuji K, et al. Gastric cancer surgery in patients aged at least 80 years old. *Hepatogastroenterology.* 1994;41(6):516–520.

66. Audisio RA, Veronesi P, Ferrario L, et al. Elective surgery in gastrointestinal tumours in the aged. *Ann Oncol.* 1997;8(4):317–327.

67. Enzinger PC, Mayer RJ. Gastrointestinal cancer in older patients. *Semin Oncol.* 2004;31(2): 206–219.

68. Gretschel S, Estevez-Schwarz L, Hünerbein M, et al. Gastric cancer surgery in elderly patients. *World J Surg.* 2006;30(8):1468–1474.

69. Coniglio A, Tiberio GA, Busti M, et al. Surgical treatment for gastric carcinoma in the elderly. *J Surg Oncol.* 2004;88(4):201–205.

70. Maehara Y, Emi Y, Tomisaki S, et al. Age-related characteristics of gastric carcinoma in young and elderly patients. *Cancer.* 1996;77(9):1774–1780.

71. Pisanu A, Montisci A, Piu S, et al. Curative surgery for gastric cancer in the elderly: treatment decisions, surgical morbidity, mortality, prognosis and quality of life. *Tumori.* 2007;93(5):478–484.

72. Otsuji E, Fujiyama J, Takagi T, et al. Results of total gastrectomy with extended lymphadenectomy for gastric cancer in elderly patients. *J Surg Oncol.* 2005;91(4):232–236.

73. Bittner R, Butters M, Ulrich M, et al. Total gastrectomy: updated operative mortality and long-term survival with particular reference to patients older than 70 years of age. *Ann Surg.* 1996;224(1):37–42.

74. Zanetti R, Crosignani P. Cancer in Italy: incidence data from cancer registries 1983–1987. Paper presented at: Lega italiana per la lotta contro i tumori; 1992; Torino, Italy.

75. Fentiman IS, Tirelli U, Monfardini S, et al. Cancer in the elderly: why so badly treated? *Lancet.* 1990;335:1020–1022.

76. Roberts JR, Chang A, Slovis B. Severely compromised pulmonary function does not increase perioperative mortality after pulmonary lobectomy in a high volume center. *Chest.* 1999;116:370S.

77. Pagni S, Federico JA, Ponn RB. Pulmonary resection for lung cancer in octogenarians. *Ann Thorac Surg.* 1997;63:785–789.

78. Castillo MD, Heerdt PM. Pulmonary resection in the elderly. *Curr Opin Anaesthesiol.* 2007;20(1): 4–9.

79. Marcantonio ER, Goldman L, Mangione CM, et al. A clinical prediction rule for delirium after elective noncardiac surgery. *J Am Med Assoc.* 1994;271:134–139.

80. Moller JT, Cluitmans P, Rasmussen LS, et al. Long-term postoperative cognitive dysfunction in the elderly ISPOCD1 study. ISPOCD investigators. International Study of Post-Operative Cognitive Dysfunction. *Lancet.* 1998;351:857–861.

81. Ginsberg RJ, Rubinstein LV. Randomized trial of lobectomy versus limited resection for T1 N0 non-small cell lung cancer: Lung Cancer Study Group. *Ann Thorac Surg.* 1995;60:615–622.

82. Landreneau RJ, Sugarbaker DJ, Mack MJ, et al. Wedge resection versus lobectomy for stage I (T1 N0 M0) non-small cell lung cancer. *J Thorac Cardiovasc Surg.* 1997;113:691–698.

83. Smythe WR. Treatment of stage I non-small cell lung carcinoma. *Chest.* 2003;123(suppl):181–187.

84. Morandi U, Stefani A, Golinelli M, et al. Results of surgical resection in patients over the age of 70 years with non small-cell lung cancer. *Eur J Cardiothorac Surg.* 1997;11:432–439.

85. Weinmann M, Jeremic B, Toomes H, et al. Treatment of lung cancer in the elderly: Part I.

Non-small cell lung cancer. *Lung Cancer.* 2003;39:233–253.

86. Jaklitsch MT, Bueno R, Swanson SJ, et al. New surgical options for elderly lung cancer patients. *Chest.* 1999;116(suppl):480–485.

87. Sioris T, Salo J, Perhoniemi V, et al. Surgery for lung cancer in the elderly. *Scand Cardiovasc J.* 1999;33:222–227.

88. Bernardi D, Barzan L, Franchin G, et al. Treatment of head and neck cancer in elderly patients: state of the art and guidelines. *Crit Rev Oncol Hematol.* 2005;53(1):71–80.

89. Muir CS, Fraumeni Jr JF, Doll R. The interpretation of time trends. *Cancer Surv.* 1994;19–20:5–21.

90. Bliss R, Patel N, Guinea A, et al. Age is no contraindication to thyroid surgery. *Age Aging.* 1999;28:363–366.

91. Magnano M, De Stefani A, Usai A. Carcinoma of the larynx in the elderly: analysis of potentially significant prognostic variables. *Aging.* 1999;11(5):316–322.

92. Boruk M, Chernobilsky B, Rosenfeld RM, et al. Age as a prognostic factor for complications of major head and neck surgery. *Arch Otolaryngol Head Neck Surg.* 2005;131(7):605–609.

93. Kowalski LP, Alcantara PS, Magrin J, et al. A case-control study on complications and survival in elderly patients undergoing major head and neck surgery. *Am J Surg.* 1994;168:485–490.

94. Morgan RF, Hirata RM, Jaques DA, et al. Head and neck surgery in the aged. *Am J Surg.* 1982;144(4):449–451.

95. Sanabria A, Carvalho AL, Vartanian JG, et al. Comorbidity is a prognostic factor in elderly patients with head and neck cancer. *Ann Surg Oncol.* 2007;14(4):1449–1457.

96. Piccirillo JF. Importance of comorbidity in head and neck cancer. *Laryngoscope.* 2000;110(4):593–602.

97. Piccirillo JF, Tierney RM, Costas I, et al. Prognostic importance of comorbidity in a hospital-based cancer registry. *J Am Med Assoc.* 2004;291(20):2441–2447.

98. Dhiwakar M, Khan NA, McClymont LG. Surgery for head and neck skin tumors in the elderly. *Head Neck.* 2007;29(9):851–856.

99. Hamel MB, Henderson WG, Khuri SF, et al. Surgical outcomes for patients aged 80 and older: morbidity and mortality from major noncardiac surgery. *J Am Geriatr Soc.* 2005;53(3):424–429.

100. Tan E, Tilney H, Thompson M, et al. The United Kingdom National Bowel Cancer Project – epidemiology and surgical risk in the elderly. Association of Coloproctology of Great Britain and Ireland. *Eur J Cancer.* 2007;43(15):2285–2294.

101. Audisio RA, Pope D, Ramesh HS. Shall we operate? Preoperative assessment in elderly cancer patients (PACE) can help – a SIOG surgical task force prospective study PACE participants. *Crit Rev Oncol Hematol.* 2008;65(2):156–163.

102. Audisio RA, Ramesh H, Longo WE, et al. Evaluating elderly patients before cancer surgery: lessons from PACE. *Oncologist.* 2005;10(4):262–268.

103. Kristjansson SR, Nesbakken A, Jordhøy MS, et al. Comprehensive geriatric assessment can predict complications in elderly patients after elective surgery for colorectal cancer: a prospective observational cohort study.

6

Principles of radiation oncology in older adults

Benjamin D. Smith and Thomas A. Buchholz

A. Introduction

Radiation therapy (RT) plays a central role in the definitive treatment and palliation of many different cancers. RT is recommended for patients across the entire spectrum of ages, from neuroblastoma diagnosed in an infant to glioblastoma diagnosed in an octogenarian. Generally speaking, the fundamental principles of radiation therapy, such as dose, fractionation, tumor targeting, and integration with systemic therapy, are similar for both young and old. In addition, the primary goal of radiation therapy – obtaining local-regional control with acceptable morbidity – is the same for all age groups. Given these similarities, there is not a coherent set of radiation therapy principles solely applicable to older adults.

Nevertheless, a nuanced understanding of the importance of age as a factor associated with tumor behavior, response to treatment, and treatment tolerance is critically important to ensure that older adults receive optimal treatment that achieves the appropriate balance of local-regional control with morbidity. For example, older age is associated with a decreased risk of local-regional recurrence in breast cancer[1,2] but an increased risk of local-regional recurrence in endometrial cancer.[3] Age-specific differences such as these may influence clinical decision making for older adults. In addition, older adults may have a decreased functional reserve that can modulate the risk of normal tissue toxicity incurred by radiotherapy. For example, the risk of clinically significant lung damage may be much greater for an older adult with abnormal pulmonary function as compared to a younger adult with normal pulmonary reserve, and such considerations may therefore influence selection of radiotherapy dose and volume in older adults. Finally, because of limited social support or impaired mobility, older adults may experience greater logistical difficulty traveling daily to a radiotherapy clinic for a protracted course of fractionated treatment. Therefore efforts to minimize overall treatment time have special appeal to this population.

To address principles of radiotherapy in older adults, this chapter will review the clinical literature pertinent to the three most common malignancies in older adults: breast cancer, prostate cancer, and lung cancer. In addition, principles of radiotherapy in the treatment of glioblastoma multiforme and non-Hodgkin's lymphoma will also be discussed as there are high-quality data regarding the role of radiotherapy for these two malignancies. Although clinical trials focusing on radiotherapy for older patients are limited,[4] such data will be reviewed when available (Table 6.1) and will also be supplemented with results from population-based and retrospective studies.

B. General considerations

When evaluating the benefits of radiation therapy in older adults, it is helpful to understand the estimated benefit of radiation therapy and place this benefit within the context of other interventions generally accepted for older adults. One particularly helpful concept is the number needed to treat (NNT), which refers to the number of patients who require an intervention to prevent one event. For example, in the treatment of hypertension, 11 men and 21 women require optimal pharmacotherapy for 10 years to prevent one cardiac event.[5] Similarly, in the treatment of osteoporosis, 39 women require treatment with a bisphosphonate to prevent one clinically relevant fracture through 3 years of follow-up.[6] When possible, this chapter will present the NNTs associated with radiation therapy for older adults, thereby helping to contextualize the discussion of treatment.

A second important consideration for older adults is the balance between the benefit of radiation therapy and the competing risk of noncancer death. Many older cancer patients have a relatively high burden of comorbidity that predisposes them to noncancer death. For such patients, radiation therapy delivered in the adjuvant setting to prevent future recurrence may not be helpful given a high risk of death prior to recurrence. Quantitative approaches to integrate this issue into

Table 6.1 Key radiotherapy randomized clinical trials for older adults.

Site	Trial name	Patient population	Clinical question	Key results
Breast				
	Cancer and Leukemia Group B 9343[20]	Women aged ≥70 with small (≤2 cm), clinically node-negative, estrogen receptor–positive breast cancer treated with margin-negative lumpectomy	Does radiation therapy to the breast improve outcomes?	At 5 years, radiation therapy lowered the risk of local-regional recurrence from 4% to 1% but did not improve overall survival or prevent subsequent mastectomy
	Danish Breast Cancer Group 82c[27]	Postmenopausal women aged <70 with breast cancer that was node-positive, large (>5 cm), or invading the skin or chest wall; all patients were treated with mastectomy and tamoxifen	Does postmastectomy radiation improve overall survival?	At 10 years, survival was 45% in the radiation group and 36% in the no-radiation group
	Canadian Hypofractionation Trial[30,31]	Women of any age (48% were aged ≥60 years) with pT1–2 N0 breast cancer treated with conservative surgery	Are the fractionation schemes of 42.5 Gy in 16 fractions and 50 Gy in 25 fractions equivalent with respect to in-breast tumor control and cosmesis?	No difference in in-breast tumor control or cosmesis with 11 years' follow-up
Prostate				
	Scandinavian Prostate Cancer Group Study no. 4[39]	Men aged <75 years with cT1–2, PSA <50 ng/mL, Gleason score 2–7 prostate cancer	Does radical prostatectomy lower the risk of prostate cancer death?	The risk of prostate cancer death at 10 years was 10% in the prostatectomy group and 15% in the watchful waiting group; however, prostatectomy did not lower risk of prostate cancer death for men aged 65 and older
	European Organization for the Research and Treatment of Cancer 22863[46,47]	Men aged <80 years (median age 70 years) with cT3–4 prostate cancer of any Gleason score or cT1–2 with Gleason score 8–10	Does the addition of goserelin acetate for 3 years beginning at the time of radiation improve overall survival?	The addition of goserelin markedly improved survival, with 10-year overall survival of 58% in the goserelin arm compared to 40% in the control arm

Lung

Trial	Patients	Question	Results
Radiation Therapy and Oncology Group 93–11[55]	Patients of any age (87% were 60 or older) with medically inoperable stage I–III non-small-cell lung cancer	What is the maximal tolerated dose using three-dimensional conformal planning?	For patients with a total lung V_{20} <25%, the maximal tolerated dose was 83.8 Gy in 39 fractions; for total lung V_{20} between 25% and 36%, the maximal tolerated dose was 77.4 Gy in 36 fractions
Radiation Therapy and Oncology Group 88–08[65]	Patients of any age with stage II or III non-small-cell lung cancer	Does the addition of two cycles of cisplatin/etoposide chemotherapy prior to radiation improve survival?	Median survival was 13 months for the chemotherapy arm compared to 11 months for the standard radiation arm; however, for patients aged 70 and older, standard radiation was the best arm owing to chemotherapy-induced toxicity and death
European Organization for the Research and Treatment of Cancer 08941[71]	Patients of any age (median age 61) with unresectable stage IIIA-N2 non-small-cell carcinoma who responded to three cycles of platinum-based chemotherapy	Does surgical excision or radiotherapy confer a better outcome?	There was no difference in survival between the two arms, with 5-year overall survival of 16% in the surgical group versus 14% in the radiotherapy group
Intergroup 0096[80]	Patients of any age (median age 62) with limited-stage small-cell lung carcinoma treated with four cycles of cisplatin/etoposide chemotherapy and prophylactic cranial radiotherapy	Does thoracic radiotherapy to a dose of 45 Gy in 30 fractions over 3 weeks improve outcomes compared to 45 Gy in 25 fractions over 5 weeks?	Survival was improved in the 45 Gy in 3-week arm, with 5-year overall survival 26% for 45 Gy in 3 weeks compared to 16% for 45 Gy in 5 weeks; although patients aged 70 and older appeared to benefit from 45 Gy in 3 weeks, the risk of fatal lung toxicity was 10% for older patients compared to 1% for younger patients

Table 6.1 (cont.)

Site	Trial name	Patient population	Clinical question	Key results
Glioblastoma multiforme				
	Association of French-Speaking Neuro-Oncologists Radiotherapy for Glioblastoma in the Elderly Study[92]	Patients aged 70 and older with newly diagnosed glioblastoma and a Karnofsky Performance Status ≥70	Does radiotherapy (50.4 Gy in 28 fractions) improve survival compared to best supportive care?	Radiotherapy improved overall survival, with a median survival of 29 weeks in the radiotherapy arm compared to 17 weeks in the best supportive care arm; there were no significant measurable differences in quality of life between the two arms
	Canadian Hypofractionation Trial[93]	Patients aged 60 and older with newly diagnosed GBM and Karnofsky Performance Status ≥50	Is there a difference in overall survival between 60 Gy in 30 fractions over 6 weeks compared to 40 Gy in 15 fractions over 3 weeks?	Median survival was 6 months in each arm, and patients who received 40 Gy in 3 weeks experienced a lower corticosteroid requirement
Non-Hodgkin's lymphoma				
	Groupe d'Etude des Lymphomes de l'Adulte Elderly Radiotherapy Trial[98]	Patients aged 61 and older with stage I or II histologically aggressive lymphoma and no adverse factors on the age-adjusted International Prognostic Index; all patients received four cycles of CHOP chemotherapy	Does involved field radiotherapy to 39.6 Gy in 22 fractions improve outcomes?	Radiotherapy did not improve event-free or overall survival

Note. CHOP = cyclophosphamide, doxorubicin, vincristine, and prednisone.

clinical decision making will be presented in the section on breast cancer.

C. Breast cancer

Approximately 50 percent of breast cancers are diagnosed in women aged 65 and older. Of importance, the risk of local-regional recurrence of breast cancer is higher for younger women and lower for older women.[1,7,8] As discussed later, this observation has important implications for the management of breast cancer in older women.

C.1. Ductal carcinoma in situ

Ductal carcinoma in situ (DCIS) is a premalignant condition of the breast characterized by cytologically malignant cells that have not yet invaded through the ductal basement membrane. If untreated, approximately 25 to 50 percent of DCIS lesions will progress to invasive breast cancer over a woman's lifetime.[9] The primary goal in the treatment of DCIS is therefore to prevent progression to invasive breast cancer; secondary goals include prevention of recurrence of DCIS and preservation of the breast, when possible.

Mastectomy is an effective local-regional treatment option for DCIS, conferring a long-term risk of invasive or in situ recurrence of approximately 1 percent.[10] Randomized trials have not compared mastectomy to other local treatment options for DCIS; rather, four randomized trials that included younger and older women have compared conservative surgery alone to conservative surgery followed by whole-breast radiation therapy in the treatment of DCIS.[11-14] Collectively, these trials have consistently demonstrated that the addition of radiation therapy lowered the relative risk for both invasive and in situ ipsilateral breast tumor recurrence (IBTR) by approximately 60 percent but did not appear to impact overall survival.[15] Furthermore, these trials suggested that age at diagnosis did not modify the relative risk reduction conferred by RT. However, because older women experienced an absolute risk of recurrence that was lower than their younger counterparts,[7] the absolute risk reduction conferred by RT was smaller for older women than younger women.

To quantitate the absolute risk reduction conferred by radiation, specifically in older women, Smith and colleagues used the observational Surveillance, Epidemiology, and End Results (SEER)-Medicare database to estimate the risk of recurrence for women treated with and without radiation therapy following conservative surgery.[16] The cohort was prospectively stratified into women with and without risk factors for local recurrence, which were defined as age 66–69 years, comedo histology, high grade, and/or tumor size over 2.5 cm. Among women without any risk factors, the 5-year estimated IBTR risk (including invasive and in situ recurrence) was 8 percent for those treated with conservative surgery alone compared to 1 percent among those treated with conservative surgery and RT. Among patients considered high risk because of the presence of at least one risk factor, the 5-year estimated IBTR risk was 14 percent for those treated with conservative surgery alone compared to 4 percent for those treated with conservative surgery and RT. Furthermore, this study estimated the NNT with radiation therapy to prevent one IBTR, adjusting for the competing risk of death from noncancer causes as estimated using the Charlson Comorbidity Index.[17] As shown in Table 6.2, the adjusted NNT increased with age at diagnosis and comorbidity. For a healthy woman in her late sixties (high risk because of an age of 66–69 years), the adjusted NNT was 11. For a healthy woman in her seventies without any risk factors for recurrence, the adjusted NNT was 15. In contrast, for a woman in her late eighties with low-risk DCIS and significant comorbidities, the NNT was 29. These results therefore suggest that the benefit of RT for healthy older women with both low- and high-risk DCIS compares favorably to other generally accepted medical interventions.

C.2. Early invasive breast cancer

In general, women with early invasive breast cancer defined as pathologic stage T1–2 N0–1 may be treated with either conservative surgery followed by radiation or mastectomy without radiation, approaches that are supported by large randomized trials with extensive follow-up.[18,19] However, only one trial has specifically examined the role of breast radiotherapy following conservative surgery exclusively in older women with early invasive breast cancer. This trial, the Cancer and Leukemia Group B (CALGB) 9343, included women aged 70 years and older with clinically node-negative, small (≤ 2 cm), estrogen receptor (ER)-positive invasive breast cancer.[20] All patients were treated with margin-negative lumpectomy

Table 6.2 Adjusted number needed to treat for older women undergoing conservative surgery for ductal carcinoma in situ.

Age (years)	Charlson Comorbidity Index	5-year overall survival (%, 95% CI)	Adjusted number needed to treat events per 100 persons (95% CI)	
			Low risk	High risk
66–69	0	96[(94–97)]	.	11[(8–16)]
	1	93[(88–97)]	.	11[(8–17)]
	2–9	77[(66–89)]	.	13[(10–20)]
70–74	0	95[(93–96)]	15[(10–29)]	11[(8–16)]
	1	88[(84–93)]	16[(10–32)]	11[(9–17)]
	2–9	69[(58–79)]	20[(13–41)]	15[(11–22)]
75–79	0	89[(86–92)]	15[(10–31)]	11[(9–17)]
	1	90[(86–95)]	15[(10–31)]	11[(8–17)]
	2–9	68[(57–78)]	20[(14–41)]	15[(11–23)]
80–84	0	81[(77–86)]	17[(11–34)]	13[(9–19)]
	1	68[(60–77)]	20[(13–41)]	15[(11–22)]
	2–9	58[(45–72)]	24[(16–48)]	17[(13–26)]
85 and older	0	65[(56–74)]	21[(14–43)]	16[(12–24)]
	1	66[(52–80)]	21[(14–42)]	15[(11–23)]
	2–9	47[(26–69)]	29[(19–59)]	22[(16–32)]

Note. Low-risk group includes patients aged ≥70 years with tumor size ≤2.5 cm, noncomedo histology, and non–high grade. High-risk group includes any of the following: aged 66–69 years, size >2.5 cm, comedo histology, and/or high grade. A Charlson comorbidity score of 0 indicates no significant comorbidity, 1 indicates mild comorbidity, and 2–9 indicates moderate to severe comorbidity. CI = (confidence interval). The adjusted number needed to treat refers to the number of women who would require whole-breast irradiation to prevent one ipsilateral in situ or invasive breast recurrence. Adapted from Smith et al.[16]

and 5 years adjuvant tamoxifen and were randomized to receive whole-breast RT or no RT. With 5 years' follow-up, the risk of local-regional recurrence was 4 percent in the no-RT group compared to 1 percent in the RT group ($p < .001$) for a NNT of 33. With 8 years' follow-up, the risk of local-regional recurrence increased modestly to 7 percent in the no-RT group versus 1 percent in the RT group.[21] RT failed to improve either mastectomy-free survival or overall survival. A similar Canadian trial also found that the benefit of radiation was quite small for women aged 60 years and older with invasive breast cancer less than 1 cm.[22] Given the small absolute local control benefit, the National Comprehensive Cancer Network (NCCN) concluded that RT may be omitted for women who meet the strict inclusion criteria of the CALGB 9343 trial.[23]

In an attempt to validate the CALGB 9343 results, Smith and colleagues used the SEER-Medicare data to conduct a retrospective cohort study that included only older women who would have been eligible for the CALGB 9343 trial.[24] The estimated 5-year risk of local-regional recurrence was 5 percent for women who did not receive RT compared to 1 percent for women who did receive RT. These results were therefore nearly identical to the CALGB 9343 trial. The NNTs, adjusted for the competing risk of noncancer death, are reported in Table 6.3. For a healthy woman in her seventies, the adjusted NNT was 21–22. In contrast, for a woman in her late eighties with significant comorbidity, the adjusted NNT exceeded 100. Finally, Smith and colleagues examined older women who would not have been eligible for the CALGB 9343 trial because of an age 66–69 years, tumor size 2.1–5.0 cm, and/or ER negativity. Older women meeting any of these criteria experienced a higher risk of local-regional recurrence and a greater benefit from radiation. Collectively, therefore, the results from both randomized trials and population-based studies suggest that older women with early invasive breast cancer who satisfy the CALGB criteria and are treated with conservative surgery and adjuvant endocrine therapy derive only a modest benefit from RT and should only be considered for RT if under the age of 80 years and generally healthy. However, for older women with invasive breast cancer who do not meet the CALGB criteria, RT confers a greater benefit and, in the authors' opinion, should remain a standard of care.

Table 6.3 Adjusted number needed to treat for older women with estrogen receptor-positive stage I invasive breast cancer.

Age	Charlson Comorbidity Index	Eight-year survival (95% CI)	Adjusted number needed to treat (95% CI)
70–74	0	84[(83–86)]	21[(16–31)]
	1	72[(68–76)]	24[(18–36)]
	2–9	47[(40–55)]	37[(28–55)]
75–79	0	79[(76–81)]	22[(17–33)]
	1	62[(58–67)]	28[(21–42)]
	2–9	43[(36–51)]	41[(31–60)]
80–84	0	61[(57–64)]	29[(22–43)]
	1	47[(40–53)]	38[(28–56)]
	2–9	29[(21–36)]	61[(46–90)]
85 and older	0	33[(29–38)]	53[(40–78)]
	1	18[(13–24)]	97[(73–143)]
	2–9	147[(2–21)]	125[(94–185)]

Note. A Charlson comorbidity score of 0 indicates no significant comorbidity, 1 indicates mild comorbidity, and 2–9 indicates moderate to severe comorbidity. CI = (confidence interval). The adjusted number needed to treat refers to the number of women who would require whole-breast irradiation to prevent one invasive breast recurrence. Adapted from Smith et al.[24]

C.3. Locally advanced breast cancer

For women with advanced breast cancer, which is generally defined as stage T3/4 and/or N2/3 disease, treatment with modified radical mastectomy followed by postmastectomy radiation therapy (PMRT) is generally considered to be a reasonable standard of care. Two randomized trials conducted in premenopausal patients[25,26] and one trial conducted in postmenopausal patients aged 70 years and under[27] have demonstrated that the addition of PMRT lowered the relative risk of local-regional recurrence from approximately 30 percent without RT to 10 percent with RT and that this local-regional control benefit translated into an absolute improvement in overall survival of approximately 9–10 percent at 10 years. However, there are no randomized data to demonstrate a benefit from PMRT for women aged 70 years and older. In lieu of randomized data, Truong and colleagues reported patterns of failure in a retrospective cohort of 939 women aged 70 years and older treated with mastectomy without PMRT.[28] With 8 years' median follow-up, the risk of local-regional recurrence for women with either T3/4 or N2/3 tumors was approximately 30 percent, a risk consistent with that reported in the control arms of the PMRT randomized trials. In addition, a population-based cohort study of 2,053 women with T3/4 or N2/3 breast cancer undergoing mastectomy reported that receipt of PMRT was associated with a 15 percent relative reduction in mortality and a 6 percent absolute improvement in 5-year overall survival,[29] although this study was limited in that cause-specific survival was not reported. Thus there are some data to support use of PMRT for older women with advanced breast cancer, although randomized trials are needed to confirm the benefit of PMRT in this setting.

C.4. Radiation dose

The most common dose-fractionation scheme used in radiation therapy clinical trials has been 50 Gy in 25 fractions delivered to the whole breast or chest wall, followed by a boost of 10–16 Gy in five to eight fractions to the lumpectomy cavity or mastectomy scar.[1] Hence a conventional course of radiotherapy may require up to 6.5 weeks of daily treatment, which may be prohibitively difficult for certain older women who may experience logistical hurdles to such protracted treatment. To address this issue, three large, multicenter trials have compared a short radiotherapy course to a protracted course following conservative surgery. The trial with the most mature results was conducted by 10 Canadian institutions and compared 50 Gy in 25 fractions to 42.5 Gy in 16 fractions in a cohort of patients with pT1–2 N0 breast cancer treated with conservative surgery with negative surgical margins. Although this trial did not specifically focus on older women, 48 percent of the study subjects were aged 60 years or older. With a median follow-up of 11 years, no significant differences with respect to IBTR or cosmesis have been noted in the two arms.[30,31] Similar results with 5 years' median follow-up have been reported by two trials conducted in the United

Kingdom.[32,33] Hence 42.5 Gy in 16 fractions is an acceptable alternative fractionation scheme that may be used to reduce overall treatment time for older women who require breast radiotherapy following conservative surgery. It is important to note that this approach has not been validated in women who require nodal radiation or radiation to the chest wall.

Recently, interest has also grown in delivery of accelerated partial-breast irradiation (APBI) for older women with small invasive or in situ breast cancers treated with conservative surgery.[34] APBI may be delivered with external-beam radiotherapy or with brachytherapy using a balloon catheter such as the MammoSite device or multiple interstitial catheters. Theoretical advantages of APBI include a shorter overall treatment time (typically 3.85 Gy twice daily for 10 treatments with external beam or 3.4 Gy twice daily for 10 treatments with brachytherapy) and decreased radiation dose to uninvolved portions of the breast. Theoretical disadvantages include possible undertreatment of clinically occult disease remote from the lumpectomy cavity and the potential for increased normal tissue toxicity. At the current time, outcome data with APBI remain preliminary, although this treatment approach is growing in popularity. In the United States, a large multicenter randomized clinical trial (Radiation Therapy Oncology Group [RTOG] 0413/National Surgical Adjuvant Breast and Bowel Project [NSABP] B-39) is comparing whole-breast irradiation with APBI, though results of this trial will likely not be available until approximately 2015.[35]

C.5. Treatment toxicity

To the authors' knowledge, there are no compelling data to demonstrate an increase in radiation toxicity for older women as compared to younger women. However, data regarding toxicity of radiation specifically in older women were documented by the CALGB 9343 trial using both physician and patient assessment.[20] As compared to older women treated with tamoxifen alone, older women treated with radiation plus tamoxifen consistently rated breast pain as worse through 4 years of follow-up. Older women treated with radiation also rated fibrosis or retraction as worse through 2 years' follow-up, but these differences resolved by 4 years' follow-up. Physicians rated overall cosmesis, breast edema, skin color changes, and fibrosis or retraction as worse in the radiation plus tamoxifen group through

2 years' follow-up, but these differences resolved at 4 years' follow-up. In general, other series that did not include prospective, patient-based assessment have concluded that radiotherapy for breast cancer is well tolerated by older women.[36,37]

D. Prostate cancer

Prostate cancer is the most common malignancy in men, with approximately 70 percent of cases diagnosed in patients aged 65 years and older. Patients with nonmetastatic disease are typically stratified into three clinical risk categories based on prostate-specific antigen (PSA), Gleason score (GS), and clinical stage. Low-risk includes patients with GS 6 or less, PSA 10 ng/mL or less, and clinical stage T1–T2a. Intermediate risk includes patients with either GS 7 or PSA more than 10 ng/mL and less than 20 ng/mL and/or clinical stage T2b. High risk includes patients with either GS 8 or more, PSA more than 20 ng/mL, and/or clinical stage T2c or higher.[38] This risk grouping strongly correlates with outcomes following definitive local therapy such as radical prostatectomy, external-beam radiation therapy, or interstitial brachytherapy.

D.1. Low and intermediate risk

Low- and intermediate-risk prostate cancer is typically a slowly progressive process, with disease-related deaths extremely unlikely within the first 5 years of diagnosis.[39] Accordingly, guidelines from the NCCN recommend consideration of definitive local therapy only for those patients with an anticipated life expectancy of at least 10 years.[40] However, although life expectancy can be accurately estimated for populations of older adults, it remains difficult to precisely estimate life expectancy for an individual older adult.[41]

There are surprisingly little randomized data to guide local treatment decisions for men of any age with low- to intermediate-risk prostate cancer. The only published, mature data derive from the Scandinavian Prostate Cancer Group Study no. 4, which enrolled 699 patients with primarily low- or intermediate-risk prostate cancer who were randomized to watchful waiting or radical prostatectomy.[39] At 10 years' follow-up, 15 percent of men in the watchful-waiting group had died from prostate cancer compared to 10 percent of men in the radical prostatectomy group. Radical prostatectomy also significantly improved overall survival and lowered the risk of local progression and distant metastasis. With respect to age, this trial only included men under the age of 75 years. In a pre-specified secondary analysis, the benefit of radical prostatectomy appeared limited to patients under the age of 65 years, thus suggesting that radical prostatectomy may not be beneficial for men aged 65–75 years.

Because the majority of patients on the Scandinavian Prostate Cancer Study had clinically detected prostate cancer, it is unclear whether the identified benefit of radical prostatectomy, or other local treatments such as radiotherapy, will extend to patients currently diagnosed with prostate cancer on the basis of a screening PSA assessment. Indeed, many physicians now advocate "active surveillance with selective delayed intervention" for the population of older men with screening-detected, low-risk prostate cancer.[42] Active surveillance with delayed intervention differs from watchful waiting in that patients undergoing a course of watchful waiting typically choose to forego any form of local therapy in favor of a palliative treatment approach, whereas patients undergoing active surveillance choose to delay local therapy until there is clinical evidence of tumor progression. Thus active surveillance typically entails quarterly PSA assessment and clinical exam, with prostate rebiopsy at 1–2 years postdiagnosis and again at 5 and 10 years postdiagnosis. Local treatment is indicated if the PSA doubling time drops below 3 years, Gleason score progresses, or there is clinical or pathologic evidence to suggest an increasing volume of disease. Using this approach in a prospective study of 299 patients, Klotz and colleagues reported that only 34 percent of patients ultimately received local therapy and less than 1 percent died from prostate cancer.[42] On the basis of these and other results, ongoing randomized trials in the United States and United Kingdom are comparing active surveillance to definitive local therapy. While these clinical trials are awaited, the authors feel that close active surveillance with selective delayed intervention is a reasonable strategy that should be strongly considered for many older men with low-risk prostate cancer.

As clinical trials to define the role of local therapy in older men with low- to intermediate-risk prostate cancer are ongoing, population-based data have also been used to explore potential benefits of local therapy in older men. For example, a population-based cohort study of nearly 45,000 men aged 65–80 years concluded that older men who received definitive local therapy experienced improved prostate cancer–specific sur-vival and overall survival after adjusting for relevant clinical-pathologic characteristics including age and comorbidity.[43] However, the difference in prostate cancer–specific survival was quite small, with 2.5 percent of men in the observation group experiencing death from prostate cancer compared to 1.9 percent of men in the treatment group, resulting in an NNT of 167, which suggests that the potential impact of local therapy for older men with low- to intermediate-risk prostate cancer is likely to be quite small.

D.2. High risk

Men with high-risk prostate cancer, even if clinically localized, experience a substantial risk of prostate cancer death if untreated. For example, a population-based study of 767 men with organ-confined prostate cancer who did not receive either surgery, radiation, or hormonal therapy at diagnosis found that prostate cancer–specific mortality for those with Gleason score 8–10 tumors was 40 percent at 5 years and 80 percent at 10 years.[44] As a result, prostate cancer therapy is typically recommended for all men with high-risk prostate cancer, regardless of age, with the exception of those with severe comorbidity resulting in a very high and immediate risk of noncancer death. Standard treatments for older men with high-risk prostate cancer typically include hormone therapy and/or radiation therapy (radical prostatectomy may also be considered in select men with clinically localized disease and minimal comorbidity). Other portions of this text will discuss hormone therapy in greater detail; this chapter will focus on the literature pertaining to radiotherapy.

Hormone therapy alone versus hormone therapy and radiation

The Scandinavian Prostate Cancer Group Study no. 7 randomized patients with locally advanced prostate cancer to indefinite antiandrogen therapy alone versus indefinite antiandrogen therapy concurrent with local radiotherapy (50 Gy to the seminal vesicles and 70 Gy to the prostate).[45] This landmark study found that radiation therapy conferred an absolute improvement in overall survival of 10 percent at 10 years, indicating an NNT of 10. The survival benefit of radiation was primarily realized between 5 and 10 years' follow-up, suggesting that antiandrogen therapy alone may be reasonable treatment for older patients with severe comorbidity resulting in a life expectancy of less than 5 years.

Radiation therapy alone versus radiation therapy plus hormone therapy

The European Organization for Research and Treatment of Cancer (EORTC) conducted a landmark randomized clinical trial (EORTC 22863) in 415 men with high-risk prostate cancer, defined as clinical stage T3–4 of any grade or clinical stage T1–2 with Gleason score 810.[46,47] Patients were randomized to either radiation alone (50 Gy to the pelvis and 70 Gy to the prostate) or radiation with androgen deprivation therapy (ADT). ADT consisted of a steroidal antiandrogen (cyproterone acetate) administered orally for 1 month beginning 1 week prior to initiation of radiation, in addition to subcutaneous injection of the gonadotropin releasing hormone agonist goserelin acetate beginning on day 1 of radiation and continued for a total of 3 years. Median follow-up for this trial is now over 9 years, and the results have remained remarkably consistent and strong, with the addition of ADT conferring a 67 percent relative improvement in 10-year overall survival from 40 percent in patients treated with radiation alone to 58 percent in patients receiving concurrent hormone therapy (NNT = 6). Notably, the median age of patients treated on this trial was 70 years, although patients over the age of 80 were excluded. Therefore this trial provides strong evidence to support a benefit from the addition of ADT to radiotherapy specifically in older adults aged 80 years and under. In a follow-up study, the EORTC sought to determine the appropriate duration of ADT for men with locally advanced prostate cancer (EORTC 22961). Although currently only available in abstract form, this study demonstrated that 6 months of total androgen blockade was inferior to 3 years of androgen deprivation, with 5-year overall survival of 80 percent for the 6-month arm compared to 85 percent for the 3-year arm.[48]

D.3. Dose escalation and age

Although the addition of ADT to radiation represents the most significant and meaningful recent advance in the treatment of prostate cancer, growing data also suggest that escalation of the radiation dose to approximately 75–80 Gy to the isocenter confers a modest improvement in biochemical disease-free survival and may also prevent development of distant metastasis.[49–51] Specifically, three trials have demonstrated a 10–19 percent absolute improvement in biochemical disease-free survival with dose escalation, but at the expense of a modest increase in rectal toxicity. With respect to older adults, the median age of patients enrolled in published randomized trials ranged from 67 to 69 years,[49–51] and the Dutch multicenter trial additionally chose to stratify by patient age.[50] Although these trials did not specifically report outcomes or toxicity by age, it is reasonable to assume that the benefit of dose escalation likely included older adults who were well represented on these studies. It is important to note that in contrast to the proven overall survival benefit of ADT when added to standard dose radiation, dose-escalation studies have not yet demonstrated a substantial improvement in overall survival. Furthermore, it is not known whether dose escalation is needed for older patients who receive concomitant ADT.

D.4. Radiation toxicity

Prostate radiotherapy is generally well tolerated, with a 5 percent risk of grade 2 or higher late gastrointestinal toxicity and a 12 percent risk of grade 2 or higher late genitourinary toxicity in patients treated with intensity-modulated radiotherapy to doses less than 80 Gy.[52] It is not known whether older adults experience a higher risk of toxicity than younger adults. Nevertheless, strategies to limit toxicity should be pursued for older patients. These include technical considerations such as daily target localization with fiducials implanted in the prostate or image guidance with daily kilovoltage cross-sectional imaging, intensity-modulated treatment to improve rectal and bladder dose volume parameters, and careful attention to adequate contouring of targets and normal tissue. In addition, because RTOG 94-13 did not demonstrate a clear survival benefit derived from whole pelvic radiotherapy,[53] the authors would recommend omission of pelvic radiotherapy in older patients, with the exception of those with known lymph node involvement, in an effort to minimize bowel and bladder toxicity from this unproven treatment approach.

E. Lung cancer

Approximately 70 percent of lung cancers are diagnosed in patients aged 65 years and older. Older lung cancer patients have a high prevalence of smoking-related comorbidities such as chronic obstructive pulmonary disease, coronary artery disease, and vascular disease. These comorbidities significantly impact decisions regarding optimal therapy. For example, although lobectomy is generally considered the standard of care for patients

Table 6.4 Late lung toxicity by radiation dose in radiation therapy and oncology group 93-11.

Dose	Fractions	Late lung toxicity				
		Grade 1	Grade 2	Grade 3	Grade 4	Grade 5
Patients with total lung $V_{20} < 25\%$						
70.9 Gy	33	30%	21%	11%	0%	0%
77.4 Gy	36	21%	21%	17%	0%	0%
83.8 Gy	39	29%	35%	0%	0%	0%
90.3 Gy	42	13%	29%	10%	3%	3%
Patients with total lung V_{20} between 25% and 36%						
70.9 Gy	33	15%	25%	15%	0%	0%
77.4 Gy	36	12%	44%	12%	4%	0%
Toxicity Definitions						
Grade 1	Asymptomatic or mild symptoms (dry cough); mild radiographic changes					
Grade 2	Moderate symptomatic fibrosis or pneumonitis (severe cough); low-grade fever; patchy radiographic appearance					
Grade 3	Severe symptomatic fibrosis or pneumonitis; dense radiographic changes					
Grade 4	Severe respiratory insufficiency; continuous oxygen or assisted ventilation required					
Grade 5	Death					

Note. Adapted from Bradley et al.[55]

with stage I or II non-small-cell lung cancer, only approximately 75 percent of older patients with early lung cancer are treated surgically because of multiple factors, including the presence of comorbid illness.[54]

E.1. Medically inoperable, stage I, non-small-cell lung cancer

For patients with medically inoperable, stage I, non-small-cell lung carcinoma, local radiotherapy represents a reasonable treatment option. Historically, such patients have received treatment with fractionated external beam techniques to doses of 66 Gy or higher, without techniques to account for respiratory motion.[55–57] A representative, retrospective study from the University of Texas M. D. Anderson Cancer Center reported treatment outcomes for 85 patients treated with three-dimensional conformal radiotherapy, of whom 85 percent were aged 65 years or older.[56] Local-regional control rates were 77 percent at 2 years and 70 percent at 5 years. It should be noted that patients in this study did not receive elective hilar or mediastinal nodal irradiation, and in a comparison to historical controls, receipt of elective nodal irradiation was associated with inferior outcomes. Omission of elective nodal irradiation markedly improves tolerance to treatment in the older adult because of the reduced dose to the uninvolved lung and esophagus and also enables safer escalation of the radiotherapy dose.

Dose

Regarding radiation dose, the RTOG conducted a prospective phase I–II dose-escalation study (RTOG 93-11) to determine the maximal tolerated dose for patients with medically inoperable stage I–III non-small-cell lung cancer.[55] Older adults aged 60 years and over comprised 87 percent of patients enrolled in this study. For those with less than 25 percent of the total volume of lung volume receiving a dose of 20 Gy (lung $V_{20} < 25\%$), the radiation dose was escalated from 70.9 Gy in 33 fractions to 77.4 Gy in 36 fractions to 83.8 Gy in 39 fractions to 90.3 Gy in 42 fractions. The 90.3-Gy dose level was considered too toxic, with two treatment-related deaths. However, toxicity in the first three dose levels was considered acceptable, with the risk of late grade 2 or higher lung toxicity (primarily pneumonitis) ranging from 31 to 39 percent (Table 6.4). Of note, although this trial included patients with very poor lung function (forced expiratory volume in 1 second [FEV1] as low as 0.42 L), no treatment-related deaths were noted in the first three dose levels. This trial was not powered to determine the optimal dose for patients with stage I, medically inoperable, non-small-cell lung cancer, although retrospective studies generally support a dose of at least 66 Gy in 33 fractions,[57] and based on the results of RTOG 93-11, a dose of 70.9 Gy in 33 fractions is not unreasonable. At present, there are few data to determine how chronologic age or physiologic aberrations in pulmonary function associated with the aging process should influence selection of radiotherapy dose because neither age nor impaired pulmonary function is closely linked to the risk of radiation-induced pulmonary toxicity.[58]

Stereotactic radiosurgery

Recent technological advances in the delivery of thoracic radiotherapy may further improve outcomes for older adults with early-stage lung cancer. For example, gating the delivery of radiation to the respiratory cycle allows for a modest reduction in the planning target volume and should therefore lower the probability of lung toxicity.[59] In addition, several centers have investigated stereotactic radiosurgery for early thoracic neoplasms, whereby very high doses are delivered over relatively few fractions. Typically, such patients are treated on linear accelerators with the capability to image the tumor prior to each fraction, thereby ensuring that setup errors are minimized. In addition, methods to account for tumor motion during the respiratory cycle – either tumor tracking, gated treatment, or inhibition with breath hold or abdominal compression – are mandatory to reduce the dose to uninvolved lung.[60] A representative clinical study of stereotactic radiosurgery was reported by Timmerman and colleagues, in whose study 70 patients with medically inoperable stage I lung cancer (median age 70 years) were enrolled in a prospective phase II study.[61] Patients were treated with 60–66 Gy in three fractions, resulting in an outstanding 2-year local control rate of 95 percent. However, this article provided a cautionary note regarding such large fraction sizes as radiotherapy was thought to contribute to six deaths (9%), and severe toxicity was noted in 46 percent of patients with central tumors and 17 percent of patients with peripheral tumors. On the basis of these results, stereotactic radiosurgery is generally contraindicated for tumors located within 2 cm of the carina but is gaining acceptance as an effective therapeutic modality for peripheral tumors,[62] and further research is ongoing to determine its role in the treatment of central tumors.[63]

E.2. Stage III (locally advanced) non-small-cell lung cancer

Sequential chemoradiotherapy

Patients of any age with stage III non-small-cell lung cancer experience a relatively poor prognosis, with only 10–20 percent experiencing long-term survival despite aggressive combined modality therapy. Historically, radiotherapy alone was used to treat stage III non-small-cell lung carcinoma, but 5-year survival was only 3–10 percent.[64,65] Over the past 25 years, a series of prospective randomized trials have demonstrated that the addition of platinum-based doublet chemotherapy substantially improves overall survival as compared to radiation alone and furthermore that concurrent chemoradiotherapy marginally improves outcomes as compared to sequential treatment. For example, the CALGB 8433 and RTOG 88-08 both demonstrated that sequential, platinum-based doublet chemotherapy followed by conventional radiotherapy improves outcomes compared to radiotherapy alone, with 5-year survival improved from 6 to 17 percent in CALGB 8433 and from 5 to 8 percent in RTOG 88-08.[64,65] Neither of these trials excluded patients solely on the basis of advanced age. However, the CALGB 8433 trial was relatively small, and age-specific outcomes were not reported.[64] In contrast, the RTOG 88-08 trial did report age-specific outcomes and noted that patients aged 70 years and older experienced the best median survival when treated with conventional radiotherapy alone (median survival of 13.1 months) compared to sequential chemoradiotherapy (median survival 10.9 months). This difference was at least partially attributable to excess chemotherapy-related toxicity and death in older patients.[65]

Concurrent chemoradiotherapy

Given the relatively small benefit of sequential chemoradiotherapy approaches, and perhaps complete lack of benefit for older adults, further clinical trials have sought to improve outcomes with the concurrent delivery of radiosensitizing chemotherapy and radiotherapy. To date, three published trials have demonstrated a 2- to 4-month improvement in median survival with the concurrent approach, but at the expense of an increased risk of esophageal toxicity and myelosuppression.[66–68] It should be noted that one of these trials excluded patients over the age of 70 years,[66] and the other two trials excluded patients over the age of 75 years.[67,68] Furthermore, none of these trials compared the benefit of concurrent therapy for older versus younger patients. Thus, at present, no evidence supports concurrent therapy for patients over the age of 75 years, and it is not known whether older adults between the ages of 65 and 75 derive a benefit from treatment that is comparable to younger patients.

Only one prospective clinical trial has rigorously evaluated the toxicity profile of concurrent therapy in older patients. This trial, the North Central Cancer Treatment Group 94-24-52, randomized patients of any age to either conventional daily radiotherapy to 60 Gy or to hyperfractionated radiotherapy (60 Gy in 40 fractions with a 2-week break after 30 Gy).[69] All patients received concurrent cisplatin and etoposide. This study did not demonstrate a benefit from hyperfractionated radiotherapy. In a post hoc analysis, outcomes for older patients aged 70 years and older were compared to younger patients under the age of 70 years. Thus this study provides the best data regarding tolerance of concurrent therapy in older patients. Older patients in this study experienced an excess risk of grade 4 plus pneumonitis (6% for older vs. 1% for younger patients) and grade 4 plus hematologic toxicity (78% vs. 56%), but no differences in overall survival were noted for older versus younger patients. It is important to note that this study was conducted prior to the era of routine three-dimensional treatment planning and that elective nodal irradiation was mandatory. It is not known whether use of three-dimensional treatment planning and omission of elective nodal irradiation might help minimize the age-specific differences noted in toxicity of concurrent chemoradiotherapy.

Trimodality therapy

The role of radiotherapy in conjunction with surgery remains controversial and unclear for older adults with stage III non-small-cell lung cancer. For patients who are medically fit and therefore candidates for concurrent chemoradiotherapy, clinical trials have sought to further improve outcomes with the addition of surgery. Specifically, the Southwest Oncology Group (SWOG) conducted an influential phase II trial (SWOG 88-05) in which patients up to the age of 75 years were treated with two cycles of cisplatin and etoposide concurrent with radiotherapy to 45 Gy followed by surgical resection.[70] Owing to a favorable 3-year survival of 26 percent noted in this phase II study, SWOG launched a phase III trial to compare definitive chemoradiotherapy (radiation dose 61 Gy) to induction chemoradiotherapy (radiation dose 45 Gy) followed by surgical resection. Although this trial has been presented in abstract form, final publication is yet awaited,

and age-specific outcomes have not been comprehensively reported. Therefore, at present, there is no conclusive phase III evidence to support trimodality therapy for older adults with stage III non-small-cell lung cancer.

For those older adults considered for sequential chemoradiotherapy, there is no clear role for surgical resection. Specifically, the EORTC conducted a prospective randomized trial of patients with stage IIIA (N2) non-small-cell lung cancer who received three cycles of platinum-based induction chemotherapy, with responders then randomized to local-regional radiotherapy or definitive surgery.[71] The median age of patients in this trial was 61 years, with a maximum age of 78, and patients were not excluded solely on the basis of chronologic age provided that they were considered physiologically fit for thoracotomy. With a median follow-up of nearly 6 years, there was no difference in survival between the two arms, with 5-year overall survival of 16 percent in the surgical group versus 14 percent in the radiotherapy group, and no subset analysis by age was reported. Thus surgery did not provide a benefit over radiotherapy for older adults who received induction chemotherapy for stage IIIA non-small-cell lung cancer.

Dose

For older adults treated with concurrent chemoradiotherapy, the optimal radiotherapy dose has yet to be established. Although most trials used relatively low doses on the order of 60–66 Gy with conventional fractionation, results of small dose-escalation trials suggested a possible benefit from higher doses,[72,73] and thus RTOG 06-17 is currently comparing 60 Gy to 74 Gy in patients treated with concurrent carboplatin and paclitaxel with or without cetuximab. For patients who will receive sequential chemoradiotherapy, the RTOG 93-11, as discussed earlier, identified 83.8 Gy in 39 fractions as the maximal tolerated dose for patients with a predicted total lung V_{20} less than 25 percent and 77.4 Gy in 36 fractions for patients with a predicted lung V_{20} ranging from 25 to 36 percent.[55] To help minimize pulmonary and esophageal toxicity, radiotherapy portals should be limited to include only sites of radiographic disease and should not include uninvolved nodal stations.[74] For older adults with a predicted total lung V_{20} over 36 percent or a predicted mean total lung dose of at least 20 Gy, high-dose radiation is thought to be prohibitively toxic, and generally a palliative approach is favored.[75]

Radioprotectors

Because radiation induces its biologic effects through the generation of highly reactive oxygen species, there has been significant interest in identification of pharmacologic agents that could selectively function as antioxidants in normal tissues, thereby protecting such tissues from radiation-induced damage. One such agent, amifostine, has been studied in the setting of concurrent chemoradiotherapy for non-small-cell lung cancer to determine whether it reduces the risk of radiation-induced esophagitis or pneumonitis. In RTOG 98-01, 243 patients with stage II–IIIA/B non-small-cell lung cancer receiving neoadjuvant chemotherapy followed by concurrent chemoradiotherapy with carboplatin and paclitaxel were randomized to amifostine 500 mg IV four times weekly or no amifostine.[76] Patient-assessed symptoms of esophagitis were reduced in the amifostine arm, but physician-reported esophagitis assessments were similar in both arms. Approximately 37 percent of patients in this study were aged 65 years and older, and age was used as a stratification variable in randomization. Interestingly, older patients appeared to garner a greater benefit from amifostine, as assessed from swallowing diaries. However, patients receiving amifostine also experienced a significantly higher risk of nausea, vomiting, cardiovascular toxicity, infection, and febrile neutropenia. Given the mixed results of this and other studies, the American Society of Clinical Oncology recently concluded that data are insufficient to recommend amifostine for the prevention of esophagitis in patients undergoing concurrent chemoradiotherapy for non-small-cell lung cancer.[77]

Staging

Owing to the potential toxicity and relatively poor outcomes of concurrent chemoradiotherapy with or without surgery, it is imperative that older adults undergo meticulous staging evaluation prior to treatment. For example, whole-body positron emission tomography has been shown to identify sites of otherwise occult distant metastasis[78] and should be routinely incorporated into the staging assessment. In addition, cross-sectional imaging of the brain is recommended to rule out occult central nervous system metastasis. It should also be noted that clinical factors, such as Karnofsky Performance less than 70, Eastern Cooperative Oncology Group (ECOG) performance status over 1, pretreatment weight loss of more than 5 percent, and the presence of pleural effusion, have been consistently associated with poor prognosis[79] and in many cases have served as exclusion criteria for randomized trials; thus older adults with these risk factors should likely be treated with palliative intent.

E.3. Small-cell lung carcinoma

The current standard of care in the treatment of limited-stage small-cell carcinoma of the lung was derived from the landmark Intergroup 0096 study that compared 45 Gy in 30 fractions over 3 weeks to 45 Gy in 25 fractions over 5 weeks. All patients received four cycles of cisplatin/etoposide starting with initiation of thoracic radiotherapy, and prophylactic cranial irradiation was recommended. Patients receiving 45 Gy in 3 weeks experienced improved overall survival, with a median survival of 23 months and a 5-year survival rate of 26 percent, compared to a median survival of 19 months and 5-year survival of 16 percent for the 45 Gy in 5 weeks arm (NNT = 10).[80] Notably, outcomes for older patients aged 70 years or older were directly compared to younger patients ages less than 70 years.[81] It appeared that both older and younger patients experienced a survival benefit from 45 Gy in 3 weeks. However, older patients treated on either study arm experienced greater toxicity, with severe hematologic toxicity of 84 percent for older patients compared to 61 percent for younger patients and fatal toxicity of 10 percent for older patients compared to 1 percent for younger patients. The principal cause of fatal toxicity in older patients was hematologic, suggesting that alternative chemotherapeutic strategies and/or growth factor support are particularly important in this older patient population. Overall survival at 5 years was 22 percent for younger patients compared to 16 percent for older patients ($p = .05$), with the difference primarily due to the increased risk of treatment-related mortality in older patients. Of note, older patients with an ECOG performance status of 2 faired quite poorly, with a median survival of only 7.6 months. Thus aggressive combined modality therapy for older small-cell lung cancer patients should be approached with caution and is unlikely to be beneficial in older adults with a poor baseline performance status.

For patients who respond to chemoradiation, prophylactic cranial irradiation (PCI) has been shown to confer an absolute overall survival benefit of 5 percent at 5 years, from 15.3 percent in untreated patients to 20.7 percent in treated patients (NNT = 19).[82] Although there is no clear consensus regarding the optimal dose of PCI, currently accepted fractionation schemes range from 24 Gy in 12 fractions to 25 Gy in 10 fractions up to 36 Gy in 18 fractions. Detailed neuropsychiatric testing has failed to identify major cognitive deficits attributable to PCI,[83,84] but relatively few older adults have been assessed, and at present it is not known how the low doses of radiotherapy used for PCI impact the aging brain.

E.4. Palliation of intrathoracic symptoms

For patients who are not candidates for potentially curative therapy, radiotherapy may provide meaningful palliation of intrathoracic symptoms such as hemoptysis, chest pain, cough, and dyspnea. However, it is important to note that palliative radiotherapy is generally not indicated in an otherwise asymptomatic patient.[85] The optimal radiotherapy dose and fractionation scheme for palliation is not clear. Several trials have compared hypofractionated regimens, such as 10 Gy in a single fraction or 16–17 Gy in 2 fractions, with a more protracted course, such as 30 Gy in 10 fractions, 42 Gy in 15 fractions, or 50 Gy in 25 fractions.[86–88] Although symptom control appears equivalent among the various fractionation schemes tested, at least some trials suggest a small but potentially meaningful improvement in duration of response and survival with a more protracted course.[86,87] Therefore the authors recommend that hypofractionation should be reserved for older adults with very limited life expectancy or who cannot travel for daily treatments.

F. Glioblastoma multiforme

Glioblastoma multiforme (GBM) is a relatively uncommon, high-grade malignancy of the central nervous system associated with a particularly poor prognosis in older adults. Current prognostic schemes for GBM from both the RTOG and the EORTC/National Cancer Institute of Canada (NCIC) include age as an important factor in risk stratification schemes.[89,90] For example, the EORTC/NCIC nomogram assigns age over 60 years as a marker of poor prognosis, with an effect size comparable to other adverse risk factors such as poor mini-mental status at diagnosis or treatment with partial resection only.[89] Similarly, the RTOG recursive partitioning analysis identified age over 50 years as the single most important prognostic factor for malignant glioma.[90]

Despite their rarity, there are surprisingly high-quality data from randomized clinical trials to define evidence-based treatment approaches in the older adult. For example, certain single-institution studies have questioned the benefit of radiation for older adults with GBM given their particularly poor prognosis.[91] However, in a recently published clinical trial, the Association of French-Speaking Neuro-Oncologists randomized 81 patients aged 70 years and older with newly diagnosed GBM and a Karnofsky Performance score of 70 or more to best supportive care or radiotherapy to 50.4 Gy in 28 fractions.[92] At a median follow-up of 21 weeks, radiotherapy was found to prolong overall survival, with a median survival of 29 weeks in the radiotherapy arm compared to 17 weeks in the supportive-care arm. Using patient-oriented health-related quality of life measures, the investigators found no significant differences between the two different treatment arms. Radiotherapy was generally well tolerated, although one patient in the radiotherapy group developed transient early delayed somnolence, and patients in both groups developed corticosteroid-induced diabetes mellitus and myopathy.

A complementary trial from four Canadian institutions attempted to define the optimal radiotherapy dose for patients with GBM.[93] Although 60 Gy in 30 fractions over 6 weeks has been commonly considered a standard treatment course for GBM,[94] the value of this prolonged treatment course has been questioned, particularly in light of the results of the French study that showed that radiotherapy only prolongs survival by approximately 12 weeks, indicating that up to half the life expectancy gained by radiotherapy can be consumed by treatment itself. As an alternative to conventional fractionation, this Canadian trial compared 60 Gy in 30 fractions over 6 weeks to 40 Gy in 15 fractions over 3 weeks in a cohort of 100 patients with newly diagnosed GBM and Karnofsky Performance score of 50 or higher.[93] With all patients followed until death, median survival was 6 months in each arm, and no differences were noted with respect to health-related quality of life or performance status. Of note, patients assigned to 40 Gy in 3 weeks required lower steroid doses than patients in the 60-Gy arm. Thus these two clinical trials provided high-quality evidence suggesting that radiotherapy prolongs survival for older adults with glioblastoma and that the best treatment approach is likely 40 Gy in 15 fractions.

One important, and to date unanswered, question regards the use of chemotherapy in older adults with glioblastoma. Although the joint EORTC/NCIC trial demonstrated that the addition of concurrent and adjuvant temozolomide to conventional radiotherapy (60 Gy in 30 fractions) substantially improved overall survival,[95] this trial excluded patients over the age of 70 years. Thus it is unknown whether temozolomide can be safely combined with radiotherapy in older adults and, furthermore, whether temozolomide may be safely combined with abbreviated, hypofractionated radiotherapy.

G. Non-Hodgkin's lymphoma

Non-Hodgkin's lymphoma (NHL) includes a diverse group of neoplasms, with approximately 58 percent diagnosed in patients aged 65 years and older. Older age has been recognized as an important adverse prognostic factor for various types of NHL. Specifically, both the International Prognostic Index (IPI) for histologically aggressive lymphoma[96] and the Follicular Lymphoma International Prognostic Index[97] identified age over 60 years as one of the five key prognostic factors associated with a poor prognosis for patients with either type of lymphoma. To date, only one published randomized trial has specifically attempted to define the role of radiotherapy in older patients with lymphoma. Specifically, the Groupe d'Etude des Lymphomes de l'Adulte conducted a randomized trial that enrolled individuals over the age of 60 with newly diagnosed stage I or II histologically aggressive lymphoma (diffuse large B-cell lymphoma, anaplastic lymphoma, nonanaplastic T/NK-cell lymphoma) with no adverse prognostic factors based on the IPI.[96,98] Patients were treated with four cycles of cyclophosphamide, doxorubicin, vincristine, and prednisone (CHOP) and were then randomized to involved field radiotherapy to 39.6 Gy in 22 fractions or observation. Fewer than 10 percent of the patients in this study had bulky disease. With a median follow-up of 7 years, no significant differences were noted with respect to event-free survival or overall survival, leading the authors to conclude that radiotherapy was not beneficial in this setting. Thus, although treatment guidelines from the NCCN continue to recommend abbreviated CHOP chemotherapy followed by involved field radiotherapy for patients with stage I or II aggressive lymphoma regardless of age,[99] the

best evidence for older patients now suggests that consolidative radiotherapy is not beneficial. In the future, additional trials are needed to confirm the lack of benefit derived from radiotherapy in older patients who receive CHOP combined with rituximab, which now represents the standard of care for systemic therapy of aggressive lymphoma. Randomized trials are also needed to define the role of radiotherapy for older patients with localized lymphoma in the presence of IPI risk factors or those with bulky disease. In addition, the role of radiotherapy for patients of any age with stage III or IV aggressive lymphoma is unclear, and randomized trials are needed in this area as well.

Older patients with advanced lymphoma frequently develop symptomatic lesions that may

A. Pretreatment

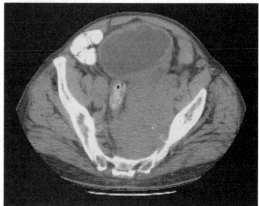

B. Posttreatment

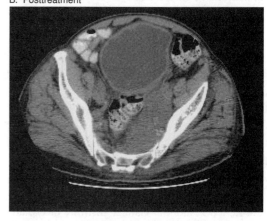

Figure 6.1 *A.* Pretreatment CAT scan showing a 14 × 8 cm biopsy-proven grade II follicular lymphoma in the pelvis of a man in his nineties. The mass produced severe bilateral lower-extremity and scrotal lymphedema and left hydronephrosis. Previous treatment with rituximab failed to induce a clinical or radiographic response. *B.* CAT scan 7 weeks after treatment with 4 Gy in two fractions. The mass decreased in size to 12 × 4 cm, and the patient's lymphedema completely resolved.

Table 6.5 Key unanswered questions regarding radiotherapy in the treatment of older adults with cancer.

	Ongoing trials
Breast	
Does postmastectomy radiation improve survival and/or quality of life for women aged 70 years and older with locally advanced breast cancer?	–
Can accelerated partial breast irradiation replace conventional whole-breast irradiation for select older women with early breast cancer?	NSABP B-39/RTOG 0413
Are there acceptable hypofractionation strategies for older women who require nodal or chest wall irradiation?	–
Prostate	
Can expected 10-year survival be accurately estimated for individual patients with newly diagnosed low- to intermediate-risk prostate cancer?	–
Does local therapy improve survival for older men with low- to intermediate-risk prostate cancer?	VA PIVOT study; U.K. Protect trial; SWOG PR11 START trial
Does active surveillance with delayed selective intervention compromise survival for older men with low- to intermediate-risk prostate cancer?	VA PIVOT study; U.K. Protect trial; SWOG PR11 START trial
Does escalation of the radiotherapy dose improve overall survival or quality of life for men with low- to intermediate-risk prostate cancer?	RTOG 0126
Is escalation of the radiotherapy dose needed for men receiving androgen deprivation therapy?	–
How does age at diagnosis impact the morbidity of prostate radiotherapy?	–
How do radical prostatectomy, external beam radiotherapy, and brachytherapy compare with respect to quality-of-life and cancer outcomes?	VA PIVOT study; U.K. Protect trial; SWOG PR11 START trial
Lung	
For stage I medically inoperable non-small-cell carcinoma, does stereotactic radiosurgery improve survival with acceptable morbidity as compared to fractionated three-dimensional conformal radiation?	–
For clinical stage I operable non-small-cell lung cancer, can stereotactic radiosurgery replace lobectomy?	RTOG 0618
For stage III non-small-cell carcinoma, are there subsets of older adults for whom concurrent chemoradiotherapy is well tolerated and beneficial?	–
What is the optimal dose of radiotherapy for older adults receiving concurrent chemoradiation?	RTOG 0617/CALGB 30609
Is prophylactic cranial irradiation in the treatment of small-cell carcinoma safe for older adults?	–
Glioblastoma multiforme	
Is temozolomide safe and effective for patients aged 70 years and older?	–
Can hypofractionated radiotherapy (such as 40 Gy in 15 fractions) be safely combined with concurrent temozolomide?	–
Non-Hodgkin's lymphoma	
Is there a role for radiotherapy in older adults with histologically aggressive stage I or II lymphoma with one or more International Prognostic Index risk factors or bulky disease?	–
What is the optimal palliative dose of radiotherapy for older adults with histologically aggressive lymphoma?	–

Note. CALGB = Cancer and Leukemia Group B; NSABP = National Surgical Adjuvant Breast and Bowel Project; RTOG = Radiation Therapy Oncology Group; SWOG = Southwest Oncology Group. A dash indicates that to the authors' knowledge, no clinical trials are currently investigating the given question. The list of clinical trials is meant to be representative rather than comprehensive.

require local therapy. For those with indolent lymphoma, there is growing evidence that low-dose, palliative radiotherapy confers a substantial benefit. For example, Haas and colleagues reported a series of 109 patients with 304 sites of symptomatic, recurrent indolent lymphoma who were treated with low-dose radiotherapy, either 4 Gy in one fraction or 4 Gy in two fractions.[100] The overall response rate was 92 percent, with 61 percent of patients achieving a complete response. Among responders, the median time to local progression was 2 years, suggesting that this low-dose, palliative approach provided durable local palliation with almost no significant toxicity. In this study, the median age was 62 years, and age was not correlated with response rates. Therefore this palliative, low-dose approach to the symptomatic management of relapsed, indolent lymphoma should be considered an important component in the armamentarium of treatment options for older adults. An example of a patient in his nineties who derived significant palliative benefit from this approach is presented in Figure 6.1. Further research is needed to define the optimal palliative dose for older patients with aggressive lymphomas.[101,102]

H. Summary

The use of radiotherapy in the treatment of older adults presents significant challenges because of the lack of studies focused on this patient population and the associated comorbidities and functional limitations that cosegregate with the aging process. Table 6.5 identifies important unanswered questions in geriatric radiation oncology. To date, patients over the age of 65 (or 70) have been underrepresented or excluded from many randomized clinical trials despite the fact that they represent a common subset of individuals who develop cancer.[4] Furthermore, as advances in medical sciences lead to gains in life expectancy, the importance of high-level evidence to guide treatment decisions in the elderly becomes even more urgent. Further randomized trials to define the risks and benefits of radiotherapy in older adults are thus urgently needed to improve care for this growing patient population.

References

1. Bartelink H, Horiot JC, Poortmans P, et al. Recurrence rates after treatment of breast cancer with standard radiotherapy with or without additional radiation. *N Engl J Med.* 2001;345(19):1378–1387.

2. Bartelink H, Horiot JC, Poortmans PM, et al. Impact of a higher radiation dose on local control and survival in breast-conserving therapy of early breast cancer: 10-year results of the randomized boost versus no boost EORTC 22881–10882 trial. *J Clin Oncol.* 2007; 25(22):3259–3265.

3. Creutzberg CL, van Putten WL, Koper PC, et al. Surgery and postoperative radiotherapy versus surgery alone for patients with stage-1 endometrial carcinoma: multicentre randomised trial. PORTEC Study Group. Post Operative Radiation Therapy in Endometrial Carcinoma. *Lancet.* 2000;355(9213):1404–1411.

4. Hutchins LF, Unger JM, Crowley JJ, et al. Underrepresentation of patients 65 years of age or older in cancer-treatment trials. *N Engl J Med.* 1999;341(27):2061–2067.

5. Wong ND, Thakral G, Franklin SS, et al. Preventing heart disease by controlling hypertension: impact of hypertensive subtype, stage, age, and sex. *Am Heart J.* 2003;145(5):888–895.

6. Black DM, Cummings SR, Karpf DB, et al. Randomised trial of effect of alendronate on risk of fracture in women with existing vertebral fractures. Fracture Intervention Trial Research Group. *Lancet.* 1996;348(9041):1535–1541.

7. Solin LJ, Fourquet A, Vicini FA, et al. Long-term outcome after breast-conservation treatment with radiation for mammographically detected ductal carcinoma in situ of the breast. *Cancer.* 2005;103(6):1137–1146.

8. Clarke M, Collins R, Darby S, et al. Effects of radiotherapy and of differences in the extent of surgery for early breast cancer on local recurrence and 15-year survival: an overview of the randomised trials. *Lancet.* 2005;366(9503):2087–2106.

9. Page DL, Dupont WD, Rogers LW, et al. Continued local recurrence of carcinoma 15–25 years after a diagnosis of low grade ductal carcinoma in situ of the breast treated only by biopsy. *Cancer.* 1995;76(7):1197–1200.

10. Fonseca R, Hartmann LC, Petersen IA, et al. Ductal carcinoma in situ of the breast. *Ann Intern Med.* 1997;127(11):1013–1022.

11. Fisher B, Land S, Mamounas E, et al. Prevention of invasive breast cancer in women with ductal carcinoma in situ: an update of the national surgical adjuvant breast and bowel project experience. *Semin Oncol.* 2001;28(4):400–418.

12. Bijker N, Meijnen P, Peterse JL, et al. Breast-conserving treatment with or without radiotherapy in ductal carcinoma-in-situ: ten-year results of European Organisation for Research and Treatment of Cancer randomized phase III trial 10853 – a study by the EORTC Breast Cancer Cooperative Group and EORTC Radiotherapy Group. *J Clin Oncol.* 2006;24(21):3381–3387.

13. Emdin SO, Granstrand B, Ringberg A, et al. SweDCIS: radiotherapy after sector resection for ductal carcinoma in situ of the breast: results of a randomised trial in a population offered mammography screening. *Acta Oncol.* 2006;45(5):536–543.

14. Houghton J, George WD, Cuzick J, et al. Radiotherapy and tamoxifen in women with completely excised ductal carcinoma in situ of the breast in the UK, Australia, and New Zealand: randomised controlled trial. *Lancet.* 2003;362(9378):95–102.

15. Viani GA, Stefano EJ, Afonso SL, et al. Breast-conserving surgery with or without radiotherapy in women with ductal carcinoma in situ: a meta-analysis of randomized trials. *Radiat Oncol.* 2007;2:28.

16. Smith BD, Haffty BG, Buchholz TA, et al. Effectiveness of radiation therapy in older women with ductal carcinoma in situ. *J Natl Cancer Inst.* 2006;98(18):1302–1310.

17. Charlson ME, Pompei P, Ales KL, et al. A new method of classifying prognostic comorbidity in longitudinal studies: development and validation. *J Chron Dis.* 1987;40(5):373–383.

18. Fisher B, Anderson S, Bryant J, et al. Twenty-year follow-up of a randomized trial comparing total mastectomy, lumpectomy, and lumpectomy plus irradiation for the treatment of invasive breast cancer. *N Engl J Med.* 2002;347(16):1233–1241.

19. Veronesi U, Cascinelli N, Mariani L, et al. Twenty-year follow-up of a randomized study comparing breast-conserving surgery with radical mastectomy for early breast cancer. *N Engl J Med.* 2002;347(16):1227–1232.

20. Hughes KS, Schnaper LA, Berry D, et al. Lumpectomy plus tamoxifen with or without irradiation in women 70 years of age or older with early breast cancer. *N Engl J Med.* 2004;351(10):971–977.

21. Hughes KS, Schnaper LA, Berry D, et al. Lumpectomy plus tamoxifen with or without irradiation in women 70 years of age or older with early breast cancer: a report of further follow-up [abstract]. *Proc San Antonio Breast Cancer Symp.* 2006;A11.

22. Fyles AW, McCready DR, Manchul LA, et al. Tamoxifen with or without breast irradiation in women 50 years of age or older with early breast cancer. *N Engl J Med.* 2004;351(10):963–970.

23. Carlson RW, Anderson BO, Burstein HJ, et al. Breast cancer. *J Natl Compr Canc Netw.* 2005;3(3):238–289.

24. Smith BD, Gross CP, Smith GL, et al. Effectiveness of radiation therapy for older women with early breast cancer. *J Natl Cancer Inst.* 2006;98(10):681–690.

25. Overgaard M, Hansen PS, Overgaard J, et al. Postoperative radiotherapy in high-risk premenopausal women with breast cancer who receive adjuvant chemotherapy. Danish Breast Cancer Cooperative Group 82b Trial. *N Engl J Med.* 1997;337(14):949–955.

26. Ragaz J, Olivotto IA, Spinelli JJ, et al. Locoregional radiation therapy in patients with high-risk breast cancer receiving adjuvant chemotherapy: 20-year results of the British Columbia randomized trial. *J Natl Cancer Inst.* 2005;97(2):116–126.

27. Overgaard M, Jensen MB, Overgaard J, et al. Postoperative radiotherapy in high-risk postmenopausal breast-cancer patients given adjuvant tamoxifen: Danish Breast Cancer Cooperative Group DBCG 82c randomised trial. *Lancet.* 1999;353(9165):1641–1648.

28. Truong PT, Lee J, Kader HA, et al. Locoregional recurrence risks in elderly breast cancer patients treated with mastectomy without adjuvant radiotherapy. *Eur J Cancer.* 2005;41(9):1267–1277.

29. Smith BD, Haffty BG, Hurria A, et al. Postmastectomy radiation and survival in older women with breast cancer. *J Clin Oncol.* 2006;24(30):4901–4907.

30. Whelan T, MacKenzie R, Julian J, et al. Randomized trial of breast irradiation schedules after lumpectomy for women with lymph node-negative breast cancer. *J Natl Cancer Inst.* 2002;94(15):1143–1150.

31. Whelan TJ, Pignol JP, Julian J, et al. Long-term results of a randomized trial of accelerated hypofractionated whole breast irradiation following breast conserving surgery in women with node-negative breast cancer. *Int J Radiat Oncol Biol Phys.* 2008;72(suppl 1): S28.

32. Bentzen SM, Agrawal RK, Aird EG, et al. The UK Standardisation of Breast Radiotherapy (START) Trial B of radiotherapy hypofractionation for treatment of early breast cancer: a randomised trial. *Lancet.* 2008;371(9618):1098–1107.

33. Bentzen SM, Agrawal RK, Aird EG, et al. The UK Standardisation of Breast Radiotherapy (START) Trial A of radiotherapy hypofractionation for treatment of early breast cancer: a randomised trial. *Lancet Oncol.* 2008;9(4):331–341.

34. Arthur DW, Vicini FA. Accelerated partial breast irradiation as a part of breast conservation therapy. *J Clin Oncol.* 2005;23(8):1726–1735.

35. NSABP Protocol B-39/RTOG Protocol 0413: a randomized phase III study of conventional whole breast irradiation (WBI) versus partial breast irradiation (PBI) for women with stage 0, I, or II breast cancer. Radiation Therapy Oncology Group Web site. Available at: http://www.rtog.org/members/protocols/0413/0413.pdf.

36. Vlastos G, Mirza NQ, Meric F, et al. Breast conservation therapy as a treatment option for the elderly. The M. D. Anderson experience. *Cancer.* 2001;92(5):1092–1100.

37. Deutsch M. Radiotherapy after lumpectomy for breast cancer in very old women. *Am J Clin Oncol.* 2002;25(1):48–49.

38. D'Amico AV, Whittington R, Malkowicz SB, et al. Predicting prostate specific antigen outcome preoperatively in the prostate specific antigen era. *J Urol.* 2001;166(6):2185–2188.

39. Bill-Axelson A, Holmberg L, Ruutu M, et al. Radical prostatectomy versus watchful waiting in early prostate cancer. *N Engl J Med.* 2005;352(19):1977–1984.

40. Mohler J, Babaian RJ, Bahnson RR, et al. Prostate cancer: clinical practice guidelines in oncology. *J Natl Compr Canc Netw.* 2007;5(7):650–683.

41. McCloskey SA, Kuettel MR. Counterpoint: prostate cancer life expectancy can not be accurately predicted from currently available tools. *J Natl Compr Canc Netw.* 2007;5(7):709–713.

42. Klotz L. Active surveillance for prostate cancer: for whom? *J Clin Oncol.* 2005;23(32):8165–8169.

43. Wong YN, Mitra N, Hudes G, et al. Survival associated with treatment vs observation of localized prostate cancer in elderly men. *J Am Med Assoc.* 2006;296(22):2683–2693.

44. Albertsen PC, Hanley JA, Fine J. 20-year outcomes following conservative management of clinically localized prostate cancer. *J Am Med Assoc.* 2005;293(17):2095–2101.

45. Widmark A, Klepp O, Solberg A, et al. Endocrine treatment, with or without radiotherapy, in locally advanced prostate cancer (SPCG-7/SFUO-3): an open randomised phase III trial. *Lancet.* 2009;373(9660):301–308.

46. Bolla M, Collette L, Van Tienhoven G, et al. Ten year results of long term adjuvant androgen deprivation with goserelin in patients with locally advanced prostate cancer treated with radiotherapy: a phase III EORTC study [abstract]. *Int J Radiat Oncol Biol Phys.* 2008;72(suppl 1):A65, S30.

47. Bolla M, Collette L, Blank L, et al. Long-term results with immediate androgen suppression and external irradiation in patients with locally advanced prostate cancer (an EORTC study): a phase III randomised trial. *Lancet.* 2002;360(9327):103–106.

48. Bolla M, van Tienhoven G, de Reijke TM, et al. Concomitant and adjuvant androgen deprivation (ADT) with external beam irradiation (RT) for locally advanced prostate cancer: 6 months versus 3 years ADT – results of the randomized EORTC phase III trial 22961 [abstract]. *J Clin Oncol.* 2007;25(suppl 18):5238s.

49. Kuban DA, Tucker SL, Dong L, et al. Long-term results of the M. D. Anderson randomized dose-escalation trial for prostate cancer. *Int J Radiat Oncol Biol Phys.* 2008;70(1):67–74.

50. Peeters ST, Heemsbergen WD, Koper PC, et al. Dose-response in radiotherapy for localized prostate cancer: results of the Dutch multicenter randomized phase III trial comparing 68 Gy of radiotherapy with 78 Gy. *J Clin Oncol.* 2006;24(13):1990–1996.

51. Zietman AL, DeSilvio ML, Slater JD, et al. Comparison of conventional-dose vs high-dose conformal radiation therapy in clinically localized adenocarcinoma of the prostate: a randomized controlled trial. *J Am Med Assoc.* 2005;294(10):1233–1239.

52. Zelefsky MJ, Levin EJ, Hunt M, et al. Incidence of late rectal and urinary toxicities after three-dimensional conformal radiotherapy and intensity-modulated radiotherapy for localized prostate cancer. *Int J Radiat Oncol Biol Phys.* 2008;70(4):1124–1129.

53. Lawton CA, DeSilvio M, Roach M III, et al. An update of the phase III trial comparing whole pelvic to prostate only radiotherapy and neoadjuvant to adjuvant total androgen suppression: updated analysis of RTOG 94-13, with emphasis on unexpected hormone/radiation interactions. *Int J Radiat Oncol Biol Phys.* 2007;69(3):646–655.

54. Bach PB, Cramer LD, Warren JL, et al. Racial differences in the treatment of early-stage lung cancer. *N Engl J Med.* 1999;341(16):1198–1205.

55. Bradley J, Graham MV, Winter K, et al. Toxicity and outcome results of RTOG 9311: a phase I–II dose-escalation study using three-dimensional conformal radiotherapy in patients with inoperable non-small-cell lung carcinoma. *Int J Radiat Oncol Biol Phys.* 2005;61(2):318–328.

56. Fang LC, Komaki R, Allen P, et al. Comparison of outcomes for patients with medically inoperable stage I non-small-cell lung cancer treated with two-dimensional vs. three-dimensional radiotherapy. *Int J Radiat Oncol Biol Phys.* 2006;66(1):108–116.

57. Sibley GS. Radiotherapy for patients with medically inoperable stage I nonsmall cell lung carcinoma: smaller volumes and higher doses – a review. *Cancer.* 1998;82(3):433–438.

58. Lind PA, Marks LB, Hollis D, et al. Receiver operating characteristic curves to assess predictors of radiation-induced symptomatic lung injury. *Int J Radiat Oncol Biol Phys.* 2002;54(2):340–347.

59. Starkschall G, Forster KM, Kitamura K, et al. Correlation of gross tumor volume excursion with potential benefits of respiratory gating. *Int J Radiat Oncol Biol Phys.* 2004;60(4):1291–1297.

60. Timmerman RD, Park C, Kavanagh BD. The North American experience with stereotactic body radiation therapy in non-small cell lung cancer. *J Thorac Oncol.* 2007;2(7 suppl 3): S101–S112.

61. Timmerman R, McGarry R, Yiannoutsos C, et al. Excessive toxicity when treating central tumors in a phase II study of stereotactic body radiation therapy for medically inoperable early-stage lung cancer. *J Clin Oncol.* 2006;24(30):4833–4839.

62. Chang JY, Dong L, Liu H, et al. Image-guided radiation therapy for non-small cell lung cancer. *J Thorac Oncol.* 2008;3(2):177–186.

63. Chang JY, Balter PA, Dong L, et al. Stereotactic body radiation therapy in centrally and superiorly located stage I or isolated recurrent non-small-cell lung cancer. *Int J Radiat Oncol Biol Phys.* 2008;72(4):967–971.

64. Dillman RO, Herndon J, Seagren SL, et al. Improved survival in stage III non-small-cell lung cancer: seven-year follow-up of cancer and leukemia group B (CALGB) 8433 trial. *J Natl Cancer Inst.* 1996;88(17):1210–1215.

65. Sause W, Kolesar P, Taylor SI, et al. Final results of phase III trial in regionally advanced unresectable non-small cell lung cancer: Radiation Therapy Oncology Group, Eastern Cooperative Oncology Group, and Southwest Oncology Group. *Chest.* 2000;117(2):358–364.

66. Fournel P, Robinet G, Thomas P, et al. Randomized phase III trial of sequential chemoradiotherapy compared with concurrent chemoradiotherapy in locally advanced non-small-cell lung cancer: Groupe Lyon-Saint-Etienne d'Oncologie Thoracique-Groupe Francais de Pneumo-Cancerologie NPC 95–01 Study. *J Clin Oncol.* 2005;23(25):5910–5917.

67. Furuse K, Fukuoka M, Kawahara M, et al. Phase III study of concurrent versus sequential thoracic radiotherapy in combination with mitomycin, vindesine, and cisplatin in unresectable stage III non-small-cell lung cancer. *J Clin Oncol.* 1999;17(9):2692–2699.

68. Huber RM, Flentje M, Schmidt M, et al. Simultaneous chemoradiotherapy compared with radiotherapy alone after induction chemotherapy in inoperable stage IIIA or IIIB non-small-cell lung cancer: study CTRT99/97 by the Bronchial Carcinoma Therapy Group. *J Clin Oncol.* 2006;24(27):4397–4404.

69. Schild SE, Stella PJ, Geyer SM, et al. The outcome of combined-modality therapy for stage III non-small-cell lung cancer in the elderly. *J Clin Oncol.* 2003;21(17):3201–3206.

70. Albain KS, Rusch VW, Crowley JJ, et al. Concurrent cisplatin/etoposide plus chest radiotherapy followed by surgery for stages IIIA (N2) and IIIB non-small-cell lung cancer: mature results of Southwest Oncology Group phase II study 8805. *J Clin Oncol.* 1995;13(8):1880–1892.

71. van Meerbeeck JP, Kramer GW, Van Schil PE, et al. Randomized controlled trial of resection versus radiotherapy after induction chemotherapy in stage IIIA-N2 non-small-cell lung cancer. *J Natl Cancer Inst.* 2007;99(6):442–450.

72. Bradley J. A review of radiation dose escalation trials for non-small cell lung cancer within the Radiation Therapy Oncology Group. *Semin Oncol.* 2005;32(2 suppl 3):S111–S113.

73. Rosenzweig KE, Fox JL, Yorke E, et al. Results of a phase I dose-escalation study using three-dimensional conformal radiotherapy in the treatment of inoperable nonsmall cell lung carcinoma. *Cancer.* 2005;103(10):2118–2127.

74. De Ruysscher D, Wanders S, van Haren E, et al. Selective mediastinal node irradiation based on FDG-PET scan data in patients with non-small-cell lung cancer: a prospective clinical study. *Int J Radiat Oncol Biol Phys.* 2005;62(4):988–994.

75. Rodrigues G, Lock M, D'Souza D, et al. Prediction of radiation pneumonitis by dose – volume histogram parameters in lung cancer – a systematic review. *Radiother Oncol.* 2004;71(2):127–138.

76. Movsas B, Scott C, Langer C, et al. Randomized trial of amifostine in locally advanced non-small-cell lung cancer patients receiving chemotherapy and hyperfractionated radiation: radiation therapy oncology group trial 98-01. *J Clin Oncol.* 2005;23(10):2145–2154.

77. Hensley ML, Hagerty KL, Kewalramani T, et al. American Society of Clinical Oncology 2008 clinical practice guideline update: use of chemotherapy and radiation therapy protectants. *J Clin Oncol.* 2009;27(1):127–145.

78. Mac Manus MP, Hicks RJ, Ball DL, et al. F-18 fluorodeoxyglucose positron emission tomography staging in radical radiotherapy candidates with nonsmall cell lung carcinoma: powerful correlation with survival and high impact on treatment. *Cancer.* 2001;92(4): 886–895.

79. Werner-Wasik M, Scott C, Cox JD, et al. Recursive partitioning analysis of 1999 Radiation Therapy Oncology Group (RTOG) patients with locally-advanced non-small-cell lung cancer (LA-NSCLC): identification of five groups with different survival. *Int J Radiat Oncol Biol Phys.* 2000;48(5):1475–1482.

80. Turrisi 3rd AT, Kim K, Blum R, et al. Twice-daily compared with once-daily thoracic radiotherapy in limited small-cell lung cancer treated concurrently with cisplatin and etoposide. *N Engl J Med.* 1999;340(4):265–271.

81. Yuen AR, Zou G, Turrisi AT, et al. Similar outcome of elderly patients in intergroup trial 0096: cisplatin, etoposide, and thoracic radiotherapy administered once or twice daily in limited stage small cell lung carcinoma. *Cancer.* 2000;89(9):1953–1960.

82. Auperin A, Arriagada R, Pignon JP, et al. Prophylactic cranial irradiation for patients with small-cell lung cancer in complete remission. Prophylactic Cranial Irradiation Overview Collaborative Group. *N Engl J Med.* 1999;341(7):476–484.

83. Arriagada R, Le Chevalier T, Borie F, et al. Prophylactic cranial irradiation for patients with small-cell lung cancer in complete remission. *J Natl Cancer Inst.* 1995;87(3):183–190.

84. Grosshans DR, Meyers CA, Allen PK, et al. Neurocognitive function in patients with small cell lung cancer: effect of prophylactic cranial irradiation. *Cancer.* 2008;112(3):589–595.

85. Falk SJ, Girling DJ, White RJ, et al. Immediate versus delayed palliative thoracic radiotherapy in patients with unresectable locally advanced non-small cell lung cancer and minimal thoracic symptoms: randomised controlled trial. *Br Med J.* 2002;325(7362):452–453.

86. Erridge SC, Gaze MN, Price A, et al. Symptom control and quality of life in people with lung cancer: a randomised trial of two palliative radiotherapy fractionation schedules. *Clin Oncol (R Coll Radiol).* 2005;17(1):61–67.

87. Kramer GW, Wanders SL, Noordijk EM, et al. Results of the Dutch national study of the palliative effect of irradiation using two different treatment schemes for non-small-cell lung cancer. *J Clin Oncol.* 2005;23(13):2962–2970.

88. Sundstrom S, Bremnes R, Aasebo U, et al. Hypofractionated palliative radiotherapy (17 Gy per two fractions) in advanced non-small-cell lung carcinoma is comparable to standard fractionation for symptom control and survival: a national phase III trial. *J Clin Oncol.* 2004;22(5):801–810.

89. Gorlia T, Van Den Bent MJ, Hegi ME, et al. Nomograms for predicting survival of patients with newly diagnosed glioblastoma: prognostic factor analysis of EORTC and NCIC trial 26981–22981/CE.3. *Lancet Oncol.* 2008;9(1):29–38.

90. Curran Jr WJ, Scott CB, Horton J, et al. Recursive partitioning analysis of prognostic factors in three Radiation Therapy Oncology Group malignant glioma trials. *J Natl Cancer Inst.* 1993;85(9):704–710.

91. Peschel RE, Wilson L, Haffty B, et al. The effect of advanced age on the efficacy of radiation therapy for early breast cancer, local prostate cancer and grade III–IV gliomas. *Int J Radiat Oncol Biol Phys.* 1993;26(3):539–544.

92. Keime-Guibert F, Chinot O, Taillandier L, et al. Radiotherapy for glioblastoma in the elderly. *N Engl J Med.* 2007;356(15):1527–1535.

93. Roa W, Brasher PM, Bauman G, et al. Abbreviated course of radiation therapy in older patients with glioblastoma multiforme: a prospective randomized clinical trial. *J Clin Oncol.* 2004;22(9):1583–1588.

94. Bleehen NM, Stenning SP. A Medical Research Council trial of two radiotherapy doses in the treatment of grades 3 and 4 astrocytoma. The Medical Research Council Brain Tumour Working Party. *Br J Cancer.* 1991;64(4):769–774.

95. Stupp R, Mason WP, Van Den Bent MJ, et al. Radiotherapy plus concomitant and adjuvant temozolomide for glioblastoma. *N Engl J Med.* 2005;352(10):987–996.

96. A predictive model for aggressive non-Hodgkin's lymphoma. The International Non-Hodgkin's Lymphoma Prognostic Factors Project. *N Engl J Med.* 1993;329(14):987–994.

97. Solal-Celigny P, Roy P, Colombat P, et al. Follicular lymphoma international prognostic index. *Blood.* 2004;104(5):1258–1265.

98. Bonnet C, Fillet G, Mounier N, et al. CHOP alone compared with CHOP plus radiotherapy for localized aggressive lymphoma in elderly patients: a study by the Groupe d'Etude des Lymphomes de l'Adulte. *J Clin Oncol.* 2007;25(7):787–792.

99. Zelenetz AD, Advani RH, Byrd JC, et al. Non-Hodgkin's lymphomas. *J Natl Compr Canc Netw.* 2008;6(4):356–421.

100. Haas RL, Poortmans P, de Jong D, et al. High response rates and lasting remissions after low-dose involved field radiotherapy in indolent lymphomas. *J Clin Oncol.* 2003;21(13):2474–2480.

101. Haas RL, Poortmans P, de Jong D, et al. Effective palliation by low dose local radiotherapy for recurrent and/or chemotherapy refractory non-follicular lymphoma patients. *Eur J Cancer.* 2005;41(12):1724–1730.

102. Murthy V, Thomas K, Foo K, et al. Efficacy of palliative low-dose involved-field radiation therapy in advanced lymphoma: a phase ii study. *Clin Lymphoma Myeloma.* 2008;8(4):241–245.

Part 2

Management of solid tumors in older adults

Management of breast cancer in older adults

Michelle Shayne and Gretchen Kimmick

A. Introduction

Increasing age is a major risk factor for the development of breast cancer. While approximately 1 in 233 women are diagnosed with breast cancer in the fourth decade of life, the risk increases to 1 in 27 in the seventh decade (Figure 7.1).[1] Thus over half the women diagnosed with breast cancer in the United States annually are 65 years of age and older.[2] With the aging of the population in the United States, and given that breast cancer represents the second leading cause of cancer death for women in the United States,[3] optimizing management of this disease in this population of patients is of utmost importance.

As a generality, less aggressive tumor biologic characteristics are associated with breast cancers in older women. For instance, several prognostic features of tumors in older women often indicate favorable prognosis: steroid receptor positivity, lower proliferative rate, diploid (vs. aneuploid), and low histologic grade. In addition, p53 is more often normal, and less expression of epidermal growth factor receptor and c-erbB2 are observed in this population of patients.[4–6] Though ductal histology remains the most common regardless of age, the more indolent histologies, such as tubular, mucinous, and papillary, are observed with greater frequency in older patients than in younger patients.[4,7]

Despite these more favorable tumor characteristics, breast cancer survival is poorer and breast cancer–specific mortality is greater for women over age 75 as compared with younger patients.[8,9] The reasons for this apparent discrepancy are varied and likely include lower rates of screening mammography; diagnosis at more advanced stage; increased comorbidities and poorer functional status, limiting management options; and reduced chemotherapy dose intensity or avoidance of chemotherapy altogether as a means of limiting treatment-related toxicity. There are fewer data to guide clinicians managing older patients with breast cancer because of a paucity of data from clinical trials; older patients were excluded from many of the landmark studies.

B. Approach to management: Weighing risks and benefits

Determining the optimal treatment approach for any cancer patient requires careful consideration of the potential risks and benefits of treatment. The treating clinician must determine the risk posed by the cancer and weigh it against the potential benefits and risks of the treatment modality. For early-stage breast cancer, there are a series of major decisions faced (Table 7.1). Initially, when a diagnosis of breast cancer is made, the patient and physician discuss breast-conserving surgery versus mastectomy. Subsequently, for older women who have undergone breast-conserving surgery for a node-negative, hormone receptor–positive tumor, a discussion often ensues regarding whether the addition of radiation is worthwhile. The physician and patient must then weigh the potential benefits of adjuvant chemotherapy and/or hormonal therapy. Within each of these major choices, additional, more subtle issues arise, which will be further discussed later.

For older patients, declining functional status and coexisting illnesses raise concern about complications from even the most routine of treatments. Most functional, healthy older women tolerate and should be offered the same standard operative, radiotherapeutic, and systemic treatment options that would be offered to younger patients. To help physicians determine who is at particularly high risk for treatment-related complications, the geriatric assessment is being tailored for use in patients with cancer. Use of a geriatric assessment has been recommended in consensus guidelines.[10] The comprehensive geriatric assessment (CGA) classifies patients with respect to functional reserve, life expectancy, and stress tolerance (see Chapter 1).[11] Currently research is under way to determine if the CGA can be used to assess the risks

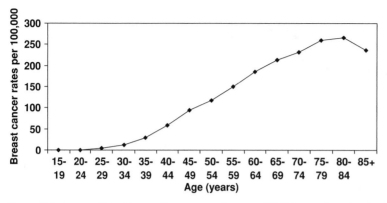

Figure 7.1 Age-specific incidence of breast cancer (rates per 100,000, age adjusted to the 2000 U.S. population).[116]

associated with cancer therapies in older patients. This will facilitate tailoring therapy for each individual patient.

C. Determining mortality and relapse risk: Standard pathologic prognostic and predictive indicators

A variety of prognostic and predictive variables are available for consideration when estimating the risk of disease recurrence (Table 7.2). Pathologic variables, such as tumor size, nodal status, histologic tumor type, and pathologic grade, are routinely evaluated for their prognostic value regardless of patient age.

Hormone receptor and HER2 status demonstrate both prognostic and predictive value in terms of potential response to endocrine therapy or trastuzumab, respectively. In addition to predicting for response to endocrine therapy, positive estrogen receptor (ER) and/or progesterone receptor (PR) status further serves as an indicator of diminished magnitude of chemotherapy benefit as compared with ER-negative disease.[12]

Presence of HER2 protein overexpression as determined by immunohistochemistry or HER2

gene amplification assessed by fluorescence in situ hybridization has also been shown to function as a predictor of heightened response to anthracyclines[13,14] and taxanes[15] as compared with HER2-negative breast cancers. Data exist to support the hypothesis that clinical benefits of a taxane- and trastuzumab-containing regimen for patients with HER2-overexpressing tumors may be similar to anthracycline/trastuzumab-containing regimens while avoiding the added cardiac toxicity of the anthracycline.[16] This is of particular importance for older patients, who are at increased risk of anthracycline-related cardiac toxicity.[17,18]

C.1. Tumor gene expression analysis

The most novel means of assessing risk for systemic breast cancer recurrence involves the analysis of individual tumor gene expression profiles. Gene expression profiles (GEP) or signatures address the inherent heterogeneity of breast cancer in terms of natural history and response to treatment. The two currently available molecular assays are the OncotypeDX and MammaPrint assays.

The MammaPrint 70-gene signature was initially conceived as a means of identifying

Table 7.1 Major management choices for early-stage breast cancer.

	Choices	
Surgery	Breast-conserving surgery versus mastectomy	The outcome, with respect to survival, is the same in women whose breast cancer is small enough to remove and leave an acceptable appearance of the breast
Radiation	Radiation after breast-conserving surgery or not	For women with clinically negative nodes and a hormone receptor–positive stage I tumor who are going to take adjuvant hormonal therapy, it may be acceptable to omit radiation after breast-conserving surgery
Chemotherapy	Adding chemotherapy or not	The additional benefits of chemotherapy are weighed against the risk of tumor recurrence and the side effects

Table 7.2 Prognostic and predictive factors for recurrence of early-stage breast cancer.

	Meaning in terms of prognosis	Meaning in terms of predicting response to treatment
Tumor size	Larger tumors have greater risk of relapse	
Node	Presence of node involvement and greater number of involved lymph nodes portend higher risk of recurrence	
Histology	– Colloid and papillary histologies have better prognosis – Medullary and inflammatory histologies have worse prognosis – Presence of lymphovascular or perineural invasion indicates worse prognosis	
Tumor grade	Higher grade portends slightly higher risk of recurrence	Higher grade predicts greater likelihood of benefit from chemotherapy
Proliferative markers	Higher proliferative rate protends worse prognosis	Higher proliferative rate indicates greater likelihood of response to chemotherapy
Hormone receptors	Better prognosis if hormone receptor positive	– Hormone receptor positivity predicts higher response likelihood of benefit from hormonal treatments – Hormone receptor negativity predicts higher response to chemotherapy
Human epidermal growth factor receptor–2 (HER2)	Presence indicates higher risk of tumor recurrence	Presence predicts response to chemotherapy with anthracyclines and taxanes and to medications that block HER2, including trastuzumab, lapatinib
Gene expression profiles (OncoytpeDX™)	Higher score indicates higher risk of recurrence	For node-negative, hormone receptor–positive HER2 negative tumors: – Lower score predicts benefit of hormone therapies – Higher score predicts benefit of chemotherapy

younger patients with breast cancer at low risk for systemic disease recurrence who might be spared systemic chemotherapy.[19] This assay has now been validated in both younger and older women. In a group of predominantly postmenopausal women with a median age of 62.5 years, MammaPrint had an excellent negative predictive value of 100 percent, which was similar to that observed in younger women.[19] In younger women, the positive predictive value was 12 percent at 5 years. This finding suggests that additional clinically relevant gene expression signatures for predicting systemic relapse in older postmenopausal women may exist.

OncotypeDX, a gene expression array obtained by multiplex reverse transcriptase polymerase chain reaction, has proven to be prognostic and predictive in early-stage breast cancer patients with hormone receptor–positive, HER2-negative, node-negative breast cancer. In the cohorts used to determine prognostic and predictive value of OncotypeDX testing, 45 and 30 percent of patients, respectively, were aged 60 years and older, though women over age 70 years were excluded from National Surgical Adjuvant Bowel and Breast (NSABP) B-14 and NSABP B-20 clinical trials, so this group is not represented.[20,21]

Prospective validation for GEP, including OncotypeDX, MammaPrint, and other assays, is ongoing. Currently active intergroup trials include the TAILORx (Trial Assigning Individualized Options for Treatment) and MINDACT (Microarray In Node-Negative and 1 to 3 positive lymph node Disease may Avoid ChemoTherapy) clinical trials, studying OncotypeDX and MammaPrint, respectively. Despite a lack of prospective validation of these assays, standard guidelines do support their use for determining prognosis and for therapeutic decision making when tumors are ER expressing and node negative.[22]

C.2. Statistical modeling to ascertain relapse risk

A validated Internet-based tool called Adjuvant-Online is available for use by clinicians to determine the level of risk from the tumor in terms of tumor relapse and mortality risk.[23] Furthermore, the tool allows estimation of absolute benefits of chemotherapy and/or hormonal therapy for reducing the risk of relapse and death. The online tool requires the following be entered to calculate risks and benefits of treatment: age, comorbidity status, tumor size, number of involved nodes, tumor grade, and hormone receptor status. The output is based on actuarial analysis derived from Surveillance Epidemiology and End Results (SEER) data and on the 1998 overviews of randomized trials on adjuvant chemotherapy. Since the statistical modeling is based on the 1998 meta-analysis of adjuvant trials, in which very few women over age 70 years had been enrolled, the accuracy of the percentage estimates for older women is not very robust.

D. Management introduction

Optimal outcomes for patients of any age with breast cancer require an integrated, multidisciplinary approach to care. Coordinated efforts of general and plastic surgery, radiation oncology, medical oncology, and social work teams optimize outcomes not only with respect to quality of life but also with respect to disease-free and overall survival. Special considerations in the management of older breast cancer patients will be described subsequently. Though breast cancer is more common in older patients, only recently has research and understanding in this area begun to evolve.

Once a better understanding is achieved regarding an older patient's risks of breast cancer relapse and mortality, within the context of the existing functional status, comorbidities, and life expectancy, decision making pertaining to management options can begin.

E. Surgery

Breast surgery, either mastectomy or breast-conserving surgery, is an essential component of curative management for early-stage breast cancer. Overall, older patients tolerate surgery well, with low preoperative mortality rates of only 1–2 percent.[24–26] In terms of treatment of local disease, survival is comparable to younger patients.[27] With respect to age, it is physiologic age rather than chronologic age that is a significant determinant of survival after surgery.[25,28,29]

E.1. Surgery and risk assessment

There are three available tools that can be used for preoperative evaluation of older patients: the American Society of Anesthesiologists (ASA) grade, the Acute Physiology and Chronic Health Evaluation (APACHE II) index, and the Preoperative Assessment of Cancer in the Elderly (PACE) tool. The ASA has been used to assess preoperative functional status and intraoperative variables as they relate to adverse postoperative outcomes in older patients.[30] Emergency surgery and intraoperative tachycardia were identified as the significant predictors of adverse postoperative outcomes for older surgical patients. The APACHE II index incorporates physiologic measures such as age; presence or absence of advanced chronic health issues; heart and respiratory rates; temperature; oxygenation; mean arterial blood pressure; arterial pH; serum concentration levels of sodium, potassium, and creatinine; packed-cell volume; white blood cell count; and Glasgow coma scale score. In one study, designed to use the APACHE II to determine risk of morbidity and mortality for patients undergoing major liver resection for primary and metastatic hepatic tumors, age was not associated with morbidity.[31] The PACE incorporates a battery of validated instruments, including the CGA, the Brief Fatigue Inventory, the Eastern Cooperative Oncology Group Performance Status, and the ASA grade, and is being developed as a means to determine surgical candidacy of older cancer patients. In a prospective study of 460 older patients undergoing elective surgery, almost half of whom had breast cancer, the PACE assessment effectively described functional and health status, and it is hoped that this tool will be useful in determining the fitness of older patients for surgery.[32]

Women 70 years of age and older, when given a choice, prefer breast conservation to mastectomy.[33] The option of breast conservation should therefore be offered to all older women when medically feasible and appropriate because body image can impact psychological health at any age.[34] Furthermore, greater functional limitations are seen after mastectomy than after lumpectomy in older breast cancer survivors.[35]

Patients with large tumors or locally advanced disease often require or benefit from systemic treatment prior to surgery. Chemotherapy may be used with appropriate patients as a means to decrease tumor burden prior to surgery. In addition, hormonal therapy has also been used for this purpose in selected older breast cancer patients with estrogen receptor–positive disease.[36]

E.2. Axillary management

Omission of axillary lymph node dissection (ALND) from breast cancer management is more commonly observed with older women.[37] While local control may be undermined slightly, an adverse impact on survival appears less likely for older women than for younger women with early-stage disease.[38] For 354 women 70 years of age and older in one study with a clinically negative axilla treated with conservative surgery and tamoxifen, omission of axillary dissection and postoperative radiation resulted in an axillary recurrence rate of 4.2 percent. The incidence rate of ipsilateral tumor recurrence and breast cancer mortality over a median follow-up of 15 years was 8.3 and 17 percent, respectively.[39]

In addition, older women may be at greater risk of developing upper extremity morbidity, including lymphedema, in the setting of axillary dissection, with a resultant negative impact on quality of life.[40] Accordingly, ALND should be reserved for situations in which the information derived from the procedure will clearly affect treatment decision making. ALND should be performed, for instance, if the information gleaned will alter decisions about use of systemic chemotherapy or postmastectomy radiation. Presently ALND is appropriate in the setting of clinically positive axillary adenopathy. Another indication for ALND is the presence of a positive sentinel lymph node (see the following discussion).

An increasingly used, less morbid, alternative approach to assessment of nodal status is the sentinel lymph node biopsy (SLNB). The prognostic value of SLNB has been studied in older breast cancer patients and deemed comparable to younger patients.[41]

Although the level of evidence on the use of SLNB in older breast cancer patients is considered limited, this procedure is recommended by the American Society of Clinical Oncology for use in this population.[42] If the sentinel node is positive for metastatic involvement, ALND is indicated.

Omission of axillary assessment has been investigated and purported as a means of reducing surgical morbidity in older patients with breast cancer because information derived from this approach often does little to influence subsequent treatment decision making. In women aged 70 years and older with clinically negative axillary nodes, and in whom tamoxifen is used as adjuvant medical management, axillary recurrence rates are similar with or without surgical axillary assessment.[39,43,44] Furthermore, the rate of distant disease recurrence, disease-specific mortality,[39] and overall survival[44] were not increased by omitting the procedure.

In summary, for older women with clinically node-negative breast cancer, SLNB is an appropriate alternative to ALND when the information gained from the procedure would change recommendations for systemic therapy. Women aged 70 years and older with hormone receptor–positive, clinically node-negative breast cancer, in which the primary tumor is 2 cm in size and smaller, can forego surgical axillary assessment when adjuvant hormonal therapy is employed. Patients with clinically involved axillary lymph nodes and/or positive SLNB should undergo ALND, providing that they are able to tolerate the surgery.

F. Radiation therapy

A standard component of breast conservation therapy for women of all ages is fractionated radiation therapy with a boost to the lumpectomy site. A treatment approach that delivers 45–50 Gy to the whole breast over the course of 4.5–5 weeks has been shown to significantly decrease the risk of local breast cancer recurrence and modestly affect survival.[45]

Breast radiation is generally well tolerated in patients regardless of age, including women over age 80 years.[46] The benefits of radiation therapy for older patients with early-stage breast cancer have been questioned, given the reported low risk of local recurrence after quadrantectomy alone – as low as 3.8 percent without radiation in women aged 55 years and older.[47] Furthermore, the benefits of local radiation appear to decline in older women with increasing comorbidity.[48] The frequency and duration of the treatment course also pose challenges for older patients with decreased mobility and limited access to transportation. These issues have formed the basis for investigation into alternative schedules and doses of radiotherapy such as hypofractionation, partial breast irradiation, and substitution of hormonal therapy for radiotherapy.

G. Hypofractionated radiation therapy

As a means of decreasing the frequency of treatments, while attempting to maintain equivalent outcomes, once weekly, also called *hypofractionated*, radiotherapy is a nonstandard alternative for select older patients. A retrospective review of 70 patients, median age of 81 years, with hormone receptor–positive, T1–4 tumors reported a local control rate of 86 percent at a median follow-up of 36 months.[49] The patients received tamoxifen at 20 mg/d along with high dose per fraction radiotherapy, which in most cases consisted of seven treatments of 6.5 Gy delivered weekly over 6 weeks. In a prospective study of 150 patients, median age 78 years, 90 percent of whom had estrogen receptor positive tumors and 72 percent of whom had breast-conserving surgery, the local recurrence rate was only 2.3 percent at a median follow-up of 65 months after treatment with once-weekly radiation therapy delivered in five fractions of 6.5 Gy to a total dose of 32.5 Gy.[50] Side effects were acceptable with mild early reactions and moderate, primarily low-grade late toxicity overall. A third report described results of hypofractionated radiation and hormonal therapy in a group of 115 women, median age 83 years, who were treated with this alternative schedule because of very old age, refusal of surgery, locally advanced disease, and/or significant comorbidity. Five-year local progression-free survival was 78 percent, leading the authors to conclude that hormonal therapy and hypofractionated radiotherapy were acceptable alternatives to surgery for patients who are not surgical candidates or who refuse surgery or standard schedules of radiation.[51] The 5-year overall survival in this study was 38 percent and was influenced primarily by T stage, nodal status, and performance status. Grade 3 toxicity was experienced in only 6 percent of patients.

G.1. Partial breast irradiation

Another alternative with a potentially more acceptable schedule and toxicity level to the standard whole-breast radiotherapy with boost to the tumor bed is partial breast irradiation (PBI). This approach is based on the premise that most local recurrences of breast cancer appear in close proximity to the original tumor site. With the radiation field limited to the tumor bed and the total dose of radiation thus reduced, the duration of treatment can likewise be reduced. In a review of phase II and III trials, feasibility, efficacy, and toxicity of PBI in elderly women was examined by Hannoun-Levi and colleagues.[52] The authors of this analysis concluded that PBI appears to be a reasonable alternative to standard 5-week adjuvant radiation therapy or no radiation in cases where older patients may be unable to otherwise tolerate the conventional approach to treatment. Large multicenter randomized phase III trials are needed to compare PBI with standard adjuvant radiation therapy, with particular attention given to quality-of-life assessments and economic analyses. In addition, longer duration of follow-up is needed before PBI can gain acceptance as a standard of care.

G.2. Omitting radiation in patients treated with hormonal therapy

Some retrospective analyses of selected older women with estrogen receptor–positive early-stage breast cancer treated with surgery followed by adjuvant hormonal therapy suggest that the addition of radiation therapy may not be necessary.[53–55] Others have shown that while adjuvant radiation therapy is of added benefit in terms of optimizing local control, the benefits are observed primarily in older patients with minimal comorbidity.[48] There are also data to support that adjuvant radiation in older women confers benefits with respect to reducing local recurrences and second primary tumors regardless of increasing age or comorbidity.[56] Thus, though there appears to be some controversy regarding which groups of older women may not derive enough additional benefits from radiation therapy to justify its use in terms of local control, there is agreement regarding the lack of survival benefit conferred by radiation therapy in this group of patients. In a study of 636 women age 70 and older with clinical stage T1 N0 M0, stage I, estrogen receptor–positive breast cancer treated with breast-conserving surgery, tamoxifen, and randomized to receive either radiation or no radiation, the only significant difference between the two groups was the 5-year rate of local or regional recurrence (1% and 4%, respectively,

$p < .001$).[57] There were no significant differences observed between the 2 groups in terms of mastectomy rates for local recurrence, distant metastases, or 5-year overall survival. Furthermore, physician and patient assessments regarding cosmesis and adverse events consistently rated tamoxifen and radiotherapy inferior to tamoxifen alone. An updated report, at a median follow-up of 7.9 years, described a 7 percent local recurrence rate for women treated with tamoxifen and no radiation vs. 1 percent for those who received tamoxifen and radiotherapy.[43]

To summarize, the standard approach to adjuvant radiation therapy, regardless of age, is whole-breast radiation daily for 5–6 weeks with a boost to the tumor bed. The primary advantage conferred by this modality is a decrease in local recurrence rates by approximately two-thirds. Because the risk of local recurrence for older patients is deemed low – approximately 5 percent – alternatives to the standard approach have been explored as a means of simplifying the treatment schedule, reducing duration of therapy, and minimizing toxicity. It must be remembered, however, that although local recurrence rates may be lower in older women as a group, factors such as hormone receptor negativity, high tumor grade, large tumor size, presence of lymphovascular invasion or nodal involvement, and close or involved margin status portend a higher risk of local recurrence and should be considered when planning local definitive therapy. Adjuvant radiation should be recommended for older women with tumors that have characteristics that put them at higher risk of local recurrence. Though approaches such as hypofractionated radiotherapy, partial breast irradiation, and substitution of hormonal therapy for radiation have been studied in older breast cancer patients, further studies are needed to better define the role of these approaches and identify ideal candidates for their use.

H. Systemic therapy by stage

Breast cancer stage is determined by the size of the invasive component of the tumor within the breast (T) and the number of involved axillary lymph nodes (N), according to the TNM staging classification shown in Table 7.3. Stage of breast cancer correlates with outcome and is therefore used as an indicator for whether systemic adjuvant therapy should be delivered. Survival by stage of breast cancer is depicted in Figure 7.2. In the following sections, we discuss treatment according to stage of the cancer.

H.1. Ductal carcinoma in situ

Ductal carcinoma in situ (DCIS) represents the earliest stage of breast cancer: stage 0. The risk of death from breast cancer in women with stage 0 disease is extremely small. The goal of systemic therapy for DCIS therefore is primarily to prevent future breast cancers.

The selective estrogen receptor modulator, tamoxifen, has demonstrated significant benefits in terms of reducing future breast disease in the ipsilateral breast in women with DCIS, regardless of age; however, the magnitude of benefit was shown to be greater in women under age 50 as compared with women 50 years of age and older. In the National Surgical Adjuvant Breast and Bowel Project B-24, a randomized controlled trial that included 1,804 women with DCIS randomized to lumpectomy plus radiation with or without tamoxifen for 5 years, the relative risk reduction for ipsilateral breast tumors was 38 percent for women younger than 50 years and 22 percent for women aged 50 years and over.[58] Though the benefits in both age groups were statistically significant, the absolute benefits for reducing ipsilateral breast tumors were 5.4 and 1.3 percent for women under and over age 50 years, respectively. Benefits from tamoxifen in this trial with respect to the contralateral breast were significant only in terms of reducing the risk of DCIS, and not invasive disease. The relative risk reduction for noninvasive, contralateral disease for all-comers, regardless of age, was 78 percent, an absolute risk reduction of 0.5 percent.

When having a balanced discussion with older patients regarding the use of tamoxifen for DCIS, treating physicians must also discuss the potential side effects. The risks of uterine cancer and thrombotic complications associated with tamoxifen are more commonly seen with postmenopausal women, particularly the elderly. This may be the result of increasing concentrations of tamoxifen and metabolites observed with increasing age.[59]

In contrast to the findings of the NSABP B-24 trial, results of a study from the United Kingdom, Australia, and New Zealand, the UK/ANZ trial, did not provide evidence to support the use of tamoxifen for women with completely excised DCIS.[60] The UK/ANZ study was a 2 × 2 randomized factorial trial in which 1,701 women

Table 7.3 AJCC staging criteria for breast cancer.[115]

Symbol (TNM system)	Meaning
Primary tumor (T)	
TX	Primary tumor cannot be assessed
T0	No evidence of primary tumor
Tis	Carcinoma in situ; intraductal carcinoma, lobular carcinoma in situ, or Paget's disease of the nipple with no tumor
T1	Tumor ≤2 cm in greatest dimension
	T1a ≤0.5 cm in greatest dimension
	T1b >0.5 cm but not >1 cm in greatest dimension
	T1c >1 cm but not >2 cm in greatest dimension
T2	Tumor >2 cm but not >5 cm in greatest dimension
T3	Tumor >5 cm in greatest dimension
T4	Tumor of any size with direct extension to chest wall or skin (includes inflammatory carcinoma)
Regional lymph nodes (N)	
NX	Regional lymph nodes cannot be assessed (e.g., previously removed)
N0	No regional lymph-node metastases
N1	Metastasis to movable ipsilateral axillary nodes
N2	– Metastases to ipsilateral axillary nodes fixed to one another or to other structures
	– N2a metastasis in ipsilateral axillary lymph nodes fixed to one another (matted) or to other structures
	– N2b metastasis only in clinically apparent ipsilateral internal mammary nodes and in the absence of clinically evident axillary lymph node metastasis
N3	Metastases to ipsilateral internal mammary lymph nodes
Distant metastasis (M)	
MX	Presence of distant metastasis cannot be assessed
M0	No evidence of distant metastasis
M1	Distant metastases (including metastases to ipsilateral supraclavicular lymph nodes)
Clinical stage	
0	Tis, N0, M0
1	T1, N0, M0
IIA	T0, N1, M0
	T1, N1, M0
	T2, N0, M0
IIB	T2, N1, M0
	T3, N0, M0
IIIA	T0 or T1, N2, M0
	T2, N2, M0
	T3, N1 or N2, M0
IIIB	T4, any N, M0
	Any T, N3, M0
IV	Any T, any N, MI

with completely excised DCIS were randomized to radiation or not and to tamoxifen or not. The use of tamoxifen decreased the risk of ipsilateral DCIS (hazard ratio 0.68 [0.49–0.96]; $p = .03$) but not invasive cancer. Use of radiotherapy was beneficial in reducing ipsilateral invasive disease (0.45 [0.24–0.85]; $p = .01$) and ductal carcinoma in situ (0.36 [0.19–0.66]; $p = .0004$). There was no evidence of interaction between radiotherapy and tamoxifen.

The IBIS II trial, ongoing presently, is seeking to answer the question of whether there is a role for the use of aromatase inhibitors in the management of DCIS in postmenopausal women.

I. Early stage

Effective systemic therapies for breast cancer include hormonal therapy, chemotherapy, and immunotherapy. Adjuvant systemic therapy for

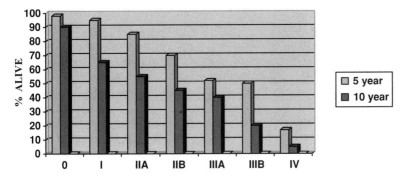

Figure 7.2 Survival by breast cancer stage information from Haskell's *Cancer Treatment*, fifth edition.[117]

early-stage disease is chosen based on the tumor characteristics: hormonal therapy for tumors that are hormone receptor positive; chemotherapy for tumors that are hormone receptor negative or high enough risk to justify its use; and the immunotherapy trastuzumab for HER2-positive cancers.

I.1. Hormonal therapy

After local definitive therapy, many early-stage breast cancers in older women can be optimally managed with adjuvant endocrine therapy only. Once the determination is made that chemotherapy is not indicated, using tools such as those delineated earlier, a decision can then be made regarding the optimal approach to endocrine therapy.

The Early Breast Cancer Trialist Collaborative Group (EBCTCG) demonstrated that tamoxifen conferred significant benefits for managing early-stage estrogen receptor–positive breast cancer regardless of age.[61] With 15 years of follow-up, tamoxifen was associated with substantial benefit. With 5 years of tamoxifen, the annual recurrence rate was reduced by 45 percent and the annual death rate by 35 percent in women ages 60–69. For women 70 years of age and older, the annual recurrence rate and the annual mortality rate were reduced by 31 and 51 percent, respectively, with 5 years of adjuvant tamoxifen. For over 30 years, tamoxifen has remained the standard agent for adjuvant endocrine therapy in women with estrogen receptor–positive breast cancer either in lieu of or following administration of chemotherapy. Use of tamoxifen, however, is not without risks, particularly an increased risk of endometrial cancer and thromboembolic complications, and increasing age has been shown to be an independent risk factor for these complications.[62]

Aromatase inhibitors block the formation of tamoxifen and have a distinctly different toxicity profile that does not include thrombotic complications or endometrial cancer. In 2002, data were published from the Arimidex, Tamoxifen, Alone or in Combination trial that demonstrated superiority of the aromatase inhibitor anastrozole for 5 years when directly compared with 5 years of tamoxifen in the adjuvant setting.[63] Anastrozole was superior to tamoxifen or the combination in terms of disease-free survival, development of distant metastatic disease, and incidence of contralateral breast cancer. No significant differences were observed between the groups in terms of overall survival. Following the publication of these data, additional clinical trials were published that solidified the role of aromatase inhibitors for postmenopausal women with estrogen receptor–positive breast cancer.[64,65]

One of the most concerning potential side effects of aromatase inhibition is that of a decline in bone mineral density with resultant heightened incidence of bone fractures. Musculoskeletal pain is also observed more frequently in patients taking aromatase inhibitors as compared with tamoxifen. Incidence of ischemic cerebrovascular events, venous thromboembolic events, endometrial cancer, vasomotor symptoms, and vaginal bleeding are less commonly experienced on an aromatase inhibitor as compared with tamoxifen.[63] Safety analysis in the BIG-98 clinical trial, which compared the aromatase inhibitor letrozole with tamoxifen, demonstrated an overall low incidence of cardiovascular adverse events for both agents but a statistically increased incidence of higher grade for these events in the letrozole arm of 2.4 percent compared to the tamoxifen arm of 1.4 percent ($p = .001$).[66] In this trial, a diagnosis of hypertension and history of prior cardiac event were risk factors for developing cardiac events while taking letrozole. The risk of cardiac events appeared to be greater for women in the 65–74 years of age range as compared with women below age 65 or women 75 years of age and older.[67]

I.2. Chemotherapy

The decision to incorporate chemotherapy into the management of breast cancer for older women is complex. The magnitude of benefit derived from chemotherapy has been shown to decrease with increasing age.[61] This may be due in part to the more favorable tumor features generally associated with breast cancer in older women.[6] Because there is some degree of physiologic decline in organ function, often accompanied by an increase in comorbidities with increasing age, the toxicity of chemotherapy can be exacerbated.[68] Clinicians also struggle with formulating estimates of life expectancy because it is more difficult to justify administration of potentially toxic therapy when competing risks for decreased survival could undermine the full benefits of the treatment in question.[69]

Data from the EBCTCG demonstrate a progressive decline in relative efficacy from adjuvant chemotherapy with increasing age.[61] Though statistically significant benefits were conferred by adjuvant polychemotherapy in terms of reduction in disease recurrence and breast cancer–specific mortality, a 10 percent absolute improvement in 15-year survival was seen in women under age 50 years as opposed to a 3 percent absolute gain in 15-year survival for women aged 50–69 years.

I.3. Determinants of increased benefit from chemotherapy

Tumor characteristics that are associated with increased risk of disease relapse are also markers of increased benefit from chemotherapy. Lymph node involvement, negative estrogen receptor status, and HER2 overexpression/amplification are tumor features associated with added survival benefits from chemotherapy in older and younger patients alike.

Women with node-positive breast cancer have a higher risk of recurrence and death from breast cancer and are therefore potential candidates for adjuvant chemotherapy. The intensity of chemotherapy has been the main question, with concern about more toxicity and less benefit from adjuvant chemotherapy in older women. This myth is dispelled by two studies from the Can-

cer and Leukemia Group B (CALGB). An analysis of data from CALGB randomized trials confirmed the benefit, with minimal additional toxicity, of more intense versus less intense adjuvant chemotherapy among women over age 70 years.[70] Even more compelling were the results of a prospective randomized trial of capecitabine, the oral pro-drug of 5-fluorouracil which was thought more tolerable and acceptable in older women, versus standard IV chemotherapy (doxorubicin/cyclophosphamide or cyclophosphamide/methotrexate/fluorouracil), which showed significantly more relapses (HR 2.09, 95% confidence interval [CI] 1.38–3.17) and higher mortality (HR 1.5, 95% CI 1.11–2.76) with capecitabine. The median follow-up in this trial was 2.4 years, and 633 women over age 65 years were randomized. Older women with high-risk breast cancer should therefore be offered standard adjuvant systemic therapy.[71]

Chemotherapy regimens of lesser toxicity have also proven beneficial and might be considered for older feeble patients or those with higher levels of comorbidity. In a trial of 338 women over age 65 years with node-positive operable breast cancer, the 6-year disease-free survival for the group that received an epirubicin-based chemotherapy regimen in addition to tamoxifen was 72.6 percent compared with 69.3 percent in the group that received tamoxifen alone ($p = .14$).[72] Multivariate analysis confirmed the beneficial effect of adding chemotherapy: the relative risk of disease relapse of 1.93 (95% CI 1.70–2.17) with tamoxifen compared to chemotherapy/tamoxifen. Compliance with the weekly regimen (six cycles of weekly epirubicin at 30 mg on days 1, 8, and 15 out of 28 days) was good and proved safe from the standpoint of hematologic, nonhematologic, and cardiac toxicities.

Two additional adjuvant trials have included patients over age 65 years.[73,74] The International Breast Cancer Study Group Trial studied 608 menopausal women with node-positive breast cancer, of whom 172 (28%) were 65 years of age and older. In this trial, tamoxifen alone was compared with tamoxifen plus three cycles of cyclophosphamide, methotrexate, and fluorouracil.[73] The overall 5-year disease-free survival was statistically superior for the group of patients who received the combination of chemotherapy and tamoxifen; however, no significant difference was observed for the older subgroup of patients. The International Collaborative Cancer Group evaluated 604 postmenopausal women with node-positive breast cancer, of whom 27 percent were 65 years of age and older.[74] The patients were randomized to receive either tamoxifen alone or a combination of tamoxifen and single-agent epirubicin at 50 mg/m^2 on days 1 and 8 of a 28-day cycle. The 5-year overall disease-free survival was significantly better for the chemotherapy/tamoxifen arm. The study was not sufficiently powered to ascertain the effect of treatment with respect to age.

Though the absolute magnitude of benefit from chemotherapy for patients with node-positive breast cancer is greater for younger women, the standard of care remains to employ chemotherapy in this setting regardless of age.

There are conflicting data regarding whether chemotherapy confers additional benefits above and beyond what is gained from 5 years of adjuvant hormonal therapy for older women with node-negative breast cancer. The NSABP B-20 trial demonstrated benefits in terms of improved disease-free survival and overall survival for cyclophosphamide, methotrexate, 5-fluorouracil (CMF) in addition to tamoxifen over that of tamoxifen alone.[75] In contrast, the International Breast Cancer Study Group enrolled 1,669 postmenopausal women with node-negative breast cancer to compare the benefits of CMF plus tamoxifen versus tamoxifen alone. The investigators in this trial concluded that only women with ER-negative tumors derived significant benefit in terms of disease-free survival and overall survival from the combination treatment. Women with ER-positive tumors had no benefit from the combination treatment compared with tamoxifen alone.

Older women are more likely to have breast cancers that are estrogen receptor positive, yet chemotherapy has been shown to be of greater benefit for estrogen receptor–negative disease. The EBCTCG showed that in women aged 50–69 years with ER-poor breast cancer, the annual breast cancer recurrence and mortality rates for those who received polychemotherapy compared with those who did not were 0.67 versus 0.84, respectively. These rates were 0.74 versus 0.95, respectively, for older women with ER-positive disease.[61,76] The CALGB also reported that benefits from adjuvant chemotherapy in 6,644 women with lymph node–positive breast cancer were significantly greater in those with estrogen receptor–negative disease as compared to those with estrogen receptor–positive tumors.[12] The 5-year improvement in disease-free survival for patients who received chemotherapy for management of ER-negative

tumors was 22.8 percent compared with 7 percent for those with ER-positive tumors. Likewise, improvements for overall survival were 16.7 percent versus 4.0 percent, respectively. The French Adjuvant Study Group has demonstrated that for patients with node-positive breast cancer, it is the subgroup of older patients with ER-negative disease that primarily account for the improvement in 6-year disease-free survival from epirubicin-based chemotherapy.[71] In addition, there are retrospective population-based analyses that demonstrate that survival benefits from adjuvant chemotherapy for women with ER-negative tumors exist regardless of age.[77,78]

The use of the 21-gene profile (OncotypeDX), described earlier, can be particularly useful in determining if chemotherapy should be added to hormone therapy in patients with node-negative, ER-positive breast cancer. If the risk of disease recurrence is significant enough to warrant the use of systemic treatment, chemotherapy remains the standard of care for women with estrogen receptor–negative breast cancer regardless of age.

J. Tools to assess benefits and toxicity from chemotherapy

Life expectancy, comorbidities, and expected benefits and toxicities from chemotherapy combine to form complex treatment decision making on behalf of older patients with breast cancer. A growing number of tools are available to clinicians as a means of assisting with this involved process.

A Markov analysis of the medical literature considering patients between the ages of 65 and 85 years with three levels of comorbidity was performed to determine a threshold risk of disease relapse at 10 years for which treatment would result in an absolute reduction of 1 percent in relapse or mortality (Figure 7.3).[79] The authors of this analysis concluded that a reduction in disease relapse from adjuvant medical management is

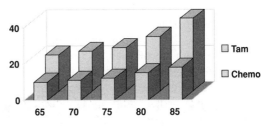

Figure 7.3 Ten-year risk in breast cancer relapse necessary to translate into a chemotherapy benefit where mortality is improved by 1% in patients with hormone receptor–positive breast cancer.[79,115]

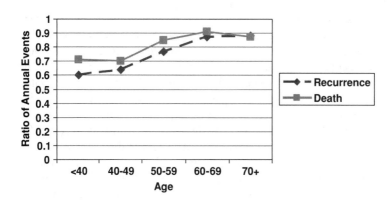

Figure 7.4 Benefit of adjuvant chemotherapy by age group.[61]

similar for older and younger patients with breast cancer. The effect on mortality, however, diverges significantly based on age and comorbidity.

An often serious dose-limiting toxicity of chemotherapy that is more commonly observed in older patients is that of neutropenic complications (see Chapter 23). Another model has been developed to assess risk of developing early neutropenic complications in older cancer patients receiving systemic chemotherapy.[80] The model was validated in 1,386 patients 65 years of age and older with a variety of malignancies, including breast cancer, and demonstrated good discrimination between older patients at decreased risk of developing chemotherapy-related neutropenic events and those at increased risk. Baseline clinical risk factors associated with increased risk of cycle number 1 neutropenic events included use of anthracycline-based chemotherapy regimens ($p < .001$), use of nonchemotherapy immune-modulatory agents ($p = .003$), elevated bilirubin ($p = .016$), and reduced glomerular filtration rate ($p < .001$). Reduced risk of cycle 1 neutropenic events was associated with myeloid growth factor prophylaxis ($p < .001$). This model requires prospective validation.

K. Available chemotherapy regimens

The EBCTCG demonstrated that adjuvant anthracycline-containing regimens are superior to non-anthracycline-containing regimens with respect to both recurrence-free survival and overall survival, with anthracyclines providing an additional 12 percent proportional reduction, and overall survival, with a significant 11 percent proportional reduction in mortality.[81] The benefits of polychemotherapy in this meta-analysis were evident for patients aged 50–69 years as well as

patients under age 50 years; however, there was insufficient evidence for patients 70 years of age and older, primarily because too few women over age 70 years had been studied (Figure 7.4).

On the basis of this study and others,[82] anthracyclines came to comprise the backbone of adjuvant chemotherapy for management of breast cancer. Nevertheless, anthracycline-containing regimens are not without significant associated toxicities, including the potential for decline in cardiac ejection fraction and myelotoxicity. Older patients are particularly susceptible to anthracycline-associated toxicities.[17,83]

For many years, the only standard alternative non-anthracycline-containing chemotherapy regimen available to patients has been cyclophosphamide, methotrexate, and 5-fluorouracil (CMF). Some clinicians choose to reduce the relative dose intensity (RDI) of standard chemotherapy regimens as a means of reducing chemotherapy-related toxicity in older breast cancer patients. Either approach (i.e., CMF or reduced RDI), particularly the latter, may result in suboptimal outcomes for these patients.[84] Furthermore, CMF has not proven to be less toxic for older breast cancer patients.[73] In one prospective study of 283 consecutive breast cancer patients 65 years of age and older treated in community oncology practices, 31 percent of patients received less than 85 percent of the standard chemotherapy dose intensity.[85] While this practice resulted in a lower rate of toxicity than that observed for older breast cancer patients enrolled in clinical trials,[67] the degree of reduction in RDI observed in the nonclinical trial setting could potentially compromise the outcome of these patients.

For older patients with high-risk breast cancer, one approach to limiting chemotherapy-related toxicity is the delivery of doxorubicin and cyclophosphamide (AC) in uncoupled sequential fashion along with paclitaxel (four cycles for each of the three drugs).[86] Although the trial that demonstrated efficacy of the regimen included only 18 percent of patients who were 60 years of age and older, the sequential 2-weekly (dose dense) administration of doxorubicin followed by paclitaxel followed by cyclophosphamide was no different in terms of efficacy as compared with 2-weekly concurrent AC followed by paclitaxel. The toxicity profile of the regimen was also acceptable.

Another alternative to standard AC is that of docetaxel and cyclophosphamide (TC).[87] This chemotherapy regimen was compared head-to-head with AC and demonstrated a significant improvement in disease-free and overall survival for the 16 percent of patients aged 65 years of age and older in the trial and was consistent with the benefits observed in the overall population of patients studied.[87]

For older patients with HER2-overexpressing breast cancers, trastuzumab should be employed in addition to a taxane with or without a prior anthracycline. If there is an existing contraindication to the use of anthracyclines such as known cardiac disease, the docetaxel, carboplatin, and trastuzumab regimen may be used.[16] This regimen also has an acceptable toxicity profile and is thus suitable for most older patients with breast cancer.

L. Metastatic disease

Five to 10 percent of breast cancer cases are stage IV at time of diagnosis, and a significant proportion of women develop recurrent or metastatic disease following primary and adjuvant treatment. When recurrent, disease that has spread outside the local-regional area is often incurable. Five-year survival for metastatic breast cancer averages 25 percent, and cure is exceptionally rare. As such, treatment is considered palliative, with the goal of controlling further spread and complications of the disease, while maintaining optimal quality of life and the best functional level possible. Treatment regimens, whether chemotherapy or endocrine based, should be continued as long as there is demonstrated effect by imaging, declining tumor markers (where applicable), and decreasing symptoms reported by the patient. In addition, to continue any treatment, it should be well tolerated, and the patient should feel comfortable with its ongoing use.

Variables associated with improved survival in the metastatic setting include positive ER status, absence of visceral involvement, disease-free interval of at least 24 months from time of completion of adjuvant therapy, and minimal disease burden (oligometastatic disease).

Although complete remissions are rare, the treating physician should not miss an opportunity to design treatment strategies with intent to cure. This should be considered particularly in the setting of oligometastatic disease where surgery and/or stereotactic body radiotherapy and systemic therapy may result in potential long-term disease-free survival.[88,89] In a small pilot study, stereotactic body radiotherapy for oligometastasis resulted in 56 percent actuarial 4-year survival and local control of 89 percent.[88] Patients with unresectable oligometastases should be offered chemotherapy. A retrospective study of 263 patients with metastatic breast cancer showed that systemic therapy resulted in 16.6 percent of patients achieving complete responses (CRs), and of those with CR, 3.1 percent remained in a CR for over 5 years.[89] Patients with oligometastases were most likely to achieve CR.

In some cases, surgery for the primary tumor should be undertaken in the metastatic setting. One study from the Geneva Cancer Registry demonstrated a survival advantage for this approach.[90] In this study, where the median age at diagnosis was 67.4 years, and 46 percent of the 300 women studied were over age 70 years, complete excision of the breast tumor with negative surgical margins resulted in a 40 percent reduction in risk of breast cancer death as compared with women who did not undergo the surgery. The benefit of the surgical intervention was particularly evident for women with metastatic disease relegated solely to bone.

For the most part, the management of metastatic disease in women 65 years of age and older is similar to that of younger patients. Because the biology of most breast cancers in older women is more indolent, as reflected by characteristics such as ER positivity, HER2 nonoverexpression, and slower growth rate, endocrine (i.e., hormonal) therapy is often selected as first-line systemic therapy. This approach also has the benefit of fewer toxicities and side effects as compared with chemotherapy. As with treatment decision making in the adjuvant setting, life expectancy, comorbidity, and functional status must be taken into consideration in treating older women with metastatic disease. CGA should be performed to facilitate decision making (see the previous discussion and Chapter 1).

L.1. Endocrine Therapy

Determination of which hormonal agent to use should depend in part on information regarding type of hormonal therapy received in the adjuvant setting, the interval between completion of adjuvant therapy and diagnosis of metastatic disease, and how well the prior therapy was tolerated. Response rates along with time to progression appear to be higher for older women who receive first-line letrozole or anastrozole in the metastatic setting as compared with tamoxifen.[91]

The first-line agent should be continued until disease progression as long as it is well tolerated. With evidence of disease progression following a period of stability or response of 4 months or longer, observation for possible withdrawal response should be initiated prior to commencing a second-line endocrine agent. A next-line choice for patients who progress after letrozole or anastrozole is either exemestane or fulvestrant. The strategy of employing successive endocrine therapies offers the longest duration of optimal quality of life.

L.2. Chemotherapy

Chemotherapy should be considered for patients whose cancer becomes refractory to endocrine therapy or who have significant symptomatic visceral disease. Chemotherapy should also be considered for patients with more life threatening or rapidly progressive disease. When compared with endocrine therapy, disease response to chemotherapy generally occurs more rapidly. The duration of objective response to chemotherapy is typically on the order of months, with the longest duration usually observed in the first-line setting and successive response durations decreasing with each subsequent regimen. Side effect and toxicity profiles of standard chemotherapy agents are generally similar for older and younger patients.[92,93] Older patients may be at increased risk of hematologic and cardiac chemotherapy-related toxicities.[94] Chemotherapy-induced nausea and vomiting is generally more common in younger patients as compared with older patients.[95]

Most antineoplastic agents are eliminated though biliary or renal excretion. Because renal function declines with age,[96,97] clearance of drugs that are renally eliminated is reduced. Reduction in glomerular filtration in older persons is not necessarily accompanied by a rising serum creatinine because of the concomitant loss in muscle mass commonly associated with increasing age.[98] Therefore creatinine clearance should be calculated for all older persons receiving renally cleared chemotherapy agents, and appropriate dose modifications should be made. Liver size and blood flow also decrease with increasing age.[99] This can result in higher plasma concentrations and decreased systemic clearance of some drugs. Nevertheless, only patients with significant liver dysfunction seem to be at increased risk of toxicity. Dose reduction is indicated for patients with liver dysfunction, particularly when manifesting with an elevation in bilirubin, when using anthracyclines, taxanes, vinorelbine, and gemcitabine.

M. Choice of chemotherapeutic regimen

The use of sequential single-agent chemotherapy is often preferable to combination chemotherapy because the former approach is far better tolerated. Furthermore, given the more indolent tumor biology of breast cancer in older patients, single-agent chemotherapy will often suffice to confer adequate disease control in the palliative setting. Combination chemotherapy should only be considered for rapidly progressive disease. Though most combinations do not yield better survival compared to sequential single agents, combinations overall do provide higher objective response rates and longer time to disease progression.[100-102] Combinations for which survival may be improved over single-agent treatment include the following: docetaxel and capecitabine versus docetaxel alone[103] and gemcitabine and paclitaxel versus paclitaxel alone; however, there was no cross-over arm included in these studies, and therefore it is not known whether single-sequential therapy would have been as effective.[104]

The most effective antineoplastic agents for management of metastatic breast cancer, at any age, include the anthracyclines (including liposomal doxorubicin, which confers less cardiotoxicity than the nonliposomal preparation); taxanes; alkylating agents such as cyclophosphamide; antimetabolites including fluorouracil, capecitabine, gemcitabine; and vinorelbine.

M.1. Targeted agents

Agents that have been developed to interfere with specific mechanisms that affect growth, proliferation, and death of cancer cells are considered targeted drugs. These drugs are developed to target a molecule or pathway specific to the cancer cell; the collateral damage to other tissue and organs is therefore less than that associated with conventional chemotherapy, and side effects are fewer.

Trastuzumab is one such drug. It is a humanized, monoclonal antibody with the "target" being the HER2 receptor, which is overexpressed in approximately 20 to 30 percent of breast cancers. The presence of HER2 is associated with increased proliferation and decreased apoptosis. Trastuzumab is associated with an increased risk for decline in cardiac left ventricular ejection fraction.[105] Accordingly, cardiac function must be monitored while patients are receiving this drug. Whereas monotherapy is associated with a response rate of approximately 15 percent, response rates and survival are significantly improved when trastuzumab is used in conjunction with chemotherapy.[106]

Lapatinib is a small-molecule dual-tyrosine kinase inhibitor that targets both HER2 and the epidermal growth factor receptor (EGFR or HER1). This oral drug taken in combination with capecitabine has demonstrated activity for patients with HER2-positive metastatic breast cancer. When capecitabine and lapatinib are employed in patients whose tumors had progressed despite use of anthracyclines, taxanes, and trastuzumab, the median time to progression was almost double that seen with capecitabine monotherapy (8.4 vs. 4.4 months).[107] Whereas the median age in this study for the patients on the combination arm was 56 years, patients up to age 80 years were included. The combination was well tolerated; diarrhea was the most common high-grade toxicity. Another common toxicity from lapatinib is skin rash. Cardiac effects of lapatinib have been studied in 3,558 patients in 18 phase I–III clinical trials, where 1.6 percent of patients experienced a decline in left ventricular ejection fraction – 1.4 percent developed asymptomatic declines in ejection fraction, and 0.2 percent of patients were symptomatic. The patients with symptomatic cardiac dysfunction responded rapidly to standard management.[108]

Bevacizumab is a monoclonal antibody that targets the vascular endothelial growth factor receptor. It is thought to exert its effects, at least in part, by inhibiting tumor angiogenesis. The drug received accelerated approval by the U.S. Food and Drug Administration (FDA) for use in the management of metastatic breast cancer in conjunction with paclitaxel. The FDA accelerated approval was based on results from a phase III clinical trial that demonstrated a significant improvement in median progression-free survival (PFS) for patients who received the bevacizumab/paclitaxel combination as compared with paclitaxel monotherapy (PFS 11.3 vs. 5.8 months, respectively; hazard ratio 0.48, $p < .0001$).[109] There was no significant difference in overall survival between the two study arms. The FDA approval, despite the lack of a difference in overall survival and significant toxicity profile, was viewed by many as controversial. Potential serious side effects from the drug include hypertension, proteinuria, bleeding, and arterial thrombotic events. The highest risk of developing arterial thombotic complications has been observed in patients over age 65 years with prior history of arterial events.[110]

N. Other supportive therapies for metastatic breast cancer

N.1. Bisphosphonates

When osseous metastases are present, bisphosphonates, such as zoledronic acid, should be incorporated into the management plan. Bisphosphonates are employed to decrease rates of pathologic fractures, pain, and hypercalcemia. Long-term administration of these drugs has not been associated with significant side effects in older cancer patients.[111] The most common side effects observed in older patients include low-grade fevers, nausea, vomiting, acute and reversible renal dysfunction, and hypocalcemia. Osteonecrosis of the jaw (ONJ) has also been associated with bisphosphonate use. Increasing age does not appear to be an independent risk factor for development of ONJ.[112] Dosing adjustments of bisphosphonates are required in patients with impaired renal function.

O. The frail elderly patient

Frailty is characterized by limited functional reserve and decreased resistance in the presence of stressors.[113] Frailty arises from a generalized decline in the body's physiologic systems that may undermine survival and, in the setting of malignancy, enhance the potential for treatment-related toxicity and complications. For frail patients, particularly those with metastatic disease, the benefits of chemotherapy are often outweighed by the potential toxicities. Hormonal therapy should be considered for women with hormone receptor–positive disease.[114] Endocrine therapies, while much better tolerated, have side effects that could potentially significantly undermine quality of life for individuals with minimal functional reserve. Careful discussions should be had with patients regarding their goals of care. The approach to patient care should be tailored accordingly. For frail patients, particularly those with advanced breast cancer the best supportive care is often a reasonable and preferred option.

References

1. Ries LAG, Melbert D, Krapcho M, et al. SEER cancer statistics review, 1975–2004. SEER Web site. Available at: http://seer.cancer.gov/csr/1975_2004/.

2. Jemal A, Siegel R, Ward E, et al. Cancer statistics, 2008. *CA Cancer J Clin*. 2008;58:71–96.

3. Jemal A, Siegel R, Ward E, et al. Cancer statistics, 2007. *CA Cancer J Clin*. 2007;57:43–66.

4. Diab SG, Clark GM, Osborne CK, et al. Tumor characteristics and clinical outcome of tubular and mucinous breast carcinomas. *J Clin Oncol*. 1999;17:1442–1448.

5. Taylor IW, Musgrove EA, Friedlander ML, et al. The influence of age on the DNA ploidy levels of breast-tumors. *Eur J Cancer Clin Oncol*. 1983;19:623–628.

6. Lyman GH, Lyman S, Balducci L, et al. Age and the risk of breast cancer recurrence. *Cancer Control*. 1996;3:421–427.

7. Honma N, Sakamoto G, Akiyama F, et al. Breast carcinoma in women over the age of 85: distinct histological pattern and androgen, estrogen, and progesterone receptor status. *Histopathology*. 2003;42:120–127.

8. Adami HO, Malker B, Holmberg L, et al. The relation between survival and age at diagnosis in breast cancer. *N Engl J Med*. 1986;315:559–563.

9. Holli K, Isola J. Effect of age on the survival of breast cancer patients. *Eur J Cancer*. 1997;33:425–428.

10. Extermann M, Aapro M, Bernabei R, et al. Use of comprehensive geriatric assessment in older cancer patients: recommendations from the task force on CGA of the International Society of Geriatric Oncology (SIOG). *Crit Rev Oncol Hematol*. 2005;55:241–252.

11. Balducci L. Geriatric oncology. *Crit Rev Oncol Hematol*. 2003;46:211–220.

12. Berry DA, Cirrincione C, Henderson IC, et al. Estrogen-receptor status and outcomes of modern chemotherapy for patients with node-positive breast cancer. *J Am Med Assoc*. 2006;295:1658–1667.

13. Gennari A, Sormani MP, Pronzato P, et al. HER2 status and efficacy of adjuvant anthracyclines in early breast cancer: a pooled analysis of randomized trials. *J Natl Cancer Inst*. 2008;100:14–20.

14. Pritchard KI, Shepherd LE, O'Malley FP, et al. HER2 and responsiveness of breast cancer to adjuvant chemotherapy. *N Engl J Med*. 2006;354:2103–2111.

15. Hayes DF, Thor AD, Dressler LG, et al. HER2 and response to paclitaxel in node-positive breast cancer. *N Engl J Med*. 2007;357:1496–1506.

16. Slamon D, Eiermann W, Robert N, et al. Phase III trial comparing AC-T with AC-TH and with TCH in the adjuvant treatment of HER2 positive early breast cancer patients: second interim efficacy analysis. Paper presented at: 29th Annual SABCS; December 14th-17th 2006; San Antonio, Texas.

17. Pinder MC, Duan Z, Goodwin JS, et al. Congestive heart failure in older women treated with adjuvant anthracycline chemotherapy for breast cancer. *J Clin Oncol*. 2007;25:3808–3815.

18. Hershman DL, McBride RB, Eisenberger A, et al. Doxorubicin, cardiac risk factors, and cardiac toxicity in elderly patients with diffuse B-cell non-Hodgkin's lymphoma. *J Clin Oncol*. 2008;26:3159–3165.

19. Buyse M, Loi S, van't Veer L, et al. Validation and clinical utility of a 70-gene prognostic signature for women with node-negative breast cancer. *J Natl Cancer Inst*. 2006;98:1183–1192.

20. Paik S, Shak S, Tang G, et al. A multigene assay to predict recurrence of tamoxifen-treated, node-negative breast cancer. *N Engl J Med*. 2004;351:2817–2826.

21. Paik S, Tang G, Shak S, et al. Gene expression and benefit of chemotherapy in women with node-negative, estrogen receptor-positive breast cancer. *J Clin Oncol*. 2006;24:3726–3734.

22. Harris L, Fritsche H, Mennel R, et al. American Society of Clinical Oncology 2007 update of recommendations for the use of tumor markers in breast cancer. *J Clin Oncol*. 2007;25:5287–5312.

23. Ravdin PM, Siminoff LA, Davis GJ, et al. Computer program to assist in making decisions about adjuvant therapy for women with early breast cancer. *J Clin Oncol*. 2001;19:980–991.

24. Pierga JY, Girre V, Laurence V, et al. Characteristics and outcome of 1755 operable breast cancers in women over 70 years of age. *Breast*. 2004;13:369–375.

25. Cutuli B, Aristei C, Martin C, et al. Breast-conserving therapy for stage I–II breast cancer in elderly women. *Int J Radiat Oncol Biol Phys*. 2004;60:71–76.

26. Wazer DE, Erban JK, Robert NJ, et al. Breast conservation in elderly women for clinically negative axillary lymph nodes without axillary dissection. *Cancer*. 1994;74:878–883.

27. Yancik R, Ries LG, Yates JW. Breast cancer in aging women: a population-based study of contrasts in stage, surgery, and survival. *Cancer*. 1989;63:976–981.

28. Singletary SE, Shallenberger R, Guinee VF. Breast cancer in the elderly. *Ann Surg*. 1993;218:667–671.

29. Bergman L, Kluck HM, van Leeuwen FE, et al. The influence of age on treatment choice and survival of elderly breast cancer patients in

south-eastern Netherlands: a population-based study. *Eur J Cancer*. 1992;28A:1475–1480.

30. Leung JM, Dzankic S. Relative importance of preoperative health status versus intraoperative factors in predicting postoperative adverse outcomes in geriatric surgical patients. *J Am Geriatr Soc*. 2001;49:1080–1085.

31. Gagner M, Franco D, Vons C, et al. Analysis of morbidity and mortality rates in right hepatectomy with the preoperative APACHE II score. *Surgery*. 1991;110:487–492.

32. Pope D, Ramesh H, Gennari R, et al. Pre-operative assessment of cancer in the elderly (PACE): a comprehensive assessment of underlying characteristics of elderly cancer patients prior to elective surgery. *Surg Oncol*. 2006;15:189–197.

33. Sandison AJ, Gold DM, Wright P, et al. Breast conservation or mastectomy: treatment choice of women aged 70 years and older. *Br J Surg*. 1996;83:994–996.

34. Figueiredo MI, Cullen J, Hwang YT, et al. Breast cancer treatment in older women: does getting what you want improve your long-term body image and mental health? *J Clin Oncol*. 2004;22:4002–4009.

35. Sweeney C, Schmitz KH, Lazovich D, et al. Functional limitations in elderly female cancer survivors. *J Natl Cancer Inst*. 2006;98:521–529.

36. Mano M, Fraser G, McIlroy P, et al. Locally advanced breast cancer in octogenarian women. *Breast Cancer Res Treat*. 2005;89:81–90.

37. Truong PT, Bernstein V, Wai E, et al. Age-related variations in the use of axillary dissection: a survival analysis of 8038 women with T1-ST2 breast cancer. *Int J Radiat Oncol Biol Phys*. 2002;54:794–803.

38. Wazer DE, Schmidt-Ullrich RK, Ruthazer R, et al. The influence of age and extensive intraductal component histology upon breast lumpectomy margin assessment as a predictor of residual tumor. *Int J Radiat Oncol Biol Phys*. 1999;45:885–891.

39. Martelli G, Miceli R, Costa A, et al. Elderly breast cancer patients treated by conservative surgery alone plus adjuvant tamoxifen: fifteen-year results of a prospective study. *Cancer*. 2008;112: 481–488.

40. Mandelblatt JS, Edge SB, Meropol NJ, et al. Sequelae of axillary lymph node dissection in older women with stage 1 and 2 breast cancer. *Cancer*. 2002;95:2445–2454.

41. Gennari R, Rotmensz N, Perego E, et al. Sentinel node biopsy in elderly breast cancer patients. *Surg Oncol*. 2004;13:193–196.

42. Lyman GH, Giuliano AE, Somerfield MR, et al. American Society of Clinical Oncology guideline recommendations for sentinel lymph node biopsy in early-stage breast cancer. *J Clin Oncol*. 2005;23:7703–7720.

43. Hughes KS, Schnaper LA, Berry D, et al. Lumpectomy plus tamoxifen with or without irradiation in women 70 years of age or older with early breast cancer. *N Engl J Med*. 2004;351:971–977.

44. Rudenstam CM, Zahrieh D, Forbes JF, et al. Randomized trial comparing axillary clearance versus no axillary clearance in older patients with breast cancer: first results of International Breast Cancer Study Group Trial 10-93. *J Clin Oncol*. 2006;24:337–344.

45. Vinh-Hung V, Verschraegen C. Breast-conserving surgery with or without radiotherapy: pooled-analysis for risks of ipsilateral breast tumor recurrence and mortality. *J Natl Cancer Inst*. 2004;96:115–121.

46. Deutsch M. Radiotherpay after lumpectomy for breast cancer in very old women. *Am J Clin Oncol*. 2002;25:48–49.

47. Veronesi U, Luini A, Del Vecchio M, et al. Radiotherapy after breast-preserving surgery in women with localized cancer of the breast. *N Engl J Med*. 1993;328:1587–1591.

48. Smith BD, Gross CP, Smith GL, et al. Effectiveness of radiation therapy for older women with early breast cancer. *J Natl Cancer Inst*. 2006;98:681–690.

49. Maher M, Campana F, Mosseri V, et al. Breast cancer in elderly women: a retrospective analysis of combined treatment with tamoxifen and once-weekly irradiation. *Int J Radiat Oncol Biol Phys*. 1995;31:783–789.

50. Ortholan C, Hannoun-Levi JM, Ferrero JM, et al. Long-term results of adjuvant hypofractionated radiotherapy for breast cancer in elderly patients. *Int J Radiat Oncol Biol Phys*. 2005;61:154–162.

51. Courdi A, Ortholan C, Hannoun-Levi JM, et al. Long-term results of hypofractionated radiotherapy and hormonal therapy without surgery for breast cancer in elderly patients. *Radiother Oncol*. 2006;79:156–161.

52. Hannoun-Levi JM, Courdi A, Marsiglia H, et al. Breast cancer in elderly women: is partial breast irradiation a good alternative? *Breast Cancer Res Treat*. 2003;81:243–251.

53. Dunser M, Haussler B, Fuchs H, et al. Tumorectomy plus tamoxifen for the treatment of breast cancer in the elderly. *Eur J Surg Oncol*. 1993;19:529–531.

54. Martelli G, DePalo G, Rossi N, et al. Long-term follow-up of elderly patients with operable breast cancer treated with surgery without axillary dissection plus adjuvant tamoxifen. *Br J Cancer*. 1995;72:1251–1255.

55. Sader C, Ingram D, Hastrich D. Management of breast cancer in the elderly by complete local

excision and tamoxifen alone. *Aust N Z J Surg.* 1999;69:790–793.

56. Geiger AM, Thwin SS, Lash TL, et al. Recurrences and second primary breast cancers in older women with initial early-stage disease. *Cancer.* 2007;109:966–974.

57. Hughes KS, Schnaper LA, Berry D, et al. Lumpectomy plus tamoxifen with or without irradiation in women 70 years of age or older with early breast cancer. *N Eng J Med.* 2004;351:971.

58. Fisher B, Dignam J, Wolmark N, et al. Tamoxifen in treatment of intraductal breast cancer: National Surgical Adjuvant Breast and Bowel Project B-24 randomised controlled trial. *Lancet.* 1999;353:1993–2000.

59. Peyrade F, Frenay M, Etienne MC, et al. Age-related difference in tamoxifen disposition. *Clin Pharmacol Ther.* 1996;59:401–410.

60. Houghton J, George WD, Cuzick J, et al. Radiotherapy and tamoxifen in women with completely excised ductal carcinoma in situ of the breast in the UK, Australia, and New Zealand: randomised controlled trial. *Lancet.* 2003;362:95–102.

61. Abe O, Abe R, Enomoto K, et al. Effects of chemotherapy and hormonal therapy for early breast cancer on recurrence and 15-year survival: an overview of the randomised trials. *Lancet.* 2005;365:1687–1717.

62. Cohen I, Azaria R, Fishman A, et al. Endometrial cancers in postmenopausal breast cancer patients with tamoxifen treatment. *Int J Gynecol Pathol.* 1999;18:304–309.

63. Baum M, Buzdar AU, Cuzick J, et al. Anastrozole alone or in combination with tamoxifen versus tamoxifen alone for adjuvant treatment of postmenopausal women with early breast cancer: first results of the ATAC randomised trial. *Lancet.* 2002;359:2131–2139.

64. Goss PE, Ingle JN, Martino S, et al. A randomized trial of letrozole in postmenopausal women after five years of tamoxifen therapy for early-stage breast cancer. *N Engl J Med.* 2003;349:1793–1802.

65. Coombes RC, Hall E, Gibson LJ, et al. A randomized trial of exemestane after two to three years of tamoxifen therapy in postmenopausal women with primary breast cancer. *N Engl J Med.* 2004;350:1081–1092.

66. Mouridsen H, Keshaviah A, Coates AS, et al. Cardiovascular adverse events during adjuvant endocrine therapy for early breast cancer using letrozole or tamoxifen: safety analysis of BIG 1-98 trial. *J Clin Oncol.* 2007;25:5715–5722.

67. Crivellari D, Sun Z, Coates AS, et al. Letrozole compared with tamoxifen for elderly patients with endocrine-responsive early breast cancer: the BIG 1-98 trial. *J Clin Oncol.* 2008;26:1972–1999.

68. Muss HB, Berry DA, Cirrincione C, et al. Toxicity of older and younger patients treated with adjuvant chemotherapy for node-positive breast cancer: the Cancer and Leukemia Group B Experience. *J Clin Oncol.* 2007;25:3699–3704.

69. Chapman JA, Meng D, Shepherd L, et al. Competing causes of death from a randomized trial of extended adjuvant endocrine therapy for breast cancer. *J Natl Cancer Inst.* 2008;100:252–260.

70. Muss HB, Woolf S, Berry D, et al. Adjuvant chemotherapy in older and younger women with lymph node-positive breast cancer. *J Am Med Assoc.* 2005;293:1073–1081.

71. Muss HB, Berry DA, Cirrincione CT, et al. Adjuvant chemotherapy in older women with early-stage breast cancer. *N Engl J Med.* 2009;360:2055–2065.

72. Fargeot P, Bonneterre J, Roche H, et al. Disease-free survival advantage of weekly epirubicin plus tamoxifen versus tamoxifen alone as adjuvant treatment of operable, node-positive, elderly breast cancer patients: 6-year follow-up results of the French adjuvant study group 08 trial. *J Clin Oncol.* 2004;22:4622–4630.

73. Crivellari D, Bonetti M, Castiglione-Gertsch M, et al. Burdens and benefits of adjuvant cyclophosphamide, methotrexate, and fluorouracil and tamoxifen for elderly patients with breast cancer: the International Breast Cancer Study Groups Trial VII. *J Clin Oncol.* 2000;18:1412–1422.

74. Wils JA, Bliss JM, Marty M, et al. Epirubicin plus tamoxifen versus tamoxifen alone in node-positive postmenopausal patients with breast cancer: a randomized trial of the International Collaborative Cancer Group. *J Clin Oncol.* 1999;17:1988–1998.

75. Fisher B, Dignam J, Wolmark N, et al. Tamoxifen and chemotherapy for lymph node-negative, estrogen receptor-positive breast cancer. *J Natl Cancer Inst.* 1997;89:1673–1682.

76. Clarke M, Coates AS, Darby SC, et al. Adjuvant chemotherapy in oestrogen-receptor-poor breast cancer: patient-level meta-analysis of randomised trials. *Lancet.* 2008;371:29–40.

77. Giordano SH, Duan Z, Kuo YF, et al. Use and outcomes of adjuvant chemotherapy in older women with breast cancer. *J Clin Oncol.* 2006;24:2750–2756.

78. Elkin EB, Hurria A, Mitra N, et al. Adjuvant chemotherapy and survival in older women with hormone receptor-negative breast cancer: assessing outcome in a population-based, observational cohort. *J Clin Oncol.* 2006;24:2757–2764.

79. Extermann M, Balducci L, Lyman GH. What threshold for adjuvant therapy in older breast cancer patients? *J Clin Oncol.* 2000;18:1709–1717.

80. Shayne M, Culakova E, Dale D, et al. A validated risk model for early neutropenic events in older cancer patients receiving systemic chemotherapy. *Proc Am Soc Clin Oncol.* 2007;25:9026.

81. Polychemotherapy for early breast cancer: an overview of the randomized trials. Early Breast Cancer Trialists' Collaborative Group. *Lancet.* 1998;352:930–942.

82. Fisher B, Brown AM, Dimitrov NV, et al. Two months of doxorubicin-cyclophosphamide with and without interval reinduction therapy compared with 6 months of cyclophosphamide, methotrexate, and fluorouracil in positive-node breast cancer patients with tamoxifen-nonresponsive tumors: results from the National Surgical Adjuvant Breast and Bowel Project B-15. *J Clin Oncol.* 1990;8:1483–1496.

83. Doyle JJ, Neugut AI, Jacobson JS, et al. Chemotherapy and cardiotoxicity in older breast cancer patients: a population-based study. *J Clin Oncol.* 2005;23:8597–8605.

84. Lyman GH, Shayne M. Granulocyte colony-stimulating factors: finding the right indication. *Curr Opin Oncol.* 2007;19:299–307.

85. Shayne M, Culakova E, Wolff DA, et al. Dose intensity and hematologic toxicity in older breast cancer patients receiving systemic chemotherapy. *Cancer.* 2009;115:5319–5328.

86. Citron ML, Berry DA, Cirrincione C, et al. Randomized trial of dose-dense versus conventionally scheduled and sequential versus concurrent combination chemotherapy as postoperative adjuvant treatment of node-positive primary breast cancer: first report of intergroup trial C9741/cancer and leukemia group B trial 9741. *J Clin Oncol.* 2003;21:1431–1439.

87. Jones SE, Savin MA, Holmes FA, et al. Phase III trial comparing doxorubicin plus cyclophosphamide with docetaxel plus cyclophosphamide as adjuvant therapy for operable breast cancer. *J Clin Oncol.* 2006;24:5381–5387.

88. Milano MT, Zhang H, Metcalfe SK, et al. Oligometastatic breast cancer treated with curative-intent stereotactic body radiation therapy. *Breast Cancer Res Treat.* 2009; 115:601–608.

89. Greenberg PA, Hortobagyi GN, Smith TL, et al. Long-term follow-up of patients with complete remission following combination chemotherapy for metastatic breast cancer. *J Clin Oncol.* 1996;14:2197–2205.

90. Rapiti E, Verkooijen HM, Vlastos G, et al. Complete excision of primary breast tumor improves survival of patients with metastatic breast cancer at diagnosis. *J Clin Oncol.* 2006;24:2743–2749.

91. Mouridsen H, Chaudri-Ross HA. Efficacy of first-line letrozole versus tamoxifen as a function of age in postmenopausal women with advanced breast cancer. *Oncologist.* 2004;9:497–506.

92. Giovanazzi-Bannon S, Rademaker A, Lai G, et al. Treatment tolerance of elderly cancer patients entered onto phase II clinical trials: an Illinois Cancer Center study. *J Clin Oncol.* 1994;12:2447–2452.

93. Christman K, Muss HB, Case LD, et al. Chemotherapy of metastatic breast cancer in the elderly: the Piedmont Oncology Association experience. *J Am Med Assoc.* 1992;268:57–62.

94. Kimmick GG, Fleming R, Muss HB, et al. Cancer chemotherapy in older adults – a tolerability perspective. *Drugs Aging.* 1997;10:34–49.

95. Booth CM, Clemons M, Dranitsaris G, et al. Chemotherapy-induced nausea and vomiting in breast cancer patients: a prospective observational study. *J Support Oncol.* 2007;5:374–380.

96. Brown WW, Davis BB, Spry LA, et al. Aging and the kidney. *Arch Intern Med.* 1986;146:1790–1796.

97. Anderson S, Brenner BM. Effects of aging on the renal glomerulus. *Am J Med.* 1986;80:435–442.

98. Swedko PJ, Clark HD, Paramsothy K, et al. Serum creatinine is an inadequate screening test for renal failure in elderly patients. *Arch Intern Med.* 2003;163:356–360.

99. Wynne HA, Cope LH, Mutch E, et al. The effect of age upon liver volume and apparent liver blood flow in healthy man. *Hepatology.* 1989;9:297–301.

100. Norris B, Pritchard KI, James K, et al. Phase III comparative study of vinorelbine combined with doxorubicin versus doxorubicin alone in disseminated metastatic/recurrent breast cancer: National Cancer Institute of Canada Clinical Trials Group Study MA8. *J Clin Oncol.* 2000;18:2385–2394.

101. Martin M, Ruiz A, Munoz M, et al. Gemcitabine plus vinorelbine versus vinorelbine monotherapy in patients with metastatic breast cancer previously treated with anthracyclines and taxanes: final results of the phase III Spanish Breast Cancer Research Group (GEICAM) trial. *Lancet Oncol.* 2007;8:219–225.

102. Carrick S, Parker S, Wilcken N, et al. Single agent versus combination chemotherapy for metastatic breast cancer. *Cochrane Database Syst Rev.* 2005;CD003372.

103. O'Shaughnessy J, Miles D, Vukelja S, et al. Superior survival with capecitabine plus docetaxel combination therapy in anthracycline-pretreated patients with advanced breast cancer: phase III trial results. *J Clin Oncol.* 2002;20:2812–2823.

104. Albain KS, Nag SM, Calderillo-Ruiz G, et al. Gemcitabine plus paclitaxel versus paclitaxel monotherapy in patients with metastatic breast cancer and prior anthracycline treatment. *J Clin Oncol.* 2008;26:3950–3957.

105. Keefe DL. Trastuzumab-associated cardiotoxicity. *Cancer.* 2002;95:1592–1600.

106. Seidman AD, Fornier MN, Esteva FJ, et al. Weekly trastuzumab and paclitaxel therapy for metastatic breast cancer with analysis of efficacy by HER2 immunophenotype and gene amplification. *J Clin Oncol.* 2001;19:2587–2595.

107. Geyer CE, Forster J, Lindquist D, et al. Lapatinib plus capecitabine for HER2-positive advanced breast cancer. *N Engl J Med* 2006;355:2733–2743.

108. Perez EA, Byne JA, Isaac W, et al. Cardiac safety experience in 3127 patients (pts) treated with lapatinib [abstract]. *Ann Oncol.* 2006;17(suppl 9):70.

109. Miller K, Wang M, Gralow J, et al. Paclitaxel plus bevacizumab versus paclitaxel alone for metastatic breast cancer. *N Engl J Med.* 2007;357:2666–2676.

110. Scappaticci FA, Skillings JR, Holden SN, et al. Arterial thromboembolic events in patients with metastatic carcinoma treated with chemotherapy and bevacizumab. *J Natl Cancer Inst.* 2007;99:1232–1239.

111. Tralongo P, Repetto L, Di Mari A, et al. Safety of long-term administration of bisphosphonates in elderly cancer patients. *Oncology.* 2004;67:112–116.

112. Wilkinson GS, Kuo YF, Freeman JL, et al. Intravenous bisphosphonate therapy and inflammatory conditions or surgery of the jaw: a population-based analysis. *J Natl Cancer Inst.* 2007;99:1016–1024.

113. Ferrucci L, Guralnik JM, Studenski S, et al. Designing randomized, controlled trials aimed at preventing or delaying functional decline and disability in frail, older persons: a consensus report. *J Am Geriatr Soc.* 2004;52:625–634.

114. Dittus K, Muss HB. Management of the frail elderly with breast cancer. *Oncology.* 2007;21:1727–1734; discussion 1737, 1740.

115. Singletary SE, Allred C, Ashley P, et al. Revision of the American Joint Committee on Cancer staging system for breast cancer. *J Clin Oncol.* 2002;20:3628–3636.

116. Horner MJ, Ries LAG, Krapcho M, et al. SEER cancer statistics review, 1975–2006. SEER Web site. Available at: http://seer.cancer.gov/csr/1975_2006/.

117. Chap LI, Barshy SH, Bassett LW, et al. Breast cancer: natural history and pretreatment assessment. In: Cancer Treatment. Philadelphia: W. B. Saunders; 2001:507.

8

Management of lung cancer in older adults

Suresh S. Ramalingam and Chandra P. Belani

A. Introduction

Lung cancer is the leading cause of cancer-related deaths in the world, with more than a million deaths reported each year.[1] In the United States, approximately 215,000 new cases of lung cancer were diagnosed in the year 2008.[2] Elderly patients (aged 70 years or more) account for about 50 percent of all lung cancers in the United States.[3] Notably, 14 percent of the patients are 80 years of age or older. Because the population older than 65 years constitutes the fastest-growing segment of the United States, the number of cases of lung cancer diagnosed in elderly patients is expected to increase in the near future.[4] Lung cancer presents at an advanced stage in a majority of the patients. Systemic therapy constitutes the mainstay of treatment for advanced-stage disease and is associated with modest survival and quality-of-life benefits.[5] Earlier stages of lung cancer are treated with combined modality treatment that consists of either surgery or radiation with systemic therapy. Though important therapeutic advances have been accomplished in a number of areas of lung cancer, including the development of molecularly targeted agents, the overall 5-year survival rate remains dismal at less than 15 percent.[2]

Non-small-cell lung cancer (NSCLC) accounts for approximately 85 percent of all cases of lung cancer.[6] It includes the histological subtypes adenocarcinoma, squamous cell carcinoma, large-cell carcinoma, and bronchioalveolar carcinoma (BAC). Small-cell lung cancer (SCLC), which is the other major histological type, has decreased in incidence in recent years. The stage distribution and the incidence of various histological subtypes of lung cancer in the elderly are comparable to those in younger patients.[3] Overall, the incidence of adenocarcinoma is increasing, whereas squamous cell tumors have decreased. This is attributed to a change in smoking habits from nonfiltered to filtered cigarettes in the past 4–5 decades. Approximately 85–90 percent of all patients with lung cancer are either current or former smokers.[7] The

biology of lung cancer in never-smokers appears to be different and is associated with a better prognosis compared to smokers. The molecular differences in the tumors of smokers and never-smokers are only beginning to be understood.

Elderly patients are underrepresented in lung cancer studies. A retrospective analysis of all patients entered in clinical trials conducted by the Southwest Oncology Group between the years 1993 and 1996 demonstrated that only 25 percent of the patients were over the age of 65 years, and an even smaller proportion of those were above 70 years.[8] Because aging is associated with changes in body fat, total body water, and renal, hepatic, and bone marrow function, the practical application of data obtained from clinical trials that include a predominantly younger population to the elderly is fraught with risk.[9] Though elderly-specific clinical trials have been conducted in advanced-stage NSCLC, retrospective analysis of outcomes for the elderly subset of patients in randomized clinical trials continue to be used to guide treatment for the older patient population in a variety of settings. A recent analysis of the Surveillance, Epidemiology, and End Results database in the United States noted a lower overall survival for elderly (aged 70 years or older) patients across sex, stages, and histological subtypes.[3] The reasons behind this observation could be the reluctance of the very elderly to receive therapy, use of less aggressive treatment approaches, and the higher prevalence of comorbid illness. These factors underscore the need for developing novel treatment options tailored only for elderly patients.

B. Non-small-cell lung cancer (NSCLC)

The treatment of NSCLC has undergone major changes in recent years. Therapeutic agents that target specific molecular events in the cancer cell and its microenvironment, such as inhibitors of the epidermal growth factor receptor (EGFR) and

Table 8.1 Prospective randomized trials in elderly patients (phase III studies).

Regimen	Median PFS	Median survival	1-year survival
Vinorelbine (N = 76)	Not reported	28 weeks	55%
Best supportive care (N = 78)[10]		21 weeks	41%
		(p = .03)	
Vinorelbine (N = 233)	18 weeks[a]	36 weeks	38%
Gemcitabine (N = 233)	17 weeks[a]	28 weeks	28%
Vinorelbine + gemcitabine	19 weeks[a]	30 weeks	30%
(N = 232)[12]		(p = .93)[b]	
		(p = 0.69)[c]	
Docetaxel (N = 90)	5.5 m	14.3 m	59%
Vinorelbine (N = 92)[11]	3.1 m	9.9 m	37%
	(p < .001)	(p = .138)	
Vinorelbine (N = 99)	2.7 m	5.9 m	33%
Gefitinib (N = 97)[93]	2.9 m	8.0 m	34%
		(HR 0.98)	

[a]Represents median TTP.
[b]Comparison of vinorelbine plus gemcitabine vs. vinorelbine.
[c]Comparison of vinorelbine plus gemcitabine vs. gemcitabine.

the vascular endothelial growth factor–mediated pathway, are currently in routine clinical use. In addition, a number of novel chemotherapeutic agents with a more favorable tolerability profile have been developed in the past 2 decades. There have also been major improvements in supportive care measures that have contributed to the improvements in outcome for NSCLC.

C. Advanced-stage NSCLC

Approximately 50 percent of all patients with lung cancer have either stage IIIB or IV disease. Patients with wet stage IIIB that have a malignant pleural or pericardial effusion have a similar prognosis as those with stage IV disease and are therefore treated along similar lines. A major determinant of outcome with advanced-stage disease is the performance status of the patient. Those with a good performance status (0 or 1 on the Eastern Cooperative Oncology Group [ECOG] Scale) have a better outcome compared to those with a poor performance status. Poor performance status also significantly affects the ability to tolerate various treatment options.

D. Systemic chemotherapy: Monotherapy

The benefit with chemotherapy in elderly patients with advanced NSCLC was established by a randomized phase III study that compared monother-apy with vinorelbine to best supportive care alone (Table 8.1).[10] The primary intent of the study was to compare quality of life (QOL), measured by the European Organization for Research and Treatment of Cancer (EORTC) QLQ-C30 and the EORTC QLQ-LC13 scales. Previously untreated elderly patients with NSCLC with an ECOG performance status of 0–2 were eligible (aged 70 years or older). The median age of the participants was 74 years (range 70–86). Though the planned sample size was 350 patients, the study was stopped after only 161 evaluable patients were enrolled because of slow accrual rate. Despite this, improvements in several symptom scores for patients treated with vinorelbine and a trend toward favorable global and cognitive function were noted. In addition, there was a statistically significant improvement in median survival (29 vs. 22 weeks, p = .04). The objective response rate was 20 percent with vinorelbine. Treatment discontinuation because of severe toxicity was noted in only 5 out of the 71 evaluable patients. This was the first prospective clinical trial that demonstrated a significant but modest benefit with chemotherapy in elderly patients with NSCLC.

The proven efficacy of vinorelbine in this setting led to a phase III study that compared its efficacy to that of single-agent docetaxel, a semisynthetic taxane.[11] Patients with advanced NSCLC, aged over 70 years, were randomized to vinorelbine or docetaxel (60 mg/m^2 every 3 weeks). There was an improvement in response rate and

Table 8.2 Outcomes for combination chemotherapy in elderly patients (selected studies).

Author	Regimen	Response rate	Median survival	1-year survival
Lilenbaum[13]	Carboplatin + paclitaxel (N = 77)	36%	8 m	35%
	Paclitaxel (N = 78)	21%	5.6 m	31%
Langer[15]	Carboplatin + paclitaxel (N = 51)		9.7 m	
	Cisplatin + gemcitabine (N = 63)	25% (all regimens combined)	7.3 m	35% (all regimens combined)
	Cisplatin + docetaxel (N = 58)		7.2 m	
	Cisplatin + paclitaxel (N = 55)	9.7 m	8.8 m	
Belani[21a]	Cisplatin + docetaxel (N = 149)	Not reported	12.6 m	52%
	Carboplatin + docetaxel (N = 118)		9 m	39%
	Cisplatin + vinorelbine (N = 134)		9.9 m	41%
Langer[14]	Cisplatin + paclitaxel (N = 64)	25%	9.2 m	Not reported
	Cisplatin + etoposide (N = 22)	18%	6.3 m	
Ramalingam[20]	Carboplatin + paclitaxel (weekly) (N = 72)	26%	9.1 m	31%
	Carboplatin + paclitaxel (3 weekly) (N = 74)	19%	7.9 m	33%

[a] Elderly defined as those with age ≥65 years.

progression-free survival with docetaxel, though the survival differences did not reach statistical significance (14.3 m vs. 9.9 m, $p = .78$). However, improvement in disease-related symptoms occurred more commonly with docetaxel. Adverse events were similar between the two agents, with the exception of neutropenia, which was more common with docetaxel (83% vs. 69%, $p = .03$). This study established a role for docetaxel as monotherapy for elderly patients with advanced-stage NSCLC.

E. Combination chemotherapy

Combination chemotherapy has not been well studied in the elderly population. The current treatment patterns are largely based on subset analysis of elderly patient data from large randomized clinical trials (Table 8.2). A phase III study randomized elderly (70 years and older) NSCLC patients to treatment with vinorelbine, gemcitabine, or the combination of the two agents.[12] Approximately 230 patients were enrolled in each treatment arm (median age 74). There was no significant difference in the median survival between the three regimens. The response rates were also similar (18%, 16%, and 21%, respectively). The combination arm was associated with a higher degree of myelosuppression and certain nonhematological toxicities such as vomiting, constipation, and fatigue. QOL, assessed at

baseline and at the time of completion of cycle 3 of therapy, also failed to demonstrate differences in functional status or symptom scores between the three treatment regimens. Taken together, the study failed to establish an advantage for a nonplatinum combination for elderly NSCLC patients.

Carboplatin-based regimens, which are commonly used for the treatment of advanced NSCLC in the United States, are well tolerated by elderly patients. The Cancer and Leukemia Group B (CALGB) investigators randomized patients with advanced NSCLC to paclitaxel as monotherapy or in combination with carboplatin.[13] In the pre-specified group of elderly patients (aged 70 years or older), the response rate (36% vs. 21%) and median survival (8 m vs. 5.8 m) were numerically higher for the combination. However, the 1-year survival rate was comparable (35% vs. 31%). The differences in efficacy between monotherapy versus combination therapy were similar between elderly and younger patients. Though toxicity was greater with the combination for the overall population, the age-specific differences were not reported.

Several other groups have reported on outcomes for elderly patients who participated in phase III studies that compared various platinum-based regimens for first-line therapy of advanced-stage NSCLC. The ECOG compared the outcomes for elderly patients (aged 70 years or older) treated in their study that compared cisplatin-etoposide combination to cisplatin-paclitaxel.[14] The elderly group constituted approximately 15 percent of the study population and harbored a higher incidence of cardiac and respiratory comorbid illness. There were no differences in efficacy outcomes between the elderly and younger patients, but certain toxicities, such as leucopenia and neurotoxicity, were more common in the elderly. An elderly subset analysis of the four-arm study conducted by ECOG also reported similar results.[15] In this study, patients with advanced-stage NSCLC were randomized to therapy with cisplatin-docetaxel, cisplatin-gemcitabine, cisplatin-paclitaxel, or carboplatin-paclitaxel.[16] Of the 1,207 patients enrolled, approximately 20 percent were aged 70 years or older. Similar to the overall outcome of the study, the four regimens were associated with comparable efficacy in the elderly. The response rate, median survival, and progression-free survival were also similar between the younger and elderly patients. There was, however, a slightly higher incidence of myelosuppression in the elderly patients.

The combination of carboplatin and paclitaxel, the most commonly used regimen in the United States, appears to have similar toxicity and efficacy between older and younger patients.[17] The subset analysis of a phase III study that compared four cycles of the combination versus continuation of therapy until progression revealed no statistically significant differences in the efficacy and toxicity between patients older or younger than the age of 70 years. Approximately 30 percent of the study participants were 70 years of age or older. Notably, there was no survival advantage with continued administration of chemotherapy beyond four cycles.[18]

In an effort to improve the tolerability profile of paclitaxel, a weekly schedule of administration has been evaluated. In a phase III study, the weekly schedule of paclitaxel was compared to the standard 3-weekly regimen in combination with carboplatin for first-line therapy of advanced NSCLC.[19] There were no differences in survival, though the incidences of arthralgia, myalgia, and neuropathy were lower with the weekly schedule. In a subset analysis of the 31 percent of elderly patients enrolled, the efficacy parameters were similar for the two schedules.[20] However, grade 3 neuropathy was lower (5.5% vs. 9.5%) in the elderly with the weekly schedule, providing a better overall therapeutic index. Taken together, these results support the use of carboplatin and paclitaxel combination in elderly patients with advanced NSCLC.

The combination of docetaxel with a platinum compound has not been tested in prospective studies for elderly patients. In the pivotal phase III study, the combination of cisplatin or carboplatin with docetaxel demonstrated similar efficacy as the reference regimen of cisplatin-vinorelbine for the overall patient population.[21] Analysis of the outcomes for patients aged 65 years or older who participated in the study demonstrated comparable efficacy with outcomes for the younger patients. There was, however, a modest increase in grade 3 toxicities, such as neutropenia, asthenia, infection, and pulmonary toxicity, in the elderly patients. In particular, the use of cisplatin-based regimens was associated with a higher degree of neurosensory toxicity and diarrhea.

Gemcitabine-based doublets also appear to be a reasonable treatment option. In a meta-analysis of studies that compared gemcitabine-based combinations to monotherapy for the elderly subset, the response rate was higher for the combination, though the survival was not superior.[22] There was a higher incidence of grades 3–4 thrombocytopenia with the combination regimens. Taken together, it is rational to treat elderly patients with carboplatin-based doublet regimens, provided they have a good performance status.

Recently, the combination of molecularly targeted agents with platinum-based doublets has emerged as a strategy to improve the outcome for advanced-stage NSCLC. Bevacizumab, a monoclonal antibody against the vascular endothelial growth factor, given in combination with carboplatin and paclitaxel, led to improvement in survival for patients with advanced nonsquamous NSCLC. This regimen was subsequently approved by the U.S. Food and Drug Administration (FDA) for this indication.[23] A subset analysis of the ECOG 4599 study was conducted to evaluate the outcome for elderly patients (Table 8.3).[24] Approximately 26 percent of the study population was aged 70 years or older. There was a trend toward improved response rate and progression-free survival with the addition of bevacizumab to chemotherapy in the elderly but without a survival advantage. Notably, certain toxicities, such as neutropenia, thrombocytopenia, bleeding, proteinuria, and hypertension, were more common among the elderly with the addition of bevacizumab to chemotherapy. A trend toward higher treatment-related deaths was noted for the combination of bevacizumab and chemotherapy in the

Table 8.3 Bevacizumab in combination with chemotherapy for elderly patients.[24]

	Carboplatin, paclitaxel + bevacizumab	Carboplatin, paclitaxel
N	111	113
Response rate (%)	29	17[a]
Median PFS (m)	5.9	4.9
Median survival (m)	11.3	12.1
Fever with Gr 3/4 neutropenia (%)	6.2	0.9[a]
Gr 3/4 proteinuria (%)	7.9	–
Gr 3/4 hypertension (%)	6.2	0.9[a]
Gr 3/4 bleeding (%)	7.9	1.7[a]
Treatment-related deaths	7	2

[a] Statistically significant differences

elderly patients (6.8% vs. 1.8%, $p = .10$). Though this was an unplanned subset analysis, the higher incidence of toxicity calls for greater caution and underscores the need for prospective studies to assess the therapeutic index of the combination of chemotherapy and a targeted agent (three-drug regimens) in the elderly.

F. Second-line therapy

Approximately 60–70 percent of the patients who experience disease progression with first-line therapy are candidates for salvage therapy. Docetaxel, pemetrexed, and erlotinib are all approved as monotherapy for second-line treatment of advanced NSCLC. Docetaxel and pemetrexed are both efficacious in the elderly subset (aged 70 years or older) to the same degree as in younger patients, based on the results of a subset analysis of the phase III randomized study that compared the efficacy of these two agents.[25,26] Recently, the benefit of pemetrexed has been found to be limited to patients with nonsquamous histology. The reasons

behind the higher sensitivity of nonsquamous histological subsets to pemetrexed therapy are under study.

Erlotinib, an inhibitor of the epidermal growth factor receptor pathway (EGFR), improved survival over placebo (median survival 6.7 m vs. 4.7 m) for patients who experienced disease progression following one or two prior regimens for advanced NSCLC.[27] Approximately 23 percent of the patients who participated in this phase III National Cancer Institute of Canada study (NCIC-BR 21) were aged 70 years or older (Table 8.4).[28] There were no differences in overall survival, progression-free survival, and response rate between the elderly and younger patients treated with erlotinib. However, there was an increase in certain adverse events, such as grades 3–4 skin rash (16% vs. 6%), fatigue (7% vs. 2%), and dehydration (4% vs. <1%), and a higher rate of treatment discontinuation in the elderly group (13% vs. 5%). The QOL benefits were similar for the younger and older patients. Thus erlotinib is a reasonable treatment option for elderly patients with advanced-stage NSCLC in the salvage setting. In the past few years, the presence of EGFR gene mutations in the tumor has emerged as a promising predictor of efficacy with EGFR tyrosine kinase inhibitors.[29,30] If such biomarkers are validated for patient selection, the magnitude of benefit with erlotinib will be optimized. It is also important to note that the incidence of mutations varies by region, ethnicity, and smoking status.[29]

Erlotinib has subsequently been tested in a prospective phase II study for elderly patients. Only patients who had not received any prior therapy for advanced NSCLC were included.[31] For the 80 patients in the study, the median survival was 10.9 months, and the disease control rate was 51 percent. Therapy was tolerated well by a majority of the patients. Given this broad efficacy of erlotinib in the first-line setting, it is likely that the benefits would be larger if molecular selection factors were utilized for treatment selection.

Table 8.4 Epidermal growth factor receptor inhibitors in elderly patients.

Regimen	Indication	Response rate	Median survival	1-year survival
Erlotinib[94] ($N = 80$)	First line	10%	10.9 m	46%
Gefitinib[95] ($N = 50$)	First line	25%	10.0 m	50%
Erlotinib[28] ($N = 112$)	Second or third line	8%	7.6 m	Not reported
Placebo ($N = 50$)		–	5.0 m	

Table 8.5 Chemotherapy in early-stage non-small-cell lung cancer: NCIC-BR 10 study.[37]

	Age ≤ 65 years	Age > 65 years
N	327	155
Chemotherapy (N)	165	77
Observation	162	78
Dose intensity		
Cisplatin (mg/m^2/week)	18	14.1
Vinorelbine (mg/m^2/week)	13.2	9.9
Hazard ratio for chemotherapy arm: survival		0.61 (0.38–0.098, $p = .04$)
Hazard ratio for chemotherapy arm: disease-specific survival		0.66 (0.39–1.13, $p = .79$)

G. Early-stage NSCLC: Surgically resectable patients

Only about 20–30 percent of patients with NSCLC present with early-stage disease that is amenable to surgical resection. Even in this subgroup, the presence of comorbid illness precludes surgery in more than one-third of the patients. The stage distribution at the time of diagnosis is similar between the younger and older patients. Overall, the outcomes for surgery and radiation therapy for early-stage disease also appear comparable between the younger and older patients in recent times. In the 1970s, the reported mortality from surgery in elderly patients (aged over 70 years) was more than 25 percent in the immediate postoperative period.[32] Subsequent studies in more recent times have shown the risk to be much lower.[33] Regardless, it is important to select elderly patients for surgery only after careful consideration of performance status, comorbid illness, and pulmonary function. The use of both radiation and surgery in patients over 80 years of age was associated with a slightly inferior outcome in a recent analysis of the Surveillance Epidemiology and End Results (SEER) database.[3] Furthermore, elderly patients who received no therapy for early-stage disease had an inferior outcome compared to a similar group of younger patients.

The use of systemic therapy in the adjuvant therapy setting has resulted in an improvement in the cure rate associated with surgery in patients with stages II and IIIA NSCLC.[34] The 5-year survival rate is improved by approximately 5–15 percent for patients treated with three to four cycles of cisplatin-based chemotherapy.[35,36] This new treatment paradigm calls for careful evaluation of the risk-benefit ratio for the use of cisplatin-based

adjuvant chemotherapy in the elderly population with lung cancer.

The NCIC-BR 10 study compared the use of cisplatin and vinorelbine (four cycles) versus observation following surgical resection for patients with stages IB and II NSCLC.[35] The study comprised a predominantly younger patient population (median age 61 years) and demonstrated a statistically significant improvement in 5-year survival rate with chemotherapy (69% vs. 54%, $p = .03$). Out of the 482 patients in the study, 155 were aged 65 years or older, but only 23 were aged 75 years or older (Table 8.5).[37] The survival benefit with chemotherapy was maintained in the elderly patient group and was similar to that in younger patients. However, the dose intensity and the number of cycles of chemotherapy administered to older patients were lower. No differences were noted in toxicity, hospitalization rate, or treatment-related deaths between the younger and older patient populations. Taken together, this study suggests that adjuvant chemotherapy is safe and beneficial to elderly patients. However, because the number of patients older than 75 years of age was very small, these conclusions cannot be broadly applied to the very elderly age group. Recently, the results of a meta-analysis that reported on the impact of adjuvant chemotherapy in elderly patients were published.[38] Data from patients enrolled in five randomized phase III studies of adjuvant cisplatin-based chemotherapy, including 414 with ages 70 years and older, were reported. The survival benefit in the elderly group was comparable to that in the younger patients. Several important differences in chemotherapy dose and the number of cycles administered between the young and elderly patient groups were noted. For instance, 42 percent of elderly versus only 19 percent of younger patients received less than 175 mg/m^2 of cisplatin, and 42 percent versus 23 percent of patients received two cycles or less of adjuvant chemotherapy, respectively. This finding is of significance because it indicates that almost half the elderly patients were not able to complete the planned course of adjuvant chemotherapy. A trend toward higher toxicity was noted in the elderly but did not reach statistical significance.

Overall, there is limited evidence supporting the use of adjuvant chemotherapy for elderly patients in the routine clinical setting. The implications of adjuvant chemotherapy on physical function, cognition, and survival should all be considered in the decision process. In particular, for patients aged over 75 years, the risk-benefit ratio has not been studied adequately.

H. Combined-modality therapy

The treatment of patients with surgically unresectable stage III disease involves a combined-modality approach that includes radiation therapy and chemotherapy. Several studies have established the superiority of concurrent chemoradiotherapy over the sequential approach.[39–41] The concurrent approach is associated with a higher incidence of toxicities such as esophagitis and pneumonitis. The suitability of the combined-modality approach for elderly patients has only been studied in subset analyses of randomized phase III studies in a post hoc manner. The North Central Cancer Treatment Group (NCCTG) group conducted a randomized study to compare once-daily versus twice-daily (split course) radiation fractions in combination with cisplatin and etoposide for locally advanced NSCLC. Approximately 26 percent of the participants were aged 70 years or older.[42] A higher proportion of elderly patients experienced toxicity of grade 4 or higher severity (81% vs. 61%). The incidences of myelosuppression and pneumonitis were also higher in the elderly group. Despite the differences in toxicity, the 2- and 5-year survival rates were comparable between younger and older patients. Similarly, the CALGB investigators evaluated the outcome for elderly patients who participated in two randomized studies of combined chemotherapy and radiation.[43] The efficacy outcomes were comparable between patients aged 70 years and older and those aged under 70 years. Myelosuppression was more common in the elderly age group, similar to the NCCTG observation. Notably, none of the patients included in these studies were older than 80 years of age.

These results have been substantiated further by the subset analysis of the RTOG 9410 study, which compared sequential chemoradiotherapy to the concurrent approach.[39] Two radiation schedules were tested with concurrent chemotherapy (once daily vs. twice daily). Overall, the study documented the superiority of one-daily radiation with concomitant chemotherapy. The twice-daily approach did not result in overall benefit. Approximately 17 percent of the patients enrolled were older than 70 years of age.[44] In addition to a higher incidence of grade 3 neutropenia, the elderly had a lower treatment completion rate with the twice-daily regimen. The long-term toxicities were similar between the elderly and younger patients. There were no differences in efficacy between the older and younger patients. This analysis concluded that the higher short-term toxicity with concurrent chemoradiation was acceptable in the elderly patients because survival was more favorable with this approach.

In the absence of elderly-specific studies to evaluate the combined modality approach, the current treatment patterns are guided by the data from these subset analyses. Because only the fittest of the elderly patients were enrolled to these phase III studies, the concurrent chemoradiotherapy approach should only be offered to the elderly patients with a good performance status and minimal comorbid illness.

I. Small-cell lung cancer (SCLC)

Small-cell lung cancer (SCLC) is a tobacco-related cancer characterized by an explosive growth rate and exquisite sensitivity to chemotherapy. The survival outcomes for patients with SCLC are generally poor. The incidence of SCLC in the United States continues to decline based on a registry survey and now constitutes about 13 percent of all lung cancer cases, but the burden of the disease remains great because of a steady increase in the absolute number of cases as the population grows.[6,45] There is emerging evidence that the incidence of SCLC in the elderly continues to increase.[45,46] Analysis of the national SEER database between 1988 and 2003 revealed that 42 percent of all cases of SCLC are diagnosed in elderly patients older than 70 years, and about 10 percent of cases occurred in very elderly patients older than 80 years of age.[45] Temporal analysis of the data, however, revealed a 10 percent increase in the proportion of SCLC diagnosed in patients 70 years or older when the decade of 1988–1997 was compared to the succeeding half decade, 1998, and 2003. Furthermore, the proportion of patients aged over 80 years rose by almost 40 percent in the same time period.[45] The treatment of SCLC is dictated by the stage of the disease. For the overall patient population, extensive-stage disease, defined as disease that cannot be confined to one radiation port, is treated with systemic chemotherapy. For patients with limited-stage disease, the combination of radiation and chemotherapy is the preferred approach.

J. Extensive-stage SCLC

The combination of a platinum compound and etoposide for four to six cycles is the standard regimen for the treatment of SCLC. Though there is a small survival advantage with the use of cisplatin-containing regimens based on meta-analyses,[47,48] the favorable toxicity profile of carboplatin-etoposide over cisplatin-etoposide supports its preferential use in elderly patients, in whom it has been extensively studied.[49–51] In a phase II study, elderly patients with predominantly extensive-stage disease received the combination of carboplatin and etoposide. The efficacy data were consistent with other front-line therapy studies with an objective response rate of 60 percent and a 1-year survival rate of 26 percent.[50] The main toxicities were hematologic (grade 4 neutropenia of 31% and grade 4 thrombocytopenia of 12%), and there was no treatment-related renal toxicity. Recently, the results of a phase III trial of cisplatin-etoposide versus carboplatin-etoposide in elderly patients or those with a poor performance score were reported.[52] The median age was 74 years, and 92 percent of all patients were older than 70 years. A very high rate of grade 3 or 4 neutropenia was recorded in both arms (95% and 90%, respectively), but the rate of grade 3 or 4 infection was relatively low (7% and 6%, $p = .78$), a reflection of the use of growth factor support in more than 50 percent of patients in each cohort. The only significant difference in the toxicity profiles of both regimens was the higher rate of thrombocytopenia in the carboplatin arm (56% vs. 16%, $p < .01$). Although mild renal impairment (grade 1 or 2) was 3 times as common with cisplatin as with carboplatin, the clinically relevant grade 3 or 4 renal impairment

was rare in both arms. Despite its limitations, such as the use of potentially suboptimal drug dosages, the study provides valuable information about the efficacy of carboplatin-etoposide combination as an alternative to split-dose cisplatin-etoposide in elderly patients with extensive-stage SCLC.[52]

The combination of cisplatin and irinotecan is used commonly in Japan for extensive-stage SCLC based on a phase III study that demonstrated superior survival over cisplatin-etoposide.[53] However, this regimen was not associated with any advantage over the standard cisplatin-etoposide in the North American patient population.[54,55] The dose-limiting toxicity of diarrhea noted with the cisplatin-irinotecan regimen is another reason not to use this regimen for elderly patients.

K. Salvage therapy

Topotecan, a topoisomerase inhibitor, is the only approved agent for the treatment of relapsed SCLC. It received FDA approval based on a favorable impact in symptom control despite the lack of a survival advantage.[56] Recently, a phase III study compared oral topotecan to best supportive care in patients with poor performance status who were deemed unsuitable for combination chemotherapy. Topotecan administration was tolerated well, with 99 percent of the patients completing more than 90 percent of their prescribed doses. Topotecan therapy was associated with improved survival (13.9 vs. 25.9 weeks, $p < .01$) and better QOL, especially in patients whose disease relapsed shortly (within 60 days) after completion of front-line chemotherapy.[57]

There have been no elderly-specific studies in the salvage therapy setting for SCLC. Because the survival advantage with salvage chemotherapy has not yet been established conclusively, the treatment is primarily meant to achieve qualitative benefits. In the absence of data with topotecan in elderly-specific SCLC studies, it should be offered only to fit elderly patients. The favorable tolerability profile of oral topotecan suggests that this would be a reasonable option for elderly patients.

L. Limited-stage SCLC

A multimodality approach consisting of radiation and platinum-etoposide chemotherapy is the recommended treatment for patients with limited-stage SCLC. The addition of thoracic radiation to platinum-based chemotherapy is associated with an approximately 30 percent increase in disease control in the chest and up to 14 percent reduction in mortality.[58-60] There was a 5.4 percent absolute improvement in 3-year survival, as demonstrated by meta-analyses of randomized studies. From subset analyses, it appears that the benefit is confined to younger patients (aged less than 55 years) with a trend toward an adverse outcome in patients aged more than 70 years.[58]

Further efforts at improving local disease control led to the evaluation of a hyperfractionated radiation schedule dose given as 45 Gy in 1.5 Gy twice daily. This approach was proven superior to conventional fractionation by a randomized study (5-year survival rate of 26% vs. 15%). Approximately 31 percent of patients randomized to the twice-daily radiation therapy were aged 65 years or older.[61] Despite the efficacy advantage, this treatment regimen has not gained a foothold in routine practice in the United States because of toxicity concerns.[62] A retrospective analysis that compared the outcomes between younger and elderly patients enrolled in the intergroup trial, INT 0096, noted adverse outcomes with the split-course regimen in the elderly.[63] For the 13 percent of the participants who were aged over 70 years, a significant increase in severe hematologic and fatal toxicities (84% vs. 61% and 10% vs. 1%, respectively) were observed. Moreover, there was a trend toward inferior overall survival (16% vs. 22%, $p = .05$) for the elderly group.[63] Similar findings were reported from a secondary analysis of the NCCTG trial, also designed to compare one versus two daily fractions of radiation in combination with chemotherapy for limited-stage SCLC patients.[64] Comparison of the elderly cohort to the younger patients showed no significant difference in survival outcome or disease control rate (2-year and 5-year survival rates of 48% vs. 33% and 22% vs. 17%, respectively, $p = .14$), but there was a significantly higher incidence of pneumonitis in the elderly (0% vs. 6%, $p = .008$) and a 10-fold greater treatment-related mortality (0.5% vs. 5.6%, $p = .03$).

Alternative strategies with once-daily therapy to a higher total dose of 70 Gy or twice-daily therapy to a higher dose with planned treatment breaks have been explored in other early-phase clinical trials for limited-stage SCLC, though they have not been tested specifically in elderly patients.[65-67] The potential for treatment breaks and consequent delays in treatment with this regimen in elderly patients is also of concern because the time interval between the initiation and completion of radiotherapy is an important predictor of outcome.[68]

In routine practice, oncologists sometimes use lower doses of chemotherapy in elderly patients to improve the tolerance of treatment regimens. While this seems like a reasonable strategy, it is important to determine if the efficacy is compromised and whether the toxicity profile is improved. Phase II clinical trials that evaluated a reduced number of cycles of chemotherapy and abbreviated radiation therapy have noted modest response rates and survival results.[69,70] In a phase II study, two cycles of chemotherapy (cyclophosphamide, doxorubicin, vincristine [CAV] followed by cisplatin and etoposide) with abbreviated concurrent thoracic irradiation to 30 Gy were given to 55 elderly patients or those with a poor performance status. The objective response rate was 88 percent, and 18 percent of participants were alive at 5 years. Although the toxicity rate was generally low, three patients died of treatment-related toxicity.[69] However, these promising results were not confirmed in larger studies that compared full- and reduced-intensity chemotherapy.[71-73]

Taken together, concurrent chemotherapy and radiation can be administered to fit elderly patients with limited-stage SCLC, with cisplatin as the preferred platinum agent. For patients with multiple comorbid illness, the sequential chemotherapy and radiation approach is a better alternative. The use of twice-daily radiation in elderly patients should be restricted to those with excellent performance status without any major comorbid illness because it is associated with increased treatment-related fatalities in the elderly.

M. Prophylactic cranial irradiation

For patients who achieve excellent response to combined-modality therapy, the brain is a common site of relapse. This prompted the evaluation of PCI to improve the outcome for limited-stage SCLC. Several small prospective studies demonstrated reduced incidence of brain metastasis following PCI but lacked enough power to detect improvement in overall survival.[74-76] This issue was laid to rest by meta-analyses using pooled individual patient data that demonstrated a survival benefit with PCI in patients who achieve complete remission with chemoradiotherapy.[77-79] There was a 54 percent relative risk reduction in the incidence of brain metastasis, which translated into a 5.4 and 8.8 percent absolute improvement in 3-year overall survival and disease-free survival, respectively.[78] The benefit was noted in all age groups, including patients older than 65 years of age. Despite the efficacy benefits, the potential for adverse events associated with PCI, such as memory loss, intellectual degradation, and motor abnormalities, has contributed to the reluctance to administer PCI to elderly patients.[80] A retrospective analysis of registry data in Vancouver, Canada, demonstrated that PCI was offered less often to patients aged over 75 years.[81] Another limitation of the current data is the lack of a standard approach for evaluation of cognitive changes across clinical trials. The prevalence of preexisting neurocognitive impairment in older patients further confounds the ability to study the effects of PCI on cognitive function. In a prospective study that evaluated neuropsychiatric function prior to PCI in 46 patients with SCLC, 80 percent had impaired memory, 38 percent had frontal lobe executive function impairment, and one-third had motor deficits.[82] A larger longitudinal study involving 432 patients with SCLC revealed that a neurologic diagnosis was established in about 65 percent of these patients on long-term follow-up, but about half of these were present at the time of diagnosis before any intervention.[83]

At the time of diagnosis, approximately 18 to 24 percent of patients with SCLC have brain metastasis,[83,84] and up to 70 percent of patients with extensive-stage disease will develop brain metastasis within 2 years of diagnosis compared with 47 percent of patients with limited-stage disease.[85] In spite of this, patients with extensive-stage disease were not considered for PCI because of the generally poor outcome in this setting. However, there is emerging evidence of the utility of PCI in patients with extensive-stage SCLC who experience a good response to chemotherapy.[86] In a phase III study in extensive-stage SCLC, patients with an initial response to four to five cycles of chemotherapy were randomized to PCI or observation only. Interestingly, in addition to a reduction in the incidence of brain metastasis in the PCI arm (17% vs. 41%, $p < .001$), there was a two fold increase in the 1-year survival rate (27% vs. 13%, $p < .003$). The results of this study have led to the use of PCI even for extensive-stage SCLC by a number of physicians. It is to be noted that the study excluded patients aged over 75 years, and the median participant age was 62 years. A careful evaluation of the risk-benefit ratio, with particular focus on cognitive changes with PCI in elderly patients, is necessary before it can be recommended for routine use in elderly patients.

N. Future perspectives

The treatment of lung cancer has undergone some major changes in recent years. The higher proportion and number of elderly patients diagnosed with lung cancer call for an urgent need to evaluate new treatment regimens in elderly-specific or enriched clinical trials. Data obtained from studies that involve predominantly younger patients or the fittest older patients cannot be used for routine practice, particularly with the newer agents. Molecularly targeted agents, which were thought to be selective to the target, were originally anticipated to have minimal effects on normal tissue and thus a favorable toxicity profile. However, it is now clear that these new agents have unique toxicities, such as skin rash, hypertension, hand-foot syndrome, proteinuria, and so on, that all require strong supportive care measures to minimize patient discomfort.

Another major area of investigation should be the use of comprehensive geriatric assessment methods in clinical trials of elderly patients. A number of useful tools that assess the baseline physical function and temporal changes with therapy are available and ready for evaluation in prospective clinical trials.[87–90] Because palliation remains the primary intent of treating patients with advanced-stage lung cancer, to be effective for the treatment of elderly patients new regimens should not only have robust efficacy but should also be associated with minimal detriment to physical and cognitive function. Studies should also evaluate the impact of comorbid illness and concomitant prescription medications on the outcome of anticancer therapies in elderly patients.

The promising results noted with EGFR inhibitors in molecularly selected patients provide a glimpse of the future of lung cancer therapy. Already, prediction of benefit (or lack of) with platinum-based chemotherapy based on markers such as ERCC1 has yielded another new approach.[91] The use of genomic profiling to identify risk of recurrent disease following surgery for early-stage disease has the potential to inform and optimize the use of chemotherapy in the adjuvant therapy setting.[92] In the upcoming era of individualized therapy, it is conceivable that more effective results can be achieved by merely selecting the patients most suited for various treatment options. These new developments hold a great deal of promise. Particularly for elderly patients, we need to be cognizant that we tailor the therapy, taking both risks and benefits into consideration.

References

1. Parkin DM, Bray F, Ferlay J, et al. Global cancer statistics, 2002. *CA Cancer J Clin.* 2005;55:74–108.

2. Jemal A, Siegel R, Ward E, et al. Cancer statistics, 2008. *CA Cancer J Clin.* 2008;58:71–96.

3. Owonikoko TK, Ragin CC, Belani CP, et al. Lung cancer in elderly patients: an analysis of the surveillance, epidemiology, and end results database. *J Clin Oncol.* 2007;25:5570–5577.

4. Edwards BK, Howe HL, Ries LA, et al. Annual report to the nation on the status of cancer, 1973–1999, featuring implications of age and aging on U.S. cancer burden. *Cancer.* 2002;94: 2766–2792.

5. Bunn PA Jr. Chemotherapy for advanced non-small-cell lung cancer: who, what, when, why? *J Clin Oncol.* 2002;20:23S–33S.

6. Govindan R, Page N, Morgensztern D, et al. Changing epidemiology of small-cell lung cancer in the United States over the last 30 years: analysis of the surveillance, epidemiologic, and end results database. *J Clin Oncol.* 2006;24:4539–4544.

7. Wakelee HA, Chang ET, Gomez SL, et al. Lung cancer incidence in never smokers. *J Clin Oncol.* 2007;25:472–478.

8. Hutchins LF, Unger JM, Crowley JJ, et al. Underrepresentation of patients 65 years of age or older in cancer-treatment trials. *N Engl J Med.* 1999;341:2061–2067.

9. McLean AJ, Le Couteur DG. Aging biology and geriatric clinical pharmacology. *Pharmacol Rev.* 2004;56:163–184.

10. Effects of vinorelbine on quality of life and survival of elderly patients with advanced non-small-cell lung cancer.The Elderly Lung Cancer Vinorelbine Italian Study Group. *J Natl Cancer Inst.* 1999;91:66–72.

11. Kudoh S, Takeda K, Nakagawa K, et al. Phase III study of docetaxel compared with vinorelbine in elderly patients with advanced non-small-cell lung cancer: results of the West Japan Thoracic Oncology Group Trial (WJTOG 9904). *J Clin Oncol.* 2006;24:3657–3663.

12. Gridelli C, Perrone F, Gallo C, et al. Chemotherapy for elderly patients with advanced non-small-cell lung cancer: the Multicenter Italian Lung Cancer in the Elderly Study (MILES) phase III randomized trial. *J Natl Cancer Inst.* 2003;95:362–372.

13. Lilenbaum RC, Herndon JE II, List MA, et al. Single-agent versus combination chemotherapy in advanced non-small-cell lung cancer: the cancer and leukemia group B (study 9730). *J Clin Oncol.* 2005;23:190–196.

14. Langer CJ, Manola J, Bernardo P, et al. Cisplatin-based therapy for elderly patients with advanced non-small-cell lung cancer: implications of Eastern Cooperative Oncology Group 5592, a randomized trial. *J Natl Cancer Inst.* 2002;94: 173–181.

15. Langer CJ, Vangel M, Schiller J, et al. Age-specific subanalysis of ECOG 1594: fit elderly patients (70–80 yrs) with NSCL do as well as younger pts (<70 years). *Proc Am Soc Clin Oncol.* 2003;22:639.

16. Schiller JH, Harrington D, Belani CP, et al. Comparison of four chemotherapy regimens for advanced non-small-cell lung cancer. *N Engl J Med.* 2002;346:92–98.

17. Hensing TA, Peterman AH, Schell MJ, et al. The impact of age on toxicity, response rate, quality of life, and survival in patients with advanced, stage IIIB or IV nonsmall cell lung carcinoma treated with carboplatin and paclitaxel. *Cancer.* 2003;98:779–788.

18. Socinski MA, Schell MJ, Peterman A, et al. Phase III trial comparing a defined duration of therapy versus continuous therapy followed by second-line therapy in advanced-stage IIIB/IV non-small-cell lung cancer. *J Clin Oncol.* 2002;20:1335–1343.

19. Belani CP, Ramalingam S, Perry MC, et al. Randomized, phase III study of weekly paclitaxel in combination with carboplatin versus standard every-3-weeks administration of carboplatin and paclitaxel for patients with previously untreated advanced non-small-cell lung cancer. *J Clin Oncol.* 2008;26:468–473.

20. Ramalingam S, Perry MC, La Rocca RV, et al. Comparison of outcomes for elderly patients treated with weekly paclitaxel in combination with carboplatin versus the standard 3-weekly paclitaxel and carboplatin for advanced nonsmall cell lung cancer. *Cancer.* 2008;113:542–546.

21. Belani CP, Fossella F. Elderly subgroup analysis of a randomized phase III study of docetaxel plus platinum combinations versus vinorelbine plus cisplatin for first-line treatment of advanced nonsmall cell lung carcinoma (TAX 326). *Cancer.* 2005;104:2766–2774.

22. Russo A, Rizzo S, Fulfaro F, et al. Gemcitabine-based doublets versus single-agent therapy for elderly patients with advanced nonsmall cell lung cancer: a literature-based meta-analysis. *Cancer.* 2009;115(9):124–131.

23. Sandler A, Gray R, Perry MC, et al. Paclitaxel-carboplatin alone or with bevacizumab for non-small-cell lung cancer. *N Engl J Med.* 2006;355:2542–2550.

24. Ramalingam SS, Dahlberg SE, Langer CJ, et al. Outcomes for elderly, advanced-stage non small-cell lung cancer patients treated with bevacizumab in combination with carboplatin and paclitaxel: analysis of Eastern Cooperative Oncology Group Trial 4599. *J Clin Oncol.* 2008;26:60–65.

25. Weiss GJ, Langer C, Rosell R, et al. Elderly patients benefit from second-line cytotoxic chemotherapy: a subset analysis of a randomized phase III trial of pemetrexed compared with docetaxel in patients with previously treated advanced non-small-cell lung cancer. *J Clin Oncol.* 2006;24:4405–4411.

26. Hanna N, Shepherd FA, Fossella FV, et al. Randomized phase III trial of pemetrexed versus docetaxel in patients with non-small-cell lung cancer previously treated with chemotherapy. *J Clin Oncol.* 2004;22:1589–1597.

27. Shepherd FA, Rodrigues Pereira J, Ciuleanu T, et al. Erlotinib in previously treated non-small-cell lung cancer. *N Engl J Med.* 2005;353:123–132.

28. Wheatley-Price P, Ding K, Seymour L, et al. Erlotinib for advanced non-small-cell lung cancer in the elderly: an analysis of the National Cancer Institute of Canada Clinical Trials Group Study BR.21. *J Clin Oncol.* 2008;26:2350–2357.

29. Paez JG, Janne PA, Lee JC, et al. EGFR mutations in lung cancer: correlation with clinical response to gefitinib therapy. *Science.* 2004;304:1497–1500.

30. Lynch TJ, Bell DW, Sordella R, et al. Activating mutations in the epidermal growth factor receptor underlying responsiveness of non-small-cell lung cancer to gefitinib. *N Engl J Med.* 2004;350:2129–2139.

31. Jackman DM, Yeap BY, Lindeman NI, et al. Phase II clinical trial of chemotherapy-naive patients > or = 70 years of age treated with erlotinib for advanced non-small-cell lung cancer. *J Clin Oncol.* 2007;25:760–766.

32. Evans EW. Resection for bronchial carcinoma in the elderly. *Thorax.* 1973;28:86–88.

33. Ginsberg RJ, Hill LD, Eagan RT, et al. Modern thirty-day operative mortality for surgical resections in lung cancer. *J Thorac Cardiovasc Surg.* 1983;86:654–658.

34. Pignon JP, Tribodet H, Scagliotti GV, et al. Lung adjuvant cisplatin evaluation: a pooled analysis by the LACE Collaborative Group. *J Clin Oncol.* 2008;26:3552–3559.

35. Winton T, Livingston R, Johnson D, et al. Vinorelbine plus cisplatin vs. observation in resected non-small-cell lung cancer. *N Engl J Med.* 2005;352:2589–2597.

36. Douillard JY, Rosell R, De Lena M, et al. Adjuvant vinorelbine plus cisplatin versus observation in patients with completely resected stage IB-IIIA non-small-cell lung cancer (Adjuvant Navelbine International Trialist Association [ANITA]): a randomised controlled trial. *Lancet Oncol.* 2006;7:719–727.

37. Pepe C, Hasan B, Winton TL, et al. Adjuvant vinorelbine and cisplatin in elderly patients: National Cancer Institute of Canada and Intergroup Study JBR.10. *J Clin Oncol.* 2007;25:1553–1561.

38. Fruh M, Rolland E, Pignon JP, et al. Pooled analysis of the effect of age on adjuvant cisplatin-based chemotherapy for completely resected non-small-cell lung cancer. *J Clin Oncol.* 2008;26:3573–3581.

39. Curran W, Scott C, Langer CJ, et al. Phase III comparison of sequential vs concurrent chemoradiation for patients (pts) with unresected stage iii non-small cell lung cancer (NSCLC): Initial report of Radiation Therapy Oncology Group (RTOG) 9410. *Proc Am Soc Clin Oncol.* 2000;19:484a.

40. Furuse K, Fukuoka M, Kawahara M, et al. Phase III study of concurrent versus sequential thoracic radiotherapy in combination with mitomycin, vindesine, and cisplatin in unresectable stage III non-small-cell lung cancer. *J Clin Oncol.* 1999;17:2692–2699.

41. Belani CP, Choy H, Bonomi P, et al. Combined chemoradiotherapy regimens of paclitaxel and carboplatin for locally advanced non-small-cell lung cancer: a randomized phase ii locally advanced multi-modality protocol. *J Clin Oncol.* 2005;23:5853–5.

42. Schild SE, Stella PJ, Geyer SM, et al. The outcome of combined-modality therapy for stage III non-small-cell lung cancer in the elderly. *J Clin Oncol.* 2003;21:3201–3206.

43. Rocha Lima CM, Herndon JE II, Kosty M, et al. Therapy choices among older patients with lung carcinoma: an evaluation of two trials of the Cancer and Leukemia Group B. *Cancer.* 2002;94:181–187.

44. Langer C, Hsu C, Curran W, et al. Elderly patients (pts) with locally advanced non-small cell lung cancer (LA-NSCLC) benefit from combined modality therapy: secondary analysis of Radiation Therapy Oncology Group (RTOG) 94-10 [abstract]. *Proc Am Soc Clin Oncol.* 2002;20:1193.

45. Owonikoko TR, Belani CP, Oton AB, et al. Lung cancer in elderly patients: an analysis of the SEER database. *J Clin Oncol.* 25(35):5570–5577.

46. Gaspar LE, Gay EG, Crawford J, et al. Limited-stage small-cell lung cancer (stages I–III): observations from the National Cancer Data Base. *Clin Lung Cancer.* 2005;6:355–360.

47. Mascaux C, Paesmans M, Berghmans T, et al. A systematic review of the role of etoposide and cisplatin in the chemotherapy of small cell lung cancer with methodology assessment and meta-analysis. *Lung Cancer.* 2000;30:23–36.

48. Pujol JL, Carestia L, Daures JP. Is there a case for cisplatin in the treatment of small-cell lung cancer? A meta-analysis of randomized trials of a cisplatin-containing regimen versus a regimen

without this alkylating agent. *Br J Cancer.* 2000;83: 8–15.

49. Fukuda M, Soda H, Soejima Y, et al. A phase I trial of carboplatin and etoposide for elderly (> or = 75 year-old) patients with small-cell lung cancer. *Cancer Chemother Pharmacol.* 2006;58:601–606.

50. Quoix E, Breton JL, Daniel C, et al. Etoposide phosphate with carboplatin in the treatment of elderly patients with small-cell lung cancer: a phase II study. *Ann Oncol.* 2001;12:957–962.

51. Larive S, Bombaron P, Riou R, et al. Carboplatin-etoposide combination in small cell lung cancer patients older than 70 years: a phase II trial. *Lung Cancer.* 2002;35:1–7.

52. Okamoto H, Watanabe K, Kunikane H, et al. Randomised phase III trial of carboplatin plus etoposide vs split doses of cisplatin plus etoposide in elderly or poor-risk patients with extensive disease small-cell lung cancer: JCOG 9702. *Br J Cancer.* 2007;97:162–169.

53. Noda K, Nishiwaki Y, Kawahara M, et al. Irinotecan plus cisplatin compared with etoposide plus cisplatin for extensive small-cell lung cancer. *N Engl J Med.* 2002;346:85–91.

54. Hanna N, Bunn PA Jr, Langer C, et al. Randomized phase III trial comparing irinotecan/cisplatin with etoposide/cisplatin in patients with previously untreated extensive-stage disease small-cell lung cancer. *J Clin Oncol.* 2006;24:2038–2043.

55. Natale NB, Lara P, Chansky K, et al. S0124: a randomized phase III trial comparing irinotecan/cisplatin (IP) with etoposide/cisplatin (EP) in patients (pts) with previously untreated extensive stage small cell lung cancer (E-SCLC) [abstract]. *J Clin Oncol.* 2008;26:7512.

56. von Pawel J, Schiller JH, Shepherd FA, et al. Topotecan versus cyclophosphamide, doxorubicin, and vincristine for the treatment of recurrent small-cell lung cancer. *J Clin Oncol.* 1999;17:658–667.

57. O'Brien ME, Ciuleanu TE, Tsekov H, et al. Phase III trial comparing supportive care alone with supportive care with oral topotecan in patients with relapsed small-cell lung cancer. *J Clin Oncol.* 2006;24:5441–5447.

58. Pignon JP, Arriagada R, Ihde DC, et al. A meta-analysis of thoracic radiotherapy for small-cell lung cancer. *N Engl J Med.* 1992;327:1618–1624.

59. Arriagada R, Pignon JP, Ihde DC, et al. Effect of thoracic radiotherapy on mortality in limited small cell lung cancer: a meta-analysis of 13 randomized trials among 2,140 patients. *Anticancer Res.* 1994;14:333–335.

60. Warde P, Payne D. Does thoracic irradiation improve survival and local control in limited-stage small-cell carcinoma of the lung? A meta-analysis. *J Clin Oncol.* 1992;10:890–895.

61. Turrisi AT III, Kim K, Blum R, et al. Twice-daily compared with once-daily thoracic radiotherapy in limited small-cell lung cancer treated concurrently with cisplatin and etoposide. *N Engl J Med.* 1999;340:265–271.

62. Movsas B, Moughan J, Komaki R, et al. Radiotherapy patterns of care study in lung carcinoma. *J Clin Oncol.* 2003;21:4553–4559.

63. Yuen AR, Zou G, Turrisi AT, et al. Similar outcome of elderly patients in intergroup trial 0096: cisplatin, etoposide, and thoracic radiotherapy administered once or twice daily in limited stage small cell lung carcinoma. *Cancer.* 2000;89:1953–1960.

64. Schild SE, Stella PJ, Brooks BJ, et al. Results of combined-modality therapy for limited-stage small cell lung carcinoma in the elderly. *Cancer.* 2005;103:2349–2354.

65. Socinski MA, Bogart JA. Limited-stage small-cell lung cancer: the current status of combined-modality therapy. *J Clin Oncol.* 2007;25:4137–4145.

66. Schild SE, Bonner JA, Hillman S, et al. Results of a phase II study of high-dose thoracic radiation therapy with concurrent cisplatin and etoposide in limited-stage small-cell lung cancer (NCCTG 95-20-53). *J Clin Oncol.* 2007;25:3124–3129.

67. Bogart JA, Herndon JE II, Lyss AP, et al. 70 Gy thoracic radiotherapy is feasible concurrent with chemotherapy for limited-stage small-cell lung cancer: analysis of Cancer and Leukemia Group B study 39808. *Int J Radiat Oncol Biol Phys.* 2004;59:460–468.

68. Pijls-Johannesma M, De Ruysscher D, Vansteenkiste J, et al. Timing of chest radiotherapy in patients with limited stage small cell lung cancer: a systematic review and meta-analysis of randomised controlled trials. *Cancer Treat Rev.* 2007;33:461–473.

69. Murray N, Grafton C, Shah A, et al. Abbreviated treatment for elderly, infirm, or noncompliant patients with limited-stage small-cell lung cancer. *J Clin Oncol.* 1998;16:3323–3328.

70. Jeremic B, Shibamoto Y, Acimovic L, et al. Carboplatin, etoposide, and accelerated hyperfractionated radiotherapy for elderly patients with limited small cell lung carcinoma: a phase II study. *Cancer.* 1998;82:836–841.

71. Girling DJ. Comparison of oral etoposide and standard intravenous multidrug chemotherapy for small-cell lung cancer: a stopped multicentre randomised trial. Medical Research Council Lung Cancer Working Party. *Lancet.* 1996;348:563–566.

72. Souhami RL, Spiro SG, Rudd RM, et al. Five-day oral etoposide treatment for advanced small-cell

lung cancer: randomized comparison with intravenous chemotherapy. *J Natl Cancer Inst.* 1997;89:577–580.

73. Ardizzoni A, Favaretto A, Boni L, et al. Platinum-etoposide chemotherapy in elderly patients with small-cell lung cancer: results of a randomized multicenter phase II study assessing attenuated-dose or full-dose with lenograstim prophylaxis – a Forza Operativa Nazionale Italiana Carcinoma Polmonare and Gruppo Studio Tumori Polmonari Veneto (FONICAP-GSTPV) study. *J Clin Oncol.* 2005;23:569–575.

74. Arriagada R, Pignon JP, Laplanche A, et al. Prophylactic cranial irradiation for small-cell lung cancer. *Lancet.* 1997;349:138.

75. Arriagada R, Le Chevalier T, Borie F, et al. Prophylactic cranial irradiation for patients with small-cell lung cancer in complete remission. *J Natl Cancer Inst.* 1995;87:183–190.

76. Gregor A, Cull A, Stephens RJ, et al. Prophylactic cranial irradiation is indicated following complete response to induction therapy in small cell lung cancer: results of a multicentre randomised trial. United Kingdom Coordinating Committee for Cancer Research (UKCCCR) and the European Organization for Research and Treatment of Cancer (EORTC). *Eur J Cancer.* 1997;33:1752–1758.

77. Meert AP, Paesmans M, Berghmans T, et al. Prophylactic cranial irradiation in small cell lung cancer: a systematic review of the literature with meta-analysis. *BMC Cancer.* 2001;1:5.

78. Auperin A, Arriagada R, Pignon JP, et al. Prophylactic cranial irradiation for patients with small-cell lung cancer in complete remission. Prophylactic Cranial Irradiation Overview Collaborative Group. *N Engl J Med.* 1999;341: 476–484.

79. Cranial irradiation for preventing brain metastases of small cell lung cancer in patients in complete remission. *Cochrane Database Syst Rev.* 2000;CD002805.

80. Arriagada R, Le Chevalier T, Riviere A, et al. Patterns of failure after prophylactic cranial irradiation in small-cell lung cancer: analysis of 505 randomized patients. *Ann Oncol.* 2002;13:748–754.

81. Ludbrook JJ, Truong PT, MacNeil MV, et al. Do age and comorbidity impact treatment allocation and outcomes in limited stage small-cell lung cancer? a community-based population analysis. *Int J Radiat Oncol Biol Phys.* 2003;55:1321–1330.

82. Meyers CA, Byrne KS, Komaki R. Cognitive deficits in patients with small cell lung cancer before and after chemotherapy. *Lung Cancer.* 1995;12:231–235.

83. Seute T, Leffers P, ten Velde GP, et al. Neurologic disorders in 432 consecutive patients with small cell lung carcinoma. *Cancer.* 2004;100: 801–806.

84. Seute T, Leffers P, Wilmink JT, et al. Response of asymptomatic brain metastases from small-cell lung cancer to systemic first-line chemotherapy. *J Clin Oncol.* 2006;24:2079–2083.

85. van Oosterhout AG, van de Pol M, ten Velde GP, et al. Neurologic disorders in 203 consecutive patients with small cell lung cancer: results of a longitudinal study. *Cancer.* 1996;77:1434–1441.

86. Slotman B, Faivre-Finn C, Kramer G, et al. Prophylactic cranial irradiation in extensive small-cell lung cancer. *N Engl J Med.* 2007;357:664–672.

87. Fillenbaum GG, Smyer MA. The development, validity, and reliability of the OARS multidimensional functional assessment questionnaire. *J Gerontol.* 1981;36:428–434.

88. Maestu I, Munoz J, Gomez-Aldaravi L, et al. Assessment of functional status, symptoms and comorbidity in elderly patients with advanced non-small-cell lung cancer (NSCLC) treated with gemcitabine and vinorelbine. *Clin Transl Oncol.* 2007;9:99–105.

89. Katz S. Assessing self-maintenance: activities of daily living, mobility, and instrumental activities of daily living. *J Am Geriatr Soc.* 1983;31:721–727.

90. Podsiadlo D, Richardson S. The timed "up & go": a test of basic functional mobility for frail elderly persons. *J Am Geriatr Soc.* 1991;39:142–148.

91. Olaussen KA, Dunant A, Fouret P, et al. DNA repair by ERCC1 in non-small-cell lung cancer and cisplatin-based adjuvant chemotherapy. *N Engl J Med.* 2006;355:983–991.

92. Potti A, Mukherjee S, Petersen R, et al. A genomic strategy to refine prognosis in early-stage non-small-cell lung cancer. *N Engl J Med.* 2006;355:570–580.

93. Crino L, Cappuzzo F, Zatloukal P, et al. Gefitinib versus vinorelbine in chemotherapy-naive elderly patients with advanced non-small-cell lung cancer (INVITE): a randomized, phase II study. *J Clin Oncol.* 2008;26:4253–4260.

94. Jackman DM, Yeap BY, Lindeman NI, et al. Phase II clinical trial of chemotherapy-naive patients >= 70 years of age treated with erlotinib for advanced non-small-cell lung cancer. *J Clin Oncol.* 2007;25;751–753.

95. Ebi N, Semba H, Tokunaga SJ, et al. A phase II trial of gefitinib monotherapy in chemotherapy-naive patients of 75 years or older with advanced non-small cell lung cancer. *J Thorac Oncol.* 2008;3:1166–1171.

9 Management of head and neck cancer in older adults

Julie A. Kish

A. Introduction/incidence

In North America, head and neck cancer, including cancer of the oral cavity, oropharynx, hypopharynx, larynx, nasopharynx, and sinuses, constitutes 3–4 percent of all cancers, with 55,000 new cases expected in 2008.[1] Deaths from head and neck cancers in the United States will approach 12,500 per year, and the peak incidence is between the ages of 50 and 70 years. Suffering with head and neck cancer is universally overwhelming. With life expectancy increasing and thus the population aging, we can anticipate more elderly patients with head and neck cancer. Unfortunately, elderly patients are often treated less aggressively than their younger counterparts. In a retrospective analysis, Bernardi and colleagues noted a lower prevalence of aggressive standard treatment in patients older than 70 years. Aggressive standard treatment would be surgery or surgery combined with radiation or chemoradiation. In an Italian Radiation Oncology Group study, only 30–74 percent of patients aged older than 70 years received aggressive standard treatment, whereas 67–91 percent of patients aged less than 70 years did.[2] Derks and colleagues also noted that only 62 percent of patients aged over 70 years received aggressive standard treatment compared to 89 percent in the 45–60 age group.[3] The management of these patients appears to be biased by chronological age.[4,5,6] The question becomes, are there objective data to support this use of age alone? Does the cancer-specific survival of these patients support this conclusion? Surveillance Epidemiology and End Results (SEER) data in 2,508 cases of cancer of the larynx, tongue, and tonsil show that cancer-specific survival curves for ages 50–69 and over 70 years are superimposable.[2] The influences on outcomes in elderly patients are the same factors that affect younger patients: functional status, comorbidities, and social support. Even accounting for comorbidities, patients over 70 years old still receive standard aggressive care less often.[3]

Treatment choice by the elderly, when corrected for comorbidity, is still substantially influenced by social factors, particularly when more than one modality is involved. Patient preferences must also be considered because many would prefer less toxic treatment therapy even if the outcome is decreased survival.[4] There also may be physician bias against an aggressive approach that includes chemotherapy.

The approach to treatment of head and neck cancer in the elderly should begin with two important assumptions: first, head and neck cancer, unlike many other cancers, will result in the patient's death within a few years while producing extensive physical and emotional morbidity if left untreated. Second, factors that are important in the treatment of younger patients are the same in older patients, with the exception of life expectancy. These include functional performance status, comorbidities, nutritional status, social support systems, and psychological coping skills. The comprehensive geriatric assessment (CGA) can help define patients' limitations and provide objective measures to define therapy.

These caveats basically address issues as noted in the National Comprehensive Cancer Network (NCCN) guidelines for treatment in senior adult oncology.[7]

B. Goals of multimodality treatment

Historically, head and neck cancer treatment has revolved around surgery and radiation. However, chemotherapy has now become an integral part of the head and neck armamentarium and treatment plan. To achieve a level of sophisticated care to include all modalities, a head and neck team approach should exist. The multimodality team should consist of a head and neck oncologic surgeon, a radiation oncologist, a medical oncologist, a head and neck nurse, a social worker, speech and swallowing therapists, a dietician, and if possible, a geriatrician. The oncologic surgeon functions in the staging of patient, determination of resectability, and management of residual disease. The radiation oncologist will design the plan incorporating intensity-modulated radiation therapy (IMRT), hyperfractionation, and possibly various protectors. The medical oncologist is the team quarterback, assessing the patient's ability to handle chemotherapy based on comorbidities and managing chemotherapy-related toxicities. A head and neck oncology nurse is invaluable in maintaining patient access to treatment and coordination of all components of care. The nutritionist is crucial because most patients will lose about 10 percent of their body weight during radiation. The speech and swallowing therapists' role is most important posttreatment. The geriatrician can have varied roles, including performing a geriatric assessment (see Chapter 1), managing comorbidities, and discussing treatment goals and preferences with the oncology team.

This team functions most effectively under the auspices of a tumor board. Once the team is assembled, its goals are as follows:

1. appropriately target intensity of treatment for desired results
2. identify potential and real complicating factors
3. prevent side effects
4. institute supportive care earlier, specifically feeding tubes, nutrition, and social support

C. Workup

To determine the appropriate therapy, accurate staging is crucial. It should include physical exam, formal endoscopy and biopsy, and appropriate radiologic imaging (computed tomography [CT] and positron emission tomography [PET] scans), including CT of the thorax because a high incidence of second primary tumors occurs.[7,8] Nodal disease will predict lifetime risk of distant disease: N_1, 10 percent; N_2, 15 percent; N_3, 30 percent.[9,10]

D. Etiology and molecular markers

In the past, tobacco and alcohol have been the major risk factors associated with head and neck cancers.[10,11] In recent times, human papillomavirus (HPV) has been identified as a risk factor for head and neck cancers. Approximately 25 percent of newly diagnosed squamous cell carcinoma of the head and neck (SCCHN) have HPV DNA. Data on percentage of patients over 70 years old are not yet available. These tend to arise in the oral cavity and pharynx, but not the larynx.[11,12] Among HPV-positive patients, 85–90 percent are HPV 16 positive.[11,12] HPV-positive SCCHN is associated with certain sexual patterns, including multiple partners, oral sex, oral anal contact, and HIV infection.[13] In addition, the HPV-positive tumors tend to have a better prognosis and increased radiosensitivity compared to HPV-negative tumors.[14] The implication of HPV positivity in the senior population is not clear. This needs to be evaluated.

As noted earlier, staging dictates treatment. It is crucial that the patient have the appropriate workup for defining treatment. Head and neck cancer is divided into early-stage disease (stages I and II), nonmetastatic locoregional advanced disease (stages III, IVA,B), and metastatic stage IVC.[15]

Single-modality surgery or radiation is utilized for early disease with curative intent. Chemotherapy alone does not provide curative treatment. It is predominantly used with concurrent radiation, either for unresectable disease and/or organ preservation or as palliative therapy in metastatic disease. All head and neck patients deserve individualized treatment. It is good clinical practice to have these decisions made at a multidisciplinary tumor board, especially in the senior adult population.[15] In addition to curative intent of treatment, functional outcomes related to speech and swallowing weigh heavily. This is clearly of substantial import in older patients who are at potential nutritional risk at baseline and may be psychosocially challenged.

Early-stage disease (stages I–II) is most effectively treated with either surgery or radiation, depending on site. Chemotherapy has no role in early-stage disease (Figure 9.1).[15] Failure rates are very low in stage I, which has a 80–90 percent 5-year survival ratio, whereas in stage II, the 5-year survival is slightly less, at 65–80 percent 5-year overall survival.[16–19]

The majority of head and neck cancer patients (60–80%) present with locally advanced nonmetastatic disease.[1] The crucial decision to be made in this potentially curable group is resectability. The oncologic goal of resectability is removal of all tumor with acceptable morbidity. Unfortunately, there is no standard definition of resectability. It varies with disease site, surgeon,

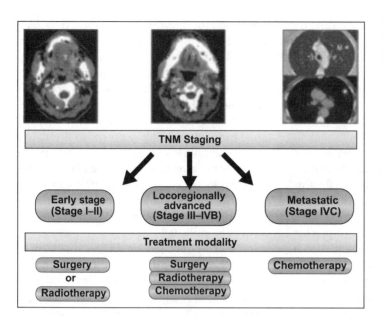

Figure 9.1 Staging of squamous cell carcinoma of the head and neck and general treatment schema. From Choong and Vokes.[15]

institution, and most important, extent of disease (Figure 9.2).

Postoperative radiation is often added to decrease locoregional recurrence. In high-risk patients, the addition of chemotherapy to radiation will also decrease recurrence.[20] Further discussion will be under combined treatment.

Unresectable tumors usually require definitive concurrent chemoradiotherapy. Even in patients who are deemed resectable, organ preservation may be a functionally better choice, and thus chemoradiation is most appropriate for base-of-tongue, larynx, and hypopharyngeal tumors.

E. Combined modality treatment

One of the major advances in treatment of head and neck cancer is the integration of chemotherapy (Figure 9.3), especially in the setting of concurrent radiation. Several randomized phase III

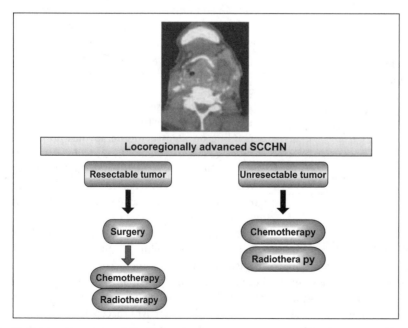

Figure 9.2 Various treatment schema utilized in squamous cell carcinoma of the head and neck therapy. From Choong and Vokes.[15]

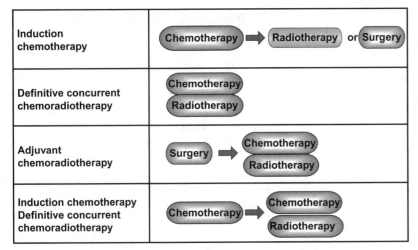

Induction chemotherapy	Chemotherapy ➡ Radiotherapy or Surgery
Definitive concurrent chemoradiotherapy	Chemotherapy / Radiotherapy
Adjuvant chemoradiotherapy	Surgery ➡ Chemotherapy / Radiotherapy
Induction chemotherapy Definitive concurrent chemoradiotherapy	Chemotherapy ➡ Chemotherapy / Radiotherapy

Figure 9.3 Treatment schema for locoregionally advanced squamous cell carcinoma of the head and neck. From Choong and Vokes.[15]

clinical trials have demonstrated improved overall and progression-free survival.[21] These trials have established single-agent high-dose cisplatin and concurrent radiation as standards of care for patients with advanced nasopharyngeal cancer and unresectable head and neck cancer, for organ preservation, and for postoperative adjuvant treatment for patients with high-risk factors.[21]

Concomitant chemoradiotherapy exploits the synergism of two independent treatment modalities, thus producing chemotherapy radiosensitization. Several mechanisms have been postulated to explain this. One is that the chemotherapy decreases tumor repopulation postradiation. Another is that chemotherapy recruits cells into a more radiosensitive state and/or inhibits repair of sublethal radiation damage.[22]

Several chemotherapy drugs have been utilized in this context, including 5-fluorouracil (5-FU) and bleomycin as well as cisplatin. Clearly cisplatin has emerged as the standard chemoradiation arm of all trials. The RTOG phase II data utilizing cisplatin at 100 mg/m² q21 days during radiation in patients with unresectable disease was the impetus for subsequent successful phase III trials.[23] Intergroup 0099 randomized patients with advanced nasopharyngeal cancer to radiation alone versus combined cisplatin and radiation followed by adjuvant cisplatin and 5-FU. This trial demonstrated a highly significant overall progression-free survival advantage and established cisplatin plus radiation followed by cisplatin and 5-FU as standard of care for nasopharyngeal cancer in North America.[24]

Subsequently, an Intergroup trial for unresectable head and neck patients randomized to radiation alone, radiation and cisplatin, or radiation plus cisplatin and 5-FU reached the same conclusion: cisplatin plus radiation improved survival and progression-free survival. The addition of 5-FU only resulted in greater toxicity.[25]

The Intergroup 91-11 laryngeal trial demonstrated similar results for organ/larynx preservation with combined cisplatin and radiation, specifically, substituting chemoradiation for surgery (involving removal of the larynx and postoperative radiation).[26] There has been a meta-analysis of 50 trials of concomitant chemoradiotherapy, and again, an absolute survival advance of 8 percent over 5 years has been noted. This was slightly higher with cisplatin as the sensitizer.[27]

The implications of this standard of care for the older patient are substantial. Patient selection for chemoradiotherapy and provision of adequate supportive care are crucial.[15] The presence of comorbidities clearly affects survival and treatment choice.[28] It has been stated that the survival benefit of chemoradiotherapy decreases with increasing age. However, this is most likely because of death from noncancer causes.[29]

The simultaneous use of two independently toxic treatments will understandably result in greater toxicity than either alone. The supportive care measures require significant interdisciplinary collaboration. Nutrition and hydration are critical. Most patients require the use of a percutaneous endoscopy gastrostomy (PEG) feeding tube to prevent radiation treatment breaks and excessive weight loss and to manage fluids and medications.[30] Aggressive physician and nurse monitoring is most beneficial. It is important to advocate for early – even pretreatment – PEG placement. This allows the patient and family time to become comfortable with usage and avoid treatment delays. However, with these therapies, there is increasing concern about posttreatment dysphagia and PEG tube dependence.[30]

Another scenario utilizing chemoradiotherapy is the postoperative setting for high-risk patients: those with positive margins, two or more positive lymph nodes, or extracapsular extension. Two studies, one from the European Organization for Research and Treatment of Cancer (EORTC) and one from Radiation Therapy Oncology Group (RTOG), utilizing high-dose cisplatin (100 mg/ m^2/q21 days) with radiation showed a survival advantage as well as locoregional control with this approach.[31,32]

The utilization of chemotherapy with postoperative radiation in the elderly requires critical planning because life expectancy is decreased in the over-70 age group and therapy is adjuvant. The standard dose of cisplatin at 100 mg/m^2/q21 days may be too toxic in patients who are aged 70 years or over and have a decreased glomerular filtration rate (GFR) and decreased hearing. It is of utmost importance to calculate the creatinine clearance for all older patients and obtain an audiogram. A normal serum creatinine often may not equal a normal creatinine clearance. Either a dose reduction of cisplatin or substitution of carboplatin can be used. A creatinine clearance of less than 50 mL/min should preclude cisplatin. Weekly carboplatin can be substituted dosed based on target area under the curve. Although advanced age itself is not an exclusion criterion from combined modality postoperative treatment, the lack of objective data from clinical trials because of noninclusion of the elderly makes treatment decision making difficult.[5] It appears that the older fit patient should be offered this treatment, after consideration of life expectancy and comorbidities. An Italian phase II trial of combined postoperative chemoradiation in patients aged 70 years or older demonstrated the feasibility of this approach in older patients. The chemotherapy utilized was carboplatin day 1–5 of weeks 1, 3, and 5.[31] This demonstrates a need for phase III trials utilizing current U.S. standard cisplatin with radiation versus other drugs in older patients. Additionally, guidelines for therapy based on renal function and tolerance are needed.

F. Induction chemotherapy

Chemotherapy in head and neck cancer has historically been relegated to palliative treatment. It is never curative alone, even when a complete response is achieved, because recurrence invariably occurs. Now that combined chemoradiotherapy has emerged as the North American standard for locally advanced head and neck cancer, new interest is being focused on induction chemotherapy as part of sequential treatment. Improvements in locoregional control have been associated with consistent (18–23%) distant disease recurrence rate in four major trials.[25,32–34] This plus the high rate of activity of docetaxol along with platinum and 5-FU has precipitated a resurgence of the assessment of induction chemotherapy.

Organ preservation with induction chemotherapy originated in the 1980s. Jacobs and colleagues utilized chemotherapy followed by radiation alone, reducing the need for laryngectomy.[35] This led to the Veterans Administration (VA) cooperative trial that randomized patients to surgery for laryngeal cancer versus induction chemotherapy, reevaluation, then radiation alone.[36] This study confirmed that organ preservation was feasible for all but T_4 laryngeal patients. Concurrent chemoradiation was evolving at the same time with the Intergroup 91-11 trial.[26] This trial utilized the VA experimental arm, induction chemotherapy (cisplatin and infusional 5-FU) followed by radiation versus radiation alone, versus concurrent cisplatin and radiation versus radiation alone. The concurrent arm showed the best laryngectomy-free survival and local regional control. As a result of this trial, induction chemotherapy followed by radiation alone has fallen out of favor.[15] The Meta-analysis of Chemotherapy in Head and Neck Cancer (MACH-NC) found only 15 induction trials that utilized effective drugs like cisplatin and 5-FU. Pooled data from these trials only demonstrated a 5 percent improvement with the use of chemotherapy on survival.[37]

The taxanes, particularly docetaxol, have substantial activity in head and neck cancer. Two trials, Tax 323 and Tax 324, attempted to exploit taxane effectiveness in an induction trial. Tax 323 was the EORTC 24971 comparing induction with cisplatin and 5-FU (PF) versus Taxotere, cisplatin, and 5-FU (TPF) followed by radiation alone in unresectable patients. No patients were older than 71 years of age. This study showed improvement overall with progression-free survival with TPF but a higher toxic death rate and hematologic toxicities.[38]

Tax 324 randomized both unresectable and organ preservation patients to similar induction regimens followed by chemoradiotherapy. The chemoradiotherapy utilizes carboplatin instead of cisplatin, as is the current standard.[39] The age range of these patients extended beyond 80 years, but there was no analysis to determine tolerability in older patients. Thus, though the TPF regimen can be used safely as an induction regimen in general, its actual role for patients over 70 is unclear, and it has not been compared to a standard chemoradiotherapy of cisplatin and radiation.

Although induction chemotherapy's role in head and neck cancer is unclear, two observations have remained true over the 30 years since its introduction. First, patients who have a complete response to induction chemotherapy have a survival advantage over patients with either partial or no response.[40–42] Second, patients who respond to cisplatin-based chemotherapy subsequently will have an improved response to radiation and ultimately survival.[40] This observation has led investigators Urba and Worden at the University of Michigan to design organ preservation trials based on response to one induction cycle of chemotherapy. A patient with a 50 percent or more response goes on to chemoradiation. Less than 50 percent response leads to surgery.[43,44] Until easily accessible reproducible markers are found and utilized, this may allow for more personalized tailored treatment. This warrants consideration in our senior patients, who, if appropriately selected, might do better with surgery rather than organ preservation and be spared the substantial toxicity (acute and chronic) of combined chemotherapy and radiation.

G. Metastatic disease/recurrent

The incidence of patients presenting at diagnosis with distant metastases is not high and can vary from 2 to 17 percent[45] and is higher in patients with bilateral neck disease. Metastases can be most effectively found with a PET scan.[46,47] Owing to the propensity for SCCHN to metastasize to the lung, PET has a high sensitivity to detect overall metastases, which can significantly alter treatment and, of course, prognosis. Most common sites of metastases are lung, liver, and bone.[45] Skin metastases, particularly stomal mets, are indicators of poor prognosis.[48.] Distant metastatic disease at presentation or recurrence portends poor outcome. Cisplatin-based combination chemotherapy does produce substantial response rates but, to date, no overall improvement in the 6–9 months median survival.[49,50] The taxanes have been utilized and produce significant response rates, as noted in Tax 323, 324,[38,39] but substantial hematologic toxicity may preclude their use in the older patient.

The role of chemotherapy in the older head and neck patient has not been specifically studied. Only a small percentage of elderly patients do participate in clinical trials.[51,52] No studies to date have an elderly patient with head and neck cancer outcome focus. Argiris and colleagues analyzed the outcome of elderly patients in two completed ECOG trials of palliative chemotherapy.[53] These studies utilized cisplatin-based combinations for patients with recurrent and/or metastatic head and neck cancer. Patients aged 70 years and over were analyzed. Fifty-three of 399 eligible patients were aged 70 years and older. The objective response rate (28% vs. 33%) was comparable to younger patients as well as median time to progression (5.3 vs. 8 months). One-year survival was 26 percent versus 33 percent. Differences between age groups were apparent in toxicities, nephrotoxicity, diarrhea, and thrombocytopenia, being more serious in older patients despite comparable antitumor effects.[53] Only 13 percent of patients were older than 70 years in these two large phase III trials. Underrepresentation in clinical trials is a result of multiple factors: comorbidities leading to exclusion, more dependence on others for social and financial support, and a therapeutic nihilism toward the elderly.[54,55] Of particular importance is the decline in GFR and hematopoetic reserve, which probably contributed to the toxicities seen. There is a lack of available pharmacokinetic data in the elderly. We must address these issues prospectively because multiple trials point out that efficacy in young and old is comparable but toxicities vary. The NCCN guidelines are helpful in identifying factors that should influence treatment.[7]

H. Locoregional nonmetastatic recurrence

An area of intense excitement is that of reirradiation and chemotherapy. The standard approach to limited-volume recurrent disease in a previously radiated area is surgical salvage. Nonresectable recurrences in a radiated field have been treated with systemic chemotherapy, which does not cure or improve overall survival.[56] The only potentially curative treatment in these patients is salvage reirradiation along with chemotherapy.[57] This should happen in a center with the reirradiation expertise and skilled head and neck medical oncology.

I. Targeted therapy in squamous cell carcinoma of the head and neck

The epidermal growth factor receptor is highly expressed in SCCHN. When these levels are high, they are associated with a decrease in survival.[58] In 2006, the U.S. Food and Drug Administration (FDA) approved cetuximab (a monoclonal antibody) in conjunction with radiation for locally advanced potentially curable SCCHN and as a single agent for incurable recurrent/metastatic disease.[59] A phase III randomized trial with 424 patients demonstrated an increase in locoregional control from 14.9 months (radiation alone) to 24.4 months (radiation + cetuximab) ($p = .005$). There was also an increase in overall survival from 29.3 to 49 months.[60]

Post hoc analysis noted that oropharyngeal cancer benefited the most, whereas no benefit was seen for hypopharynx or larynx cancer. This study provides proof of principle regarding activity of cetuximab and radiation in SCCHN. This may provide an alternative for patients who are not candidates for high-dose cisplatin with radiation.[59] This could have particular relevance to the older patient. The toxicity is predominantly skin rash, but later toxicities with concomitant radiation are yet to be determined. A phase III randomized trial combining cisplatin, cetuximab, and radiation versus cisplatin and radiation is currently under way in the RTOG.[61] It is important to encourage seniors to participate; unfortunately, they may not meet the renal function requirement. Cetuximab is FDA approved as monotherapy in cisplatin failures with recurrent/metastatic disease. In a phase II trial, the response rate was 12.6 percent with a disease control rate of 46 percent and median duration of response of 6 months.[62] Continuing evaluation of cetuximab is ongoing. This is a viable alternative for the older patient who is cisplatin averse.

J. Quality-of-life toxicity outcomes

The toll of head and neck cancer treatment is enormous, particularly with combined chemotherapy and radiation. The majority of patients with SCCHN will be treated at some point with combined chemotherapy and radiation. Historically, early toxicity was reported as more severe, but the increased efficacy compared to a single modality is the apparent result. Subsequent phase IV trials pointed out that late toxicities, such as swallowing dysfunction, aspiration, and sensorineural hearing loss, seem to be increased with combined cisplatin and radiation, emphasizing the need for baseline audiograms that may predict for patients at high risk.[63,64] Repeat audiograms can be done during treatment if any change in hearing is reported by the patient. So one must ask, has organ preservation gone too far? Have we produced more organ dysfunction? Long-term quality-of-life follow-up may provide the answers.

The burden of long-term treatment-related side effects among cancer survivors, especially head and neck patients, is poorly documented with the newer combined-modality therapy.[63] Of note are swallowing difficulties, PEG tube dependence, aspiration, skin changes, radiation fibrosis, sensorineural hearing loss, dysgeusia, fatigue, and emotional distress. Patients with head and neck cancer are more likely to experience emotional distress than patients with cancer in other anatomic sites.[65] In addition, patients with cancer of the oral cavity, pharynx, and larynx are at higher risk of suicide than patients with lung and stomach cancers.[66]

K. Conclusion

The challenges of treating older patients with SCCHN are many, but there are significant rewards of improved progression-free and overall survival, most important, with combined chemotherapy and radiation. On the basis of currently available data, the following approach is recommended:

1. multimodality team and tumor board
2. proactive supportive care

   a. nutrition
   b. social work
   c. exercise
   d. CGA screening and proactive addressing of problems that may be decompensated by the oncologic treatment or interfere with it

3. vigilant assessment: weekly radiation and medical oncology visits and labs during therapy

4. consistent long-term follow-up every month for the first year, every 2 months the second year, and every 3 months the third year
5. participation in clinical trials, either elder specific or generic head and neck

Elder-specific trials could specifically address the pharmacokinetic issues of older patients. For example, most senior patients will not be able to tolerate 100 mg/m^2 of cisplatin because of renal or hearing impairments. Pharmacokinetic parameters should be established. Evaluation of the long-term effect of decreased dosing is important. Elder-specific clinical trials can develop algorithms for dosing. If the number of older patients is increasing, so should the number of those patients in clinical trials to provide objective data regarding treatment of the elderly with SCCHN.

References

1. Jemal A, Siegel R, Ward E, et al. Cancer statistics, 2008. *CA Cancer J Clin.* 2008;58(2):71–96.

2. Bernardi D, Barzan L, Franchin G, et al. Treatment of head and neck cancer in elderly patients: state of the art and guidelines. *Crit Rev Oncol Hematol.* 2005;53(1):71–80.

3. Derks W, de Leeuw JR, Hordijk GJ, et al. Reasons for non-standard treatment in elderly patients with advanced head and neck cancer. *Eur Arch Otorhinolaryngol.* 2005;262(1):21–26.

4. Yellen SB, Cella DF, Leslie WT. Age and clinical decision making in oncology patients. *J Natl Cancer Inst.* 1994;86(23):1766–1770.

5. Balducci L, Extermann M. Cancer and aging. An evolving panorama. *Hematol Oncol Clin North Am.* 2000;14(1):1–16.

6. Bhattacharyya N. A matched survival analysis for squamous cell carcinoma of the head and neck in the elderly. *Laryngoscope.* 2003;113(2):368–372.

7. National Comprehensive Cancer Network (NCCN) Clinical Practice Guidelines in Oncology™ senior adult oncology V.2.2007. National Comprehensive Cancer Network Web site. Available at: http://www.nccn.org/ professionals/physician_gls/f_guidelines.asp.

8. Greene FL, Page DL, Fleming ID, et al. *AJCC Cancer Staging Manual.* 6th ed. New York: Springer; 2002.

9. Leon X, Quer M, Orus C, et al. Distant metastases in head and neck cancer patients who achieved loco-regional control. *Head Neck.* 2000;22: 680–686.

10. Ellis ER, Mendenhall WM, Rao PV, et al. Does node location affect the incidence of distant metastases in head and neck squamous cell carcinoma? *Int J Radiat Oncol Biol Phys.* 1989;17:293–297.

11. Blot WJ, McLaughlin JK, Winn DM, et al. Smoking and drinking in relation to oral and pharyngeal cancer. *Cancer Res.* 1988;48(11): 3282–3287.

12. Kreimer AR, Clifford GM, Boyle P, et al. Human papillomavirus types in head and neck squamous cell carcinomas worldwide: a systematic review. *Cancer Epidemiol Biomarkers Prev.* 2005;14: 467–475.

13. Kreimer AR, Albert AJ, Daniel R, et al. Oral human papillomavirus infection in adults is associated with sexual behavior and HIV serostatus. *J Infect Dis.* 2004;189(4):686–698.

14. Gillison ML. Human papillomavirus and prognosis of oropharyngeal squamous cell carcinoma: implications for clinical research in head and neck cancers. *J Clin Oncol.* 2006;24(36): 5623–5625.

15. Choong N, Vokes E. Expanding role of the medical oncologist in the management of head and neck cancer. *CA Cancer J Clin.* 2008;58(1): 32–53.

16. Spector JG, Sessions DG, Chao KS, et al. Management of stage II (T2N0M0) glottic carcinoma by radiotherapy and conservation surgery. *Head Neck.* 1999;21:116–123.

17. Spector JG, Sessions DG, Chao KS, et al. Stage I (Tl N0 M0) squamous cell carcinoma of the laryngeal glottis: therapeutic results and voice preservation. *Head Neck.* 1999;21:707–717.

18. Sessions DG, Lenox J, Spector GJ. Supraglottic laryngeal cancer: analysis of treatment results. *Laryngoscope.* 2005;115:1402–1410.

19. Sessions DG, Lenox J, Spector GJ, et al. Analysis of treatment results for base of tongue cancer. *Laryngoscope.* 2003;113:1252–1261.

20. Cooper JS, Pajak TF, Forastiere AA, et al. Postoperative concurrent radiotherapy and chemotherapy for high-risk squamous-cell carcinoma of the head and neck. *N Engl J Med.* 2004;350:1937–1944.

21. Adelstein DJ, Rodriguez CP. Current and emerging standards of concomitant chemoradiotherapy. *Semin Oncol.* 2008;35(3): 211–220.

22. Seiwert TY, Salama JK, Vokes EE. The concurrent chemoradiation paradigm – general principles. *Nat Clin Pract Oncol.* 2007;4(2):86–100.

23. Marcial VA, Pajak TF, Mohiuddin M, et al. Concomitant cisplatin chemotherapy and radiotherapy in advanced mucosal squamous cell carcinoma of the head and neck: long-term results of the Radiation Therapy Oncology Group study 81–17. *Cancer.* 1990;66(9):1861–1868.

24. Al-Sarraf M, LeBlanc M, Giri PG, et al. Chemoradiotherapy versus radiotherapy in patients with advanced nasopharyngeal cancer: phase III randomized Intergroup study 0099. *J Clin Oncol.* 1998;16(4):1310–1317.

25. Adelstein DJ, Li Y, Adams GL, et al. An intergroup phase III comparison of standard radiation therapy and two schedules of concurrent chemoradiotherapy in patients with unresectable squamous cell head and neck cancer. *J Clin Oncol.* 2003;21(1):92–98.

26. Forastiere AA, Goepfert H, Maor M, et al. Concurrent chemotherapy and radiotherapy for organ preservation in advanced laryngeal cancer. *N Engl J Med.* 2003;349(22):2091–2098.

27. Bourhis J, Amand C, Pignon J-P. Update of MACH-NC (Meta-Analysis of Chemotherapy in Head & Neck Cancer) database focused on concomitant chemoradiotherapy [abstract]. *Proc Am Soc Clin Oncol.* 2004;22:14s.

28. Sanabria A, Carvalho AL, Vartanian JG, et al. Comorbidity is a prognostic factor in elderly patients with head and neck cancer. *Ann Surg Oncol.* 2007;14(4):1449–1457.

29. Bourhis J, Maitre A, Pignon J, et al. Impact of age on treatment effect in locally advanced head and neck cancer (HNC): two individual patient data meta-analyses [abstract]. *Proc Am Soc Clin Oncol.* 2006;24(suppl):280s.

30. Mekhail TM, Adelstein DJ, Rybicki LA, et al. Enteral nutrition during the treatment of head and neck carcinoma: is a percutaneous endoscopic gastrostomy tube preferable to a naogastric tube? *Cancer.* 2001;91(9):1785–1790.

31. Airoldi M, Cortesina G, Giordan C, et al. Postoperative adjuvant chemoradiotherapy in older patients with head and neck cancer. *Arch Otolaryngol Head Neck Surg.* 2004;130(2): 161–166.

32. Bernier J, Domenge C, Ozsahin M, et al. European Organization for Research and Treatment of Cancer Trial 22931: Postoperative irradiation with or without concomitant chemotherapy for locally advanced head and neck cancer. *N Engl J Med.* 2004;350(19):1945–1952.

33. Cooper JS, Pajak TF, Forastiere AA, et al. Radiation Therapy Oncology Group 9501/Intergroup: postoperative concurrent radiotherapy and chemotherapy for high-risk squamous-cell carcinoma of the head and neck. *N Engl J Med.* 2004;350(19):1937–1944.

34. Calais G, Alfonsi M, Bardet E, et al. Randomized trial of radiation therapy versus concomitant chemotherapy and radiation therapy for advanced-stage oropharynx carcinoma. *J Natl Cancer Inst.* 1999;91(24):2081–2086.

35. Jacobs C, Goffinet DR, Goffinet L, et al. Chemotherapy as a substitute for surgery in the treatment advanced respectable head and neck cancer: a report from the Northern California Oncology Group. *Cancer.* 1987;60(6):1178–1183.

36. Induction chemotherapy plus radiation compared with surgery plus radiation in patients with advanced laryngeal cancer. The Department of Veterans Affairs Laryngeal Cancer Study Group. *N Engl J Med.* 1991;324(24):1685–1690.

37. Pignon JP, Bourhis J, Domenge C, et al. Chemotherapy added to locoregional treatment for head and neck squamous-cell carcinoma: three meta-analyses of updated individual data. MACH-NC Collaborative Group. Meta-Analysis of Chemotherapy on Head and Neck Cancer. *Lancet.* 2000;355(9208):949–955.

38. Vermorken JB, Remenar E, van Herpen C, et al. EORTC 24971/TAX 323 Study Group Cisplatin, fluorouracil, and docetaxel in unresectable head and neck cancer. *N Engl J Med.* 2007 Oct 25;357(17):1695–1704.

39. Posner MR, Hershock DM, Blajman CR, et al. TAX 324 Study Group. Cisplatin and fluorouracil alone or with docetaxel in head and neck cancer. *N Engl J Med.* 2007 Oct 25;357(17):1705–1715.

40. Ervin TJ, Clark JR, Weichselbaum RR, et al. An analysis of induction and adjuvant chemotherapy in the multidisciplinary treatment of squamous-cell carcinoma of the head and neck. *J Clin Oncol.* 1987;5:10–20.

41. Kies MS, Gordon LI, Hauck WW, et al. Analysis of complete responders after initial treatment with chemotherapy in head and neck cancer. *Otolaryngol Head Neck Surg.* 1985;93:199–205.

42. Rooney M, Kish J, Jacobs J, et al. Improved complete response rate and survival in advanced head and neck cancer after three-course induction therapy with 120-hour 5-FU infusion and cisplatin. *Cancer.* 1985;55:1123–1128.

43. Urba S, Wolf G, Eisbruch A, et al. Single-cycle induction chemotherapy selects patients with advanced laryngeal cancer for combined chemoradiation: a new treatment paradigm. *J Clin Oncol.* 2006;24:593–598.

44. Worden FP, Kumar B, Lee JS, et al. Chemoselection as a strategy for organ preservation in advanced oropharynx cancer: response and survival positively associated with HPV16 copy number. *J Clin Oncol.* 2008;26: 3138–3146

45. Ferlito A, Shaha AR, Silver CE, et al. Incidence and sites of distant metastases from head and neck cancer. *ORL J Otorhinolaryngol Relat Spec.* 2001;63:202–207.

46. Teknos TN, Rosenthal EL, Lee D, et al. Positron emission tomography in the evaluation of stage III and IV head and neck cancer. *Head Neck.* 2001;23:1056–1060.

47. Schwartz DL, Rajendran J, Yueh B, et al. Staging of head and neck squamous cell cancer with extended-field FDG-PET. *Arch Otolaryngol Head Neck Surg.* 2003;129:1173–1178.

48. Pitman KT, Johnson JT. Skin metastases from head and neck squamous cell carcinoma: incidence and impact. *Head Neck.* 1999;21: 560–565.

49. Forastiere AA, Metch B, Schuller DE, et al. Randomized comparison of cisplatin plus fluorouracil and carboplatin plus fluorouracil versus methotrexate in advanced squamous-cell carcinoma of the head and neck: a Southwest Oncology Group study. *J Clin Oncol.* 1992;10(8): 1245–1251.

50. Jacobs C, Lyman G, Velez-Garcia E, et al. A phase III randomized study comparing cisplatin and fluorouracil as single agents and in combination for advanced squamous cell carcinoma of the head and neck. *J Clin Oncol.* 1992;10(2):257–263.

51. Hutchins LF, Unger JM, Crowley JJ, et al. Underrepresentation of patients 65 years of age or older in cancer-treatment trials. *N Engl J Med.* 1999;341(27):2061–2067.

52. Lewis JH, Kilgore ML, Goldman DP, et al. Participation of patients 65 years of age or older in cancer clinical trials. *J Clin Oncol.* 2003;21(7): 1383–1389.

53. Argiris A, Li Y, Murphy BA, et al. Outcome of elderly patients with recurrent or metastatic head and neck cancer treated with cisplatin-based chemotherapy. *J Clin Oncol.* 2004;22(2):262–268.

54. Kornblith AB, Kemeny M, Peterson BL, et al. Cancer and Leukemia Group B: survey of oncologists' perceptions of barriers to accrual of older patients with breast carcinoma to clinical trials. *Cancer.* 2002;95(5):989–996.

55. Trimble EL, Carter CL, Cain D, et al. Representation of older patients in cancer treatment trials. *Cancer.* 1994;74(7 suppl): 2208–2214.

56. Argiris A, Li Y, Forastiere A. Prognostic factors and long-term survivorship in patients with recurrent or metastatic carcinoma of the head and neck. *Cancer.* 2004;101(10):2222–2229.

57. Salama JK, Vokes EE. Concurrent chemotherapy and re-irradiation for locoregionally recurrent head and neck cancer. *Semin Oncol.* 2008;35(3): 251–261.

58. Egloff AM, Grandis JR. Targeting epidermal growth factor receptor and SRC pathways in head and neck cancer. *Semin Oncol.* 2008;35(3): 286–297.

59. Mehra R, Cohen RB, Burtness BA. The role of cetuximab for the treatment of squamous cell carcinoma of the head and neck. *Clin Adv Hematol Oncol.* 2008;6(10):742–750.

60. Mell LK, Weichselbaum RR. More on cetuximab in head and neck cancer. *N Engl J Med.* 2007;357(21):2201–2202; author reply 2202–2203.

61. RTOG 0522; NCT 00265941. U.S. National Institutes of Health Web site. Available at: http://www.clinicaltrials.gov.

62. Vermorken JB, Trigo J, Hitt R, et al. Open-label, uncontrolled, multicenter phase II study to evaluate the efficacy and toxicity of cetuximab as a single agent in patients with recurrent and/or metastatic squamous cell carcinoma of the head and neck who failed to respond to platinum-based therapy. *J Clin Oncol.* 2007;25(16):2171–2177.

63. Bentzen SM, Trotti A. Evaluation of early and late toxicities in chemoradiation trials. *J Clin Oncol.* 2007;25(26):4096–4103.

64. Low WK, Toh ST, Wee J, et al. Sensorineural hearing loss after radiotherapy and chemoradiotherapy: a single, blinded, randomized study. *J Clin Oncol.* 2006;24(12):1904–1909.

65. Haman KL. Psychologic distress and head and neck cancer: part 1 – review of the literature. *J Support Oncol.* 2008;6(4):155–163.

66. Misono S, Weiss NS, Fann JR, et al. Incidence of suicide in persons with cancer. *J Clin Oncol.* 2008;26(29):4731–4738.

10 Management of esophageal and gastric cancer in older adults

Shahzad Siddique and Jimmy Hwang

A. Esophageal cancer

A.1. Epidemiology

Esophageal cancer is a relatively uncommon but extremely lethal malignancy in the United States. It is estimated that 16,470 cases were diagnosed in 2008 (12,970 men and 3,500 women), with 14,280 deaths (11,250 men and 3,030 women).[1] Esophageal cancer is the seventh leading cause of death from cancer among American men, with black men having a higher incidence of disease (10 cases per 100,000 persons).[2,3] The overall 5-year survival rate from 1996 to 2004 for esophageal cancer from 17 Surveillance Epidemiology and End Results (SEER) geographic areas was 15.8 percent.[2] These cancers are more common in the elderly. A review of the SEER database from 2001 to 2005 shows that the median age of diagnosis of esophageal cancer was 69 years, with 32.7 percent of cases in patients over the age of 75 years.[2]

A.2. Pathology

The vast majority of esophageal cancers are classified histologically as squamous cell carcinomas or adenocarcinomas. Historically, squamous cell carcinomas accounted for the majority of the cancers of the esophagus in the United States, but the proportion of adenocarcinomas is increasing, and the latter are now more commonly diagnosed in the United States.[4] Other rare subtypes of esophageal cancers include melanoma, leiomyosarcomas, lymphomas, and carcinoids, but these will not be the topic of discussion in this chapter.[3] Adenocarcinoma of the esophagus occurs more commonly in the distal esophagus and at the gastroesophageal junction. In contrast, squamous cell carcinoma of the esophagus often occurs in the proximal and midesophagus. However, squamous cell carcinoma still predominates among squamous cell carcinomas in other parts of the world such as China, Japan, Russia, Iran, and Turkey.[5]

A.3. Risk factors

The major risk factors for developing adenocarcinomas of the esophagus include gastroesophageal reflux, Barrett's esophagus, and obesity. Barrett's esophagus is an acquired condition that is characterized by the replacement of the stratified squamous epithelium of the distal esophagus with the columnar epithelium most commonly seen in the stomach or intestine. It develops in 5–8 percent of patients with gastroesophageal reflux and is associated with a 40- to 125-fold relative risk of developing cancer.[6] Drugs that relax the lower esophageal sphincter, such as beta-blockers and anticholinergics, and markers for reflux, such as a hiatal hernia and esophageal ulcer, have been linked to an increased risk of the development of adenocarcinoma. A number of studies suggest that *Helicobacter pylori* correlates inversely with the risk of adenocarcinoma of the esophagus.[7]

The major risk factors for squamous cell carcinoma of the esophagus include smoking and alcohol use. The incidence of squamous cell carcinoma is increased by chronic irritation of the esophagus in conditions such as achalasia, lye ingestion, consumption of scalding beverages, and chemical irritants.[3] Exposure to smoking and radiation therapy to the chest or mediastinum are risk factors for both subtypes of cancer.

A.4. Evaluation and staging

The most common presenting symptom for esophageal cancer is dysphagia. Esophageal cancer can present as a polypoid, infiltrating, varicoid, or ulcerated mass initially detected by barium studies or endoscopies done for the evaluation of dysphagia. Endoscopic ultrasound (EUS) and computed tomography (CT) scan of the chest, abdomen, and pelvis are also part of the standard staging procedures. The accuracy of CT scan in diagnosing mediastinal invasion ranges from 59 to 82 percent.[8] EUS using high-frequency probes may be the best method to assess the depth of esophageal wall invasion. The reported accuracy of EUS in detecting local lymph node metastasis ranges from 65 to 80 percent.[9] A positron emission tomography (PET)/CT with fludeoxyglucose F-18 (FDG) is being increasingly used for the initial staging of esophageal cancer, assessment of response after neoadjuvant therapy, and detection of recurrent disease. PET/CT has a sensitivity of 51 percent and a specificity of 84 percent in the detection of nodal metastasis. Although EUS may be superior in the detection of locoregional nodal metastasis with a reported sensitivity up to 80 percent, PET/CT may detect distant metastases that are not identifiable by any other modality.[10] Moreover, FDG-PET has been shown to be superior to CT and EUS in determining postchemoradiation response, and FDG-PET response has been associated with histologic response and improved overall survival in some studies.[11]

The tumor-node-metastasis (TMN) staging system established by the 2002 version of the American Joint Committee on Cancer is used for staging esophageal cancer. The two most important prognostic factors are the depth of tumor invasion and nodal involvement. Therefore T1 lesions invade into the submucosa or lamina propria, T2 lesions penetrate into the muscularis propria, T3 lesions extend to the adventitia, and T4 lesions invade into adjacent structures. N1 disease indicates the presence of nodal metastasis, and M1 disease represents distant metastasis. Once a tumor invades into the submucosa, the likelihood of nodal disease increases to 50 percent.[8] Most patients present with locally advanced disease, and 20–30 percent of patients have distant metastasis on presentation.[10] The most common sites of metastasis include lymph nodes, liver, lung, bone, and peritoneum.

A.5. Treatment-localized disease

Primary surgery

Surgical resection has traditionally been the mainstay of therapy for localized esophageal cancer. The two main surgical approaches for resection are transthoracic esophagectomy (Ivor-Lewis technique) and transhiatal esophagectomy (THE). The transthoracic approach combines a right-sided thoracotomy with laporatomy and allows for a more extended lymph node dissection.[5] The transthoracic approach is associated with a higher perioperative morbidity secondary to cardiopulmonary complications. In a review of 944 THEs from 1998 to 2006, Orringer and colleagues found an in-hospital mortality rate

of 1 percent and a low rate of major complications, including wound infections/dehiscence (3%), atelectasis/pneumonia (2%), intrathoracic hemorrhage (<1%), recurrent laryngeal nerve paralysis (<1%), chylothorax (<1%), and tracheal laceration (<1%).[12] Supporting this finding is another study by Hulscher and colleagues that randomized 220 patients with middle to distal adenocarcinoma of the esophagus or adenocarcinoma of the gastric cardia to either THE or extended transthoracic resection. The median age was 69 years in the transhiatal esophagectomy arm ($N = 106$) with a range of 23–70 and the median age was 64 years in the THE arm ($N = 114$) with a range of 35–78. After a median follow-up of 4.7 years, there were no statistically significant differences between overall, disease-free, or quality-adjusted survival. However, THE was associated with lower morbidity, and there was a trend toward improved long-term survival at 5 years with extended transthoracic approach.[13] These data are applicable only in a patient population deemed healthy enough to undergo thoracic surgery, however.

Esophageal resection has not been extensively studied in an exclusively elderly population. The available data are limited to retrospective reviews and limited case series. Karl and colleagues reported a series of 18 patients who were aged 70 years or over and underwent esophagectomy mostly by the Ivor-Lewis technique and compared outcomes to 30 patients under the age of 70 at the same institution. Even though complication rates were higher in the group of patients aged 70 years or older, the difference was not statistically significant (30% vs. 22%, $p > .05$). The median survival was also not statistically different (28.6 vs. 28.4 months).[14] Another series examined 1,000 patients with esophageal cancer who underwent esophagectomy between 1964 and 2006. Outcomes were compared between patients in group 1 who were 75 and older ($n = 107$) and patients in group 2 who were younger than 75 ($n = 893$). Patients in group 1 were noted to have a higher rate of pulmonary complications but similar 5-year overall survivals (OS 20 vs. 31%, $p = .15$). The 30-day mortality rate for patients in group 1 over three consecutive time periods was 6.2 percent (1964–1980), 5.2 percent (1981–1983), and 0 percent (1993–2006).[15] The general conclusion from both series is that esophagectomy is a safe and effective procedure in elderly patients, though perhaps with more complications than a younger population.

Primary radiation therapy

The use of definitive radiation therapy alone for the primary treatment of esophageal cancer is limited to patients whose general condition prohibits surgical therapy or concurrent chemotherapy and radiation therapy (CRT). The advantage of primary radiation therapy is a lower morbidity compared to surgical therapy or CRT. Radiation therapy may not be as effective in the palliation of dysphagia or odynophagia as surgery and can lead to serious complications such as the development of tracheoesophageal fistulas.[5] In a review of 101 patients with a median age of 69 (range 39–86) with esophageal cancer treated with primary radiation therapy, the 3- and 5-year survival rates were 27 percent and 21 percent, respectively. The dosage of radiation used ranged from 45 to 52.5 Gy in 15 or 16 fractions delivered over 3 weeks. Therapy was well tolerated, but 5 of 20 patients surviving over 3 years developed esophageal stenosis. Interestingly, patients with adenocarcinomas had better survival.[16]

Primary chemoradiation

CRT may allow for long-term survival without the use of surgery. The Radiation Therapy Oncology Group (RTOG) 85-01 trial compared definitive radiation therapy (6,400 cGy) in 62 patients to lower-dose radiation therapy (5,000 cGy) combined with four cycles of cisplatin and 5-fluorouracil (5-FU) in 61 patients. Despite higher toxicity, such as myelosuppression, nausea, and vomiting, the overall survival was 26 percent in the combined modality arm after 5 years of follow-up compared to 0 percent in the radiation-only arm.[17] Thus CRT represents a standard therapy in the treatment of localized or locally advanced esophageal cancer. Attempts to improve the outcomes with CRT have not proven successful. The Intergroup 0123 trial attempted to increase the dose of radiation in the combined-modality arm to 6,480 cGy without an increase in efficacy.[18] Other clinical trials have looked at the combination of paclitaxel with radiation or cisplatin and irinotecan without any direct randomized comparisons to cisplatin and 5-FU-based CRT.[19,20]

There are no prospective randomized studies of CRT in elderly patients, though small retrospective analyses have been reported. A French single-institution study retrospectively reviewed all 109 patients older than 70 who underwent CRT, mostly with cisplatin and 5-FU. About one-third (38.5%) completed therapy as planned. About 26 percent of patients had severe or life-threatening toxicities, and overall, 30 percent required a dose reduction because of toxicities. A clinical complete response was reported in 57.8 percent of patients. The median survival in the patient population was 15.2 months, with 12.8 percent alive at 5 years.[21] Another study retrospectively reviewed treatment outcomes in 33 patients over the age of 71 and compared them to outcomes in 145 patients under the age of 70 treated with definitive CRT. The complete response rate was similar between the two groups (63.6% vs. 63.4%, respectively), but recurrence after an initial complete remission was higher in the elderly patients. There was also a significantly inferior overall survival rate in the elderly group (14.7 vs. 35.1 months, $p = .01$). The reason for this was uncertain, but elderly patients were more likely to discontinue therapy and have severe hematologic toxicities.[22] Taken together, these data suggest that CRT can be administered successfully and effectively to elderly patients but should be administered with close monitoring because of potential toxicities, especially hematologic.

Preoperative and perioperative chemotherapy

Studies evaluating the use of perioperative cisplatin and 5-FU compared to surgery alone have shown conflicting results. The Intergroup 113 trial in the United States randomized 440 patients to surgery alone or three cycles of cisplatin and infusional 5-FU followed by surgery and two additional adjuvant cycles of chemotherapy. There was no significant difference in survival in the two groups, with a median survival in the chemotherapy arm of 16.1 months compared to 14.9 months in the surgical arm.[23] However, the Medical Research Council randomized 802 British patients with esophageal cancer to surgery alone or two cycles of cisplatin and 5-FU, followed by surgery. The outcomes were better in the chemotherapy arm, with a median survival of 16.8 months compared to 13.3 months in the arm using surgery alone.[24] The Medical Research Council Adjuvant Gastric Infusional Chemotherapy (MAGIC) trial randomly assigned patients with potentially resectable adenocarcinomas of the stomach, esophagogastric junction, and lower esophagus to surgery alone or surgery combined with perioperative epirubicin, cisplatin, and infusional 5-FU (ECF). Thirty-seven patients (14.8%) in the perioperative chemotherapy group and 36

(14.2%) patients in the surgery-only group had esophageal cancer. Nevertheless, the use of perioperative ECF was associated with an improvement in 5-year survival (36% vs. 23%) and superior progression-free survival (hazard ratio for progression 0.66).[25] A meta-analysis that analyzed eight studies comparing neoadjuvant chemotherapy versus surgery alone ($n = 1{,}724$) found a 2-year absolute survival benefit of 7 percent.[26] However, few data are available in elderly patients assessing the efficacy of this approach.

Preoperative CRT

This approach toward the treatment of localized esophageal cancer is widely used in North America. A number of randomized trials have evaluated the use of neoadjuvant CRT in esophageal cancer with mixed results. Bosset and colleagues conducted a trial with 282 patients randomized to surgery alone or neoadjuvant CRT with cisplatin in patients with resectable squamous cell carcinoma of the esophagus. After a median follow-up of 55.2 months, there was no significant difference in overall survival, with a median survival of 18.6 months for both groups. The group treated with neoadjuvant CRT had a longer disease-free survival, a lower rate of cancer-related deaths, and a higher frequency of curative resection but a higher rate of postoperative death.[27] An Australian study randomized 128 patients with resectable esophageal cancer to surgery or neoadjuvant CRT with cisplatin and infusional 5-FU. There was no significant difference between the two groups in overall or progression-free survival. The combined-modality therapy group had a higher rate of complete resection and lower rates of positive lymph nodes.[28] A study reported by Walsh and colleagues randomized 58 patients to multimodality therapy and 55 patients to surgery. This was the only study evaluating only patients with adenocarcinomas. The patients in the multimodality arm were treated with neoadjuvant CRT with cisplatin and 5-FU. In contrast to the other studies, there was a significant difference in overall survival favoring the multimodality arm (16 vs. 11 months).[29] A meta-analysis that evaluated 10 randomized studies with 1,209 patients comparing CRT and surgery to surgery alone found a 13 percent absolute difference in survival at 2 years favoring combination therapy.[26] Given the prognosis of esophageal adenocarcinomas, preoperative CRT is often employed in this disease.

Trimodality therapy is not commonly used in the elderly population because of concerns about its toxicity. In a study that evaluated the use of multimodality therapy in 695 veterans with operable esophageal cancer, 161 patients (23%) were treated with induction CRT followed by surgery. The median age for patients selected for multimodality therapy was 60.8 years, and the median age for patients treated with surgery alone was 65.6 years. The median survival was 15.2 months, with no effect on survival by the type of treatment used. However, favorable prognostic factors included younger age, a distal esophageal tumor, and the absence of metastatic disease. There was no significant increase in perioperative mortality (13.7%) in the trimodality group.[30] Moreover, an analysis of a SEER-Medicare cohort from 1992 to 2002 of 2,626 patients aged 65 years and older suggested that patients who underwent CRT and surgery – only 7 percent of the population – had similar postoperative mortality and morbidity as those undergoing surgery alone (30% of the population).[31] As a result, preoperative CRT may be a consideration in selected elderly patients with excellent functional status.

A.6. Treatment-metastatic disease

Metastatic esophageal cancer is incurable and has a median survival ranging from 4 to 10 months. Chemotherapy is used for palliative purposes and can lead to improvement in quality of life and dysphagia in 60–80 percent of patients.[32] Chemotherapy can be used as a single agent or as a cisplatin-based combination. Agents with reports of activity include bleomycin, mitomycin, vindesine, methrotrexate, cisplatin, 5-FU, paclitaxel, docetaxel, irinotecan, etoposide, and vinorelbine. Single-agent response rates range from 15 to 30 percent, with higher responses in newer agents such as vinorelbine and taxanes.[32,33] Combination chemotherapy, traditionally with infusional 5-FU and cisplatin, has reported response rates ranging from 25 to 50 percent.[34–36] Other reported active combinations include cisplatin-irinotecan and gemcitabine-cisplatin.[34,36] More recent studies have focused on triplet combinations, including ECF, epirubicin-cisplatin-capecitabine (ECX), epirubicin-oxaliplatin-capecitabine (EOX), epirubicin-oxaliplatin-5-FU (EOF), and docetaxel-cisplatin-5-FU (DCF). These combinations are associated with response rates ranging from 29 to 47 percent and median survival ranging from 8.1 to 11.2 months.[37,38] Cunningham and colleagues randomized 1,002 patients with advanced esophageal cancer in a study with a 2 × 2 factorial design to chemotherapy with ECF, ECX, EOF, or EOX. The substitution of capecitabine-oxaliplatin for 5-FU-cisplatin allowed for easier administration and less toxicity. The regimens containing oxaliplatin and capecitabine were found to be noninferior in terms of overall survival compared to the other regimens.[37] Combination chemotherapy regimens led to higher response at the expense of higher toxicity.

The role of chemotherapy in the treatment of elderly patients with metastatic esophageal cancer was addressed by a pooled analysis of eight consecutive North Central Cancer Treatment Group trials. The study included 367 patients and compared treatment outcomes between 152 (42%) patients older than age 64 to 213 patients younger than age 64. The median survival was similar between the two groups (6 and 6.7 months, respectively), and progression-free survival was 3.3 months for both groups. The rates of severe hematologic and nonhematologic toxicities were higher among the elderly patients.[39] A British study evaluated the effects and tolerability of chemotherapy in elderly patients through a pooled analysis of three clinical trials. The trials contained 1,080 patients, of which 257 (23.8%) were over the age of 69. Patients were treated with a cisplatin-containing combination such as ECF/MCF (mitomycin C, cisplatin, and infusional 5-FU), protracted infusional 5-FU with or without mitomycin C, or FAMTX (methotrexate, 5-FU, and doxorubicin). There were no significant differences between toxicity, objective response rates, symptomatic response rates, failure-free survival, or overall survival. Independent prognostic factors for survival included performance status and locally advanced disease.[40] Thus the available data suggest that chemotherapy should be considered in elderly patients with metastatic esophageal cancer as they seem to derive similar benefits as the overall population.

A.7. Treatment-palliative measures

Beyond chemotherapy, a number of interventions can be employed for the palliation of dysphagia in the setting of esophageal cancer, including stents, laser ablation, and photodynamic therapy. These techniques are often employed in patients who are not suitable candidates for surgery, chemotherapy, or CRT. Self-expanding metallic stents are easy to deploy and have been shown to provide effective intermediate-term palliation of dysphagia. The main complications include stent migra-

tion and severe reflux in stents that extend beyond the gastroesophageal junction.[41-43] In addition, solid foods cannot typically be eaten, though pureed foods and liquids are often well tolerated. Laser therapy can be used to debulk endoscopically accessible tumor but often requires multiple treatments. The major limitations include the expense of therapy and limited long-term efficacy. Long-term efficacy of laser therapy can be augmented with the use of brachytherapy.[41,44] Photodynamic therapy (PDT) is an endoscopic procedure that uses light to activate photosensitizing compounds incorporated into tissue. The light absorbed by the photosensitizer results in tumor destruction via oxidative damage. PDT has been studied in the treatment of high-grade dysplasia and for the palliation of dysphagia in patients with advanced disease with obstruction.[45,46]

A.8. Treatment conclusion

Esophageal cancer is diagnosed commonly in elderly patients. The typical treatment for esophageal cancer often incorporates multimodality therapy, including chemotherapy, radiation, and/or surgery. Data for the treatment of elderly patients are limited to retrospective reviews or pooled analysis across multiple trials. These studies suggest that elderly patients with good performance status and limited comorbidities can often be treated like their younger counterparts, with similar outcomes. However, some studies have also shown that elderly patients have higher toxicities.

B. Gastric cancer

B.1. Epidemiology

Gastric cancer is one of the leading causes of cancer-related death worldwide. Gastric cancer exhibits remarkable geographic variation, with a majority of cases arising in Japan, eastern Asia, South America, and eastern Europe. The incidence rates are lowest in western Europe and North America. The prevalence of gastric cancer in Japan is about 8 times higher than in the United States.[47,48] The incidence rates of gastric cancer are highest in Asian/Pacific Islanders, blacks, and American Indian/Alaska Natives. The American Cancer Society estimates that there will be 21,500 new cases of gastric cancer in the United States in 2008, and 10,880 deaths.[1] Both globally and in the United States, there has been a general overall decrease of both incidence and mortality rates for gastric cancer, despite a marked increase in the incidence of tumors of the gastroesophageal junction and gastric cardia.[49] The median age of diagnosis for cancer of the stomach was 71 years from 2001 to 2005, with 39.9 percent of cases occurring in patients over the age of 74. The median age of death in the United States from cancer of the stomach was 73 years from 2001 to 2005.[2]

B.2. Pathology

The majority of gastric cancers are adenocarcinomas. Other histologic subtypes are relatively uncommon and include lymphoma, leiomyosarcoma, carcinoid, and squamous cell carcinoma.[50] The Lauren classification system describes gastric tumors on the basis of microscopic and gross pathologic features. It stratifies gastric adenocarcinoma into diffuse and intestinal subtypes.[47,48,50] The intestinal type is characterized by cohesive neoplastic cells that form glandlike structures. It may be preceded by a prolonged precancerous phase, tends to arise in the background of chronic atrophic gastritis, occurs in high-risk countries (such as Japan), occurs more often distally, is ulcerative in nature, and is more common in men. In the diffuse type, individual cells infiltrate into the wall of the stomach and cause thickening without formation of a discrete mass. The diffuse type shows more geographic variation, has a poor prognosis, and occurs more often in younger patients with a family history of gastric cancer.[48,51,52] However, not all gastric tumors can be classified as either intestinal or diffuse. Gastric cancer can also be subdivided by the site of origin. Global trends show a decrease in distal gastric cancer and intestinal-type lesions.[47,48,51] It is not clear that there is a difference in outcomes by these classifications.

B.3. Risk factors

Risk factors for gastric cancer can be separated into precursor lesions, environmental factors, and genetic conditions. Chronic atrophic gastritis and intestinal metaplasia have been closely linked to the intestinal type of gastric cancer and are noted to be more prevalent in regions of the world with the highest rates of gastric cancer.[53,54] Corea's model of gastric carcinogenesis postulates the progression of the gastric mucosa through stages of chronic active gastritis, glandular atrophy, intestinal metaplasia, and dysplasia before development of gastric adenocarcinoma.[54,55] Observational and case studies have found an increased risk of gastric cancer in patients with pernicious anemia, hypertrophic gastropathy, adenomatous polyps of the stomach, and who have had a distal gastrectomy for benign disorders.[51]

Epidemiologic studies have found a consistent association between *Helicobacter pylori* infection and the risk of gastric cancer. Prospective studies in high-risk populations with *H. pylori* infection have found increased rates of gastric cancer, particularly in patients with severe gastric atrophy, corpus-predominant gastritis, and intestinal metaplasia.[47,56,57] *H. pylori* treatment does not decrease the risk of development of cancer, and some data suggest that treatment for *H. pylori* decreases the risk of second gastric cancers.[55] An increase in gastric cancer risk has been noted with smoking, obesity, and low socioeconomic status.[47,58–60] Studies that have evaluated the relationship between diet and gastric cancer have shown a protective effect of fruits and vegetables. Diets that are rich in salted, smoked, or poorly preserved foods have an increased risk of disease. Foods rich in nitrates, nitrites, and secondary amines have also been shown to induce gastric tumors in animals.[58,59,61]

The majority of gastric cancers occur sporadically, but 8–10 percent have been associated with an inherited component. Gastric cancer is associated with germ line mutations of p53, BRCA2, and familial cancer syndromes such as hereditary nonpolyposis colon cancer, familial adenomatous polyposis, and Peutz-Jeghers syndrome.[47,62] E-cadherin mutations are autosomal dominant and have been found in families with hereditary diffuse gastric cancer with a penetrance of approximately 70 percent.[47,52]

B.4. Evaluation and staging

Gastric cancer in early stages of the disease often presents without any specific symptoms. Consequently, the disease is detected in locally advanced or advanced stages in 80 to 90 percent of patients.[47] The most common presenting symptoms included anorexia, nausea, vomiting, weight loss, dyspepsia, and melena.[49] Findings on physical exam are also indicative of advanced disease. Lymphatic dissemination can present as supraclavicular adenopathy (Virchow's node), axillary adenopathy (Irish's node), or intra-abdominal adenopathy. The disease can disseminate through the abdominal cavity and result in a periumbilical nodule (Sister Mary Joseph's node), ovarian metastasis (Krukenberg's tumor), a mass in the cul-de-sac (Blumer's shelf), peritoneal carcinomatosis, or malignant ascites.[50,51] Laboratory abnormalities can include anemia, abnormal liver function tests, and fecal occult blood. Paraneoplastic manifestations of gastric cancer include microangiopathic hemolytic anemia, acanthosis nigricans, the sudden appearance of seborrheic keratoses (Leser-Trélat sign), and chronic hypercoagulability leading to excessive intravascular clotting (Trousseau's syndrome).[5,51]

The diagnosis of gastric cancer is often made after an upper gastrointestinal series and through endoscopy with biopsy. EUS is effective in determining the depth of invasion. Contrast-enhanced CT scan of the abdomen/pelvis and chest radiograph are the recommended staging studies. Diagnostic laparoscopy is a more sensitive and accurate method for the diagnosis of peritoneal disease than either CT scans or ultrasound. FDG-PET scans have a less well defined role in the staging of gastric cancer in comparison to esophageal cancer because of the propensity to develop peritoneal metastases.

The TMN staging system of the American Joint Committee on Cancer incorporates the depth of tumor invasion into the abdominal wall, extent of lymph node involvement, and the presence of distal metastasis. The depth of invasion and extent of nodal involvement are the most important factors in predicting disease-free and overall survival. T1 lesions penetrate into the lamina propria or submucosa, T2 lesions invade into the muscularis propria, T3 lesions penetrate into the serosa, and T4 lesions invade into adjacent structures. It is important to note that N1 disease represents metastasis in 1–6 regional nodes, N2 disease indicates metastasis in 7–15 regional nodes, N3 disease involves more than 15 nodes, and M1 disease represents distant metastasis.

B.5. Treatment-localized disease

Primary surgery

Surgery is the primary treatment for localized gastric cancer. For distal tumors, partial gastrectomy can be performed. Total gastrectomy may be required for proximal lesions and larger mid-gastric lesions. A randomized trial comparing subtotal versus total gastrectomy in 618 Italian patients with distal gastric cancer found similar survival but a better nutritional status and quality of life with the subtotal procedure.[63]

The extent of the resection, the level of lymph node dissection, and the necessity of splenectomy or distal pancreatectomy remain areas of controversy.[5,51,64] The nomenclature used for surgery for gastric cancer uses the R classification to indicate the extent of residual tumor after resection and the D classification to designate the extent of lymph node dissection. The goal of surgery is to achieve an R0 resection (no residual disease) with at least a D1 lymph node dissection (i.e., resection of the N1 or perigastric lymph nodes). In Western countries, D1 dissections are used, whereas the Japanese have long favored a more extended D2 or D3 dissection, which involves resection of more distant lymph nodes such as those along the splenic artery or para-aortic lymph nodes. Evaluating whether there is a true difference in surgical approaches is difficult. For example, in Japan, there are more patients with gastric cancer, and a higher proportion of patients have early-stage disease, but interestingly, they also have an increased stage-specific survival.[52] Several clinical trials have compared D1 and D2 lymph node dissections in Western populations.[65–70] The largest of these trials, by the Dutch Gastric Cancer Group (711 patients) and the Medical Research Council (737 patients), have shown no survival advantage with a D2 dissection and increased morbidity.[65,67] In the Dutch study, morbidity and mortality were higher with D2 dissection, splenectomy, pancreatectomy, and in patients over the age of 70.[66] An Italian study showed that D2 resection with pancreas preservation did not show a significantly higher morbidity or mortality compared to a D1 resection.[68] A randomized trial in Taiwan compared D1 and D3 lymph node dissection and found more complications with more extended lymphadenectomy but also an improved survival with the D3 procedure.[69,70] A recent trial evaluating the role of the addition of para-aortic lymph node dissection to D2 lymphadenectomy showed no benefit.[71]

The mortality and morbidity of gastric resection has been the topic of retrospective studies in the elderly population. In a review of 502 patients with gastric cancer treated surgically in England and Wales, the average age of the patient population was 70 years. The risk of postoperative death was higher in patients with major comorbid diseases and patients who underwent more extensive surgery.[72] In the Dutch study comparing D1 and D2 dissection, 230 patients were over the age of 70. The mortality rate in patients over 70 getting a D2 resection was significantly higher than younger patients (17% vs. 5.9%).[66] Laparoscopically assisted distal gastrectomy has also been evaluated in elderly patients (over age 70) with early-stage gastric cancer and was associated with more rapid return of gastric function, fewer complications, and a shorter hospital stay.[73] In addition, palliative resection has been shown to increase survival in elderly patients with advanced disease.[74]

Perioperative therapy

The 5-year survival rates for patients treated with curative surgical resection in Western countries are disappointing, ranging from 10 to 50 percent. The prognosis is significantly worse once there is nodal involvement, and patients with stage III disease treated surgically have 5-year survivals ranging from 10 to 20 percent.[75–77] Multimodality therapy is now generally accepted to provide the best chances for cure for the treatment of gastric cancer. However, the treatment paradigms vary based on geographic location. In the United States, 5-FU-based CRT is the standard, whereas Europeans favor perioperative chemotherapy, based on the MAGIC study, and the Japanese have accepted the adjuvant use of S-1 (an oral fluoropyrimidine not approved in the United States).

Adjuvant therapy

Adjuvant chemotherapy with single- or multiagent regimens has been extensively studied in gastric cancer with widely varying results likely dependent on patient population, surgery, and chemotherapy evaluated. At least five meta-analyses addressing the topic have been published and show a marginal survival benefit.[77–81] Modern studies have focused on the use of combination chemotherapy regimens with anthracyclines/platinum drugs and have shown increased toxicity without significant advantages in disease-free or overall survival.[82–84] The largest adjuvant chemotherapy trial evaluated the use of S-1 in 1,059 Japanese patients with stage II and III gastric cancer after a D2 resection. The trial was stopped early, after 1 year of enrollment, when a survival benefit was observed in the treatment arm. The drug was well tolerated, and extended follow-up showed a 3-year overall survival of 80.1 percent in the S-1 group versus 70.1 percent in the surgery-only group.[85] Currently S-1 is not available for use in the United States outside of clinical trials.

In the United States, adjuvant CRT is the standard. It was evaluated in a landmark study (INT 116), reported by Macdonald and colleagues, including 556 American patients with stage IB–IV (M0) resected gastric cancer. The experimental CRT arm consisted of bolus 5-FU-leucovorin, followed by chemotherapy combined with 4,500 cGy of radiation delivered over 5 weeks, then two further cycles of chemotherapy. The median overall survival was 27 months in the surgery-only group and 36 months in the combined-modality arm ($p = .005$). However, only 10 percent of patients were treated with the recommended D2 resection, and the majority of patients (54%) underwent a D0 or incomplete lymph node resection.[86] This trial has led to the standard use of adjuvant chemoradiation therapy in the United States, despite what some consider the suboptimal use of surgery.

Perioperative chemotherapy or CRT

Neoadjuvant, or preoperative, therapy allows for downstaging of tumors and theoretical elimination of micrometastatic disease prior to surgical resection. A study evaluated induction chemotherapy (5-FU, leucovorin, and cisplatin) followed by 5-FU-based CRT and, finally, surgery in 34 patients. This preoperative regimen resulted in an R0 resection rate of 70 percent and a pathologic complete response rate of 30 percent.[87] The largest study to evaluate perioperative therapy is the MAGIC trial, which used the ECF regimen and resulted in an improvement in overall and progression-free survival, as noted earlier. About 20 percent of the patients who were enrolled on this study were age 70 years or older.[25]

B.6. Treatment-advanced disease

The prognosis for metastatic gastric cancer is dismal, with a median survival of 7–10 months. The standard of care in both Europe and the United states is combination chemotherapy, as several regimens have been demonstrated to be superior to supportive care alone. Studies in advanced gastric cancer often combine esophageal cancer, gastroesophageal junction cancer, and gastric cancer. Consequently, the regimens used to treat gastric cancer and esophageal cancer are similar. Common regimens used include ECF, DCF, EOX, EOF, and ECX. The substitution of oxalipatin-capecitabine for cisplatin-5-FU allows for equivalent efficacy with reduced toxicity.[37] A meta-analysis that examined the use of chemotherapy in advanced gastric cancer found that combination chemotherapy regimens with 5-FU, anthracycline, and platinum achieved the best survival results. Bolus 5-FU was associated with higher toxicity than infusional 5-FU. In addition, combination chemotherapy resulted in a small but statistically significant survival advantage of approximately 1 month.[88] Another phase II–III study in untreated advanced gastric cancer compared DCF to CF and found longer time to progression (TTP) and overall survival. Two-year survival was longer in DCF (18%) over CF (9%) at the price of increased grade III and IV toxicity.[89] The Japanese have studied the combination of S-1 and cisplatin versus S-1 alone in a phase III clinical trial in first-line treatment of advanced gastric cancer. Combination therapy was associated with improved overall survival (13 vs. 11 months) and significantly improved progression-free survival. There were also increased grade III and IV events in the combination arm, including neutropenia, anemia, nausea, and anorexia.[90] A phase III German study compared the use of the FLO regimen (infusional 5-FU, leucovorin, and oxaliplatin) to the FLP regimen (infusional 5-FU, leucovorin, and cisplatin) in patients with previously untreated advanced gastric cancer. There was a trend toward improved median progression-free survival with the FLO regimen but no significant difference in overall survival. The FLO regimen was associated with a significant decrease of toxicity of any grade. In 94 patients over the age of 65 years, treatment with FLO resulted in superior response rates, time to treatment failure, progression-free survival, and overall survival compared to FLP.[91]

Combination chemotherapy regimens have been studied in elderly patients, primarily in small, nonrandomized studies. The combination of weekly oxaliplatin, fluorouracil, and folinic acid (OXALF) was evaluated in 17 Italian patients aged 70 years and older. The overall response rate was 47 percent, the time to disease progression was 5.9 months, and overall survival was 7.5 months. There were no grade III–IV toxicities or toxicity-related mortalities reported.[92] Another study evaluated the combination of oxaliplatin, infusional fluorouracil, and folinic acid (FOLFOX 4) in 31 elderly patients over the age of 65 years. The overall response rate was 32 percent, and the median time to progression was 6.8 months. There were eight episodes of grade III neutropenia, three episodes of grade IV neutropenia, two episodes of grade III emesis, seven episodes of grade III oral mucositis, and one episode of grade III neuropathy.[93] A third study evaluated a combination of oxaliplatin, 5-FU, and folinic acid in 24 Asian patients over the age of 64 years. The overall response rate was 50 percent, the median progression-free sur-

vival was 5.4 months, and the median overall survival was 7.4 months. The main toxicities were anemia and leucopenia, observed in 39.8 percent and 19 percent of patients, respectively.[94] A retrospective study evaluating oral fluoropyrimidines (capecitabine or S-1) and cisplatin in first-line treatment of 72 patients over the age of 70 has been published. The combination of capecitabine and cisplatin was associated with a slightly higher response rate and higher toxicity (hand-foot syndrome and diarrhea).[95] All four studies concluded that combination chemotherapy was efficacious and well tolerated in an elderly population.

B.7. Treatment-palliative care

Palliative measures for the treatment of gastric cancer are similar to modalities used for esophageal cancer. Self-expanding metallic stents can be used to alleviate gastric outlet obstruction and malignant small bowel strictures.[96,97] The neodymium-yttrium laser has been used to palliate dysphagia and bleeding in unresectable carcinomas of the gastric cardia.[98] Intraperitoneal chemotherapy has also been evaluated with agents such as mitomycin-C, cisplatin, and 5-FU. Results have been promising but associated with significant toxicity, and such therapy is still considered experimental.[99,100]

B.8. Treatment conclusion

Gastric cancer is more common in elderly patients. Surgical therapy is used to treat gastric cancer in its early stages. The extent of resection required is an area of controversy. A number of series have shown that elderly patients can be successfully treated with either a D1 or D2 resection. In general, older patients with more comorbidities have worse outcomes with more extensive surgeries. Combined-modality therapy is used to treat more advanced gastric cancer. There are limited data concerning the use of combined-modality therapy in elderly patients. Combination chemotherapy is widely used to treat metastatic gastric cancer, though there is no single standard regimen. A number of combination chemotherapy regimens have demonstrated activity in elderly populations. Combination chemotherapy can result in higher toxicity in elderly patients in comparison to younger patients, particularly regimens that include agents with bone marrow toxicity, so patients should be carefully monitored.

References

1. American Cancer Society. *Cancer Facts and Figures, 2008*. Atlanta, GA: American Cancer Society; 2008.

2. Reis LA, Melbert D, Krapcho M, et al., eds. *SEER Cancer Statistics Review, 1975–2005*. Bethesda, MD: National Cancer Institute; 2008.

3. Enzinger PC, Mayer RJ. Esophageal cancer. *N Engl J Med*. 2003;349(23):2241–2252.

4. Sial SH, Catalano MF. Gastrointestinal tract cancer in the elderly. *Gastroenterol Clin*. 2001;30(2):565–590.

5. Khushalani N. Cancer of the esophagus and stomach. *Mayo Clin Proc*. 2008;83(1):712–722.

6. Shaheen N, Ransohoff DF. Gastroesophageal reflux, Barrett esophagus, and esophageal cancer: scientific review. *J Am Med Assoc*. 2002;287(15): 1972–1981.

7. Lagergren J. Adenocarcinoma of oesophagus: what exactly is the size of the problem and who is at risk? *Gut*. 2005;54(suppl 1):1–5.

8. Iyer RB, Silverman PM, Tamm EP, et al. Diagnosis, staging, and follow-up of esophageal cancer. *AJR Am J Roentgenol*. 2003;181(3): 785–793.

9. Pech O, May A, Günter E, et al. The impact of endoscopic ultrasound and computed tomography on the TNM staging of early cancer in Barrett's esophagus. *Am J Gastroenterol*. 2006;101(10):2223–2229.

10. Bruzzi JF, Munden RF, Truong MT, et al. PET/CT of esophageal cancer: its role in clinical management. *Radiographics*. 2007;27(6):1635–1652.

11. Levine EA, Farmer MR, Clark P, et al. Predictive value of 18-fluoro-deoxy-glucose-positron emission tomography (18F-FDG-PET) in the identification of responders to chemoradiation therapy for the treatment of locally advanced esophageal cancer. *Ann Surg*. 2006;243(4):472–478.

12. Orringer MB, Marshall B, Chang AC, et al. Two thousand transhiatal esophagectomies: changing trends, lessons learned. *Ann Surg*. 2007;246(3): 363–372; discussion 372–374.

13. Hulscher JB, van Sandick JW, de Boer AG, et al. Extended transthoracic resection compared with limited transhiatal resection for adenocarcinoma of the esophagus. *N Engl J Med*. 2002;347(21): 1662–1669.

14. Audisio RA, Veronesi P, Ferrario L, et al. Elective surgery for gastrointestinal tumours in the elderly. *Ann Oncol*. 1997;8(4):317–326.

15. Morita M, Yoshida R, Ohgaki K, et al. Clinical significance of an esophagectomy in patients 75 years of age or older based on an analysis of 1,000 operative cases with esophageal cancer. Paper presented at: 2008 Gastrointestinal Cancer Symposium; January 25–27, 2008; Orlando, FL.

16. Sykes AJ, Burt PA, Slevin NJ, et al. Radical radiotherapy for carcinoma of the oesophagus: an effective alternative to surgery. *Radiother Oncol*. 1998;48(1):15–21.

17. Cooper JS, Guo MD, Herskovic A, et al. Chemoradiotherapy of locally advanced esophageal cancer: long-term follow-up of a prospective randomized trial (RTOG 85–01). *J Am Med Assoc*. 1999;281(17):1623–1627.

18. Minsky BD, Pajak TF, Ginsberg RJ, et al. INT 0123 (Radiation Therapy Oncology Group 94-05) phase III trial of combined-modality therapy for esophageal cancer: high-dose versus standard-dose radiation therapy. *J Clin Oncol*. 2002;20(5):1167–1174.

19. Adelstein DJ, Rice TW, Rybicki LA, et al. Does paclitaxel improve the chemoradiotherapy of locoregionally advanced esophageal cancer? A nonrandomized comparison with fluorouracil-based therapy. *J Clin Oncol*. 2000;18(10):2032–2039.

20. Ilson DH, Bains M, Kelsen DP, et al. Phase I trial of escalating-dose irinotecan given weekly with cisplatin and concurrent radiotherapy in locally advanced esophageal cancer. *J Clin Oncol*. 2003;21(15):2926–2932.

21. Tougeron D, DiFiore F, Thureau S, et al. Safety and outcome of definitive chemoradiotherapy in elderly patients with oesophageal cancer. *Br J Cancer*. 2008;99:1586–1592.

22. Takeuchi S, Ohtsu A, Doi T, et al. A retrospective study of definitive chemoradiotherapy for elderly patients with esophageal cancer. *Am J Clin Oncol*. 2007;30(6):607–611.

23. Kelsen DP, Winter KA, Gunderson LL, et al. Long-term results of RTOG trial 8911 (USA Intergroup 113): a random assignment trial comparison of chemotherapy followed by surgery compared with surgery alone for esophageal cancer. *J Clin Oncol*. 2007;25(24): 3719–3725.

24. Medical Research Council Oesophageal Cancer Working Party. Surgical resection with or without preoperative chemotherapy in oesophageal cancer: a randomized controlled trial. *Lancet*. 2002;359:1723–1733.

25. Cunningham D, Allum WH, Stenning SP, et al. Perioperative chemotherapy versus surgery alone for resectable gastroesophageal cancer. *N Engl J Med*. 2006;355(1):11–20.

26. Gebski V, Burmeister B, Smithers BM, et al. Australasian Gastro-Intestinal Trials Group. Survival benefits from neoadjuvant chemoradiotherapy or chemotherapy in

oesophageal carcinoma: a meta-analysis. *Lancet Oncol.* 2007;8(3):226–234.

27. Bosset JF, Gignoux M, Triboulet JP, et al. Chemoradiotherapy followed by surgery compared with surgery alone in squamous-cell cancer of the esophagus. *N Engl J Med.* 1997;337(3):161–167.

28. Burmeister BH, Smithers BM, Gebski V, et al. Surgery alone versus chemoradiotherapy followed by surgery for resectable cancer of the oesophagus: a randomised controlled phase III trial. *Lancet Oncol.* 2005;6(9):659–668.

29. Walsh TN, Noonan N, Hollywood D, et al. A comparison of multimodal therapy and surgery for esophageal adenocarcinoma. *N Engl J Med.* 1996;335(7):462–467.

30. Billingsley KG, Maynard C, Schwartz DL, et al. The use of trimodality therapy for the treatment of operable esophageal carcinoma in the veteran population: patient survival and outcome analysis. *Cancer.* 2001;92(5):1272–1280.

31. Smith GL, Smith BD, Buchholz TA, et al. Patterns of care and locoregional treatment outcomes in older esophageal cancer patients: The SEER-Medicare cohort. *Int J Radiat Oncol Biol Phys.* 2009;74:482–489.

32. Tew WP, Kelsen DP, Ilson DH. Targeted therapies for esophageal cancer. *Oncologist.* 2005;10(8):590–601.

33. Sandler AB, Kindler HL, Einhorn LH, et al. Phase II trial of gemcitabine in patients with previously untreated metastatic cancer of the esophagus or gastroesophageal junction. *Ann Oncol.* 2000;11(9):1161–1164.

34. Ilson DH, Saltz L, Enzinger P, et al. Phase II trial of weekly irinotecan plus cisplatin in advanced esophageal cancer. *J Clin Oncol.* 1999;17(10):3270–3275.

35. Muro K, Hamaguchi T, Ohtsu A, et al. A phase II study of single-agent docetaxel in patients with metastatic esophageal cancer. *Ann Oncol.* 2004;15(6):955–959.

36. Kroep JR, Pinedo HM, Giaccone G, et al. Phase II study of cisplatin preceding gemcitabine in patients with advanced esophageal cancer. *Ann Oncol.* 2004;15(2):230–235.

37. Cunningham D, Starling N, Rao S, et al. Upper Gastrointestinal Clinical Studies Group of the National Cancer Research Institute of the United Kingdom. Capecitabine and oxaliplatin for advanced esophagogastric cancer. *N Engl J Med.* 2008;358(1):36–46.

38. Lorenzen S, Hentrich M, Haberl C, et al. Split-dose docetaxel, cisplatin and leucovorin/fluorouracil as first-line therapy in advanced gastric cancer and adenocarcinoma of the gastroesophageal junction: results of a phase II trial. *Ann Oncol.* 2007;18(10):1673–1679.

39. Jatoi A, Foster NR, Egner J, et al. Elderly patients with metastatic esophageal/gastric cancer: a pooled analysis of age-based outcomes from 8 consecutive North Central Cancer Treatment Group (NCCTG) therapeutic trials. Paper presented at: 44th American Society of Clinical Oncology Annual Meeting; May 30–June 3, 2008; Chicago, IL.

40. Trumper M, Ross PJ, Cunningham D, et al. Efficacy and tolerability of chemotherapy in elderly patients with advanced oesophago-gastric cancer: a pooled analysis of three clinical trials. *Eur J Cancer.* 2006;42(7):827–834.

41. Clements WD, Johnston LR, McIlwrath E, et al. Self-expanding stents for malignant dysphagia. *J R Soc Med.* 1996;89(8):454–456.

42. Cwikiel W, Tranberg KG, Cwikiel M, et al. Malignant dysphagia: palliation with esophageal stents – long-term results in 100 patients. *Radiology.* 1998;207(2):513–518.

43. Laasch HU, Marriott A, Wilbraham L, et al. Effectiveness of open versus antireflux stents for palliation of distal esophageal carcinoma and prevention of symptomatic gastroesophageal reflux. *Radiology.* 2002;225(2):359–365.

44. Spencer GM, Thorpe SM, Blackman GM, et al. Laser augmented by brachytherapy versus laser alone in the palliation of adenocarcinoma of the oesophagus and cardia: a randomised study. *Gut.* 2002;50(2):224–227.

45. Gossner L, May A, Sroka R, et al. Photodynamic destruction of high grade dysplasia and early carcinoma of the esophagus after the oral administration of 5-aminolevulinic acid. *Cancer.* 1999;86(10):1921–1928.

46. Thomas RJ, Abbott M, Bhathal PS, et al. High-dose photoirradiation of esophageal cancer. *Ann Surg.* 1987;206(1):193–199.

47. Dicken BJ, Bigam DL, Cass C, et al. Gastric adenocarcinoma. *Ann Surg.* 2005;241(1):27–39.

48. Lochhead P, El-Omar EM. Gastric cancer. *Br Med Bull.* 2008;85:87–100.

49. Allum WH, Griffin SM, Colin-Jones D. Guidelines for the management of oesophageal and gastric cancer. *Gut.* 2002;50(suppl 5):1–23.

50. Gunderson LL, Donohue JH, Alberts SR. Cancer of the stomach. In: Abeloff MD, Armitage JO, Niederhuber JE, et al., eds. *Clinical Oncology.* Philadelphia: Elsevier; 2004:1819–1875.

51. Fuchs CS, Mayer RJ. Gastric carcinoma. *N Engl J Med.* 1995;333(1):32–41.

52. Huntsman DG, Carneiro F, Lewis FR, et al. Early gastric cancer in young, asymptomatic carriers of germ-line E-cadherin mutations. *N Engl J Med.* 2001;344(25):1904–1909.

53. El-Serag HB, Mason AC, Petersen N, et al. Epidemiological differences between

adenocarcinoma of the oesophagus and adenocarcinoma of the gastric cardia in the USA. *Gut*. 2002;50:368–372.

54. Naylor GM, Gotoda T, Dixon M, et al. Why does Japan have a high incidence of gastric cancer? Comparison of gastritis between UK and Japanese patients. *Gut*. 2006;55:1545–1552.

55. Wong BC, Lam SK, Wong WM, et al. Helicobacter pylori eradication to prevent gastric cancer in a high-risk region of China. *J Am Med Assoc*. 2004;291(2):187–194.

56. Uemura N, Okamoto S, Yamamoto S, et al. *Helicobacter pylori* infection and the development of gastric cancer. *N Engl J Med*. 2001;345(11): 784–789.

57. You W, Zhang L, Gail MH, et al. Gastric dysplasia and gastric cancer: *Helicobacter pylori*, serum vitamin C, and other risk factors. *J Natl Cancer Inst*. 2000;92(19):1607–1612.

58. Huang X, Tajima K, Hamajima N, et al. Effects of dietary, drinking, and smoking habits on the prognosis of gastric cancer. *Nutr Cancer*. 2000;38(1):30–36.

59. Devesa SS, Blot WJ, Fraumeni FJ. Changing patterns in the incidence of esophageal and gastric carcinoma in the United States. *Cancer*. 1998;83(10):2049–2053.

60. Souza RF, Spechler SJ. Concepts in the prevention of adenocarcinoma of the distal esophagus and proximal stomach. *CA Cancer J Clin*. 2005;55:334–351.

61. Ramon JM, Serra L, Cerdo C, et al. Dietary factors and gastric cancer risk. *Cancer*. 1993;71(5):1731–1735.

62. Vecchia CL, Negri E, Franceschi S, et al. Family history and risk of stomach and colorectal cancer. *Cancer*. 1992;70(1):50–55.

63. Bozzetti F, Marubini E, Bonfanti G, et al. Subtotal versus total gastrectomy for gastric cancer. *Ann Surg*. 1999;230(2):170–178.

64. Van de velde CJ. Gastric cancer: staging and surgery. *Ann Oncol*. 2002;13:3–6.

65. Bonenkamp JJ, Hermans J, Sasako M, et al. Extended lymph-node dissection for gastric cancer. *N Engl J Med*. 1999;340:908–914.

66. Hartgrink HH, Van De Velde CJ, Putter H, et al. Extended lymph node dissection for gastric cancer: who may benefit? Final results of the randomized Dutch gastric cancer group trial. *J Clin Oncol*. 2004;22(11):2069–2077.

67. Cuschieri A, Weeden S, Fielding J, et al. Patient survival after D1 and D2 resections for gastric cancer: long-term results of the MRC randomized surgical trial. *Br J Cancer*. 1999;79(9/10): 1522–1530.

68. Degiuli M, Sasako M, Calgaro M, et al. Morbidity and mortality after D1 and D2 gastrectomy for

69. Wu CW, Hsiung CA, Lo SS, et al. Randomized clinical trial of morbidity after D1 and D3 surgery for gastric cancer. *Brit J Surg*. 2004;91:283–287.

70. Wu C, Hsiung CA, Lo S, et al. Nodal dissection for patients with gastric cancer: a randomised controlled trial. *Lancet*. 2006;7:309–315.

71. Sasako M, Sano T, Yamamoto S, et al. D2 lymphadenectomy alone or with para-aortic nodal dissection for gastric cancer. *N Engl J Med*. 2008;359(5):453–462.

72. McCulloch P, Ward J, Tekkis PP. Mortality and morbidity in gastro-oesophageal cancer surgery: initial results of ASCOT multicentre prospective cohort study. *Br Med J*. 2003;327(22):1–6.

73. Yasuda K, Sonoda H, Shiroshita H, et al. Laparoscopically assisted distal gastrectomy for early gastric cancer in the elderly. *Brit J Surg*. 2004;91:1061–1065.

74. Hartgrink HH, Putter H, Kranenbarg EK, et al. Value of palliative resection in gastric cancer. *Brit J Surg*. 2002;89:1438–1443.

75. Shimada K, Ajani J. Adjuvant therapy for gastric carcinoma patients in the past 15 years. *Cancer*. 1999;86(9):1657–1668.

76. De Vita F, Giuliani F, Galizia G, et al. Neo-adjuvant and adjuvant chemotherapy of gastric cancer. *Ann Oncol*. 2007;18(suppl 6): 120–123.

77. Hermans J, Bonenkamp JJ, Boon MC, et al. Adjuvant therapy after curative resection for gastric caner: meta-analysis of randomized trials. *J Clin Oncol*. 1993;11(8):1441–1447.

78. Earle CC, Maroun JA. Adjuvant chemotherapy after curative resection for gastric cancer in non-Asian patients: revisiting a meta-analysis of randomized trials. *Eur J Cancer*. 1999;35(7): 1059–1064.

79. Mari E, Floriani I, Tinazzi A, et al. Efficacy of adjuvant chemotherapy after curative resection for gastric cancer: a meta-analysis of published randomized trials. *Ann Oncol*. 2000;11:837–843.

80. Januger K, Halstrom L, Glimelius B. Chemotherapy in gastric cancer: a review and updated meta-analysis. *Eur J Surg*. 2002;168: 597–608.

81. Liu TS, Wang Y, Chen SY, et al. An updated meta-analysis of adjuvant chemotherapy after curative resection for gastric cancer. *Eur J Surg Oncol*. 2008;34:1208–1216.

82. Costanzo FD, Gasperoni S, Manzione L, et al. Adjuvant chemotherapy in completely resected gastric cancer: a randomized phase III trial conducted by GOIRC. *J Natl Cancer Inst*. 2008;100(6):388–398.

cancer: interim analysis of Italian gastric cancer study group (IGCSG) randomized surgical trial. *Eur J Surg Oncol*. 2004;30(3):303–308.

83. Cascinu S, Labianca R, Barone C, et al. Adjuvant treatment of high-risk, radically resected gastric cancer patients with 5-fluorouracil, leukovorin, cisplatin, and epidoxorubicin in a randomized controlled trial. *J Natl Cancer Inst.* 2007;99(8): 601–607.

84. De Vita F, Giuliani F, Orditura M, et al. Adjuvant chemotherapy with epirubicin, leucovorin, 5-fluorouracil and etoposide regimen in resected gastric cancer patients: a randomized phase III trial by the Gruppo Oncologico Italia Meridionale (GOIM 9602 study). *Ann Oncol.* 2007;18: 1354–1358.

85. Sakuramoto S, Sasako M, Yamaguchi T, et al. Adjuvant chemotherapy for gastric cancer with S-1, and oral fluoropyrimidine. *N Engl J Med.* 2007;357(18):1810–1820.

86. Macdonald JS, Smalley SR, Benedetti J, et al. Chemoradiotherapy after surgery compared with surgery alone for adenocarcinoma of the stomach or gastroesophageal junction. *N Engl J Med.* 2001;345(10):725–730.

87. Ajani JA, Mansfield PF, Janjan N, et al. Multi-institutional trial of preoperative chemoradiotherapy in patients with potentially resectable gastric carcinoma. *J Clin Oncol.* 2004;22(14):2774–2780.

88. Wagner AD, Grothe W, Haerting J, et al. Chemotherapy in advanced gastric cancer: a systemic review and meta-analysis based on aggregate date. *J Clin Oncol.* 2006;24(18): 2903–2909.

89. Van Cutsem E, Moiseyenko VM, Tjulandin S, et al. Phase III study of docetaxel plus fluorouracil compared with cisplatin and fluorouracil as first-line therapy for advanced gastric cancer: a report of the V325 study group. *J Clin Oncol.* 2006;24(31):4991–4997.

90. Koizumi W, Narahara H, Hara T, et al. S-1 plus cisplatin versus S-1 alone for first-line treatment of advanced gastric cancer (SPIRITS trial): a phase III trial. *Lancet Oncol.* 2008;9:215–221.

91. Al-Batran S, Hartmann JT, Probst S, et al. Phase III trial in metastatic gastroesophogeal adenocarcinoma with fluorouracil, leucovorin plus either oxaliplatin or cisplatin: a study of the Arbeitsgemeinschaft Internistische Onkologie. *J Clin Oncol.* 2008;26(9):1435–1442.

92. Santini D, Graziano F, Catalano V, et al. Weekly oxaliplatin, fluorouracil and folinic acid (OXALF) as first-line chemotherapy for elderly patient with advanced gastric cancer. Paper presented at: 40th American Society of Clinical Oncology Annual Meeting; June 5–8, 2004; New Orleans, LA.

93. Azzarello D, Giuffre C, Panuccio V, et al. First line chemotherapy with FOLFOX 4 in elderly patients (>65 years) with advanced or metastatic gastric cancer: a pilot study. Paper presented at: 42nd American Society of Clinical Oncology Annual Meeting; June 2–6, 2006; Atlanta, GA.

94. Choi I, Lee K, Oh D, et al. Oxaliplatin, 5-fluorouracil and folinic acid as first-line chemotherapy for elderly patients with advanced gastric cancer. Paper presented at: 42nd American Society of Clinical Oncology Annual Meeting; June 2–6, 2006; Atlanta, GA.

95. Seol YM, Song MK, Choi YJ, et al. Oral fluoropyrimidines (capecitabine or S-1) and cisplatin as first line treatment in elderly patients with advanced gastric cancer: a retrospective study. *Jpn J Clin Oncol.* 2009;39(1):43–48.

96. Yates MR, Morgan DE, Baron TH. Palliation of malignant gastric and small intestinal strictures with self-expandable metal stents. *Endoscopy.* 1998;30(3):266–272.

97. Telford JJ, Carr-Locke DL, Baron TH, et al. Palliation of patients with malignant gastric outlet obstruction with the enteral Wallstent: outcomes from a multicenter study. *Gastrointestinal Endosc.* 2004;60(6):916–920.

98. Norberto L, Ranzato R, Marino S, et al. Endoscopic palliation of esophageal and cardial cancer: neodymium-yttrium aluminum garnet laser therapy. *Dis Esophagus.* 1999;12(4): 294–296.

99. Sayag-Beaujard AC, Francois Y, Glehen O, et al. Intraperitoneal chemo-hyperthermia with mitomycin C for gastric cancer patients with peritoneal carcinomatosis. *Anticancer Res.* 1999;19(2B):1375–1382.

100. Leichman L, Silberman H, Leichman CG, et al. Preoperative systemic chemotherapy followed by adjuvant postoperative intraperitoneal therapy for gastric cancer: a University of Southern California pilot program. *J Clin Oncol.* 1992;10(12): 1933–1942.

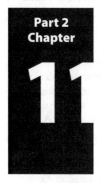

Management of colon and rectal cancer in older adults

Supriya Gupta Mohile, Harman P. Kaur, and Richard M. Goldberg

A. Introduction

With improving life expectancy, the population of patients aged 65 years and over is rapidly expanding. As a result, increasing numbers of persons aged 65 years and older will require evaluation and treatment for cancer. In Western countries, over 60 percent of new cancers and over 70 percent of cancer deaths occur in those persons aged 65 years and older.[1] More than half of these patients are over 70 years old, and one-fourth of them are over 80 years old.[2]

Colorectal cancer (CRC) can be considered a disease of the elderly, with a median age of diagnosis of 72 years.[3] There is considerable variation within the elderly subpopulation with regard to receipt of screening, surgery, and chemotherapy for early- or advanced-stage disease. These differences in patterns of care may be a result of underlying differences in the health status of older persons that preclude some from receiving aggressive standard-of-care approaches for their disease. Comprehensive geriatric assessment (CGA) could be used to help with differentiating the older fit persons who have been shown to benefit as much as their younger counterparts for treatment of CRC from those who are more vulnerable or frail.

The majority of patients with early-stage colon cancer are cured with surgery. Adjuvant chemotherapy improves outcomes for those persons who present with higher-risk stage II or stage III cancers. The standard treatment for advanced CRC includes chemotherapy either alone or in combination with targeted therapies. Surgical removal of the primary lesion or metastatic lesions in the advanced-disease setting is an option for those who are fit and have limited metastatic disease. A multidisciplinary team, preferably including a trained geriatrician or geriatric oncologist to help determine underlying fitness for treatment, should define each patient's treatment plan at presentation. In general, if treatment is deemed palliative, the most active chemotherapy option with the least toxicity should be considered to improve quality of life and prolong survival. However, if cure is a possibility, higher levels of toxicity because of more aggressive chemotherapy approaches may be deemed acceptable.[1] This approach to treatment is similar for those with stage II or III rectal cancer where a combination of pre- or postoperative radiation in combination with chemotherapy, surgery, and adjuvant chemotherapy may be offered for curative intent.

In this chapter, we provide an approach to the assessment of the older patient for CRC screening and treatment along with an overview of management options for colorectal treatment along the full clinical continuum of the disease.

B. Epidemiology of colorectal cancer in the older patient

In 2008, approximately 150,000 men and women were diagnosed with and 50,000 men and women died from cancer of the colon and rectum.[3] CRC is the third most common cancer and the second leading cause of cancer-related death in both men and women.[3] The incidence increases with advancing age, doubling every 7 years for patients aged 50 years and over.[4] Approximately one-third of CRC patients present with rectal cancer. Between the years 2000 and 2005, approximately 0.1 percent of CRCs were diagnosed under age 20 years; 1.0 percent between 20 and 34 years; 3.7 percent between 35 and 44 years; 11.6 percent between 45 and 54 years; 18.3 percent between 55 and 64 years; 25.1 percent between 65 and 74 years; 28.2 percent between 75 and 84 years; and 12.2 percent in those aged 85 years or older.[5] Figure 11.1 illustrates incidence rates of CRC by age in the years 2000–2005. Over 65 percent of patients with CRC are aged 65 years or older.[6]

The medical and societal burdens of CRC will only worsen over the coming decades as the demographic proportion and life expectancy of elderly individuals continue to grow. Women and men in

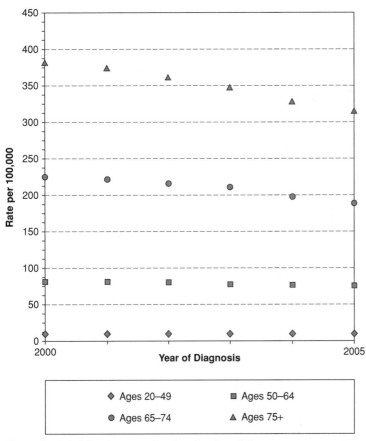

Cancer sites include invasive cases only unless otherwise noted.
Incidence source: SEER 17 areas (San Francisco, Connecticut, Detroit, Hawaii, Iowa, New Mexico, Seattle, Utah, Atlanta, San Jose-Monterey, Los Angeles, Alaska Native Registry, Rural Georgia, California excluding SF/SJM/LA, Kentucky, Louisiana and New Jersey).
Rates are per 100,000 and are age-adjusted to the 2000 US Std Population (19 age groups – Census P25-1130). Regression lines are calculated using the Joinpoint Regression Program Version 3.3, April 2008, National Cancer Institute.

Figure 11.1 Age-adjusted SEER incidence rates by age at diagnosis/death, colon and rectum, all races, both sexes, 2000–2005 (SEER 17). From SEER data (http://seer.cancer.gov/).

the United States aged 60, 70, and 80 years can expect to live an additional 24 and 20.8, 16.2 and 13.7, and 9.8 and 8.2 years, respectively.[7] Despite the rise in numbers of older adults with CRC, there is a deficiency of evidence-based data to guide decision making.[6] Elderly and poor performance status patients have historically not been included in many of the definitive clinical trials, thus making clinical decision making a difficult process for the practicing oncologist.[7] Although CRC primarily affects the elderly, pivotal trials establishing evidence-based care for this disease have tended to include patients with a median age of 60–65 years, with fewer than 20 percent of persons aged 70 years and over.[8–10] Oncologists often must extrapolate data from these small subsets of patients to our generalized popula-

tion of older patients who are vulnerable because of very advanced age, comorbidity, or decreased function. The reasons for underrepresentation of older persons in CRC are likely multifold and include strictness of protocol entry criteria as well as a clinical assumption that an older person is at higher risk of treatment-related toxicity. One study that surveyed physicians found that 50 percent did not offer clinical trial entry based on age alone.[11] Another study evaluating barriers to clinical trial participation found that both physician perceptions and protocol restrictions with regard to functional status and comorbidity were important factors that contributed to the exclusion of older adults in clinical trials.[12] Other barriers include a lack of financial, logistic, and social support. As a result of the underlying differences

Table 11.1 Physiologic changes that occur with aging that affect chemotherapy pharmacokinetics and pharmacodynamics.[130–132]

Organ system	Age-related changes
Endocrine	Hypothyroidism Hyperthyroidism Glucose intolerance and diabetes
Neurological	Decrease in cerebral blood flow Cognitive decline Peripheral and autonomic dysfunction
Immune	Weakening of adaptive immunity (decreased phagocytic activity, radical formation, and increase in cytokines) Diminished T- and B-cell proliferation and antigen-expressing surface molecules
Cardiovascular	Decline in cardiac reserves Development of cardiovascular diseases with alteration of myocardial perfusion Conduction delay
Pulmonary	Reduction in oxygen saturation capacity Impairment of response to hypoxia Decline in pulmonary reserves Chronic pulmonary diseases Decrease of respiratory muscle strength
Musculoskeletal	Reduction in skeletal muscle mass Disproportional body fat distribution Age-related bone loss
Gastrointestinal	Age-related decline in absorption, secretion, and neuromuscular function Vascular and mucosal alterations Polypharmacy with agents that depend on hepatic metabolism
Renal	Renal function declines with age Impact of hypertension, diabetes, and atherosclerosis on renal function Use of nephrotoxic drugs can add further insult to age-related physiologic changes

between clinical trial participants and the general population, dose reductions and delays are much more common in the community compared to the clinical trial setting. In one study of community oncology practices, older patients with CRC showed that 46 percent of older patients received dose reductions.[13] Dose reductions occurred even for those patients with curable disease, which potentially impacted outcomes.

Despite underrepresentation within clinical trials, we are making improvements in the care of older patients with colon cancer. CRC death rates decreased by about 6 percent from 2003 to 2004, compared with a 3 percent decrease from 2004 to 2005.[3] A recent model analyzing long-term cancer survival in the United States also showed an increase in the 5-year relative survival rate from 1998 to 2003 among patients aged 65 years and older with colon cancer (61.9% vs. 65.8%, respectively, p for trend $< .001$); this increase was greater than that demonstrated by patients aged less than 65 years in the same period (64.6% vs. 67%, respectively, p for trend $< .06$) and was

attributed to improved screening and treatment modalities.[14] Another study of 838 rectal patients aged 80 years and over showed an improvement in 5-year survival from 18 percent in 1978–1981 to 42 percent in 1994–1997.[15]

C. Selection of elderly colorectal cancer patients for screening and treatment

The aging process is associated with a number of physiologic changes that may influence underlying health status and tolerance to cancer treatment. Therefore, before discussing options for screening or treatment, the first step in evaluating older colorectal patients is to better understand the physiologic aging process and its impact on toxicity from treatment. There is a gradual loss of physiologic reserve and decline in normal organ function with aging such as decreases in the glomerular filtration rate, gastrointestinal motility, cardiac reserve, and immune and hematologic function (Table 11.1).

Table 11.2 Definitions of terms of geriatric conditions that impact life expectancy in older patients.[133,134]

Comorbidity	The concurrent presence of two or more conditions (or one severe), usually chronic in nature
Disability	Condition that causes dependency in performing tasks allowing for self-care and living in the community; can also include difficulties with mobility
Frailty	– A "stage of aging" that places an older person at high risk of physical or functional decline or death over a defined period of time – An index from the Cardiovascular Health Study where persons were frail if they had three of the following characteristics: low physical activity, weight loss, slow walking speed, low grip strength, or fatigue[134]
Functional dependence	– A condition in which an older person is unable to survive without the help of others; usually associated with deficits in activities and instrumental activities of daily living
Geriatric syndromes	– Conditions that are more likely to occur in older vulnerable and frail individuals: dementia, severe depression, falls, delirium, osteoporosis and fractures, neglect and abuse, failure to thrive
Vulnerability	– A "stage of aging" that places an older person at moderate risk of physical or functional decline or death over a defined period of time – Vulnerability generally precedes frailty – Also refers to a score of 3 or more on the Vulnerable Elders Survey, a score that is associated with a 4 times higher risk of decline or death than lower scores over a period of 2 years[135]

These changes are associated with increased toxicity and decreased tolerance to chemotherapy drugs. Along with the physical changes, there are often social support or financial concerns and more of an unwillingness to accept significant adverse effects despite the relative effectiveness of the treatments in older populations.[12] There is a need to find tools to help with decision making for therapy in older colorectal patients. These tools should clearly identify the fit older patients who will benefit from treatment for CRC without undue toxicity and should help with the evaluation of factors that may impact treatment tolerance in older, more vulnerable patients. The criteria used in the young and elderly to select or deny treatment may be different as changes that occur with the aging process may affect an older person's tolerance to treatment.[16] Patients should not be denied treatment based on their chronological age. Instead, therapeutic decision making should be individualized to the elderly patient. Various tools like the CGA, which takes into account a variety of factors known to affect morbidity and mortality in the older person, have been utilized to help determine fitness for treatment.[17] Elderly patients who are considered fit are readily identifiable and should be offered the same treatment strategies as those used in younger patients. On the opposite end of the spectrum, physicians can easily identify patients who are frail and in whom

less intensive, reduced-dose, or no chemotherapy is preferred. The intermediate or vulnerable category is much harder to define and even to recognize as these elderly may have hidden physical and/or functional deficiencies. For patients who are vulnerable, issues of life expectancy and treatment tolerance become particularly relevant.[7] (See Table 11.2) These issues will be discussed in the remainder of the book (see Chapter 1).

D. Screening for colorectal cancer in the elderly patient

With the rapidly aging population and an increasing prevalence of cancer in older adults, heath care providers are faced with opportunities and challenges in the prevention and early detection of CRC in this population. The highest incidence of CRC is in persons aged 70 years and older. Because there is a 5- to 10-year lead time for the development of carcinoma from precancerous adenomas, screening should be undertaken in persons between the ages of 60 and 70 years. Older patients (i.e., aged 70–80 years) should also be considered for screening given the high prevalence of CRC in this age group and increasing life expectancy. When considering the benefits and risks of cancer screening in the elderly, physiologic age based on underlying fitness rather than chronologic age should be assessed to estimate life expectancy. The potential improvement in life expectancy derived from a particular cancer screening test should be weighed against the current physiologic status of the patient, the potential harms of screening, and the individual's values and preferences.

Improvement in screening techniques has made a significant impact on the early detection of CRC and has reduced morbidity and mortality from this disease. Most guidelines advocate screening for CRC in adults over age 50 years with average risk.[18,19] The U.S. Preventive Services Task Force (USPSTF) recommends screening for CRC through yearly fecal occult blood testing, flexible sigmoidoscopy, double-contrast barium enema every 5 years, or colonoscopy every 10 years.[20] Until 2008, the USPSTF recommended that routine screening for persons of average risk begin at 50 years of age, and no age limit was set at which to stop screening. In a recent revision to the 2002 guidelines, USPSTF no longer recommends routine CRC screening in those aged 75–85 years old and recommends against any form of screening in patients older than 85 years.[21] These limits are only guidelines, and other consensus groups recommend more individualized decisions, of which expected longevity or remaining life expectancy (RLE) and screening history are important additional variables.[22] One criticism of the USPSTF guidelines is that these guidelines continue to center on chronologic rather than physiologic age. For example, a healthy 75-year-old may have more than 10 years of life expectancy and therefore may benefit from colorectal screening. Use of the CGA may help better individualize screening decisions for those older than 75 years.

The number of screening colonoscopies for CRC in elderly persons is increasing. An analysis of a population-based database, the National Health Interview Survey, showed that in the United States, the proportion of persons reporting up-to-date CRC testing increased from 39.5 percent in 2000 to 47.1 percent in 2005.[23] By 2005, endoscopy had become more common than home fecal occult blood testing for CRC screening. Data for cancer screening in the oldest subgroups of the population are lacking because few cancer screening clinical trials have included patients aged 70 years and over.[24] Therefore clinicians are forced to extrapolate potential benefits of screening for the elderly population.[25] Screening colonoscopy in very elderly persons (i.e., aged 80 years or older) should be performed only after careful consideration of potential benefits, risks, tolerance of eventual antineoplastic treatments, and patient prefer-

ences.[26,27] In one study that compared the impact of screening colonoscopy on outcomes of over 1,200 elderly persons,[27] the prevalence of precancerous and cancerous lesions was 13.8 percent in the 50- to 54-year-old group, 26.5 percent in the 75- to 79-year-old group, and 28.6 percent in the group aged 80 years or older. Despite higher prevalence of neoplasia in elderly patients, mean extension in life expectancy was much lower in the group aged 80 years or older than in the 50- to 54-year-old group (0.13 vs. 0.85 years). Even though prevalence of cancer increases with age, screening colonoscopy in very elderly persons (aged 80 years or older) results in only 15 percent of the expected gain in life expectancy in younger patients. Given the more limited survival benefit to older patients, the risks of the procedure should be discussed with the patient. Even though it is a relatively safe procedure, a higher risk of complications is seen in elderly patients. These risks include dehydration because of bowel preparation, electrolyte disturbances, and hypoxic complications or delirium from conscious sedation.[26] Risk of perforation of the colon was less than 0.5 percent in those aged 75 and above but was still 4 times higher than in the 65–69 age group, and the risk increased with higher numbers of comorbid conditions.[28] Failure to reach the cecum is also more common in older patients because of inadequate bowel prep and likelihood of strictures.

The decision of screening for CRC should be individualized based on RLE and the likelihood of finding polyps that would have adequate time needed for transformation into cancer. Polyps transform in about 10 years to cancer; therefore screening may not be necessary in someone with a life expectancy of 7–10 years to detect and remove polyps if the person has been undergoing routine screening previously.[29] Calculation of RLE is based on various tools like comorbidity index and functional status such as those used within the CGA.[30] In general, vulnerable or frail older adults who have difficulties performing activities of daily living and/or physical performance tests or who have one or more geriatric syndromes should forego screening colonoscopy unless they have increased risk of developing cancer over a short period of time because of their already limited life expectancy.[26] Even if the decision to forego screening in a person of advanced age or significant comorbidity is made, it is important to note that colonoscopies performed in patients with gastrointestinal symptoms (e.g., bleeding, constipation) are more likely to find CRCs compared to asymptomatic patients and should be considered for diagnostic workup rather than screening.[31]

E. Surgery for colorectal cancer in the elderly patient

Surgery is the cornerstone for treatment of localized CRC. Surgical resection of the primary tumor in the absence of metastatic disease is the main curative treatment approach for CRC. Curative options also exist for selected patients with advanced disease, including resection of liver or pulmonary metastasis, although there are limited data evaluating outcomes in elderly patients. Over the last decade, the numbers of surgeries for CRC in the elderly have increased, mainly because of improvements in surgical and anesthesia techniques.[32] Improvement in survival from CRC has been attributed to the decrease in operative mortality and possibly the inclusion of surgery in the treatment plan for local or distant metastatic disease.[1] Studies have shown that over 60 percent of patients requiring surgical intervention are aged 70 years and over.[33]

Elderly patients are also often viewed as high-risk surgical candidates with high rates of emergency presentations and perioperative mortality. One registry study evaluated outcomes of 6,457 patients with CRC from the Rotterdam Cancer Registry and found a disparity in treatment patterns between elderly and younger patients.[34] Resection rates were significantly lower in patients aged 89 or over and in patients with rectal cancer. Operative risk was greater than 10 percent for patients aged 80 and over compared to only 1 percent for those under the age of 60. Age was an independent prognostic factor for postoperative mortality in multivariate analysis. The CRC Collaborative Group published a systematic review of data from 28 independent studies that included 34,194 patients.[35] Of the 28 studies, 22 included patients with colon cancer and rectal cancer, 5 included only patients with rectal cancer, and 1 included only patients with colon cancer. Outcomes of patients aged 65–74 years, 75–84 years, 75–84 years, and 85 or more years were compared with those for patients aged less than 65 years. Older patients with an increased number of comorbid conditions were more likely to undergo emergency surgery and present with later-stage disease than younger patients. The relative risks for postoperative morbidity and mortality rose with increased age. For example, the relative risk of postoperative death was 1.8 for the 65–74 group compared to the reference incidence for the group aged less than 65 years, rising to 6.2 for those aged 85 years and over. Respiratory, cardiovascular, cerebrovascular, and thromboembolic complications were more common in those with advanced age. Although overall survival was lower for the patients of more advanced age at 2 years after surgery, cancer-specific survival differences were similar in all age groups, and differences were less pronounced if only persons who underwent curative resection were evaluated. The investigators concluded that other factors associated with age, such as comorbidities, may confound the relationship between age and surgical outcomes and that age alone should not preclude a curative surgical approach in elderly patients who are otherwise good risk.

Another study evaluated perioperative morbidity, perioperative mortality, and survival of 1,120 consecutive patients who underwent pelvic surgery for rectal cancer.[36] Outcomes of 157 patients aged 75 and older were compared to 174 younger patients randomly selected from the remaining 963 patients. There were no significant differences in perioperative complications between the two age groups. Although overall 5-year survival was lower in the older group (51% vs. 66%, $p = .02$), cancer-specific survival was not significantly different between the two groups (69% vs. 71%, $p = .75$). Basili and colleagues retrospectively studied 248 patients who underwent surgery for CRC and found that old age itself was not found to be an independent negative prognostic factor for CRC surgery.[37] These studies suggest that whenever possible, curative intent should be applied in CRC patients with good fitness, irrespective of age.[37,38] Other studies have also demonstrated that age did not significantly influence 5-year survival rates, the rates of local and distant recurrence, and complications from elective CRC surgery, although previous comorbidity did influence type of resection (emergency vs. elective).[39–42]

Outcomes of the elderly who undergo palliative surgery in the metastatic setting have not been as well studied. Although palliative surgery is recommended for patients with bowel obstruction or bleeding, the benefits of surgery for removal of the primary tumor in asymptomatic stage IV CRC patients are uncertain, and this approach has been debated. CRC patients aged 70 and over may benefit from liver resection for metastases and can achieve significant progression-free and 5-year survival from this aggressive approach.[43,44]

However, mortality from the procedure is also higher in elderly patients compared to their younger counterparts.[45] A population-based analysis utilizing the Medicare-SEER database reported that 72 percent of elderly patients ($n = 9,011$) with stage IV cancer underwent primary-cancer-directed surgery within 4 months of diagnosis.[46] Postoperative mortality at 30 days was 10 percent. Patients with left-sided colonic lesions or rectal tumors and those older than age 75 years, black, or of lower socioeconomic status were less likely to undergo surgery. Only 3.9 percent of patients underwent metastectomy, although it is unclear how many patients were eligible for this procedure.

Experts have advocated the use of the Preoperative Assessment of Cancer in the Elderly (PACE), a composite of validated questionnaires that includes the CGA, performance status, and assessments of surgical and anesthesia risks, to estimate risk for an individual elderly patient who is to undergo CRC surgery.[1] In a pilot study, PACE took approximately 20 minutes to complete and was acceptable to patients.[47,48] Performance status, activities of daily living, instrumental activities of daily living, and fatigue were significantly associated with general morbidity.

In summary, both short- and long-term outcomes are similar for the fit elderly compared to their younger counterparts. However, even in fit elders, advancing age is associated with reduced overall survival likely because of other comorbid conditions. An assessment such as PACE should be undertaken to evaluate risk from CRC surgery, and as much as possible, emergency surgery should be avoided because of an increase in morbidity and mortality compared to elective CRC procedures.[1]

F. Radiotherapy for rectal cancer in the elderly patient

Radiotherapy for rectal cancer is administered to facilitate resection in tumors considered unresectable, to prevent local recurrences, and to relieve pain or bleeding. Radiotherapy is an important consideration for all stages of rectal cancer, from curing superficial T1 disease to the palliative treatment of inoperable T4 tumors. Postoperative radiotherapy should be considered for all patients considered at high risk for local relapse after surgery if preoperative chemotherapy was not administered. This would include those patients with microscopic disease after surgery, those with node-positive disease, those with positive margins

on surgical pathology, and those who had tumor spillage during surgery.[49] Preoperative radiotherapy is generally recommended over postoperative therapy as this approach has been shown to increase efficacy of radiotherapy and reduce toxicity. Long-course radiotherapy prior to surgery (6–8 weeks later) leads to increased sphincter preservation and can downsize the primary rectal cancer.[50,51] Short-course preoperative therapy (5 Gy daily for 5 days with surgery 1 week later) has been shown to result in favorable pathological responses, overall survival, and toxicity.[52]

Dharma-Wardene and colleagues, from Alberta, Canada, evaluated patients with rectal adenocarcinoma and demonstrated that though a significant number of elderly patients were fit enough to tolerate major surgery, they were denied neoadjuvant or adjuvant therapies, presumably based on the risk for high treatment-related complication rates, with worry about a potential subsequent reduction in survival.[53] Another study that evaluated implantation of adjuvant guidelines (RT plus fluoropyrimidine chemotherapy) in 73 centers in the United States showed that only 5 percent of all patients received standard recommended schedules for combined chemoradiation.[49] An analysis of rectal cancer patients aged 80 and over in France revealed a wide variety of different treatment approaches, with only 54 percent of patients undergoing curative resection and 17 percent receiving radiotherapy.[15] A review of the clinical characteristics of these patients illustrated that more than 50 percent were eligible for pre- or postoperative radiotherapy.[1,15] Undertreatment of older persons is likely a result of the fact that there are very few patients aged 70 years and over in the radiotherapy trials that have established evidence-based approaches to the treatment of rectal cancer.[1,52,54,55]

Although fit elderly persons have been shown to derive a similar survival benefit from radiotherapy as their younger counterparts, older persons are more likely to experience toxicity from treatment.[35,56] Persons aged 75 and older had greater postoperative mortality after preoperative radiotherapy combined with TME (total mesorectal excision) in the Stockholm I trial. Toxicity and mortality are associated with higher dose and greater volume of area covered. Several studies have suggested equivalent benefit of preoperative short-course radiotherapy (5 × 5 Gy over 5 days) compared to the longer-course protocol (45–50 Gy over 4–5 weeks). Although preoperative chemoradiation has been shown to reduce pelvic recurrences more than radiotherapy alone, the overall benefit is small, survival advantage has not been proven, and few elders were included within these trials. Experts have proposed that radiotherapy be offered to all eligible older persons with rectal cancer, with short-course radiotherapy offered to older, more unfit patients. Studies have suggested that incorporating a 6- to 8-week delay after short-course radiation in older, unfit patients can help with tolerability of the radiotherapy and surgery and reduce postoperative mortality.[57,58] Further improved techniques in radiotherapy, such as intensity-modulated radiotherapy, may also improve toxicity in older patients. Despite the general consensus that radiotherapy improves outcomes for rectal cancer patients, the importance and role of radiotherapy must continue to be clarified, particularly with evaluation of overall toxicity survival benefit of preoperative chemoradiotherapy in more vulnerable populations.

G. Chemotherapy for the older patient with colorectal cancer

Approximately two-thirds of patients who are diagnosed with colon cancer are eligible to receive chemotherapy, either in the adjuvant setting or for treatment of metastatic disease. Approximately 50 percent of patients will have metastatic or unresectable cancers at the time of diagnosis or will develop metastatic disease after their initial treatment.[59] After a review of the evidence at a National Institutes of Health consensus conference in 1990, adjuvant chemotherapy for node-positive colon cancer became standard of care.[60] Prospective studies have also shown that chemotherapy for patients with metastatic disease improves quality of life and extends survival. Evidence has shown that the tolerability and efficacy of chemotherapy is similar for fit older persons compared to their younger counterparts.

G.1. Adjuvant chemotherapy for colorectal cancer

Adjuvant therapy is administered to eradicate potential residual micrometastatic disease following surgical resection. Adjuvant chemotherapy is considered the standard of care for patients with stage III colon cancer based on improvement in the overall 5-year survival rate from approximately 50 percent without adjuvant therapy to 65 percent with fluorouracil-based therapy after

surgical removal of the primary tumor.[61] More recently, the addition of a third agent, oxaliplatin, to fluorouracil plus leucovorin–based therapy has become the standard for stage III disease.[62] Table 11.3 summarizes results of studies that evaluate adjuvant chemotherapy in the elderly.

Numerous studies have demonstrated that receipt of adjuvant chemotherapy varies substantially with age. Ayanian and colleagues conducted a population-based study in California and found significantly different rates of administration of chemotherapy to stage II and III colon cancer patients based on age alone. Though 88 percent of patients aged 55 years and younger received chemotherapy, only 11 percent of those aged 85 years and older did.[63] In another study by Jessup and colleagues, the proportion of patients receiving surgery and adjuvant chemotherapy declined significantly with age. In 2001–2002, adjuvant chemotherapy was utilized in 82 percent of patients younger than 60 years but declined to 77.2 percent of those aged 60–69 years, 69 percent of those aged 70–79 years, and 39.2 percent of those aged 80 years or older.[64] A SEER database retrospective analysis by Schrag and colleagues evaluated 6,262 patients aged 65 years and older with resected stage III colon cancer and found that age at diagnosis correlated more than any other factor to receipt of chemotherapy. Overall, 55 percent received adjuvant chemotherapy within 3 months of colon cancer resection. The rates of receipt of chemotherapy were 78 percent, 74 percent, 58 percent, 34 percent, and 11 percent in the age range 65–69 years, 70–74 years, 75–79 years, 80–84 years, and 85–89 years, respectively.[65] When comparing overall survival with colon cancer-specific survival for 75- to 84-year-olds with stage III colon cancer, the investigators showed that cancer was a primary cause of death in this age group, warranting consideration for use of chemotherapy in patients with sufficient life expectancy.[65] A systematic review of 22 reports of the community rates of chemotherapy administration to patients with stage III colon cancer found significant variations in use with rates of chemotherapy use ranging from 39 to 71 percent.[66] Age and comorbidity were found to be the most significant patient factors. Older age was found to be a significant predictor of lack of evaluation by medical oncologists and/or failure to initiate chemotherapy. Nine studies analyzed the effect of comorbidity on the likelihood of receiving chemotherapy. Seven studies found higher comorbidity to be associated with a lower likelihood of receiving adjuvant

Table 11.3 Adjuvant chemotherapy for colorectal cancer in the elderly.

Study	Regimen	Study design	Sample size	Patient age	Disease-free survival	Overall survival	Toxicity (grade 3 or 4)
Monotherapy							
Popescu et al.[75a]	5-FU/LV	Prospective	543	124 aged ≥70	NR	NR	9% diarrhea 19% stomatitis 35% neutropenia
Sargent et al.[2]	5-FU/LV	Pooled	3,341	506 aged ≥70	69% disease free at 5 years	71% alive at 5 years	15% diarrhea 15% stomatitis 8% leucopenia
Haller et al.[71]	5-FU/LV	RCT	3,561	883 aged ≥70	53% disease free at 5 years	58% alive at 5 years	Older age increased the risk of stomatitis and leucopenia
QUASAR study group[72]	5-FU/LV	RCT for stage II disease	3,239	663 aged ≥70	Relative risk of recurrence at 2 years: 1.13 (0.74–1.75)	Relative risk of death at 2 years: 1.02 (0.70–1.48)	Impact of age on toxicity not reported
Fata et al.[74]	5-FU/LV	Retrospective	120	64 aged ≥65	70% disease free at 5 years	77% alive at 5 years	22% of older patients experienced grade 3 or 4 toxicity versus 16% of younger patients
Twelves et al.[80]	Capecitabine	RCT	1,984	20% aged ≥70	65.5% at 3 years in the total sample[b]	81.3% at 3 years in the total sample[b]	11% diarrhea 17% hand-foot 2% neutropenia 20% hyperbilirubinemia
Combination chemotherapy							
Andre et al.[62] Goldberg et al.[86]	FOLFOX		3,742	315 aged ≥70	Hazard ratio for recurrence-free survival at 3 years was 0.77; 78.2% disease free at 3 years; no impact of age on outcome	Hazard ratio for death at 3 years was 0.90; 87.7% alive at 3 years; no impact of age on outcome	49% neutropenia 5% thrombocytopenia 12% neuropathy[c]

Note. Efficacy and toxicity results reported for the elderly subsample. NR = not reported; RCT = randomized controlled trial.
[a] Included adjuvant and metastatic patients; adjuvant results reported in this table.
[b] No impact of age in multivariate analysis.
[c] Older age significantly associated with higher hematologic toxicity.

chemotherapy. Although the nine studies controlled for age, the interaction between age and comorbidity was not investigated. Gross and colleagues found that specific comorbidities were associated with decreased likelihood of receiving chemotherapy, including congestive heart failure (adjusted odds ratio [AOR] 0.49), chronic obstructive pulmonary disease (AOR 0.81), and diabetes (AOR 0.83).[67] In addition to receiving less chemotherapy, elders are more likely to have adjuvant chemotherapy discontinued before completion, possibly decreasing its effectiveness. Dobie and colleagues analyzed 3,193 patients using the SEER-Medicare database and found that only 2,497 (78.2%) completed the course of adjuvant chemotherapy.[68] Patients who were female, widowed, increasingly elderly, hospitalized, and living in certain regions were less likely to complete adjuvant chemotherapy than other patients.

The use of adjuvant treatment for those aged 70 years and over remains controversial because of concerns over increased toxicity and increased rates of death owing to noncancer causes in this population.[1] As life expectancy decreases, the absolute benefit of chemotherapy also decreases. Thus, for patients who are older and have comorbid illness, the absolute benefit of adjuvant chemotherapy may be small, and decisions to forego treatment may be appropriate given the patient's overall health status.[69] Data in elders, although limited, suggest that older patients derive significant benefit from adjuvant therapies provided they have life expectancies of 5 years or more.[70] Older patients entered into clinical trials are a selected group with minimal comorbidities. These persons represent a selected fit group that represents the healthiest of the older adults in the general population. Analyses of clinical trials that compare the outcomes of these generally fit patients aged 70 and over with those younger than age 70 demonstrate similar efficacy and tolerability of adjuvant chemotherapy.

Multiple studies have shown that adjuvant 5-fluorouracil (5-FU) with or without leucovorin has good tolerability and efficacy in fit older patients (Table 11.3). A pooled analysis of 3,351 elderly patients from seven clinical trials evaluated 5-fluorouracil-based adjuvant therapy for stage II–III disease.[2] Chemotherapy was associated with a statistically significant effect on overall survival (hazard ratio [HR] 0.76) and time to recurrence (HR 0.68) when compared to surgery alone. Toxicity was not found to be significantly higher for those aged 70 years and over. However,

probability of death from causes other than cancer was strongly associated with higher age. Patients aged 70 and over had a 13 percent higher probability of death owing to causes other than cancer compared to 2 percent in those aged 50 years or younger. Various adjuvant 5-FU regimens were compared in 3,561 patients with high-risk stage II and III colon cancer in the Intergroup 0089 phase III clinical trial.[71] Persons aged 70 years and older made up 24.8 percent of the patient sample. Older age (65 years or older) was significantly associated with decreased 5-year disease-free survival (61% vs. 53%, $p < .0001$) and overall survival (66% vs. 58%, $p < .0001$). Within a proportional hazard regression model, older age (over 65 years) was associated with a significantly higher risk of dying at 5 years (HR 1.47, 95% confidence interval [CI] 1.33–1.64). Older patients also had significantly higher rates of stomatitis and leucopenia, although toxicity-related mortality was not different between the older and younger patients. The QUASAR trial evaluated whether 5-FU-leucovorin improved outcomes for stage II cancer patients.[72] The trial involved 3,239 patients, and 663 (20%) were aged 70 years and over. The absolute survival benefit for the whole group was small (3.6%), and chemotherapy did not decrease the relative risk of disease recurrence or death in the older patients. Other investigations have confirmed the efficacy and tolerability of 5-FU used in the adjuvant setting to treat elderly patients with stage III CRC.[73–75] However, the impact of adjuvant chemotherapy on overall survival in elderly patients, especially those who are vulnerable, requires further research.

Studies utilizing population-based registries provide additional information on the efficacy of adjuvant therapy in a more heterogeneous population. Two population-based studies utilizing the SEER-Medicare linked database found improved survival for those patients receiving adjuvant chemotherapy. In a study by Sundararajan and colleagues,[76] 52 percent of patients received 5-FU therapy. The hazard ratio for death associated with 5-FU therapy was 0.66 (95% CI 0.60–0.73). Iwashyna and Lamont[77] found that 5-FU reduced the hazard of death by 27 percent (HR 0.73, 95% CI 0.65–0.82) and that the survival benefit did not diminish with older age.

The optimal duration of adjuvant chemotherapy in patients with node-positive disease has been controversial. Clinical trials varied with duration of treatment ranging from 6 to 12 months of treatment with 5-FU. Randomized clinical trials have also shown similar benefits in patients who received 6 months of therapy as compared to 12 months.[78] A retrospective study done by Neugut and colleagues with SEER-Medicare data on patients older than 65 years receiving adjuvant treatment for stage III disease showed a significant decrease in mortality in the group receiving 5–7 months of treatment compared to those who discontinued therapy before 5 months.[79] Older age and comorbidity were associated with early discontinuation of therapy. Therefore experts recommend that adjuvant therapy be given for at least 5 months, with the optimal duration being 6 months.[1]

Capecitabine, an oral pro-drug of 5-FU, has been studied in the clinical trial setting for use as an adjuvant treatment. Capecitabine has been shown to be an effective and safe alternative for use in the adjuvant setting. A randomized study (X-ACT trial) conducted by Twelves and colleagues in 1,987 patients showed similar disease-free and overall survival using capecitabine or bolus fluorouracil-leucovorin in patients with resected stage III colon cancer.[80] Approximately 20 percent of patients were aged 70 years or over. Disease-free survival in the capecitabine group was at least equivalent to that in the fluorouracil plus leucovorin group (in the intention-to-treat analysis, $p < .001$, for the comparison of the upper limit of the hazard ratio with the noninferiority margin of 1.20). Capecitabine improved relapse-free survival (HR 0.86, 95% CI 0.74–0.99, $p = .04$) and was associated with significantly fewer adverse events than fluorouracil plus leucovorin. Age was not independently associated with adverse outcome in multivariate analysis. Capecitabine was subsequently approved as a single agent for adjuvant therapy. Data from the X-ACT trial were analyzed retrospectively for safety. Patients randomized to capecitabine had less diarrhea ($p = .002$), nausea ($p = .005$), and neutropenia ($p < .00001$). All grades of hand-foot syndrome and grade 3 or 4 hyperbilirubinemia were seen more with capecitabine.[81] Owing to its oral use and superior overall safety profile, capecitabine can be considered a preferred drug for use in the adjuvant setting for the elderly population. However, care must be taken in elderly patients who have comorbidities, such as renal dysfunction or cardiovascular disease, and are receiving warfarin. Capecitabine-related toxicity is higher in patients with renal dysfunction likely because of higher systemic concentrations of catabolites

of the drug.[82] Therefore capecitabine should be dose reduced in patients with renal dysfunction, and dosing should be based on creatinine clearance. Capecitabine increases the risk of internal bleeding when utilized with warfarin. There is a significant pharmacokinetic interaction between capecitabine and warfarin. In a small study ($n = 4$) during capecitabine treatment, the area under the plasma concentration time curve of warfarin increased by 57 percent (90% CI 32–88) with a 51 percent prolongation of the elimination half-life ($t[1/2]$, 90% CI 32–74).[83] A retrospective study ($n = 77$) showed that close to 30 percent of patients who received capecitabine were also using warfarin and that those who received the two drugs experienced more episodes of gastrointestinal bleeding within 130 days (18% vs. 2%).[84] In a larger retrospective study ($n = 883$), 11 percent of patients received capecitabine concurrent with warfarin.[85] These authors found no increased risk of bleeding when warfarin was carefully managed. Therefore, for those who have manageable comorbidities, capecitabine as adjuvant therapy is an option and may be more convenient and acceptable than intravenous chemotherapy. In older patients, adherence to capecitabine should be carefully monitored.

The adjuvant treatment of elderly patients using combination chemotherapy has not been as well studied as 5-FU-leucovorin monotherapy. Although clinical trials investigating combination therapies have included elderly patients, the numbers were few, and the older patients included were likely healthier than those in the general population. A retrospective analysis of 3,742 colorectal patients (614 aged 70 and over) from four randomized clinical trials who received FOLFOX 4 (bolus and infusional 5-FU, leucovorin, and oxaliplatin) in the adjuvant, first-, and second-line settings found that the relative benefit of chemotherapy versus control was not affected by age for progression or recurrence-free survival.[86] The hazard ratios for overall survival for FOLFOX versus a comparator group were similar in older patients (0.82, 95% CI 0.63–1.06) compared to younger patients (0.77, 95% CI 0.67–0.88, $p = .79$). Although hematologic (both neutropenia and thrombocytopenia) toxicity was higher in older patients, other toxicities, such as neurologic events, diarrhea, nausea/vomiting, infection, and overall grade 3 events, were not significantly increased in the older patients. Dose intensity was similar in both age groups. Although these data were promising, the older patients were a highly

Table 11.4 Initial chemotherapy received for advanced colorectal cancer in 10 community practices.

	Age ≤65 ($n = 239$)	Age >65 ($n = 281$)	p value
Irinotecan plus fluoropyrimidine	26%	15%	<.01
Oxaliplatin plus fluoropyrimidine	58%	43%	<.001
Fluoropyrimidine alone	14%	39%	<.001
Number of chemotherapy cycles (median, range)	7 (4–11)	4 (3–8)	<.001
Bevacizumab plus chemotherapy[a]	63%	44%	.001

Note. Adapted from McKibbin et al.[87]
[a]For patients treated after May 1, 2004.

select group, representing only 16 percent of those enrolled within the clinical trials.

Overall the data support the use of adjuvant therapy for older patients deemed fit enough to tolerate treatment.[70] The survival benefit in vulnerable older patients is difficult to assess because of the higher risk in this population of dying from noncancer causes. More information is needed on the appropriate treatment strategies for those who are more vulnerable (i.e., have comorbidity or functional limitations) that may affect life expectancy. No population-based analyses are available that evaluate the use of combination adjuvant therapies for older patients, and there is limited information regarding the survival benefit of adjuvant therapy for patients aged 75 years and older.[1] Most persons aged 75 years and older are independent, have good organ function, and have a life expectancy without cancer of greater than 10 years. Eighty percent of patients with stage III colon cancer who recur do so within 3 years and, after recurrence, have a life expectancy with cancer of less than 5 years. Therefore it is reasonable to consider adjuvant chemotherapy even in selected older patients aged 75 years and over.

G.2. Chemotherapy for metastatic colorectal cancer

Until recently, bolus 5-FU and leucovorin was the standard of care for treatment of metastatic CRC. Current standard first-line therapies for fit elders with good performance status include FOLFOX (bolus/infusional 5-FU with oxaliplatin) and/or FOLFIRI (bolus/infusional 5-FU with irinotecan) with or without bevacizumab. Although evidence suggests that these regimens are tolerable and efficacious for older persons with a good performance status, studies have shown that elderly patients are

less likely to receive chemotherapy. One study that evaluated the management of advanced CRC in 10 community practices found that only 56 percent of elderly patients received first-line therapy.[87] Of the younger patients, 84 percent received doublet chemotherapy first line compared with 58 percent of elderly patients ($p < .001$). The use of irinotecan, oxaliplatin, and bevacizumab was lower in elderly patients ($p < .001$) (Table 11.4). Independent predictors of a higher risk for mortality were age under 65 (HR 1.19) and performance status of 2 or higher (HR 1.65). Though toxicity-related hospitalizations, numbers of clinic visits, and delays in therapy were significantly higher in elderly patients, other toxicity-related end points did not differ significantly between older and younger patients.

Chemotherapy strategies and options for CRC have evolved rapidly in the past few years. Table 11.5 summarizes results from selected studies that evaluate single-agent palliative chemotherapy for use in elderly patients. For some decades, 5-FU was the only drug available with activity in CRC. Palliative treatment with the combination of fluorouracil with levamisole or leucovorin has been shown to improve response rates, time to progression, and overall survival in elderly patients with metastatic CRC with acceptable toxicity.[75,88,89] In a trial by Popescu and colleagues of patients with colon cancer,[75] 844 received first-line therapy with various fluorouracil regimens or ralitrexed, and 543 received adjuvant treatment with protracted infusion of fluorouracil or bolus fluorouracil/folinic acid. Of all patients, 310 were aged 70 years or over. Of those with advanced disease, there was no difference in response rates (24% vs. 29%, $p = .19$) or median progression-free survival (164 vs. 168 days) between younger and older patients. There was no difference in overall or severe toxicity between the two age groups,

Table 11.5 Studies of single-agent chemotherapy for metastatic colorectal cancer in the elderly.

Study	Drugs	Response rate	Overall survival	Grade 3 or 4 toxicity
Mattioli et al.[91]	FU/LV	18%	13 months	No grade 3 or 4 toxicity
Popescu et al.[75]	FU/LV	24%	292 days	10% neutropenia 9% diarrhea 6% somatitis
Daniele et al.[90]	FU/LV	21%	12.6 months	3% diarrhea
Chau et al.[95]	Irinotecan	11%	9.1 months	35% neutropenia 15% diarrhea 21% lethargy
Rosati et al.[96]	Irinotecan	13%	8.3 month	39% neutropenia 13% diarrhea 9% lethargy
Feliu et al.[113]	Capecitabine	24%	11 months	2% neutropenia 6% diarrhea 6% hand-foot syndrome

Note. Patients generally aged 70 or over and fit.

except for increased grade 1 or 2 mucositis in older patients receiving bolus fluorouracil. Folprecht and colleagues carried out a retrospective analysis using source data of 3,825 patients who received 5-FU-containing treatment in 22 European trials.[89] The trials included 629 patients who were aged 70 years or older. Response rate (23.9% and 21.1%, respectively, $p = .14$) and progression-free survival (5.5 months, 95% CI 5.2–5.8; compared with 5.3 months, 95% CI 5.1–5.5, $p = .01$) were similar between older and younger patients. In addition, the investigators found an equal overall survival in elderly patients (10.8 months, 95% CI 9.7–11.8) and in younger patients (11.3 months, 95% CI 10.9–11.7, $p = .31$). In both age groups, infusional 5-FU resulted in significantly increased response rates, overall survival, and progression-free survival compared with bolus 5-FU. The investigators concluded that fit elderly patients benefited to the same extent from palliative chemotherapy with 5-FU as younger patients. Other studies that have evaluated palliative treatment with 5-FU-leucovorin in elderly populations have also shown this regimen to be tolerable and have efficacy comparable to what is expected for the younger patient population.[75,90,91]

More recently, several other cytotoxic and biologic agents have been used with improvements in survival in the metastatic setting.[7] Irinotecan, as a single agent, has demonstrated clinical benefit as second-line treatment after fluorouracil failure in patients with metastatic CRC.[92,93] A phase II study by Rothenberg and colleagues evaluated the efficacy and toxicity of irinotecan in patients

with metastatic CRC that had progressed after fluorouracil-based chemotherapy.[94] Patients aged 65 years and older were twice as likely as younger patients (38.6% vs. 18.8%, $p < .008$) to develop grade 3 and 4 diarrhea. A study by Chau and colleagues evaluated outcomes of 339 patients who received irinotecan as a single agent (350 mg/m^2 once every 3 weeks) after progression with first-line 5-FU-based chemotherapy.[95] No differences were seen between patients aged under 70 and those aged 70 years and older in response rates (9% vs. 11%) and median survival time (9 vs. 9.4 months). In this study, the proportion of older patients who experienced irinotecan-specific toxicity was similar to younger patients (45.8% vs. 37.8%). Another study prospectively evaluated 23 older patients who received weekly irinotecan (80 mg/m^2 per week for 2 weeks of a 3-week cycle).[96] There was one objective partial response and stable disease noted in another 10 patients. Approximately 40 percent experienced grade 3 or 4 neutropenia, although there was only one episode of febrile neutropenia. Grade 3 diarrhea occurred in 13 percent of patients. In other studies, irinotecan was shown to be associated with a high rate of diarrhea in elderly patients in the second-line setting, especially when given with bolus 5-FU rather than infusional administration.[97,98] In a study of 291 patients (98 who were aged 70 or over), patients were randomized to receive weekly irinotecan (125 mg/m^2 weekly for 4 weeks of a 6-week cycle) or every-3-week dosing (350 mg/m^2). Patients aged 70 years or over who received previous pelvic radiation or who had a performance status of 2 or more were further stratified to receive a lower dose of 3-weekly irinotecan (300 mg/m^2). In multivariate regression analysis, age 70 or over independently predicted grade 3 or 4 diarrhea. Older age did not influence time to progression or overall survival. Because of a potentially higher risk of diarrhea, dose modification should therefore be considered in elderly patients who are to receive irinotecan, although more research is necessary.

In elderly patients, specific drug combinations have not been studied within phase III randomized studies that evaluate efficacy or establish a safety profile; however, various phase II studies and subgroup analyses provide some evidence about therapeutic choices for this population (Table 11.5). The IFL regimen (bolus irinotecan-5-FU-leucovorin) was approved for first-line treatment of metastatic CRC in 2000. Response rates ranged from 31 to 39 percent, with median overall survival of approximately 15 months.[9,99] Combined analysis of 2,691 patients (599 who were aged 70 years or over) showed similar efficacy in older and younger patients.[100] However, older patients had a higher incidence of grade 3 or 4 neutropenia (24.3% vs. 16.1%). Vomiting, diarrhea, and dehydration are also more likely to be experienced by older patients receiving IFL.[99] FOLFIRI (bolus irinotecan with bolus/infusional 5-FU) has largely replaced IFL because of its better safety profile. FOLFIRI as first-line therapy was examined by Sastre and colleagues[101] and Souglakos and colleagues.[102] Both studies showed response rates (33–35%) and median overall survival (7–8 months) in patients older than 70 years that were comparable to the outcomes expected for younger patients. Toxicity was also similar, with grade 3 or 4 diarrhea occurring in approximately 20 percent of patients. Neutropenia was also observed in approximately 20 percent of patients.

A multivariate analysis that included 602 patients from two phase III studies of irinotecan (one in the first-line and one in the second-line setting) examined predictive factors of survival and found that elderly age was not associated with decreased survival.[103] A second pooled analysis utilized data from three randomized studies[9,104,105] of 5-FU-leucovorin versus irinotecan-5-FU-leucovorin to evaluate outcomes in elderly (70 years and older, $n = 249$) compared to nonelderly ($n = 1,010$).[100] Response rates, time to progression, and survival were comparable between the two groups. For those treated with the irinotecan combination, there was no increase in

grade 3 or 4 toxicity rates in the elderly compared to nonelderly groups.

Of note, polymorphisms in the UDP glucuronosyltransferase 1 family polypeptide A1 (UGT1A1) enzyme have been strongly associated with toxicity.[106] Prospective screening of patients for a dinucleotide repeat polymorphism in the UGTA1A1 promotor region, which has been correlated with severe neutropenia from irinotecan, may decrease the frequency of severe toxicities by avoiding irinotecan in elderly at risk.[32] In summary, although the efficacy and safety of irinotecan as a single agent or in combination therapy should be an option for elderly patients with good performance status, underlying factors that predict increased risk of toxicity (especially diarrhea) need to be further investigated. Randomized clinical trials focusing on irinotecan treatment regimens in the elderly are awaited.

Combination chemotherapy with oxaliplatin has also been shown to be effective and safe for older patients. The FOLFOX regimen resulted in better response rates and prolonged time to progression than the 5-FU (bolus plus 22-hour infusion every 2 weeks) regimen for first-line treatment in patients with metastatic CRC.[8] The dose-limiting toxicity of oxaliplatin was neurotoxicity, characterized by acute dysthesias and a cumulative peripheral neurotoxicity that is generally reversible with discontinuation of therapy. Sensory neuropathy generally occurs after cumulative doses of oxaliplatin of 700 mg/m^2 and often requires discontinuation of the drug.[107,108] Goldberg and colleagues conducted a retrospective, age-based, pooled analysis of data from three clinical trials using the FOLFOX 4 regimen for metastatic disease and one adjuvant trial, including de Gramont and colleagues,[8] Goldberg and colleagues,[99] Rothenberg and colleagues,[109] and MOSAIC.[62] These four trials formed the basis of U.S. Food and Drug Administration approval of this regimen in adjuvant and metastatic settings. In total, there were 314 patients (16%) older than 70 years, and age was not associated with differences in disease-free survival.[86] All patients regardless of age had improved disease-free survival ($p < .0001$). Hematologic toxicity was more common in elderly, specifically neutropenia ($p = .04$) and thrombocytopenia ($p = .04$). Other toxicity rates were similar in elderly and nonelderly persons. FOLFOX improved cancer outcomes in all four trials compared to control regardless of age,[86] although there were a few patients in this study older than 80 years, thus making it very difficult to extrapolate data to the very elderly. Phase II and subgroup analyses have evaluated standard FOLFOX,[110] with oxaliplatin fractionated over 2 days[111] and with dose reduction in older patients,[112] and have found comparable efficacy. In the trial with bifractionated oxaliplatin, the overall response rate was 51 percent (95% CI 41–63) with a median duration of response of 9 percent. Grade 3 neuropathy was only seen in 6 percent of patients, and grade 3 and 4 diarrhea occurred in 10.2 percent of patients. Activity of daily living and instrumental activity of daily living scores were maintained through 12 cycles of treatment. Although the toxicity rates of this regimen were higher in the very elderly utilizing standard treatment, there were fewer adverse events associated with fractionated oxaliplatin or dose reductions. More information is needed to determine which elderly patients should be considered for treatment with these alternative administration options. In addition, more information is needed regarding the impact of neurotoxicity on quality of life indices important to the elderly such as physical and functional performance.

For elderly patients with advanced CRC who are deemed ineligible for combination approaches, capecitabine has been shown to be an effective and safe option.[113] Dose-limiting side effects include diarrhea and hand-foot syndrome. In one study of 51 patients, disease control (CR + PR + stable disease) was achieved in 67 percent of patients, and treatment-related adverse events of grade 3 or 4 were observed in only 12 percent of patients (diarrhea, hand-foot syndrome, thrombocytopenia). Median overall survival was 11 months (95% CI 8.6–13.3). Capecitabine dose was reduced from 1,250 mg/m^2 twice daily for 2 weeks of a 3-week cycle to 950 mg/m^2 twice daily in those with reduced creatinine clearance (30–50 mL/min). Cassidy and colleagues performed an analysis evaluating efficacy and toxicity of capecitabine in the elderly using data from two phase III studies ($n = 1,207$) that randomized 1,207 patients to oral capecitabine versus intravenous fluorouracil/folinic acid as first-line chemotherapy for metastatic CRC.[114] A poor safety profile was demonstrated in patients aged 80 years and over, mainly because of a higher incidence of grade 3 and 4 gastrointestinal events. However, multivariate analysis revealed that age was not independently associated with adverse events from capecitabine. The toxicity of capecitabine in older patients was thought to be caused by age-related decline in renal function.[115]

Capecitabine has been used in combination with irinotecan and oxaliplatin and has shown similar efficacy and tolerability in elderly patients.[16] The combination of capecitabine plus oxaliplatin (CapOX regimen) represents an option for first-line treatment of metastatic disease in elderly patients.[116,117] In a phase II study of 50 patients[117] receiving capecitabine-oxaliplatin, overall response rate was 36 percent with an additional 36 percent of patients with stable disease. The median times to disease progression and overall survival were 5.8 months (95% CI 3.9–7.8) and 13.2 months (95% CI 7.6–16.9), respectively. Capecitabine was well tolerated overall; grade 3–4 adverse events were observed in 14 (28%) patients, and there was one treatment-related death. The FOCUS2 trial, published in abstract form,[118] was designed to evaluate the use of 5-FU or capecitabine with or without capecitabine in elderly and frail patients using a 2 × 2 factorial design. Eligible patients were considered unfit for standard full-dose combination chemotherapy. Patients were deemed unfit if they were unwilling or unsuitable for undergoing full-dose combination chemotherapy. Starting doses were 80 percent standard, with an option to escalate to full dose at 6 weeks. Patients ($n = 460$) were randomized with 43 percent of patients who were aged more than 75 years. The conclusions of the study were that quality-of-life data did not favor capecitabine over 5-FU and that comparison of progression-free survival favored the addition of oxaliplatin but did not reach significance (HR 0.87, 95% CI 0.71–1.06, $p = .16$). Capecitabine was similar to 5-FU in efficacy, but it increased the risk of grade 3 toxicity. The investigators concluded that in this frail elderly population, substituting capecitabine for 5-FU did not improve overall quality of life or efficacy and significantly increased toxicity.

The use of biologic agents, including cetuximab and bevacizumab, in combination with chemotherapy has not been well studied in the elderly population.[16] Use of cetuximab, an epidermal growth factor inhibitor (EGFR), combined with chemotherapy has shown improvement in response rates and progression-free survival when given as first-line treatment or after chemotherapy failure for metastatic CRC in patients with K-RAS wild-type tumors. It is fairly well tolerated, with the side effects being acnelike rash, infusion-related toxicity, and diarrhea.[119] In patients with metastatic CRC, combination chemotherapy with cetuximab can prolong median survival to 24 months in selected patients.[120,121] No prospective studies have evaluated cetuximab solely in a population of elderly patients. However, subgroup analyses from randomized studies and retrospective analysis suggest that the efficacy of chemotherapy with cetuximab is maintained in fit elderly patients, with slightly increased but acceptable toxicity. In a planned subgroup analysis, there were no differences in progression-free or overall survival between patients aged 65 years or older and younger patients.[122] In a retrospective study evaluating the efficacy of cetuximab in mostly pretreated elderly patients (median age 76 years, range 70–84), response rate was still 21 percent, median progression-free survival was over 4 months, and median overall survival was 16 months.[123] These studies also showed that the toxicity profile of cetuximab is similar in elderly patients compared to younger patients. Response to cetuximab has been shown to be related to the K-RAS mutation status, with response being almost exclusively seen in tumors with wild-type K-RAS as opposed to mutated K-RAS. Several trials of anti-EGFR therapies have shown higher objective response rates to cetuximab in patients with wild-type K-RAS.[124] Thus the current available data support the use of cetuximab in fit elderly patients whose tumors are wild-type K-RAS.

Bevacizumab, a recombinant humanized monoclonal antibody to the vascular EGFR, has demonstrated statistically significant improvements in response rates, progression-free survival, and overall survival when used with chemotherapy in various trials.[125] Generally, studies have found that bevacizumab with chemotherapy is as safe and effective for elderly colorectal patients as in younger patients. However, bevacizumab is associated with side effects that require careful consideration in the elderly, including hypertension, proteinuria, bleeding, wound-healing complications, and bowel perforation. Of particular importance is the risk of arterial thrombembolic events following bevacizumab, which may be more likely to occur in the elderly, especially in those who have had a previous history of such events such as stroke or myocardial infarction.[1,126] Kabbinavar and colleagues examined the clinical benefit of bevacizumab plus fluorouracil–based chemotherapy in first-line metastatic CRC treatment in patients aged 65 years and over, using data from two placebo-controlled clinical trials.[127] Efficacy and safety data were analyzed for 439 patients aged 65 years and older randomized to bevacizumab plus chemotherapy or placebo plus chemotherapy. The median age of patients was between 71 and 75 years old, and ages ranged from 65 to 90 years. However, approximately 27 percent of patients were older than 70 years, and a few patients were aged 80 years and over. Median overall survival was 19.3 months in the bevacizumab arm versus 14.3 months in the placebo plus chemotherapy arm. Toxicity was deemed to be similar to that expected in younger patients. Deaths and rates of study discontinuation were similar between the two arms. The incidence of arterial thromboembolic events of any grade was 7.6 percent in the bevacizumab plus chemotherapy group compared to 2.8 percent in the placebo plus chemotherapy group. Recently, the TREE[128] studies have evaluated the effect of the addition of bevacizumab to FOLFOX, 5-FU alone, and CapeOX regimens and have shown improvement in median survival, making it to almost 2 years. The CapeOX regimen when dose reduced was tolerated much better with less toxicity. Although this study was not designed for older patients, the study included patients older than 70 years, and there was not an increase in rates of adverse events in the available data. An analysis of data from 1,745 patients who received bevacizumab plus chemotherapy for metastatic cancer found that older age and history of atherosclerosis were independent risk factors for the development of arterial thrombotic events.[126] Overall, though benefits of bevacizumab are comparable in older patients to what is expected in younger patients, the toxicity profile differs slightly, and the risk of arterial thrombotic events with bevacizumab-containing regimens, while relatively low, may be higher in older patients than in younger patients, especially in those who have comorbidities.

In summary, given the current evidence, combination chemotherapy with FOLFOX, FOLFIRI, or capecitabine-oxaliplatin should be considered for fit, older patients. With little exception, fit elderly patients benefit to the same degree as younger patients from systemic chemotherapy. Bevacizumab can be used in elderly patients as first-line therapy in combination with chemotherapy with careful selection of patients. Bevacizumab should be avoided in patients with history of a recent vascular thrombotic event such as stroke or myocardial infarction or severe hypertension. For those who are more vulnerable, single-agent 5-FU or capecitabine can be considered. Special attention to renal function with dose reduction of capecitabine according to creatinine clearance should be undertaken. 5-FU continuous infusion has been shown to be more effective and less toxic than bolus 5-FU. For those without contraindications, 5-FU-leucovorin plus bevacizumab may be a good therapeutic option for vulnerable elderly patients.[127] If tolerated after one or two cycles, irinotecan or oxaliplatin can be added.

It is important, before initiating chemotherapy, to understand the preferences and values of the patient to appropriately individualize treatment decision making. In a study conducted by Elkins and colleagues to determine patient and physician preferences for chemotherapy, patients aged 70–89 years were interviewed within 16 weeks of metastatic CRC diagnosis. Most patients (96%) decided to receive chemotherapy, although a few (44%) wanted prognostic information. Preference for prognostic information was more common among men than women (56% vs. 29%, $p < .05$). About half of the patients (52%) preferred a passive role in the treatment decision-making process. Physician perceptions were similar to patient preferences for information in 44 percent and for decision control in 41 percent of patient-physician pairs. The investigators concluded that detailed discussion of preferred decision-making styles could potentially improve the physician-patient relationship by helping to identify patients who would benefit from shared decision making.[129]

H. Conclusion

Although half of all CRC patients are aged 70 years and over, elderly patients have been underrepresented in clinical trials. As a result, evidence-based data regarding the appropriate therapeutic strategies in this age group are sparse.[1,6] Underlying health status and life expectancy should be carefully considered prior to consideration of screening for CRC or treatment of elderly patients who are already diagnosed. Although data are limited, a comprehensive geriatric assessment for older patients with CRC can help stratify patients according to comorbidity and functional status. Values and preferences of the patient should be carefully assessed in addition. Aggres-

sive standard-of-care treatment is advocated for the fit elderly. For example, for fit older patients with metastatic CRC, combination treatment with FOLFOX or FOLFIRI has been show to be as safe and effective as in younger patients. The choice of regimen should be based on the patient's preference and specific toxicity profile. On the other hand, in frail older patients with limited life expectancy, the risk of chemotherapy is high, and palliative or supportive care should be considered. The majority of older patients are neither fit nor frail. These patients are vulnerable to increased toxicity because of underlying comorbidity or impaired functional, physical performance, or cognitive status. In addition, poor performance status may be caused by the cancer in these patients.[6] Older patients, even those who are vulnerable, can undergo surgical resection without a significant increase in morbidity or mortality from the procedure. The risks and benefits of adjuvant treatment for those who have stage III disease should be carefully considered and balanced with estimated life expectancy. For vulnerable older patients with metastatic disease, single-agent treatment with 5-FU, preferably infusional, could be undertaken, and if tolerated, addition of irinotecan or oxaliplatin could be considered. Bevacizumab is also an option in combination with chemotherapy for those without significant cardiovascular disease or a history of stroke or thromboembolic disease. Older patients, especially those with metastatic disease, may also benefit from drug holidays that allow for recovery from cumulative toxicity to allow for resumption of chemotherapy later.[108] In summary, information regarding the most appropriate treatment for CRC in elderly patients has been mainly based on extrapolation of data or pooled analyses from clinical trials. Because clinical trials tend to enroll the most healthy and motivated of older individuals, these data may not be applicable to older patients in the general population. Clinical trials that incorporate the principles of geriatric assessment are necessary to determine the best management strategies for vulnerable older adults with CRC.

References

1. Papamichael D, Audisio R, Horiot JC, et al. Treatment of the elderly colorectal cancer patient: SIOG expert recommendations. *Ann Oncol.* 2009;20(1):5–16.

2. Sargent DJ, Goldberg RM, Jacobson SD, et al. A pooled analysis of adjuvant chemotherapy for resected colon cancer in elderly patients. *N Engl J Med.* 2001;345(15):1091–1097.

3. Jemal A, Siegel R, Ward E, et al. Cancer statistics, 2008. *CA Cancer J Clin.* 2008;58(2):71–96.

4. Donald JJ, Burhenne HJ. Colorectal cancer: can we lower the death rate in the 1990s? *Can Fam Physician.* 1993;39:107–114.

5. National Cancer Institute homepage. Available at: http://seer.cancer.gov/.

6. Raftery L, Sanoff HK, Goldberg R. Colon cancer in older adults. *Semin Oncol.* 2008;35(6): 561–568.

7. Kohne CH, Folprecht G, Goldberg RM, et al. Chemotherapy in elderly patients with colorectal cancer. *Oncologist.* 2008;13(4):390–402.

8. de Gramont A, Figer A, Seymour M, et al. Leucovorin and fluorouracil with or without oxaliplatin as first-line treatment in advanced colorectal cancer. *J Clin Oncol.* 2000;18(16): 2938–2947.

9. Saltz LB, Cox JV, Blanke C, et al. Irinotecan plus fluorouracil and leucovorin for metastatic colorectal cancer. Irinotecan Study Group. *N Engl J Med.* 2000;343(13):905–914.

10. Arkenau HT, Chua YJ, Cunningham D. Current treatment strategies in elderly patients with metastatic colorectal cancer. *Clin Colorectal Cancer.* 2007;6(7):508–515.

11. Trimble EL, Carter CL, Cain D, et al. Representation of older patients in cancer treatment trials. *Cancer.* 1994;74(7 suppl): 2208–2214.

12. Townsley CA, Selby R, Siu LL. Systematic review of barriers to the recruitment of older patients with cancer onto clinical trials. *J Clin Oncol.* 2005;23(13):3112–3124.

13. Shayne M, Culakova E, Poniewierski MS, et al. Dose intensity and hematologic toxicity in older cancer patients receiving systemic chemotherapy. *Cancer.* 2007;110(7):1611–1620.

14. Brenner H, Gondos A, Arndt V. Recent major progress in long-term cancer patient survival disclosed by modeled period analysis. *J Clin Oncol.* 2007;25(22):3274–3280.

15. Bouvier AM, Launoy G, Lepage C, et al. Trends in the management and survival of digestive tract cancers among patients aged over 80 years. *Ailment Pharmacol Ther.* 2005;22:233–241.

16. Sanoff HK, Bleiberg H, Goldberg RM. Managing older patients with colorectal cancer. *J Clin Oncol.* 2007;25(14):1891–1897.

17. Balducci L, Tam-McDevitt J, Hauser R, et al. Long overdue: phase II studies in older cancer patients: where does the FDA stand? *J Clin Oncol.* 2008; 26(8):1387–1388.

18. Losey R, Messinger-Rapport BJ. At what age should we discontinue colon cancer screening in the elderly? *Cleve Clin J Med.* 2007;74(4):269–272.

19. Smith RA, von Eschenbach AC, Wender R, et al. American Cancer Society guidelines for the early detection of cancer: update of early detection guidelines for prostate, colorectal, and endometrial cancers. Also: update 2001 – testing for early lung cancer detection. *CA Cancer J Clin.* 2001;51(1):38–75; quiz 77–80.

20. Screening for colorectal cancer: recommendation and rationale. *Ann Intern Med.* 2002;137(2): 129–131.

21. Screening for colorectal cancer: U.S. Preventive Services Task Force recommendation statement. *Ann Intern Med.* 2008;149(9):627–637.

22. Smith RA, Cokkinides V, Brawley OW. Cancer screening in the United States, 2009: a review of current American Cancer Society guidelines and issues in cancer screening. *CA Cancer J Clin.* 2009;59(1):27–41.

23. Chen X, White MC, Peipins LA, et al. Increase in screening for colorectal cancer in older Americans: results from a national survey. *J Am Geriatr Soc.* 2008;56(8):1511–1516.

24. Parks SM, Hsieh C. Preventive health care for older patients. *Prim Care.* 2002;29(3):599–614.

25. Walter LC, Lewis CL, Barton MB. Screening for colorectal, breast, and cervical cancer in the elderly: a review of the evidence. *Am J Med.* 2005;118(10):1078–1086.

26. Pasetto LM, Monfardini S. Colorectal cancer screening in elderly patients: when should be more useful? *Cancer Treat Rev.* 2007;33(6): 528–532.

27. Lin OS, Kozarek RA, Schembre DB, et al. Screening colonoscopy in very elderly patients: prevalence of neoplasia and estimated impact on life expectancy. *J Am Med Assoc.* 2006;295(20): 2357–2365.

28. Gatto NM, Frucht H, Sundararajan V, et al. Risk of perforation after colonoscopy and sigmoidoscopy: a population-based study. *J Natl Cancer Inst.* 2003;95(3):230–236.

29. Stryker SJ, Wolff BG, Culp CE, et al. Natural history of untreated colonic polyps. *Gastroenterology.* 1987;93(5):1009–1013.

30. Walter LC, Covinsky KE. Cancer screening in elderly patients: a framework for individualized

decision making. *J Am Med Assoc.* 2001;285(21): 2750–2756.

31. Duncan JE, Sweeney WB, Trudel JL, et al. Colonoscopy in the elderly: low risk, low yield in asymptomatic patients. *Dis Colon Rectum.* 2006;49(5):646–651.

32. Meulenbeld HJ, Creemers GJ. First-line treatment strategies for elderly patients with metastatic colorectal cancer. *Drugs Aging.* 2007;24(3): 223–238.

33. Arbman G, Nilsson E, Storgren-Fordell V, et al. Outcome of surgery for colorectal cancer in a defined population in Sweden from 1984 to 1986. *Dis Colon Rectum.* 1995;38(6):645–650.

34. Damhuis RA, Wereldsma JC, Wiggers T. The influence of age on resection rates and postoperative mortality in 6457 patients with colorectal cancer. *Int J Colorectal Dis.* 1996;11(1): 45–48.

35. Surgery for colorectal cancer in elderly patients: a systematic review. Colorectal Cancer Collaborative Group. *Lancet.* 2000;356(9234): 968–974.

36. Puig-La Calle Jr J, Quayle J, Thaler HT, et al. Favorable short-term and long-term outcome after elective radical rectal cancer resection in patients 75 years of age or older. *Dis Colon Rectum.* 2000;43(12):1704–1709.

37. Basili G, Lorenzetti L, Biondi G, et al. Colorectal cancer in the elderly: is there a role for safe and curative surgery? *ANZ J Surg.* 2008;78(6):466–470.

38. Schiffmann L, Ozcan S, Schwarz F, et al. Colorectal cancer in the elderly: surgical treatment and long-term survival. *Int J Colorectal Dis.* 2008;23(6):601–610.

39. Zingmond D, Maggard M, O'Connell J, et al. What predicts serious complications in colorectal cancer resection? *Am Surg.* 2003;69(11):969–974.

40. Chiappa A, Zbar AP, Bertani E, et al. Surgical outcomes for colorectal cancer patients including the elderly. *Hepatogastroenterology.* 2001;48(38): 440–444.

41. Manfredi, S, Bouvier AM, Lepage C, et al. Incidence and patterns of recurrence after resection for cure of colonic cancer in a well defined population. *Br J Surg.* 2006;93(9): 1115–1122.

42. Fallahzadeh H, Mays ET. Preexisting disease as a predictor of the outcome of colectomy. *Am J Surg.* 1991;162(5):497–498.

43. Mazzoni G, Tocchi A, Miccini M, et al. Surgical treatment of liver metastases from colorectal cancer in elderly patients. *Int J Colorectal Dis.* 2007;22(1):77–83.

44. Menon KV, Al-Mukhtar A, Aldouri A, et al. Outcomes after major hepatectomy in elderly patients. *J Am Coll Surg.* 2006;203(5):677–683.

45. de Liguori Carino N, van Leeuwen BL, Ghaneh P, et al. Liver resection for colorectal liver metastases in older patients. *Crit Rev Oncol Hematol.* 2008;67(3):273–278.

46. Temple LK, Hsieh L, Wong WD, et al. Use of surgery among elderly patients with stage IV colorectal cancer. *J Clin Oncol.* 2004;22(17): 3475–3484.

47. Audisio RA, Pope D, Ramesh HS, et al. Shall we operate? Preoperative assessment in elderly cancer patients (PACE) can help. A SIOG surgical task force prospective study. *Crit Rev Oncol Hematol.* 2008;65(2):156–163.

48. Pope D, Ramesh H, Gennari R, et al. Pre-operative assessment of cancer in the elderly (PACE): a comprehensive assessment of underlying characteristics of elderly cancer patients prior to elective surgery. *Surg Oncol.* 2006;15(4):189–197.

49. Zampino MG, Labianca R, Beretta GD, et al. Rectal cancer. *Crit Rev Oncol Hematol.* 2009;70(2):160–182.

50. Minsky BD, Cohen AM, Kemeny N, et al. The efficacy of preoperative 5-fluorouracil, high-dose leucovorin, and sequential radiation therapy for unresectable rectal cancer. *Cancer.* 1993;71(11): 3486–3492.

51. Minsky BD. Preoperative combined modality treatment for rectal cancer. *Oncology.* 1994;8(5):53–58, 61; discussion 61, 64–68.

52. Improved survival with preoperative radiotherapy in resectable rectal cancer. Swedish Rectal Cancer Trial. *N Engl J Med.* 1997;336(14):980–987.

53. Dharma-Wardene MW, de Gara C, Au HJ, et al. Ageism in rectal carcinoma? Treatment and outcome variations. *Int J Gastrointest Cancer.* 2002;32(2–3):129–138.

54. Folkesson J, Birgisson H, Pahlman L, et al. Swedish Rectal Cancer Trial: long lasting benefits from radiotherapy on survival and local recurrence rate. *J Clin Oncol.* 2005;23(24): 5644–5650.

55. O'Connell JB, Maggard MA, Liu JH, et al. Are survival rates different for young and older patients with rectal cancer? *Dis Colon Rectum.* 2004;47(12):2064–2069.

56. Marijnen CA, Kapiteijn E, van de Velde CJ, et al. Acute side effects and complications after short-term preoperative radiotherapy combined with total mesorectal excision in primary rectal cancer: report of a multicenter randomized trial. *J Clin Oncol.* 2002;20(3):817–825.

57. Radu C, Berglund A, Pahlman L, et al. Short-course preoperative radiotherapy with delayed surgery in rectal cancer – a retrospective study. *Radiother Oncol.* 2008;87(3):343–349.

58. Widder J, Herbst F, Dobrowsky W, et al. Preoperative short-term radiation therapy (25 Gy, 2.5 Gy twice daily) for primary resectable rectal cancer (phase II). *Br J Cancer.* 2005;92(7): 1209–1214.

59. Thirion P, Michiels S, Pignon JP, et al. Modulation of fluorouracil by leucovorin in patients with advanced colorectal cancer: an updated meta-analysis. *J Clin Oncol.* 2004;22(18):3766–3775.

60. NIH consensus conference. Adjuvant therapy for patients with colon and rectal cancer. *J Am Med Assoc.* 1990;264(11):1444–1450.

61. Moertel CG, Fleming TR, Macdonald JS, et al. Levamisole and fluorouracil for adjuvant therapy of resected colon carcinoma. *N Engl J Med.* 1990;322(6):352–358.

62. Andre T, Boni C, Mounedji-Boudiaf L, et al. Oxaliplatin, fluorouracil, and leucovorin as adjuvant treatment for colon cancer. *N Engl J Med.* 2004;350(23):2343–2351.

63. Ayanian JZ, Zaslavsky AM, Fuchs CS, et al. Use of adjuvant chemotherapy and radiation therapy for colorectal cancer in a population-based cohort. *J Clin Oncol.* 2003;21(7):1293–1300.

64. Jessup JM, Stewart A, Greene FL, et al. Adjuvant chemotherapy for stage III colon cancer: implications of race/ethnicity, age, and differentiation. *J Am Med Assoc.* 2005;294(21): 2703–2711.

65. Schrag D, Cramer LD, Bach PB, et al. Age and adjuvant chemotherapy use after surgery for stage III colon cancer. *J Natl Cancer Inst.* 2001;93(11): 850–857.

66. Etzioni DA, El-Khoueiry AB, Beart Jr RW. Rates and predictors of chemotherapy use for stage III colon cancer: a systematic review. *Cancer.* 2008;113(12):3279–3289.

67. Gross CP, McAvay GJ, Guo Z, et al. The impact of chronic illnesses on the use and effectiveness of adjuvant chemotherapy for colon cancer. *Cancer.* 2007;109(12):2410–2419.

68. Dobie SA, Baldwin LM, Dominitz JA, et al. Completion of therapy by Medicare patients with stage III colon cancer. *J Natl Cancer Inst.* 2006;98(9):610–619.

69. Arias E. United States life tables, 2004. *Natl Vital Stat Rep.* 2007;56(9):1–39.

70. Muss HB, Biganzoli L, Sargent DJ, et al. Adjuvant therapy in the elderly: making the right decision. *J Clin Oncol.* 2007;25(14):1870–1875.

71. Haller DG, Catalano PJ, MacDonald JS, et al. Phase III study of fluorouracil, leucovorin, and levamisole in high-risk stage II and III colon cancer: final report of Intergroup 0089. *J Clin Oncol.* 2005;23(34):8671–8678.

72. Quasar Collaborative Group, Gray R, Barnwell J, et al. Adjuvant chemotherapy versus observation in patients with colorectal cancer: a randomised study. *Lancet.* 2007;370(9604):2020–2029.

73. Gill S, Loprinzi CL, Sargent DJ, et al. Pooled analysis of fluorouracil-based adjuvant therapy for stage II and III colon cancer: who benefits and by how much? *J Clin Oncol.* 2004;22(10):1797–1806.

74. Fata F, Mirza A, Craig G, et al. Efficacy and toxicity of adjuvant chemotherapy in elderly patients with colon carcinoma: a 10-year experience of the Geisinger Medical Center. *Cancer.* 2002;94(7):1931–1938.

75. Popescu RA, Norman A, Ross PJ, et al. Adjuvant or palliative chemotherapy for colorectal cancer in patients 70 years or older. *J Clin Oncol.* 1999;17(8): 2412–2418.

76. Sundararajan V, Mitra N, Jacobson JS, et al. Survival associated with 5-fluorouracil-based adjuvant chemotherapy among elderly patients with node-positive colon cancer. *Ann Intern Med.* 2002;136(5):349–357.

77. Iwashyna TJ, Lamont EB. Effectiveness of adjuvant fluorouracil in clinical practice: a population-based cohort study of elderly patients with stage III colon cancer. *J Clin Oncol.* 2002;20(19):3992–3998.

78. O'Connell MJ, Laurie JA, Kahn M, et al. Prospectively randomized trial of postoperative adjuvant chemotherapy in patients with high-risk colon cancer. *J Clin Oncol.* 1998;16(1):295–300.

79. Neugut AI, Matasar M, Wang X, et al. Duration of adjuvant chemotherapy for colon cancer and survival among the elderly. *J Clin Oncol.* 2006;24(15):2368–2375.

80. Twelves C, Wong A, Nowacki MP, et al. Capecitabine as adjuvant treatment for stage III colon cancer. *N Engl J Med.* 2005;352(26): 2696–2704.

81. Diaz-Rubio E. New chemotherapeutic advances in pancreatic, colorectal, and gastric cancers. *Oncologist.* 2004;9(3):282–294.

82. Poole C, Gardiner J, Twelves C, et al. Effect of renal impairment on the pharmacokinetics and tolerability of capecitabine (Xeloda) in cancer patients. *Cancer Chemother Pharmacol.* 2002;49(3):225–234.

83. Camidge R, Reigner B, Cassidy J, et al. Significant effect of capecitabine on the pharmacokinetics and pharmacodynamics of warfarin in patients with cancer. *J Clin Oncol.* 2005;23(21):4719–4725.

84. Shah HR, Ledbetter L, Diasio R, et al. A retrospective study of coagulation abnormalities in patients receiving concomitant capecitabine and warfarin. *Clin Colorectal Cancer.* 2006;5(5):354–358.

85. Yood MU, Quesenberry CP Jr, Alford SH, et al. An observational study examining the impact of capecitabine on warfarin antithrombotic activity and bleeding complications. *Curr Med Res Opin.* 2006;22(2):307–314.

86. Goldberg RM, Tabah-Fisch I, Bleiberg H, et al. Pooled analysis of safety and efficacy of oxaliplatin plus fluorouracil/leucovorin administered bimonthly in elderly patients with colorectal cancer. *J Clin Oncol.* 2006;24(25):4085–4091.

87. McKibbin T, Frei CR, Grene RE, et al. Disparities in the use of chemotherapy and monoclonal antibody therapy for elderly advanced colorectal cancer patients in the community oncology setting. *Oncologist.* 2008;13(8):876–885.

88. Simmonds PC. Palliative chemotherapy for advanced colorectal cancer: systematic review and meta-analysis. Colorectal Cancer Collaborative Group. *Br Med J.* 2000;321(7260): 531–535.

89. Folprecht G, Cuningham D, Ross P, et al. Efficacy of 5-fluorouracil-based chemotherapy in elderly patients with metastatic colorectal cancer: a pooled analysis of clinical trials. *Ann Oncol.* 2004;15(9):1330–1338.

90. Daniele B, Rosati G, Tambaro R, et al. First-line chemotherapy with fluorouracil and folinic acid for advanced colorectal cancer in elderly patients: a phase II study. *J Clin Gastroenterol.* 2003;36(3): 228–233.

91. Mattioli R, Lippe P, Recchia F, et al. Advanced colorectal cancer in elderly patients: tolerance and efficacy of leucovorin and fluorouracil bolus plus continuous infusion. *Anticancer Res.* 2001;21(1A): 489–492.

92. Cunningham D, Pyrhonen S, James RD, et al. Randomised trial of irinotecan plus supportive care versus supportive care alone after fluorouracil failure for patients with metastatic colorectal cancer. *Lancet.* 1998;352(9138):1413–1418.

93. Rougier P, Van Cutsem E, Bajetta E, et al. Randomised trial of irinotecan versus fluorouracil by continuous infusion after fluorouracil failure in patients with metastatic colorectal cancer. *Lancet.* 1998;352(9138):1407–1412.

94. Rothenberg ML, Cox JV, DeVore RF, et al. A multicenter, phase II trial of weekly irinotecan (CPT-11) in patients with previously treated colorectal carcinoma. *Cancer.* 1999;85(4): 786–795.

95. Chau I, Norman AR, Chunningham D, et al. Elderly patients with fluoropyrimidine and thymidylate synthase inhibitor-resistant advanced colorectal cancer derive similar benefit without excessive toxicity when treated with irinotecan monotherapy. *Br J Cancer.* 2004;91(8):1453–1458.

96. Rosati G, Cordio S. Single-agent irinotecan as second-line weekly chemotherapy in elderly patients with advanced colorectal cancer. *Tumori.* 2006;92(4):290–294.

97. Fuchs C, Mitchell EP, Hoff PM. Irinotecan in the treatment of colorectal cancer. *Cancer Treat Rev.* 2006;32(7):491–503.

98. Fuchs CS, Marshall J, Mitchelle E, et al. Randomized, controlled trial of irinotecan plus infusional, bolus, or oral fluoropyrimidines in first-line treatment of metastatic colorectal cancer: results from the BICC-C Study. *J Clin Oncol.* 2007;25(30):4779–4786.

99. Goldberg RM, Sargent DJ, Morton RF, et al. A randomized controlled trial of fluorouracil plus leucovorin, irinotecan, and oxaliplatin combinations in patients with previously untreated metastatic colorectal cancer. *J Clin Oncol.* 2004;22(1):23–30.

100. Folprecht G, Seymour MT, Saltz L, et al. Irinotecan/fluorouracil combination in first-line therapy of older and younger patients with metastatic colorectal cancer: combined analysis of 2,691 patients in randomized controlled trials. *J Clin Oncol.* 2008;26(9):1443–1451.

101. Sastre J, Marcuello E, Masutti B, et al. Irinotecan in combination with fluorouracil in a 48-hour continuous infusion as first-line chemotherapy for elderly patients with metastatic colorectal cancer: a Spanish Cooperative Group for the Treatment of Digestive Tumors study. *J Clin Oncol.* 2005;23(15):3545–3551.

102. Souglakos J, Pallis A, Kakolyris S, et al. Combination of irinotecan (CPT-11) plus 5-fluorouracil and leucovorin (FOLFIRI regimen) as first line treatment for elderly patients with metastatic colorectal cancer: a phase II trial. *Oncology.* 2005;69(5):384–390.

103. Mitry E, Douillard JY, Van Cutsem E, et al. Predictive factors of survival in patients with advanced colorectal cancer: an individual data analysis of 602 patients included in irinotecan phase III trials. *Ann Oncol.* 2004;15(7):1013–1017.

104. Douillard JY, Cunningham D, Roth AD, et al. Irinotecan combined with fluorouracil compared with fluorouracil alone as first-line treatment for metastatic colorectal cancer: a multicentre randomised trial. *Lancet.* 2000;355(9209): 1041–1047.

105. Kohne CH, van Cutsem E, Wils J, et al. Phase III study of weekly high-dose infusional fluorouracil plus folinic acid with or without irinotecan in patients with metastatic colorectal cancer: European Organisation for Research and Treatment of Cancer Gastrointestinal Group Study 40986. *J Clin Oncol.* 2005;23(22):4856–4865.

106. de Jong FA, Kehrer DF, Mathijssen RH, et al. Prophylaxis of irinotecan-induced diarrhea with neomycin and potential role for UGT1A1*28 genotype screening: a double-blind, randomized, placebo-controlled study. *Oncologist.* 2006;11(8): 944–954.

107. Park SB, Goldstein D, Lin CS, et al. Acute abnormalities of sensory nerve function associated with oxaliplatin-induced neurotoxicity. *J Clin Oncol.* 2009;27(8):1243–1249.

108. Pasetto LM, D'Andrea MR, Rossi E, et al. Oxaliplatin-related neurotoxicity: how and why? *Crit Rev Oncol Hematol.* 2006;59(2):159–168.

109. Rothenberg ML, Oza AM, Bigelow RH, et al. Superiority of oxaliplatin and fluorouracil-leucovorin compared with either therapy alone in patients with progressive colorectal cancer after irinotecan and fluorouracil-leucovorin: interim results of a phase III trial. *J Clin Oncol.* 2003;21(11): 2059–2069.

110. Figer A, Perez-Staub N, Carola E, et al. FOLFOX in patients aged between 76 and 80 years with metastatic colorectal cancer: an exploratory cohort of the OPTIMOX1 study. *Cancer.* 2007;110(12):2666–2671.

111. Mattioli R, Massacesi C, Recchia F, et al. High activity and reduced neurotoxicity of bi-fractionated oxaliplatin plus 5-fluorouracil/leucovorin for elderly patients with advanced colorectal cancer. *Ann Oncol.* 2005;16(7): 1147–1151.

112. Kim JH, Oh DY, Kim YJ, et al. Reduced dose intensity FOLFOX-4 as first line palliative chemotherapy in elderly patients with advanced colorectal cancer. *J Kor Med Sci.* 2005;20(5): 806–810.

113. Feliu J, Escudero P, Llosa F, et al. Capecitabine as first-line treatment for patients older than 70 years with metastatic colorectal cancer: an oncopaz cooperative group study. *J Clin Oncol.* 2005;23(13):3104–3111.

114. Cassidy J, Twelves C, Van Cutsem E, et al. First-line oral capecitabine therapy in metastatic colorectal cancer: a favorable safety profile compared with intravenous 5-fluorouracil/leucovorin. *Ann Oncol.* 2002;13(4):566–575.

115. Golfinopoulos V, Pentheroudakis G, Pavlidis N. Treatment of colorectal cancer in the elderly: a review of the literature. *Cancer Treat Rev.* 2006;32(1):1–8.

116. Cassidy J, Clarke S, Diaz-Rubio E, et al. Randomized phase III study of capecitabine plus oxaliplatin compared with fluorouracil/folinic acid plus oxaliplatin as first-line therapy for metastatic colorectal cancer. *J Clin Oncol.* 2008;26(12):2006–2012.

117. Feliu J, Salud A, Escudero P, et al. XELOX (capecitabine plus oxaliplatin) as first-line treatment for elderly patients over 70 years of age with advanced colorectal cancer. *Br J Cancer.* 2006;94(7):969–975.

118. Seymour MT, Maughan TS, Wasan HS, et al. Capecitabine (Cap) and oxaliplatin (Ox) in elderly and/or frail patients with metastatic colorectal cancer: the FOCUS2 trial [abstract]. *J Clin Oncol.* 2007;25(suppl):9030.

119. Bouchahda M, Macarulla T, Spano JP, et al. Cetuximab efficacy and safety in a retrospective cohort of elderly patients with heavily pretreated metastatic colorectal cancer. *Crit Rev Oncol Hematol.* 2008; 67(3):255–262.

120. Cunningham D, Humblet Y, Siena S, et al. Cetuximab monotherapy and cetuximab plus irinotecan in irinotecan-refractory metastatic colorectal cancer. *N Engl J Med.* 2004;351(4): 337–345.

121. Saltz LB, Meropol NJ, Loehrer PJ, et al. Phase II trial of cetuximab in patients with refractory colorectal cancer that expresses the epidermal growth factor receptor. *J Clin Oncol.* 2004;22(7): 1201–1208.

122. Jonker DJ, O'Callaghan CJ, Karapetis CS, et al. Cetuximab for the treatment of colorectal cancer. *N Engl J Med.* 2007;357(20):2040–2048.

123. Bouchahda M, Macarulla T, Spano JP, et al. Cetuximab efficacy and safety in a retrospective cohort of elderly patients with heavily pretreated metastatic colorectal cancer. *Crit Rev Oncol Hematol.* 2008;67(3):255–262.

124. Amado RG, Wolf M, Peeters M, et al. Wild-type KRAS is required for panitumumab efficacy in patients with metastatic colorectal cancer. *J Clin Oncol.* 2008;26(10):1626–1634.

125. Kabbinavar FF, Hambleton J, Mass RD, et al. Combined analysis of efficacy: the addition of bevacizumab to fluorouracil/leucovorin improves survival for patients with metastatic colorectal cancer. *J Clin Oncol.* 2005;23(16): 3706–3712.

126. Scappaticci FA, Skillings JR, Holden SN, et al. Arterial thromboembolic events in patients with metastatic carcinoma treated with chemotherapy and bevacizumab. *J Natl Cancer Inst.* 2007;99(16): 1232–1239.

127. Kabbinavar FF, Hurwitz HI, Yi J, et al. Addition of bevacizumab to fluorouracil-based first-line treatment of metastatic colorectal cancer: pooled analysis of cohorts of older patients from two randomized clinical trials. *J Clin Oncol.* 2009;27(2):199–205.

128. Hochster HS, Hart LL, Ramanathan RK, et al. Safety and efficacy of oxaliplatin and fluoropyrimidine regimens with or without

bevacizumab as first-line treatment of metastatic colorectal cancer: results of the TREE Study. *J Clin Oncol.* 2008;26(21):3523–3529.

129. Elkin EB, Kim SH, Casper ES, et al. Desire for information and involvement in treatment decisions: elderly cancer patients' preferences and their physicians' perceptions. *J Clin Oncol.* 2007;25(33):5275–5280.

130. Balducci L. Aging, frailty, and chemotherapy. *Cancer Control.* 2007;14(1):7–12.

131. Lichtman SM, Balducci L, Aapro M. Geriatric oncology: a field coming of age. *J Clin Oncol.* 2007;25(14):1821–1823.

132. Lichtman SM. Pharmacokinetics and pharmacodynamics in the elderly. *Clin Adv Hematol Oncol.* 2007;5(3):181–182.

133. Mohile SG, Lachs M, Dale W. Management of prostate cancer in the older man. *Semin Oncol.* 2008;35(6):597–617.

134. Fried LP, Ferrucci L, Darer J, et al. Untangling the concepts of disability, frailty, and comorbidity: implications for improved targeting and care. *J Gerontol A.* 2004;59(3):255–263.

135. Saliba D, Elliott M, Rubenstein LZ, et al. The Vulnerable Elders Survey: a tool for identifying vulnerable older people in the community. *J Am Geriatr Soc.* 2001;49(12):1691–1699.

Management of renal and bladder cancer in older adults

Matthew I. Milowsky and Dean F. Bajorin

A. Introduction

Genitourinary malignancies, including renal and bladder cancer, account for approximately one-third of cancers in men and typically occur in older adults.[1] Multimodality treatment plans are increasingly utilized in the management of patients with cancer, often with curative intent. These complex treatment algorithms have generally been developed in younger patients or older adults without significant comorbidities. Bladder and renal cancers require complicated multidisciplinary treatment plans and prospective studies to guide the management in older adults with coexisting medical illnesses. This chapter will review the current evidence-based literature related to the management of bladder and renal cancers in older adults.

B. Bladder cancer

Bladder cancer is a common malignancy with an estimated 70,980 cases (men, 52,810; women, 18,170) and 14,336 deaths (men, 10,180; women, 4,150) for the year 2009 in the United States.[2] The median age at diagnosis is 68 years, and bladder cancer was the fourth leading cause of death in men 80 years of age and older in the year 2005, with an estimated 3,985 bladder cancer–related deaths.[1] The predominant histology in the United States is urothelial or transitional cell carcinoma (TCC); however, squamous cell carcinoma as related to bilharziasis had been more common in other regions of the world, with recent reports demonstrating a decline in the relative frequency of squamous cell cancers and a rise in the rates of TCC.[3] In addition to bilharziasis, risk factors for bladder cancer include tobacco use, occupational exposures, urinary tract diseases, and pharmaceutical drug use.[4] The majority of patients present with superficial disease (i.e., disease limited to the epithelium, Ta; lamina propria, T1; or carcinoma in situ, Tis); however, approximately 20–40 percent of patients either present with more advanced disease or progress after treatment

for superficial disease. Patients with superficial disease are typically managed with complete removal of the tumor by transurethral resection with or without intravesical therapy, whereas patients with recurrent T1 or more invasive disease (i.e., invasion of the muscularis propria) are managed with radical cystectomy and bilateral pelvic lymphadenectomy. Prognosis is associated with pathological stage and lymph node involvement. In a series of 1,054 patients undergoing radical cystectomy and pelvic lymphadenectomy, the overall recurrence-free survival rates at 5 and 10 years were 68 and 66 percent, respectively.[5] Patients with non-organ-confined lymph node–negative tumors had a significantly higher probability of recurrence compared with those who had organ-confined bladder cancers. The 5- and 10-year recurrence-free survival rates for the patients with lymph node involvement were 35 and 34 percent, respectively. Although there is a survival benefit associated with combination cisplatin-based chemotherapy in patients with metastatic disease, the median survival is only 15 months, with a 5-year survival rate of 15 percent.[6] Bladder cancer is too often a devastating disease requiring a multidisciplinary approach with different therapies over the course of many years (Figure 12.1). This is particularly challenging in older adults with coexisting medical problems, such as cardiovascular or pulmonary disease as related to tobacco use, and requires treatment programs tailored to this older population.

B.1. Superficial bladder cancer

Approximately 70 percent of patients with newly diagnosed bladder cancer will present with superficial disease, with 70 percent confined to the mucosa (Ta or Tis) and 30 percent involving the submucosa (T1). The treatment of superficial disease involves complete removal of the lesion by a transurethral resection followed by rigorous surveillance with cystoscopy and urine cytology at 3-month intervals for recurrence and/or

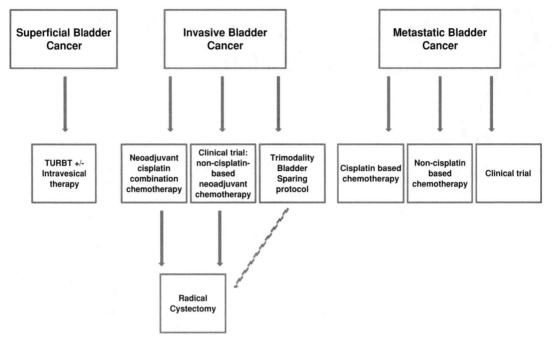

Figure 12.1 Treatment options for older adults with bladder cancer.

progression to a more advanced stage. In a population-based study evaluating the impact of age and comorbidity on surgery in patients with bladder cancer, there were no significant treatment differences noted with regard to age among patients with superficial disease.[7] Although hypertension, chronic pulmonary disease, arthritis, and heart disease affected at least 15 percent of the study population and approximately 38 percent of patients were current or former smokers, greater than 90 percent of patients with superficial disease were treated with transurethral resection alone.

The use of intravesical therapy with bacillus Calmette-Guérin (BCG) has been demonstrated to delay tumor progression and death from bladder cancer in patients who present with superficial disease.[8] Aging may be associated with a diminished response to intravesical immunotherapy. In an analysis of data from a national phase II multicenter trial of BCG plus interferon-alfa intravesical therapy for superficial bladder cancer, recurrence-free survival 2 years after the initiation of therapy was examined in patients by incremental age decade.[9] In all patients, the greatest difference in response was between the 289 patients who were 61–70 years old and the 123 who were older than 80 years, with a 22 percent difference in cancer-free survival at a median follow-up of 24 months (61% vs. 39%, $p = .0002$). On multi-

variate analysis, age was an independent risk factor for response. The authors suggest that a potential explanation may be related to a depressed baseline immune status and inability to mount an immune reaction to BCG or IFN-alpha. In another reported analysis of 805 patients with multiple or recurrent high-grade Ta, T1, and/or Tis bladder cancer who received BCG therapy, no difference was observed in the first response to BCG or cancer-free survival at 2 years among patients less than 50, 50–59, 60–69, 70–79, or 80 years or older.[10] After 5 years, 27 percent of patients older than 70 years were cancer-free compared with 37 percent younger than 70 years ($p = .005$). Although these data do support a cancer-specific survival difference in older patients receiving intravesical therapy, the magnitude and mechanism remain unclear.

Owing to the high rate of recurrence of non-muscle invasive bladder cancer, intensive and invasive surveillance strategies including periodic cystoscopy are required. In one study evaluating patients' perceived burden of cystoscopic and urinary surveillance of bladder cancer, older patients reported significantly less pain and discomfort from cystoscopy, and this was unrelated to having more previous cystoscopies performed.[11] Ongoing studies are evaluating noninvasive tests for detecting recurrent disease with the goal of limiting the need for cystoscopic surveillance in all patients.

Studies performed to date suggest that age does not appear to represent a major factor in the management of patients with superficial bladder cancer aside from a small but measurable inferior outcome with intravesical therapy as compared to younger patients. A major issue that is not well addressed in the current literature is the burden related to the need for frequent medical visits and testing for older patients with bladder cancer. Additional studies are needed to evaluate issues related to comorbidities, functional status, cognition, social functioning, and support as well as others that may affect an older patient's ability to participate in such a rigorous surveillance and treatment program.

B.2. Invasive bladder cancer

Radical cystectomy

Muscle-invasive bladder cancer has a very different biology than superficial disease. These high-grade invasive tumors are characterized by defects in the p53 and retinoblastoma protein pathways, and more than 50 percent progress to life-threatening metastases.[12] Radical cystectomy represents the gold standard for the treatment of muscle-invasive bladder cancer. This is a major surgery including removal of the bladder, regional pelvic lymph nodes, and distal ureters as well as the prostate gland, seminal vesicles, and proximal urethra in men and the urethra, uterus, fallopian tubes, anterior vaginal wall, and surrounding fascia in women. With this in mind, the safety of radical cystectomy in older patients has been questioned, with a growing body of literature supporting that the procedure can be safely performed in older adults, including those with coexisting medical illnesses. In a retrospective review of 1,054 patients who underwent radical cystectomy for bladder cancer between 1971 and 1997 stratified into four age groups – under 60 years at the time of cystectomy ($n = 309$ patients), age 60–69 years ($n = 381$ patients), age 70–79 years ($n = 314$ patients), and age 80 years or older ($n = 50$ patients) – the operative mortality rates were 1 percent, 3 percent, 4 percent, and 0 percent, respectively ($p = .14$).[13] Older patients (over 70 years) did have a higher rate of early complications ($p = .002$), whereas younger patients (under 70 years) had a higher rate of late complications ($p < .001$). The authors reported decreased overall survival and worse disease recurrence-free survival rates for the older population, which may have been in part related to a higher incidence of extravesical

disease and lower likelihood of receiving adjuvant chemotherapy in the older patients.[14]

In an attempt to examine the impact of various treatment modalities on survival among patients with bladder cancer who were 80 years or older compared with younger patients, 13,796 patients diagnosed with bladder cancer between 1988 and 1999 were identified using the Surveillance, Epidemiology, and End Results database, 24 percent of whom were older than 80 years.[15] Of patients aged 80 years and older, management included watchful waiting (7%), radiotherapy alone (1%), full or partial cystectomy (12%), and transurethral resection (79%). Patients aged 80 years and older were less likely to be treated with extirpative surgery than their younger counterparts ($p < .0001$). Among patients aged 80 years and older, radical cystectomy/partial cystectomy had the greatest risk reduction in death from bladder cancer (hazard ratio = 0.3) and death from any cause (hazard ratio = 0.4) among the primary treatment modalities (both $p < .0001$).

In a single-institution series, the role for radical cystectomy in octogenarians was evaluated by reviewing complications within 90 days of radical cystectomy in 1,142 consecutive patients entered into a prospective complication database between 1995 and 2005.[16] Octogenarians (117/1,142, 10%) were more likely to experience a postoperative complication (72% vs. 64%) than younger patients, with cardiac and neurologic complications more common ($p = .006$ and $p = .01$, respectively). Overall, the incidence of major complications was low (13%). Although the rates were slightly higher in octogenarians than in younger patients (17% vs. 13%), the difference was not statistically significant ($p = .3$) despite higher preoperative comorbidity indexes ($p < .001$) in patients aged 80 years and older. The 90-day mortality was 6.8 percent in octogenarians versus 2.2 percent ($p = 0.01$) in younger patients. There was no significant difference in disease-specific survival compared to younger patients; however, octogenarians were more likely to die of causes unrelated to bladder cancer.

Although these data lend support to the efficacy and safety of radical cystectomy in older patients, both age and comorbidity have been associated with treatment selection and survival after radical cystectomy and need to be considered when comparing outcomes after cystectomy. In a single-institution study using the age-adjusted Charlson comorbidity index (ACCI), the authors characterized the impact of age and comorbidity on disease progression, overall survival, and clinicopathologic and treatment characteristics after radical cystectomy.[17] Despite a higher prevalence of extravesical disease, patients with higher ACCI were less likely to have lymph-node dissection, and when it was performed, fewer lymph nodes were evaluated. Patients with higher ACCI were also less likely to have postoperative chemotherapy. Higher ACCI was significantly associated with lower overall ($p < .005$) but not recurrence-free ($p = .17$) survival after radical cystectomy.

Assessment tools are needed to assist in surgical decision making for older patients with invasive bladder cancer. In one study, common components of geriatric assessment were reviewed in 152 consecutive patients 70 years or older (mean age 76 years) presenting with muscle-invasive bladder cancer between 1995 and 2004.[18] Seventy-five percent had a cystectomy, including 25 percent with planned neoadjuvant chemotherapy. In a multivariate analysis, patients with a Karnofsky Performance Status (KPS) of 80 or less had 1.8 times the risk of death compared to patients with a KPS of 90 or greater (95% confidence interval [CI] 1.0–3.2, $p = .05$). Prospective studies incorporating comprehensive geriatric assessment tools are needed to better define the role for radical cystectomy in individual older adults with invasive bladder cancer.

Bladder preservation

Numerous studies over the years have determined that selective trimodality bladder preservation represents a potential alternative to radical cystectomy (Figure 12.2).[19–25] Such an approach results in approximately 50 percent long-term disease-free survival, which is comparable to the results of modern cystectomy series.[26] Bladder preservation protocols generally include as complete a transurethral resection as possible, followed by chemoradiotherapy with cisplatin-based chemotherapy.[27] The majority of bladder preservation protocols have included only patients who were candidates for salvage cystectomy. After combined modality therapy, approximately 20–30 percent of patients will have residual tumor at a restaging transurethral resection, and an additional 20–30 percent will develop new or recurrent disease in the bladder.[27] Salvage cystectomy is required for patients with muscle-invasive persistent or recurrent tumors. Because many patients treated for muscle-invasive bladder cancer are older, with comorbidities including renal dysfunction, salvage cystectomy may not be possible. On the basis of the success of bladder preservation therapy, it may be reasonable to consider definitive nonsurgical treatment in patients who are not candidates for cystectomy.

The optimal combined-modality bladder-sparing regimen has not been defined; however, the most common approaches studied to date have involved a transurethral resection of tumor followed by concurrent chemoradiation with or without perioperative chemotherapy. Cisplatin is among the most active agents in bladder cancer. As a result, the majority of chemoradiation trials in bladder cancer have utilized concurrent cisplatin with complete response rates in the 59–75 percent range and 5-year survival of approximately 50 percent.[26] A phase I study of combined-modality therapy with gemcitabine and radiotherapy in patients with muscle-invasive bladder cancer demonstrated a high rate of bladder preservation.[28] At 5 years, bladder-intact survival was 62 percent, overall survival was 76 percent, and disease-specific survival was 82 percent.[29] There was no statistical difference in quality-of-life data collected (FACT-BL and FACT-G) before, during, or after concurrent gemcitabine and radiotherapy aside from those patients who received higher gemcitabine doses with dose-limiting toxicities.[30] There have been no randomized trials comparing the results of bladder sparing with radical cystectomy. Compared with historical controls, the use of a combined-modality approach in appropriately selected patients has yielded similar outcomes. Five-year survival rates of 50–60 percent have been reported, with approximately 70 percent of these patients maintaining an intact bladder.[27] In a recent analysis of urodynamic studies and quality of life in patients treated with bladder preservation, the majority of patients with an intact bladder preserved normal bladder function, and low rates of bowel symptoms and urinary incontinence were reported.[31] Studies evaluating bladder-preservation strategies in older adults who are not candidates for salvage cystectomy are needed. An ongoing Radiation Therapy Oncology Group trial is evaluating concurrent paclitaxel and daily radiation for noncystectomy candidates with muscle-invasive bladder cancer. Patients with tumors overexpressing HER-2/neu also receive concurrent trastuzumab. An additional study targeting older adults using gemcitabine in combination with radiation therapy and incorporating a comprehensive geriatric assessment tool is planned.

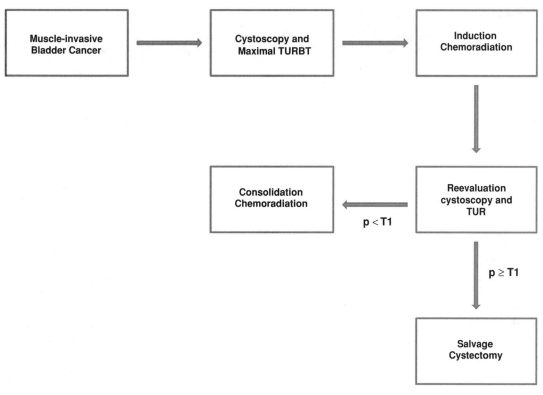

Figure 12.2 Trimodality bladder preservation schema.

B.3. Chemotherapy

Bladder cancer is a chemosensitive malignancy with an overall survival benefit associated with cisplatin combination chemotherapy in the metastatic and perioperative settings (Table 12.1). Two large randomized trials compared the four-drug regimen of methotrexate, vinblastine, doxorubicin, and cisplatin (M-VAC) to cisplatin alone and the three-drug combination of cisplatin, doxorubicin, and cyclophosphamide (CISCA) with both studies, demonstrating a response and survival advantage for M-VAC.[32,33] Despite these results, the median survival for patients treated with M-VAC is only 11–13 months, with a 6-year progression-free survival of only 3 percent.[34] Treatment with M-VAC is also associated with significant toxicity, including febrile neutropenia, mucositis, and a toxic death rate of 3–4 percent.[32,35]

On the basis of a randomized trial comparing M-VAC to the combination of gemcitabine and cisplatin (GC), the doublet regimen of GC has become a standard of care in patients with locally advanced or metastatic transitional cell carcinoma (TCC).[6,36] Although this study was not designed as a noninferiority trial, the results demonstrated a similar response rate (GC 49% and M-VAC 46%, $p = .51$), progression-free survival (GC 7.7 months and M-VAC 8.3 months, $p = .63$), and median survival (GC 14 months and M-VAC 15.2 months, $p = .66$), with a better safety profile and tolerability for the GC-treated patients.

Prospective randomized trials as well as a large meta-analysis have demonstrated a survival benefit for the use of cisplatin combination chemotherapy in the neoadjuvant setting.[37–39] The survival benefit associated with neoadjuvant chemotherapy has been associated with tumor downstaging to pT0. A U.S. phase III intergroup trial that randomized patients with invasive bladder cancer to neoadjuvant M-VAC plus cystectomy or to cystectomy alone demonstrated an 85 percent 5-year survival for patients who experienced a complete pathologic response (38% in those patients who received M-VAC compared to 15% for those undergoing cystectomy alone).[37] A systematic review and meta-analysis of 3,005 individual patient data from 11 randomized controlled trials of neoadjuvant platinum-based combination chemotherapy in invasive bladder cancer was performed.[40] Neoadjuvant platinum-based combination chemotherapy showed a significant overall survival benefit (hazard ratio [HR] 0.86, 95%

Table 12.1 Selected trials of cisplatin-based chemotherapy in bladder cancer.

Trial	Neoadjuvant or metastatic	n	Chemotherapy	Primary treatment	pCR	Outcome
Loehrer et al.[32]	Metastatic	246	M-VAC vs. cisplatin	NA	NA	Median survival: M-VAC, 12.5 months vs. cisplatin, 8.2 months
Logothetis et al.[33]	Metastatic	110	M-VAC vs. CISCA	NA	NA	Median survival: M-VAC, 11.2 months vs. CISCA, 8.3 months
von der Maase et al.[36]	Metastatic	405	M-VAC vs. GC	NA	NA	Median survival: GC, 14 months vs. M-VAC, 15.2 months
International Collaboration[39, 87]	Neoadjuvant	976	CMV	Cystectomy or RT	32.5%	6% absolute survival benefit in favor of CMV arm
Grossman et al.[37]	Neoadjuvant	307	M-VAC	Cystectomy	38%	Median survival: M-VAC arm, 77 months vs. cystectomy-alone arm, 46 months

Note. RT = radiation therapy; M-VAC = methotrexate, vinblastine, doxorubicin, cisplatin; CISCA = cisplatin, doxorubicin, cyclophosphamide; CMV = cisplatin, methotrexate, vinblastine; GC = gemcitabine, cisplatin; NA = not applicable.

CI 0.77–0.95, $p = .003$) with a 14 percent reduction in the risk of death and a 5 percent absolute benefit at 5 years (95% CI 1–7), with overall survival increasing from 45 to 50 percent. On the basis of the survival benefit seen in the randomized trials of cisplatin combination chemotherapy and the meta-analysis, neoadjuvant cisplatin-based chemotherapy now represents a standard of care in the management of patients with muscle-invasive bladder cancer. There have been several prospective trials designed to evaluate adjuvant chemotherapy; however, all have significant limitations in their interpretations.[41–45] An individual patient data meta-analysis of 491 patients from six trials, representing 90 percent of all patients randomized in cisplatin-based combination chemotherapy trials and 66 percent from all eligible trials, demonstrated a 25 percent relative reduction in the risk of death in favor of chemotherapy (HR 0.75, 95% CI 0.60–0.96, $p = .019$).[46] This meta-analysis is clearly limited by its size and the shortcomings in the adjuvant studies from which it is derived.

Although cisplatin-based combination chemotherapy is associated with a survival benefit in both the metastatic and perioperative settings, cisplatin is often problematic in older patients with coexisting medical problems (Table 12.2). The most commonly used non-cisplatin-based combination chemotherapy regimen in patients with advanced bladder cancer is gemcitabine plus carboplatin. There are no substantial data to support the use of non-cisplatin-based regimens in the perioperative setting, and trials in the metastatic setting suggest inferior response rates and survival outcomes with carboplatin-based chemotherapy.[47–50] Cisplatin-related side effects, including nephrotoxicity, neurotoxicity, ototoxicity, and vascular complications, represent a major challenge in the treatment of older patients with comorbidities.

The normal physiologic decline in renal function with aging must be considered when using

Table 12.2 Potential cisplatin-related toxicities in older adults.

Nephrotoxicity

Ototoxicity

Neurotoxicity

Vascular toxicity
- Cardiovascular
- Cerebrovascular
- Thrombotic microangiopathy
- Raynaud's phenomenon

cisplatin-based chemotherapy in older adults. Using the iohexol technique in 52 elderly healthy persons aged 70–110 years, glomerular filtration rate (GFR) showed a strong correlation with age ($p = .0002$), with an annual decline of 1.05 mL/min in patients aged 70 years and older.[51] In a retrospective study designed to determine the proportion of patients ineligible for cisplatin-based chemotherapy in the adjuvant setting using a cutoff of creatinine clearance (CrCl) < 60 mL/min or GFR < 60 mL/min/1.73 m^2, the overall proportion of patients ineligible for cisplatin-based chemotherapy using the three most commonly used formulas for calculating CrCl ranged between 24 and 52 percent.[52] With all formulas, the probability of ineligibility increased with age: by the Cockroft-Gault equation, over 40 percent of patients aged over 70 years were ineligible. The authors concluded that the widespread use of cisplatin-based perioperative chemotherapy in patients with bladder cancer may be significantly limited by the high prevalence of baseline renal insufficiency, which is most striking in the elderly.

An evaluation of high-frequency hearing loss performed as part of the National Health and Nutrition Examination Survey among 5,742 U.S. adults aged 20–69 years demonstrated the association of hearing loss with age, smoking, noise exposure, and cardiovascular risk.[53] Hearing loss after cisplatin therapy occurs mainly at high frequencies and at cisplatin dosages more than 60 mg/m^2.[54] Baseline audiometry is certainly warranted when considering cisplatin-based chemotherapy in older adults with bladder cancer, who often have a smoking history as well as coexisting cardiovascular disease. Decision making for using cisplatin in patients with significant baseline hearing dysfunction is determined by assessing the risk versus benefit in the individual patient.

Motor performance decline is associated with disability, institutionalization, and death.[55,56] In a subsample of the Italian Longitudinal Study of Aging (ages 64–84) with 1,052 subjects analyzed with normal motor performance at baseline and then assessed at 3 years using six tests of motor performance, 166 (15.8%) subjects had a decline at 3 years.[57] Age and distal symmetrical neuropathy were independent predictors of motor decline, with distal symmetrical neuropathy underestimated in the clinical and epidemiological evaluation of motor decline in older people. An adequate assessment of baseline neuropathy is necessary in older adult patients, with

bladder cancer being considered for cisplatin-based chemotherapy.

In spite of the potential for complications related to cisplatin-based chemotherapy in older patients, a retrospective analysis of four prospective clinical trials in patients with locally advanced, metastatic, or recurrent urothelial cancer stratified by age (under 70 years vs. 70 years or older) suggested that elderly patients with advanced urothelial cancer are able to tolerate platinum-based chemotherapy with comparable responses as compared to the younger patients.[58] Elderly patients with Eastern Cooperative Oncology Group performance status 2 or 3 or hemoglobin less than 10 g/dL had a median survival of 5 months compared with 14 months for older patients without these prognostic factors ($p < .001$).

Few studies designed to evaluate chemotherapy in older patients with bladder cancer with the incorporation of geriatric assessment tools have been performed to date. One prospective study aiming to evaluate the activity and toxicity of gemcitabine monotherapy in elderly patients with advanced bladder cancer incorporating a comprehensive geriatric assessment (CGA) demonstrated that gemcitabine could be safely administered, was effective, and did not worsen the functional status of elderly patients with bladder cancer.[59] A second study evaluated the safety and efficacy of first-line gemcitabine plus carboplatin in patients with advanced urothelial carcinoma who were "unfit for cisplatin." The effect of treatment on the quality of life and functional status of elderly patients (aged over 70 years) was also examined.[60] Elderly patients were stratified into group 1 (no activities of daily living [ADLs] or instrumental ADL dependency and no comorbidities), group 2 (instrumental ADL dependency or one to two comorbidities), and group 3 (ADL dependency or more than two comorbidities). Thirty-four patients were enrolled, with those in geriatric assessment groups 1 and 2 having a significantly longer median progression-free survival compared to group 3 (6.9 months, 95% CI 1.3–12.4 vs. 1.9 months, 95% CI 0.5–3.2, $p = .005$).

Prospective clinical trials in older adults with bladder cancer are desperately needed, including non-cisplatin-based chemotherapy trials in the perioperative setting. Novel agents with new toxicity profiles, such as those targeting angiogenesis, are also being actively investigated in patients with advanced bladder cancer. These clinical trials must be designed to understand the activity and toxicity profile in older adults. This may be accomplished in several ways, including the development of clinical trials specifically for older patients with comorbidities; pretreatment stratification by age and/or coexisting medical conditions; and incorporation of comprehensive geriatric assessment tools within the clinical trial design.

C. Kidney cancer

Kidney cancer typically affects individuals in the sixth and seventh decades with a median age of 65 years. An estimated 57,760 cases (men, 35,430; women, 22,330) and 12,980 deaths (men, 8,160; women, 4,820) will occur in the year 2009 in the United States.[2] Conventional or clear-cell carcinoma and papillary carcinoma are the most common subtypes, accounting for 75 percent and 12 percent of new cases, respectively.[61] Less common subtypes include chromophobe, oncocytoma, collecting duct, medullary, and unclassified tumors. Risk factors for kidney cancer include smoking, obesity, and hypertension as well as acquired cystic kidney disease associated with end-stage renal disease.[61] A minority of patients present with the classic triad of flank pain, hematuria, and a palpable abdominal mass. Approximately 50 percent of patients are diagnosed with an incidental renal mass detected on imaging performed for other reasons. Approximately 25 percent of patients present with advanced disease, including locally invasive or metastatic, and one-third of those who undergo resection of localized disease will ultimately recur.

Advanced kidney cancer has historically been an extremely difficult disease to treat; however, recent insights into the biology of the disease have led to the rapid development of multiple novel targeted therapies. The majority of conventional renal cell carcinomas are characterized by loss of the tumor suppressor gene von Hippel–Lindau (*VHL*).[62] Under normal conditions, *VHL* encodes the VHL protein targeting hypoxia-inducible factor (HIF) for proteolysis. When the *VHL* gene is inactivated, the VHL protein is defective, and HIF is not targeted for degradation. In this way, an activated HIF translocates to the nucleus, leading to the transcription of a series of genes, including vascular endothelial growth factor (VEGF), a potent promoter of angiogenesis. The VEGF and mammalian target of rapamycin (mTOR) pathways merge at the level of HIF and have become the most important targets for novel agents in

the treatment of advanced kidney cancer. This has led to an exciting and rapidly changing landscape for physicians treating patients with kidney cancer and also will represent a challenge in the application of these novel therapies with a new spectrum of side effects to older adults with coexisting medical problems.

C.1. Localized kidney cancer

Surgical management of localized kidney cancer includes radical or partial nephrectomy performed using open or laparoscopic approaches. A retrospective study evaluated whether age and comorbidity were predictors of perioperative complications and/or mortality in patients aged over 75 years who underwent surgery for renal cancer. In this series, 1,023 radical nephrectomies or nephron-sparing surgeries were performed in 115 consecutive patients aged 75 years and older and in 908 consecutive patients aged under 75 years.[63] The preoperative American Society of Anesthesiologists (ASA) score was used for risk stratification. Operative mortality and early complications within 30 days of surgery were reviewed. The younger patients had significantly lower ASA scores than the older patients. Perioperative mortality was higher in the older than in the younger patients (1.7% vs. 0.3%, $p = .29$). Overall morbidity and mortality correlated with increasing ASA score but not with age ($p < .05$). The authors concluded that advanced age alone should not be used as a criterion to deny surgery for kidney cancer, with the caveat that older patients should be counseled regarding a tendency for increased comorbidity-related perioperative mortality.

In a single-institution retrospective series comparing young patients with renal cell carcinoma and their older counterparts, 1,720 patients 18–79 years old who were treated with partial or radical nephrectomy for renal cell cancer between 1989 and 2005 were identified. Of the 1,720 patients, 89 (5%), 672 (39%), and 959 (56%) were younger than 40, 40–59, and 60–79 years old, respectively.[64] Patients younger than 40 years were significantly more likely to present with symptomatic tumors ($p = .028$). There were also significant differences in histology by age ($p < .001$); chromophobe histology decreased, whereas papillary histology increased with age. Despite similar tumor sizes in each age group, the percentage of patients treated with partial nephrectomy decreased with age. Of patients younger than 40 years, 49 percent were treated with partial nephrectomy, compared with 35 percent and 30 percent of those 40–59 and 60–79 years old, respectively ($p < .001$). There were no significant differences in cancer-specific survival according to age ($p = .17$).

Radical nephrectomy is a significant risk factor for the development of chronic kidney disease, with retrospective data demonstrating that approximately 25 percent of patients have preexisting chronic kidney disease prior to surgery.[65] The less frequent use of nephron-sparing surgery certainly deserves attention because older patients may have a greater decline in kidney function both prior to and after radical nephrectomy as related to their normal physiologic decline in renal function with aging and then having a solitary kidney.[51] Aging, proteinuria, hypertension, and diabetes mellitus appear to be the predominant risk factors for renal deterioration following radical nephrectomy.[66]

C.2. Metastatic kidney cancer

A prognostic model predicting the survival of patients with metastatic kidney cancer was derived from 670 patients (median age of 58 years) with advanced disease treated in 24 Memorial Sloan-Kettering Cancer Center clinical trials between 1975 and 1996.[67] Pretreatment features associated with a shorter survival in multivariate analysis were low KPS (less than 80%), high serum lactate dehydrogenase (more than 1.5 times the upper limit of normal), low hemoglobin (under the lower limit of normal), high "corrected" serum calcium (under 10 mg/dL), and absence of prior nephrectomy. The median time to death for patients with zero risk factors (favorable risk), one or two risk factors (intermediate risk), and three or more risk factors (poor risk) were 20, 10, and 4 months, respectively. Additional prognostic models have been developed in the era of targeted therapy, and age has not been a significant variable for outcome in patients with advanced kidney cancer.[68]

Renal cell cancer is highly resistant to chemotherapy, and alternative treatment strategies have been investigated over the years. Cytokine therapy including interferon alfa (IFNa) and interleukin-2 (IL-2) has been associated with modest response rates. Two randomized trials have demonstrated a small survival advantage for IFNa as compared to vinblastine or medroxyprogesterone.[69,70] High-dose IL-2 results in higher response rates as compared to low-dose cytokine therapy, with approximately 5–7 percent of patients achieving a durable response.[71–73] High-dose IL-2 is associated with a capillary leak syndrome necessitating hospitalization for administration, thus limiting its applicability to many patients with metastatic renal cell cancer. In a retrospective analysis of outcome in 259 patients treated with high-dose IL-2 at the National Cancer Institute between 1986 and 2006, the majority were between the ages of 40 and 60 years.[72] Older adults with coexisting medical problems are most often not candidates for high-dose IL-2 therapy.

An understanding of the biology of renal cell cancer has led to the development of several novel targeted agents with significant activity associated with a new spectrum of side effects (Table 12.3). The increased expression of VEGF in renal cancers led to a randomized phase II trial comparing placebo to the humanized VEGF-neutralizing antibody bevacizumab in patients with metastatic renal cell cancer.[74] There was a significant prolongation of the time to progression of disease in the patients receiving high-dose bevacizumab as compared with the placebo group (HR 2.55, $p = <.001$). Hypertension and asymptomatic proteinuria were the most common adverse events. Bevacizumab in combination with IFNa has demonstrated an overall response and progression-free survival advantage over IFNa monotherapy in treatment-naive patients with metastatic renal cancer.[75,76] Two small molecules, sorafenib and sunitinib, inhibit a series of receptor tyrosine kinases, including the vascular endothelial growth factor receptor (VEGFR), and have demonstrated significant activity in patients with advanced kidney cancer. Sunitinib has shown a benefit in cytokine-refractory patients as well as a progression-free and overall survival benefit versus IFNa in treatment-naive patients.[77–79] Sorafenib has demonstrated a progression-free survival benefit as compared to placebo in previously treated patients with advanced kidney cancer.[80]

The mTOR inhibitor temsirolimus has demonstrated an improved survival as compared to IFNa in modified poor-risk patients with metastatic disease.[81] Most recently, the orally administered mTOR inhibitor everolimus has shown a progression-free survival benefit as compared to placebo in patients having previously received sunitinib, sorafenib, or both.[82] Although no trials have specifically focused on older patients, the

Table 12.3 Selected trials of targeted agents in kidney cancer.

Trial	Agent	Mechanism	Setting	Outcome
Motzer et al.[79]	Sunitinib	Small-molecule tyrosine kinase inhibitor of VEGF and related receptors	First line	PFS: sunitinib, 11 months vs. IFNa, 5 months ($p < .001$)
Escudier et al.[80]	Sorafenib	Small-molecule tyrosine kinase inhibitor of VEGFR and raf kinase	Second line	PFS: sorafenib, 5.5 months vs. placebo, 2.8 months ($p < .01$)
Hudes et al.[81]	Temsirolimus	mTOR inhibitor	First line (poor risk)	MS: temsirolimus, 10.9 months vs. IFNa, 7.3 months ($p = .008$)
Motzer et al.[82]	Everolimus	mTOR inhibitor	Second line	PFS: everolimus, 4 months vs. placebo, 1.9 months ($p < .0001$)

Note. VEGF = vascular endothelial growth factor; mTOR = mammalian target of rapamycin; PFS = progression-free survival; MS = median survival; IFNa = interferon alfa.

safety and efficacy of sorafenib in elderly patients aged 65 years and older was evaluated in a subset analysis of the Advanced Renal Cell Carcinoma Sorafenib (ARCCS) Expanded Access Program in North America.[83] Sorafenib was associated with similar rates of side effects in elderly patients as compared to younger patients, and response rates were comparable to results for the total ARCCS population.

In addition to side effects including fatigue, diarrhea, rashes, and mucositis, these novel targeted agents are associated with a new spectrum of side effects that will in part guide treatment decisions in older adults with coexisting medical problems (Table 12.4). Hypertension is a major side effect of the VEGF targeted agents, including sunitinib, sorafenib, and bevacizumab.[62] Patients with a prior history of hypertension and coronary artery disease are at an increased risk of cardiotoxicity related to sunitinib.[84] These patients should be monitored for worsening hypertension and left ventricular ejection fraction decline during treatment. Sorafenib and sunitinib are also associated with hypothyroidism. The mTOR inhibitors temsirolimus and everolimus are associated with hyperglycemia and hyperlipidemia as well as the less common side effect of pneumonitis. Physicians will need to become familiar with this new side effect profile, and studies must be done to determine the best management strategies in older adult patients with baseline organ dysfunction.

An analysis according to age of the efficacy and toxicity data from phase III trials of the targeted agents sorafenib, sunitinib, temsirolimus, and bevacizumab and from a study of expanded access to sunitinib and sorafenib suggests that the progression-free and overall survival benefits seen in metastatic renal cell cancer patients aged 65 years and over are similar to those in the younger age groups.[85] In addition, the frequency of major toxicities in elderly patients treated with targeted agents is no greater than in younger patients, although such toxicities may have greater impact on quality of life. No meaningful data are available for patients aged over 85 years. The authors call for prospective studies in the elderly; however, at the current time, they recommend individual patient decision making be based on the toxicity profiles of the

Table 12.4 Common toxicities of targeted agents for kidney cancer.[62]

Agent	Toxicities
Sunitinib	Fatigue, hypertension, diarrhea, hand-foot skin reaction, mucositis, neutropenia, thrombocytopenia, hypothyroidism
Sorafenib	Fatigue, hypertension, diarrhea, hand-foot skin reaction, mucositis, dyspnea, hypothyroidism
Bevacizumab	Fatigue, hypertension, proteinuria
Temsirolimus	Fatigue, dyspnea, neutropenia, thrombocytopenia, hyperglycemia, hyperlipidemia
Everolimus	Fatigue, dyspnea, neutropenia, thrombocytopenia, hyperglycemia, hyperlipidemia

individual targeted agents, taking into account any implications related to specific comorbidities. This being said, older age has been associated with an increased risk of severe toxicity when using sunitinib.[86]

The significant progress in the development of effective therapies for patients with advanced kidney cancer must continue with clinical trials specifically targeting older patients and with special attention given to the management of side effects in these patients with baseline organ dysfunction. This will provide the framework for developing guidelines for the management of advanced kidney cancer in older adults.

References

1. Jemal A, Siegel R, Ward E, et al. Cancer statistics, 2008. *CA Cancer J Clin.* 2008;58(2):71–96.

2. Jemal A, Siegel R, Ward E, et al. Cancer Statistics, 2009. *CA Cancer J Clin.* 2009; 59(4):225–249.

3. Gouda I, Mokhtar N, Bilal D, et al. Bilharziasis and bladder cancer: a time trend analysis of 9843 patients. *J Egypt Natl Canc Inst.* 2007;19(2): 158–162.

4. Pelucchi C, Bosetti C, Negri E, et al. Mechanisms of disease: the epidemiology of bladder cancer. *Natl Clin Pract Urol.* 2006;3(6):327–340.

5. Stein JP, Lieskovsky G, Cote R, et al. Radical cystectomy in the treatment of invasive bladder cancer: long-term results in 1,054 patients. *J Clin Oncol.* 2001;19(3):666–675.

6. von der Maase H, Sengelove L, Roberts JT, et al. Long-term survival results of a randomized trial comparing gemcitabine plus cisplatin, with methotrexate, vinblastine, doxorubicin, plus cisplatin in patients with bladder cancer. *J Clin Oncol.* 2005;23(21):4602–4608.

7. Prout Jr GR, Wesley MN, Yancik R, et al. Age and comorbidity impact surgical therapy in older bladder carcinoma patients: a population-based study. *Cancer.* 2005;104(8):1638–1647.

8. Herr HW, Schwalb DM, Zhang ZF, et al. Intravesical bacillus Calmette-Guerin therapy prevents tumor progression and death from superficial bladder cancer: ten-year follow-up of a prospective randomized trial. *J Clin Oncol.* 1995;13(6):1404–1408.

9. Joudi FN, Smith BJ, O'Donnell MA, et al. The impact of age on the response of patients with superficial bladder cancer to intravesical immunotherapy. *J Urol.* 2006;175(5):1634–1639; discussion 1639–1640.

10. Herr HW. Age and outcome of superficial bladder cancer treated with bacille Calmette-Guerin therapy. *Urology.* 2007;70(1):65–68.

11. Van Der Aa MN, Steyerberg EW, Sen EF, et al. Patients' perceived burden of cystoscopic and urinary surveillance of bladder cancer: a randomized comparison. *BJU Int.* 2008;101(9): 1106–1110.

12. Wu XR. Urothelial tumorigenesis: a tale of divergent pathways. *Nat Rev Cancer.* 2005;5(9): 713–725.

13. Clark PE, Stein JP, Groshen SG, et al. Radical cystectomy in the elderly: comparison of clinical outcomes between younger and older patients. *Cancer.* 2005;104(1):36–43.

14. Clark PE, Stein JP, Groshen SG, et al. Radical cystectomy in the elderly: comparison of survival between younger and older patients. *Cancer.* 2005;103(3):546–552.

15. Hollenbeck BK, Miller DC, Taub D, et al. Aggressive treatment for bladder cancer is associated with improved overall survival among patients 80 years old or older. *Urology.* 2004;64(2): 292–297.

16. Donat SM, Siegrist T, Cronin A, et al. Radical cystectomy in octogenarians–does morbidity outweigh the potential survival benefits? *J Urol.* 2010;183:2171–2177.

17. Koppie TM, Serio AM, Vickers AJ, et al. Age-adjusted Charlson comorbidity score is associated with treatment decisions and clinical outcomes for patients undergoing radical cystectomy for bladder cancer. *Cancer.* 2008;112(11):2384–2392.

18. Weizer AZ, Joshi D, Diagnault S, et al. Performance status is a predictor of overall survival of elderly patients with muscle invasive bladder cancer. *J Urol.* 2007;177(4):1287–1293.

19. Hagan MP, Winter KA, Kaufman DS, et al. RTOG 97-06: initial report of a phase I–II trial of selective bladder conservation using TURBT, twice-daily accelerated irradiation sensitized with cisplatin, and adjuvant MCV combination chemotherapy. *Int J Radiat Oncol Biol Phys.* 2003;57(3):665–672.

20. Rodel C, Grabenbauer GG, Kuhn R, et al. Combined-modality treatment and selective organ preservation in invasive bladder cancer: long-term results. *J Clin Oncol.* 2002;20(14): 3061–3071.

21. Shipley WU, Kaufman DS, Zehr E, et al. Selective bladder preservation by combined modality protocol treatment: long-term outcomes of 190 patients with invasive bladder cancer. *Urology.* 2002;60(1):62–67.

22. Kaufman DS, Winter KA, Shipley WU, et al. The initial results in muscle-invading bladder cancer of RTOG 95-06: phase I/II trial of transurethral surgery plus radiation therapy with concurrent cisplatin and 5-fluorouracil followed by selective bladder preservation or cystectomy depending on the initial. *Oncologist.* 2000;5(6):471–476.

23. Sauer R, Birkenhake S, Kuhn R, et al. Efficacy of radiochemotherapy with platin derivatives compared to radiotherapy alone in organ-sparing treatment of bladder cancer. *Int J Radiat Oncol Biol Phys.* 1998;40(1):121–127.

24. Tester W, Caplan R, Heaney J, et al. Neoadjuvant combined modality program with selective organ preservation for invasive bladder cancer: results of Radiation Therapy Oncology Group phase II trial 8802. *J Clin Oncol.* 1996;14(1):119–126.

25. Tester W, Porter A, Asbell S, et al. Combined modality program with possible organ preservation for invasive bladder carcinoma: results of RTOG protocol 85-12. *Int J Radiat Oncol Biol Phys.* 1993;25(5):783–790.

26. Fernando SA, Sandler HM. Multimodality bladder preservation therapy for muscle-invasive bladder tumors. *Semin Oncol.* 2007;34(2): 129–134.

27. Rodel C, Weiss C, Sauer R. Trimodality treatment and selective organ preservation for bladder cancer. *J Clin Oncol.* 2006;24(35):5536–5544.

28. Kent E, Sandler H, Montie J, et al. Combined-modality therapy with gemcitabine and radiotherapy as a bladder preservation strategy: results of a phase I trial. *J Clin Oncol.* 2004;22(13):2540–2545.

29. Oh KS, Soto DE, Smith DC, et al. Combined-modality therapy with gemcitabine and radiation therapy as a bladder preservation strategy: long-term results of a phase I trial. *Int J Radiat Oncol Biol Phys.* 2009;74(2):511–517.

30. Herman JM, Smith DC, Montie J, et al. Prospective quality-of-life assessment in patients receiving concurrent gemcitabine and radiotherapy as a bladder preservation strategy. *Urology.* 2004;64(1):69–73.

31. Zietman AL, Sacco D, Skowronski U, et al. Organ conservation in invasive bladder cancer by transurethral resection, chemotherapy and radiation: results of a urodynamic and quality of life study on long-term survivors. *J Urol.* 2003;170(5):1772–1776.

32. Loehrer Sr PJ, Einhorn LH, Elson PJ, et al. A randomized comparison of cisplatin alone or in combination with methotrexate, vinblastine, and doxorubicin in patients with metastatic urothelial carcinoma: a cooperative group study. *J Clin Oncol.* 1992;10(7):1066–1073.

33. Logothetis CJ, Dexeus FH, Finn L, et al. A prospective randomized trial comparing CISCA to MVAC chemotherapy in advanced metastatic urothelial tumors. *J Clin Oncol.* 1990;8:1050–1055.

34. Saxman SB, Propert KJ, Einhorn LH, et al. Long term follow-up of a phase III intergroup study of cisplatin alone or in combination with methotrexate, vinblastine and doxorubicin in patients with metastatic urothelial cancer: a cooperative group study. *J Clin Oncol.* 1997;15:2564–2569.

35. Sternberg CN, Yagoda A, Scher HI, et al. Methotrexate, vinblastine, doxorubicin, and cisplatin for advanced transitional cell carcinoma of the urothelium: efficacy and patterns of response and relapse. *Cancer.* 1989;64(12): 2448–2458.

36. von der Maase H, Hansen SW, Roberts JT, et al. Gemcitabine and cisplatin versus methotrexate, vinblastine, doxorubicin, and cisplatin in advanced or metastatic bladder cancer: results of a large, randomized, multinational, multicenter, phase III study. *J Clin Oncol.* 2000;18(17): 3068–3077.

37. Grossman HB, Natale RB, Tangen CM, et al. Neoadjuvant chemotherapy plus cystectomy compared with cystectomy alone for locally advanced bladder cancer. *N Engl J Med.* 2003;349(9):859–866.

38. Neoadjuvant chemotherapy in invasive bladder cancer: a systematic review and meta-analysis. *Lancet.* 2003;361(9373):1927–1934.

39. Neoadjuvant cisplatin, methotrexate, and vinblastine chemotherapy for muscle-invasive bladder cancer: a randomised controlled trial. International Collaboration of Trialists. *Lancet.* 1999;354(9178):533–540.

40. Neoadjuvant chemotherapy for invasive bladder cancer. *Cochrane Database Syst Rev.* 2005;CD005246.

41. Studer U, Bacchi M, Biederman C, et al. Adjuvant cisplatin chemotherapy following cystectomy for bladder cancer: results of a prospective randomized trial. *J Urol.* 1994;152:81–84.

42. Skinner DG, Daniels JR, Russell CA, et al. The role of adjuvant chemotherapy following cystectomy for invasive bladder cancer: a prospective comparative trial. *J Urol.* 1991;145(3):459–464; discussion 464–467.

43. Freiha F, Reese J, Torti FM. A randomized trial of radical cystectomy versus radical cystectomy plus cisplatin, vinblastine and methotrexate chemotherapy for muscle invasive bladder cancer. *J Urol.* 1996;155(2):495–499; discussion 499–500.

44. Stockle M, Meyenburg W, Wellek S, et al. Advanced bladder cancer (stages pT3b, pT4a, pN1 and pN2): improved survival after radical cystectomy and 3 adjuvant cycles of chemotherapy: results of a controlled prospective study. *J Urol.* 1992;148(2 Pt 1):302–066; discussion 306–307.

45. Stockle M, Meyenburg W, Wellek S, et al. Adjuvant polychemotherapy of nonorgan-confined bladder cancer after radical cystectomy revisited: long-term results of a controlled prospective study and further experience. *J Urol.* 1995;153:47–52.

46. Adjuvant chemotherapy in invasive bladder cancer: a systematic review and meta-analysis of individual patient data. Advanced Bladder Cancer (ABC) Meta-analysis Collaboration. *Eur Urol.* 2005;48(2):189–199; discussion 199–201.

47. Milowsky MI, Stadler WM, Bajorin DF. Integration of neoadjuvant and adjuvant chemotherapy and cystectomy in the treatment of muscle-invasive bladder cancer. *BJU Int.* 2008;102(9 Pt B):1339–1344.

48. Bellmunt J, Ribas A, Eres N, et al. Carboplatin-based versus cisplatin-based chemotherapy in the treatment of surgically incurable advanced bladder carcinoma. *Cancer*. 1997;80(10):1966–1972.

49. Petrioli R, Frediani B, Manganelli A, et al. Comparison between a cisplatin-containing regimen and a carboplatin-containing regimen for recurrent or metastatic bladder cancer patients: a randomized phase II study. *Cancer*. 1996;77(2): 344–351.

50. Dogliotti L, Carteni G, Siena S, et al. Gemcitabine plus cisplatin versus gemcitabine plus carboplatin as first-line chemotherapy in advanced transitional cell carcinoma of the urothelium: results of a randomized phase 2 trial. *Eur Urol*. 2007;52(1):134–141.

51. Fehrman-Ekholm I, Skeppholm L. Renal function in the elderly (>70 years old) measured by means of iohexol clearance, serum creatinine, serum urea and estimated clearance. *Scand J Urol Nephrol*. 2004;38(1):73–77.

52. Dash A, Galsky MD, Vickers AJ, et al. Impact of renal impairment on eligibility for adjuvant cisplatin-based chemotherapy in patients with urothelial carcinoma of the bladder. *Cancer*. 2006;107(3):506–513.

53. Agrawal Y, Platz EA, Niparko JK. Prevalence of hearing loss and differences by demographic characteristics among US adults: data from the National Health and Nutrition Examination Survey, 1999–2004. *Arch Intern Med*. 2008; 168(14):1522–1530.

54. Rademaker-Lakhai JM, Crul M, Zuur L, et al. Relationship between cisplatin administration and the development of ototoxicity. *J Clin Oncol*. 2006;24(6):918–924.

55. Guralnik JM, Ferrucci L, Simonsick EM, et al. Lower-extremity function in persons over the age of 70 years as a predictor of subsequent disability. *N Engl J Med*. 1995;332(9):556–561.

56. Guralnik JM, Simonsick EM, Ferrucci L, et al. A short physical performance battery assessing lower extremity function: association with self-reported disability and prediction of mortality and nursing home admission. *J Gerontol*. 1994;49(2):M85–M94.

57. Inzitari M, Carlo A, Baldereschi M, et al. Risk and predictors of motor-performance decline in a normally functioning population-based sample of elderly subjects: the Italian Longitudinal Study on Aging. *J Am Geriatr Soc*. 2006;54(2): 318–324.

58. Bamias A, Efstathiou E, Moulopoulos LA, et al. The outcome of elderly patients with advanced urothelial carcinoma after platinum-based combination chemotherapy. *Ann Oncol*. 2005;16(2):307–313.

59. Castagneto B, Zai S, Marenco D, et al. Single-agent gemcitabine in previously untreated elderly patients with advanced bladder carcinoma: response to treatment and correlation with the comprehensive geriatric assessment. *Oncology*. 2004;67(1):27–32.

60. Bamias A, Lainakis G, Kastritis E, et al. Biweekly carboplatin/gemcitabine in patients with advanced urothelial cancer who are unfit for cisplatin-based chemotherapy: report of efficacy, quality of life and geriatric assessment. *Oncology*. 2007;73(5–6):290–297.

61. Cohen HT, McGovern FJ. Renal-cell carcinoma. *N Engl J Med*. 2005;353(23):2477–2490.

62. Rini BI. Metastatic renal cell carcinoma: many treatment options, one patient. *J Clin Oncol*. 2009; 27(19):3225–3234.

63. Berdjis N, Hakenberg OW, Novotny V, et al. Treating renal cell cancer in the elderly. *BJU Int*. 2006;97(4):703–705.

64. Thompson RH, Ordonez MA, Lasonos A, et al. Renal cell carcinoma in young and old patients – is there a difference? *J Urol*. 2008;180(4): 1262–1266; discussion 1266.

65. Huang WC, Levey AS, Serio AM, et al. Chronic kidney disease after nephrectomy in patients with renal cortical tumours: a retrospective cohort study. *Lancet Oncol*. 2006;7(9):735–740.

66. Shirasaki Y, Tsushima T, Nasu Y, et al. Long-term consequence of renal function following nephrectomy for renal cell cancer. *Int J Urol*. 2004;11(9):704–708.

67. Motzer RJ, Mazumdar M, Bacik J, et al. Survival and prognostic stratification of 670 patients with advanced renal cell carcinoma. *J Clin Oncol*. 1999;17(8):2530–2540.

68. Motzer RJ, Bukowski RM, Figlin RA, et al. Prognostic nomogram for sunitinib in patients with metastatic renal cell carcinoma. *Cancer*. 2008;113(7):1552–1558.

69. Pyrhonen S, Salminen E, Ruutu M, et al. Prospective randomized trial of interferon alfa-2a plus vinblastine versus vinblastine alone in patients with advanced renal cell cancer. *J Clin Oncol*. 1999;17(9):2859–2867.

70. Interferon-alpha and survival in metastatic renal carcinoma: early results of a randomised controlled trial. Medical Research Council Renal Cancer Collaborators. *Lancet*. 1999;353(9146): 14–17.

71. Fyfe G, Fisher RI, Rosenberg SA, et al. Results of treatment of 255 patients with metastatic renal cell carcinoma who received high-dose recombinant interleukin-2 therapy. *J Clin Oncol*. 1995;13(3):688–696.

72. Klapper JA, Downey SG, Smith FO, et al. High-dose interleukin-2 for the treatment of

metastatic renal cell carcinoma: a retrospective analysis of response and survival in patients treated in the surgery branch at the National Cancer Institute between 1986 and 2006. *Cancer*. 2008;113(2):293–301.

73. McDermott DF, Atkins MB. Immunotherapy of metastatic renal cell carcinoma. *Cancer J*. 2008;14(5):320–324.

74. Yang JC, Haworth L,Sherry RM, et al. A randomized trial of bevacizumab, an anti-vascular endothelial growth factor antibody, for metastatic renal cancer. *N Engl J Med*. 2003;349(5): 427–434.

75. Rini BI, Halabi S, Rosenberg JE, et al. Bevacizumab plus interferon alfa compared with interferon alfa monotherapy in patients with metastatic renal cell carcinoma: CALGB 90206. *J Clin Oncol*. 2008;26(33):5422–5428.

76. Escudier B, Pluzanska A, Koralewski P, et al. Bevacizumab plus interferon alfa-2a for treatment of metastatic renal cell carcinoma: a randomised, double-blind phase III trial. *Lancet*. 2007; 370(9605):2103–2111.

77. Motzer RJ, Michaelson MD, Redman BG, et al. Activity of SU11248, a multitargeted inhibitor of vascular endothelial growth factor receptor and platelet-derived growth factor receptor, in patients with metastatic renal cell carcinoma. *J Clin Oncol*. 2006;24(1):16–24.

78. Motzer RJ, Rini BI, Bukowski RM, et al. Sunitinib in patients with metastatic renal cell carcinoma. *J Am Med Assoc*. 2006;295(21):2516–2524.

79. Motzer RJ, Hutson TE, Tomczak P, et al. Sunitinib versus interferon alfa in metastatic renal-cell carcinoma. *N Engl J Med*. 2007;356(2): 115–124.

80. Escudier B, Eisen T, Stadler WM, et al. Sorafenib in advanced clear-cell renal-cell carcinoma. *N Engl J Med*. 2007;356(2):125–134.

81. Hudes G, Carducci M, Tomczak P, et al. Temsirolimus, interferon alfa, or both for advanced renal-cell carcinoma. *N Engl J Med*. 2007;356(22):2271–2281.

82. Motzer RJ, Escudier B, Oudard S, et al. Efficacy of everolimus in advanced renal cell carcinoma: a double-blind, randomised, placebo-controlled phase III trial. *Lancet*. 2008;372(9637):449–456.

83. Bukowski RM, Stadler WM, Figlin RA, et al. Safety and efficacy of sorafenib in elderly patients (pts) ≥ 65 years: a subset analysis from the Advanced Renal Cell Carcinoma Sorafenib (ARCCS) Expanded Access Program in North America. *J Clin Oncol* 26: 2008 (May 20 suppl; abstr 5045).

84. Di Lorenzo G, Autorino R, Bruni G, et al. Cardiovascular toxicity following sunitinib therapy in metastatic renal cell carcinoma: a multicenter analysis. *Ann Oncol*. 2009; 20(9):1535–1542.

85. Bellmunt J, Negrier S, Escudier B, et al. The medical treatment of metastatic renal cell cancer in the elderly: position paper of a SIOG Taskforce. *Crit Rev Oncol Hematol*. 2009;69(1):64–72.

86. Van Der Veldt AA, Boven E, Helgason HH, et al. Predictive factors for severe toxicity of sunitinib in unselected patients with advanced renal cell cancer. *Br J Cancer*. 2008;99(2):259–265.

87. Hall R. Updated results of a randomised controlled trial of neoadjuvant cisplatin (C), methotrexate (M) and vinblastine (V) chemotherapy for muscle-invasive bladder cancer [abstract]. *Proc Am Soc Clin Oncol*. 2002;21:178a.

13 Management of prostate cancer in older adults

Andrew Liman and Gurkamal Chatta

A. Epidemiology

Prostate cancer is the most common malignancy and the second leading cause of cancer-related death among men in the United States. An estimated 186,000 men were diagnosed with prostate cancer in 2008, and there were 28,660 deaths.[1] In Europe in the same year, there were 190,000 new cases diagnosed and 80,000 prostate cancer–related deaths.[2] The incidence of prostate cancer in Asia is significantly lower, with the total worldwide burden of prostate cancer thought to be in the 650,000–700,000 range. In part, the geographical differences are a reflection of widely disparate screening practices.

Prostate cancer is primarily a disease of the elderly, with the median age at diagnosis being 71 years and the median age at death being 78 years. In the United States, the lifetime risk of prostate cancer diagnosis and prostate cancer–related death is 16.7 percent and 2.8 percent, respectively (Table 13.1). Thus more men will die with, rather than of, prostate cancer. This discrepancy between incidence and death continues to fuel controversies pertaining to screening and treatment of prostate cancer. On the basis of the Surveillance, Epidemiology, and End Results (SEER) program database of the National Cancer Institute, the number of all cancer patients is expected to more than double from 1.36 million in 2000 to almost 3.0 million in 2050, because of both the aging and the growth of the U.S. population. For ages 65–84 years, the projected incidence for prostate cancer is expected to increase from 133 cases per 100,000 population to 305 cases in 2050; for age above 85 years, from 10 to 63 cases; and in aggregate, the total prostate cancer incidence in 2050 is anticipated to be 495 cases per 100,000 population.[3]

B. Etiology

As for most solid tumors, complex gene–environment interactions account for most prostate cancers. Aging, a positive family history (index case less than 60 years of age), and African American race are the best-defined risk factors for developing prostate cancer. With aging, the testosterone (T) level declines, and relatively speaking, men have higher estrogen (E) levels. This increase in the E:T ratio has been invoked as a possible transforming event in prostate epithelium.[4] Men with a first-degree relative with prostate cancer (particularly under 60 years of age) are at higher risk, with the risk increasing exponentially with more than one relative with the disease. Genetic linkage studies in these families have identified the hereditary prostate cancer locus-1 (HPC1) and single-nucleotide polymorphisms (SNPs) at three chromosomal loci – 8q24, 17q12, and 17q24.3 – as conferring increased risk. Zheng and colleagues have recently examined the association between prostate cancer risk and these loci: possession of these high-risk loci increases the risk of prostate cancer by a factor of about 4 to 5.[5] However, these risk factors do not distinguish between indolent or clinically relevant cancer. An important breakthrough in prostate cancer is the finding of fusion oncogenes: the high frequency of the TMPRSS2-ERG fusions in aggressive cancers may help with risk stratification.[6] Genetic polymorphisms have also been reported in genes for the androgen receptor, for 5α-reductase type 2, and for steroid hydroxylase, the notion being that altered androgen metabolism may confer different risk levels. Ross and colleagues suggest a difference in 5α-reductase activity between Western and Asian men owing to a polymorphism of the SRD5A2 gene.[7] A variant of the CYP3A4 gene involved in the oxidation of testosterone as well as its variant allele form, G, has been linked to a higher Gleason grade in African American men.[8] Finally, the HPC1 locus codes for RNase-L, a protein involved in interferon regulation and immune surveillance, thereby suggesting a link between inflammation and prostate cancer.[9] Thus the genetics of prostate cancer risk is complex and multifactorial.[5]

Table 13.1 Epidemiology of prostate cancer.

- Median age at diagnosis: 71 years
- Median age at death: 78 years
- Lifetime risk of CaP diagnosis: 16.7%
- Lifetime risk of CaP death: 2.8%
- More men will die with prostate cancer than from prostate cancer

Note. From Ries and Harris.[46]

African American men have the highest prostate cancer incidence rates, followed by Caucasians, Hispanics, and Asians. Data suggest that racial/ethnic variation in prostate cancer is partly because of underlying differences in androgen secretion and metabolism and perhaps more important because of environmental factors like diet, hormones, and inflammation. The role of diet is supported by the observation that Chinese Americans and Japanese Americans have much higher cancer incidence rates than their non-Westernized Asian counterparts because of the increased amount of dietary fat. Furthermore, Asian men also consume a low-fat diet with high content of soy products that have high concentrations of phytoestrogens. Phytoestrogens can affect several intracellular processes in cancer cells, so they are candidates for natural cancer-protective agents. Long-term survival analysis from the Physicians' Health Study reported that obese men are more likely to be diagnosed with metastatic prostate cancer.[10] In early-stage disease, obese men had a twofold higher risk of dying from prostate cancer than men of normal weight. The strong antioxidants lycopenes, found in tomatoes, have also been examined as protective agents for preventing prostate cancer. In a meta-analysis, the intake of tomatoes was negatively correlated with the risk of cancer. Intake of micronutrients and vitamins such as selenium, vitamin E, and vitamin D have all been proposed to reduce the risk of prostate cancer but have failed to show benefit in proof-of-principle clinical trials and formed the basis of the recently concluded, randomized prostate cancer prevention study, the Selenium and Vitamin E Cancer Prevention Trial (SELECT). The study failed to show a reduction in the incidence of prostate cancer.[11] In summary, although the role of diet is well established in prostate cancer risk, other than dietary fat, the role of other constituents – causative or protective – remains to be proven.

C. Prevention

Chemoprevention is an area of active research and potentially has huge implications in an elderly population with an increasing incidence of prostate cancer. The recently completed Prostate Cancer Prevention Trial (PCPT) showed that chemoprevention is possible with the 5α-reductase inhibitor finasteride. The PCPT began in 1993, accrued 18,882 men, and randomly assigned them to oral finasteride or oral placebo. The trial was halted at 7 years as the finasteride arm revealed a 24.8 percent reduced risk of prostate cancer[12] However, Gleason score 7–10 tumors were more common in the finasteride arm, possibly a finasteride-induced histological artifact as opposed to a true biologically aggressive tumor. The study proved that inhibiting 5α-reductase, the major target of finasteride, would block the conversion of testosterone into the more potent androgen dihydrotestosterone and reduce the risk of prostate cancer. The study also revealed that 25 percent of men with a PSA level 4.0 ng/mL or less had a normal digital rectal exam (DRE) at the time of prostate cancer diagnosis. Another trial, Reduction by Dutasteride of Prostate Cancer Events (REDUCE), is under way to ascertain whether dutasteride, another 5α-reductase inhibitor, can prevent prostate cancer.

Prior to this, two randomized controlled trials, the Nutritional Prevention of Cancer (NPC) study and the Alpha-Tocopherol, Beta-Carotene Cancer Prevention (ATBC) study, showed prostate cancer risk reductions of 43 percent for selenized yeast and 32 percent for α-tocopherol (or vitamin E). These clinical data led to the multigroup SELECT trial (see the earlier discussion). A total of 35,533 men were randomized to either placebo or selenium or vitamin E or a combination of selenium and vitamin E at 427 participating sites between 2001 and 2004. At a median follow-up of 5.46 years, there were no statistically significant differences in the rates of prostate cancer between the four groups, with a 5-year rate of 4.43 percent, 4.56 percent, 4.93 percent, and 4.56 percent for the placebo, selenium, vitamin E, and selenium plus vitamin E arms, respectively.[11] Thus, at the current time, there are no firm recommendations about prevention. Finasteride may be beneficial, but its potential benefits have to be weighed against its sexual side effects and the possibility of inducing higher-grade tumors.

D. Screening, diagnosis, and risk stratification

D.1. Screening

Given the huge discrepancy between prostate cancer incidence and prostate cancer–related mortality, screening for prostate cancer continues to be controversial. It is typically done with a combination of the serum tumor marker prostate-specific antigen (PSA) and a DRE. A DRE has low predictive value and is of limited use as over 70 percent of the tumors currently diagnosed in the United States are classified as clinical stage T1: impalpable tumors characterized by a normal DRE (Table 13.2a). The PSA is a prostate-specific serine protease (33Kd), the levels of which correlate with prostate volume and/or tumor burden – particularly at higher levels of PSA.[13] Normal PSA is reported as being under 4 ng/mL; however, on the basis of information from the PCPT, almost 25 percent of the currently diagnosed cancers have a normal PSA at presentation (Table 13.2b).

The level of the PSA is also influenced by age (increases with age); presence or absence of benign prostate hypertrophy (BPH); and presence or absence of lower urinary tract infection, inflammation, and/or obstruction. In the absence of obvious confounders, in the elderly, a PSA of over 7–8 ng/mL should be viewed with suspicion, and a PSA of less than 20 ng/dL is highly suggestive of cancer. The positive predictive value of a PSA in the 4–10 ng/mL range is 25 to 30 percent, and to improve on this, attempts have been

Table 13.2a Clinical staging of prostate cancer.

T1	*Clinically inapparent tumor (not palpable)*
T1a	Tumor incidental finding in 5% or less of tissue
T1b	Tumor incidental finding in more than 5% of tissue
T1c	Tumor identified by needle biopsy (elevated PSA)
T2	***Tumor confined within the prostate (palpable)***
T2a	Tumor involves less than one-half of one lobe
T2b	Tumor involves more than one-half of one lobe
T2c	Tumor involves both lobes
T3	***Tumor is extracapsular***
T3a	Unilateral or bilateral extracapsular extension
T3b	Involvement of seminal vesicles
T4	Involvement of adjacent organs

Note. PSA = prostate-specific antigen.

Table 13.2b Prostate cancer in patients with a prostate-specific antigen value of less than 4.0 ng/mL.

PSA value (ng/mL)	Number of patients	Prostate cancer incidence (%)
0–0.5	486	6.6
0.6–1.0	791	10.1
1.1–2.0	998	17.0
2.1–3.0	482	23.9
3.1–4.0	193	26.9

Note. PSA = prostate-specific antigen. Adapted from Thompson et al.[12]

made at (1) developing age-specific normal levels, (2) evaluating percentage free PSA – the lower the percentage free PSA, the higher the likelihood of cancer; and (3) plotting PSA velocity – a PSA rise of over 1 ng/mL/yr is indicative of underlying cancer. Thus use of age-adjusted PSA of 6.5 ng/mL in the over 70-year-olds may appropriately increase the threshold for biopsy in older men. Similarly, a 25 percent free PSA cutoff is 95 percent sensitive and results in 20 percent fewer biopsies, with only 5 percent of cancers going undetected. Biopsy is recommended for a free PSA of 10 percent or less and should be deferred for a free PSA over 25 percent. A free PSA over 10 percent and 25 percent or less is considered to be indeterminate.

Screening for prostate cancer has yet to conclusively demonstrate a reduction in prostate cancer–related mortality.[14] The controversy has been fueled further by the recently published interim results from two large, ongoing randomized trials: the Prostate, Lung, Colorectal, and Ovary (PLCO) trial in the United States and the European Randomized Screening for Prostate Cancer (ERSPC). The main end point of both these trials is differences in prostate-cancer mortality. The PLCO randomized 78,000 patients to screening or usual care, and at 7 years, there was no difference in deaths between the two arms. The ERSPC is a pan-European screening trial in which more than 250,000 men were randomly assigned to PSA screening or no active testing. At 9 years, there was a 20 percent reduction in deaths because of prostate cancer in the screened arm. The final results of these trials are eagerly awaited, but some of the reasons for the different results from these two trials include the following: (1) 7 years being insufficient time to demonstrate a survival benefit in the PLCO for a disease with a long natural history; (2) the differences in the stage at diagnosis – earlier in the PLCO versus later in the ERSPC; and

(3) the high rate of screening (~50%) even in the usual care arm in the PLCO. Interestingly, neither of the trials enrolled men over the age of 75 years.

Concerns regarding overdiagnosis and overtreatment resulting from prostate cancer screening are particularly germane in the elderly, given (1) the high prevalence of indolent disease, (2) the long and variable natural history of prostate cancer, (3) increasing comorbidities and decreasing life expectancy with aging, (4) the high risk of iatrogenic harm, and (5) the lack of demonstrated benefit of screening. Thus screening is not recommended in men over the age of 75 years or in men with a life expectancy of less than 10 years. The U.S. Preventive Services Task Force (USPSTF) recently concluded that "the current evidence is insufficient to assess the balance of benefits and harms of prostate cancer screening in men younger than age 75 years," but it now "recommends against screening for prostate cancer in men age 75 years or older."[15] The American Cancer Society recommends screening in men between the ages of 40 and 74 years, after a detailed discussion between the provider and the patient, in the context of individual risk factors and patient preferences, using the *shared decision-making model*.[16] The only published randomized trial comparing the effect of radical prostatectomy with a strategy of watchful waiting for men with clinically localized prostate cancer[17] demonstrated benefit in men aged less than 65 years and excluded men aged over 75 years. Two other completed trials, the results of which are eagerly awaited, are the Prostate Cancer Intervention versus Observation Trial (PIVOT) in the United States and the Prostate Testing for Cancer and Treatment (PROTECT) trial in the United Kingdom, which, if positive, may argue for screening and early intervention.

D.2. Diagnosis

The gold standard for a diagnosis of prostate cancer continues to be a transrectal ultrasound (TRUS)-guided needle biopsy. The false negative rate of sextant biopsies is approximately 20 to 25 percent. A second set of sextant biopsies improves the detection rate by 25 percent. Currently biopsies are recommended for patients older than 50 years with a PSA over 2.5 ng/mL or with a mean PSA velocity over 0.35 ng/mL/yr, a negative DRE, and life expectancy over 10 years. Biopsies are also recommended for individuals with a family history of prostate cancer and for African Americans using the same criteria, if they are over 40 years of age. At least 10 biopsy samples should be obtained, and many should be laterally directed.

Over 98 percent of prostate cancers are adenocarcinomas, with the rest being neuroendocrine variants, large ductal cell tumors, carcinosarcomas, and even small-cell cancer (<1%). The most commonly used system for grading adenocarcinoma of the prostate is the Gleason score. The score ranges from 2 to 10 and is a sum of the primary and secondary pattern, with each pattern being graded from 1 to 5, depending on the degree of dedifferentiation. Clinical staging (the T stage) of the tumor is done with a DRE, and at PSA levels below 20 ng/mL, the value of imaging is very limited. Nevertheless, in the higher-grade tumors (Gleason score 8 and above), prior to definitive therapy, a metastatic workup is prudent as occasionally the PSA level and the amount of tumor burden may be discordant. Over the last 3 decades, the Gleason score has been repeatedly validated as the single most reliable independent variable and drives a great deal of the therapeutic decision making. Hence, ideally, histological verification of the Gleason score should be obtained from a genitourinary (GU) pathologist. It is also important to point out that prostate cancer and BPH are two distinct and separate diseases that may coexist. Both are common in the elderly, both are androgen-dependent, they afflict different regions of the prostate, and one does not influence the risk of the other.

D.3. Risk stratification

The three clinical variables that are commonly used for risk stratification at the time of diagnosis include the serum PSA, the clinical T stage, and the Gleason score.[18] These three variables also form the basis of most of the predictive nomograms currently used in prostate cancer. A detailed discussion on nomograms is beyond the scope of this chapter; however, the ones in common use include Partin's tables, D'Amico criteria, and the Kattan nomograms. More information on these can be found online (http://www.nomogram.org).

A commonly employed stratification strategy following diagnosis is outlined in Table 13.3, whereby the tumor burden is categorized as being low, intermediate, or high. Thus patients with low tumor burden require only local therapy, and those in the latter two categories require systemic therapy in addition to local therapy. Posttreatment nomograms can help quantitate the risk of

Table 13.3 A common patient stratification.

Low risk	Intermediate risk	High risk
Must meet all	Any one factor	Any one factor
PSA $\leq$10	PSA 10–20	PSA >20
Gleason $\leq$6	Gleason 7	Gleason $\geq$8
T2a or smaller	T2b	T3 or greater

Note. PSA = prostate-specific antigen. Adapted from Kattan et al.[47]

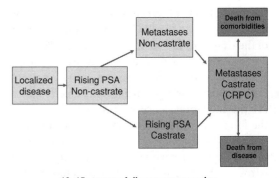

10–15+ years of disease progression

Figure 13.1 The clinical states of prostate cancer. Adapted from Scher et al.[54]

relapse and/or the possible benefits of additional therapy.

D.4. Stage migration and natural history of prostate cancer

The widespread availability of PSA testing has compressed the time from diagnosis to treatment, changing both the pattern of disease at presentation and the presentation at the time of treatment failure. As illustrated in Figure 13.1, the natural history of prostate cancer can be extremely variable, depending on disease biology. In the pre-PSA era (early 1990s), over 50 percent of patients had metastatic disease at presentation. Currently fewer than 5 percent of patients present with metastatic disease, and the largest subpopulation of men with active cancer have PSA-only disease. Our understanding of the stage migration in prostate cancer has been aided by two large longitudinal databases that each enrolls well over 10,000 prostate cancer patients regardless of stage at diagnosis. The first one, the Cancer of the Prostate Strategic Urologic Research Endeavor (CaPSURE) database, was initiated in 1995 and collects data from 31 community-based urologic practice sites. In CaPSURE, the proportion of patients presenting with low-risk disease (i.e., PSA less than 10 ng/mL, Gleason grade less than 7, and clinical stage T1 or T2a) increased from 31 percent of patients in 1990 to 47 percent in 2002. Conversely, high-risk diagnoses (PSA over 20 ng/mL, Gleason grade of 8–10, or stage T3–T4) had decreased from 41 to 15 percent.[19] The second one is the Department of Defense Center for Prostate Disease Research (CPDR), which has collected data on men with prostate cancer at Walter Reed Army Medical Center and eight other military sites around the country since 1997. In the CPDR registry, the percentage of patients presenting with locally advanced disease fell from 19.2 percent in 1988 to 4.4 percent in 1998. The rates of metastatic disease at diagno-

sis likewise declined from 14.11 to 3.3 percent in the same time period.[20]

The PSA era has also popularized the use of PSA kinetics for predicting outcome in multiple clinical settings. Thus a PSA velocity of 0.75 ng/mL per year can identify men who will develop prostate cancer; an increase of 2.0 ng/mL per year or more before prostatectomy predicts not only biochemical recurrence after primary therapy but also cancer-specific survival and overall mortality. A recent study also recommended a PSA velocity of 0.35 ng/mL or more per year at PSA levels of under 4.0 ng/mL as a trigger for doing a prostate biopsy.[21] In the setting of recurrent disease, the PSA doubling time (PSA-DT) is increasingly being used to decide on the timing of therapy. Thus, in men who are hormone sensitive, a PSA-DT of under 3 months suggests aggressive disease and should prompt treatment with androgen ablation. On the contrary, in men with PSA-only disease and a PSA-DT of over 12 months, observation is a reasonable strategy. Men with an intermediate PSA-DT are ideal candidates for clinical trials with novel agents.[22–23]

E. Treatment

Following a diagnosis of prostate cancer, it is useful to categorize patients as having (1) localized disease or (2) locally advanced disease or (3) advanced disease. The distinction between the first and last categories is relatively straightforward. However, it is often difficult to distinguish between the first two.

F. Localized disease

The three standard therapeutic approaches for men with localized or organ-confined prostate cancer are radical prostatectomy (RP), radiation therapy (RT) – either external-beam RT (EBRT), brachytherapy, or both – and active surveillance. The best treatment for localized prostate cancer remains unclear. Deciding which treatment modality to use depends on a number of factors, including patient preferences, the spectrum of patient comorbidities, and patient life expectancy. Given that the majority of cancers diagnosed are indolent, it is reasonable to recommend active surveillance in patients with (1) low-risk disease and (b) a life expectancy of less than 10 years. This is supported by a recent report from the Connecticut Tumor Registry database of 767 men, in which over a 20-year period, men with low-risk disease had very low prostate cancer–specific mortality (Figure 13.2).[24]

In patients who are appropriate candidates for intervention, RP or EBRT is equivalent. Although there has never been a head-to-head comparison of the two modalities, 15-year outcomes from either modality tend to be equivalent. In general, younger patients undergo RP more frequently, based on the notion that an RP provides more accurate staging, thereby facilitating the earlier use of adjuvant therapy, if indicated.

F.1. Radical prostatectomy

There have been studies comparing expectant management versus RP, and in the Swedish randomized trial of watchful waiting versus radical prostatectomy, 695 men with prostate cancer were accrued. Radical prostatectomy significantly reduced disease-specific mortality, overall mortality, and the risks of metastasis and local progression. However, this benefit was only observed in men who were less than 65 years of age.[17] At diagnosis, the median PSA in these patients was 12.8, and only 5 percent of these tumors were T1c. Given the more advanced nature of cancer in this population, the results may not be applicable to the U.S. population, where the incidence of T1c disease at diagnosis is 60–70 percent. Data from both the PIVOT trial in the United States and the PROTECT trial in the United Kingdom are awaited to evaluate the survival benefit of immediate intervention versus expectant management.

Radiotherapy

Radiotherapy techniques have evolved to allow higher doses of radiation to be administered safely. Conventional radiotherapy has largely been replaced by more sophisticated forms of external-beam radiotherapy called three-dimensional conformal radiotherapy (3DCRT) and intensity-modulated radiotherapy (IMRT). The standard dose of 70–77 Gy in 35–41 fractions to the prostate remains appropriate for patients with low-risk prostate cancer. However, a dose of 78 Gy results in better control rates than a dose of 70 Gy. Thus intermediate-risk and high-risk patients should receive doses between 75 and 80 Gy.[25] The advantage of IMRT techniques includes a very low risk of urinary incontinence and stricture as well as a good chance of short-term preservation of erectile function.

High–dose rate (HDR) brachytherapy represents an alternative strategy for delivering high-dose interstitial radiation therapy to the prostate. When compared with standard fractionated EBRT, HDR has a higher dose rate and fraction size per treatment. Brachytherapy as monotherapy has become a popular treatment option for early, clinically organ-confined prostate cancer (T1c–T2a, Gleason score 2–6, PSA less than 10 ng/mL). The cancer-control rates appear comparable to surgery for low-risk prostate cancer with medium-term follow-up. The risk of incontinence is minimal in patients without a previous transurethral resection of the prostate, and erectile function is preserved in the short term. Patients with high-risk cancers are generally considered poor candidates for permanent brachytherapy.

Incontinence and erectile dysfunction (ED) continue to be the two main complications associated with RP and ERBT. Incontinence rates with ERBT are under 1–2 percent; with RP, they can vary between 5 and 25 percent. With time, ED is invariable with ERBT. If a nerve-sparing RP is feasible, sexual function may be preserved; however, age over 70 years and the presence of vascular disease invariably result in ED even after a nerve-sparing RP. Similar outcomes have been reported with RP and a laparoscopic procedure. Treatment options like high-intensity focused ultrasound and cryosurgery may have a role in elderly men with localized disease, but at this point, they remain solely investigational.

Active surveillance

Active surveillance is being increasingly used in the elderly, and the general approach is outlined in Table 13.4. Klotz and colleagues recently reported an overall survival of 85 percent and disease-specific survival of 99.2 percent at 8 years.[26] The median PSA-DT in their cohort of 299 patients was 7 years. A PSA-DT of less than 3 years is associated with a more aggressive phenotype. Using

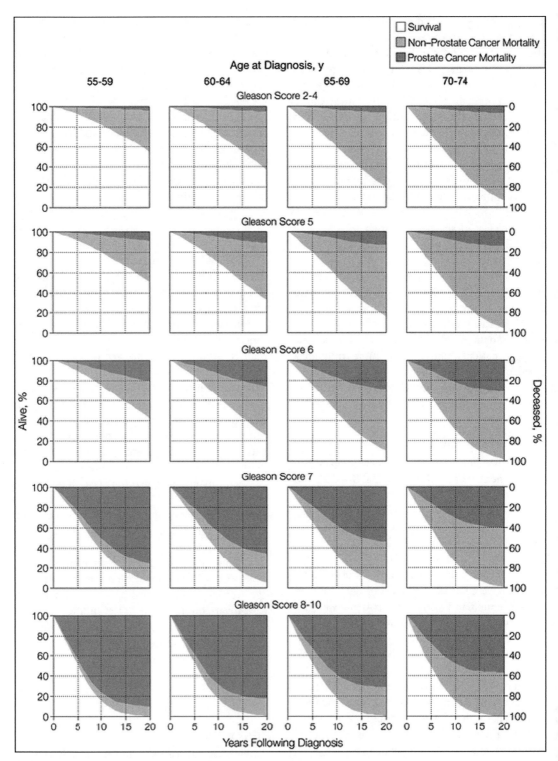

Figure 13.2 Survival and cumulative mortality from prostate cancer and other causes up to 20 years after diagnosis. Adapted from Albertsen et al.[24]
20-Year Outcomes Following Conservative Management of Clinically Localized Prostate Cancer
Peter C. Albertsen; James A. Hanley; Judith Fine *JAMA*. 2005;293:2095–2101.

Table 13.4 Active surveillance: Algorithm for eligibility, follow-up schedule, and intervention.

Eligibility:

1. Less than 70 years: PSA ≤ 10, Gleason score ≤ 6, and T1c to T2a
2. Older than 70 years: PSA < 15, Gleason score ≤ 7, and T1c to T2a
3. Men with >15-year life expectancy, <3 cores involved, and <50% of any one core

Follow-up schedule:

1. PSA, DRE every 3 months × 2 years, then every 6 months if PSA stable
2. 10–12 core biopsies at 1 year and then every 3 years until age 80 years
3. Optional: TRUS on alternate visits

Intervention:

1. For PSA doubling time <3 years (in most cases, based on at least eight determinations; approximately 20% of patients)
2. For grade progression to Gleason score ≥7 (4 + 3); approximately 5% of patients

Note. PSA = prostate-specific androgen; DRE = digital rectal examination; TRUS = transrectal ultrasound. Adapted from Klotz.[26]

these data, about 20 percent of good-risk patients will be treated for a rapid PSA doubling time, and 5 to 10 percent will be treated for grade progression while 70 percent will remain stable and avoid unnecessary aggressive treatment. In summary, watchful waiting is a reasonable treatment option, especially for elderly men with low-grade prostate cancer and low PSA values. The best available data suggest that there is no significant difference in quality of life between treated and untreated patients.[27] Active surveillance is also being evaluated in the multigroup Standard Treatment Against Restricted Treatment (START) trial. The trial opened for accrual in June 2007, will enroll 2,130 men, and has a planned completion of April 2023.

G. Locally advanced disease

Men with locally advanced disease can be thought of as intermediate or high risk (Table 13.3), and in addition to local therapy (EBRT or RP), they also require systemic therapy when treated with curative intent.[28-30] With the exception of the Messing study, survival advantage with combined-modality treatment has only been noted when EBRT is the local modality used. The combination of short-term and long-term neoadjuvant, concurrent, and adjuvant androgen-deprivation therapy (ADT) with EBRT has been proven to increase local control, disease-free survival, and overall survival for certain patient groups (Table 13.5). There are still questions pertaining to the sequencing and duration of ADT. However, the current NCCN recommendations call for patients with high-risk disease to be treated with EBRT and ADT for a total of 2–3 years: 2 years of combined androgen blockade or 3 years of leutinizing hormone-releasing hormone (LHRH) agonist monotherapy. Patients with intermediate-risk cancers may be candidates for 6 months of EBRT and concurrent ADT.[31] There are no specific guidelines for the elderly, and at the present time, decision making should solely be driven by disease biology, risk stratification, and life expectancy (Figure 13.2).

Adjuvant treatment following surgery (RP) is less clear. Current evidence-based guidelines call for (1) ADT in men who are node positive and (2) possibly EBRT in men who are margin positive. If there is a persistent PSA level following RP, patients should have their PSA-DT evaluated periodically and treated with systemic therapy

Table 13.5 Benefit of androgen-deprivation therapy (ADT) in locally advanced prostate cancer.

Duration of ADT + XRT/surgery	Source	Outcome	Control arm, % (95% CI)	ADT arm, % (95% CI)	*p* value
3 years ADT + XRT	Bolla et al.[48]	Increase in 7-year survival	62 (52–72)	78 (72–84)	.0002
Permanent ADT + XRT	Pilepich[49]	Increase in 10-year survival	38	53	<.004
6 months ADT + XRT	D'Amico et al.[31]	Increase in 5-year survival	78 (68–88)	88 (80–95)	.04
Permanent ADT + surgery	Messing et al.[29, 50]	Increase in 10-year survival	49	72.4	.025

Note. ADT = androgen-deprivation therapy; XRT = radiation therapy; CI = confidence interval. Adapted from Sharifi et al.[51]

(preferably on protocol) as their PSA-DT shortens to less than 10 months. Men who develop a PSA relapse following an RP should be considered for EBRT, provided that the PSA was undetectable for at least 6–12 months following the RP and provided that the PSA at relapse is under 2 ng/mL.[32] The threshold PSA value to qualify as a PSA relapse is considered to be over 0.4 ng/mL following a prostatectomy and over 2.0 ng/mL following radiation therapy.

H. Advanced disease

Given the trend toward increased screening, early diagnosis, and early intervention, the spectrum and presentation of advanced disease has changed dramatically in the last two decades. In the past, over 50 percent of men at the time of presentation had abdominal lymphadenopathy and/or bone metastasis. Now it is not uncommon for men to present with normal scans and a rising PSA after having failed both primary therapy and hormonal therapy. In the United States, the subpopulation of men with PSA-only disease – either hormone-naive or castrate-resistant – represents the largest subset of patients with prostate cancer.

The cornerstone for the treatment of advanced disease continues to be androgen ablation, with the goal of treatment being to lower the serum testosterone.[33] Recent advances point to persistently high levels of androgens at the tissue level (in the tumor and in metastasis), despite castrate levels of testosterone in the serum. Thus current research is focused on developing even more effective means of androgen blockade.[34] However, there is increasing recognition that there is considerable morbidity associated with the use of hormonal therapy, and great effort is being expended in developing strategies to mitigate some of the side effects associated with androgen ablation and/or androgen blockade. These issues are even more relevant in the elderly, where the risk-benefit ratio of when and how to institute hormonal therapy needs to be carefully weighed. Recently, for the first time, chemotherapy has also been shown to confer a survival advantage in men with advanced prostate cancer.

Workup of a patient with advanced disease should include serum PSA and serum testosterone levels, a bone scan, and a CT scan of the abdomen and pelvis. Ninety percent of men with prostate cancer eventually develop bone metastasis. These are primarily osteoblastic in nature and may be associated with considerable pain. Particular vigilance is needed when a positive bone scan correlates with either new localized back pain or pain in a weight-bearing area of the skeleton. These patients should be worked up with appropriate imaging (magnetic resonance imaging and/or plain films) for impending cord compression and/or an impending pathological fracture. Patients should be made non-weight-bearing and be immediately referred for both surgical and radiation consultation. Patients with suspected cord compression should be initiated and maintained on steroids until compression is ruled out.

H.1. Hormonal therapy or androgen-deprivation therapy (ADT)

ADT is any treatment that blocks the interaction of androgens with the androgen receptor (AR). Testosterone (T) and dihydrotestosterone (DHT) are the two major androgens in men, with T present mainly in circulation and DHT the primary androgen in prostatic tissues. The production of T is under the control of the hypothalamic-pituitary axis (HPA). As shown in Figure 13.3, the HPA can be perturbed in several ways to block the production of T. At the tissue level, T is converted to DHT by two isoforms of the enzyme 5α-reductase. Compared with testosterone, DHT binds the AR in a more stable manner, making DHT the primary ligand and effector of AR-mediated signaling at the tissue level. The goal of ADT is to inhibit the growth of prostate cancer by dropping the level of serum testosterone to castrate levels: less than 50 ng/dL or less than 1.7 nmol/L. This is typically achieved either with bilateral orchiectomy (surgical castration) or with LHRH agonists (chemical castration). The LHRH agonists (e.g., leuprolide and goserelin) are available as depot preparations, being administered every month or every 3 months or every 4 months. In the majority of men with prostate cancer, over 95 percent of the testosterone is produced by the testes. In men with significant testosterone output from other sources (adrenals and peripheral tissue), in addition to LHRH agonists or orchiectomy, one of the nonsteroidal antiandrogens (bicalutamide, flutamide) also needs to be used. Thus the majority of men on ADT are treated with LHRH agonists alone (monotherapy) or in combination with an antiandrogen (combined androgen blockade). Although some physicians routinely use combination therapy, a meta-analysis of 27 different trials did not show an advantage to using combined blockade in men who achieved

Figure 13.3 Endocrine therapy of prostate cancer.

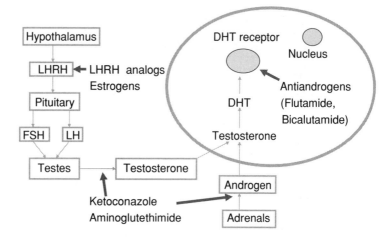

castrate testosterone levels with monotherapy. However, men with known metastatic disease who are being initiated on ADT need to be on combined blockade for the first 15–30 days to avoid the initial testosterone flare associated with LHRH therapy. After 6–8 weeks of LHRH agonist therapy, testosterone levels should be checked and, if not at castrate levels, should prompt the addition of an antiandrogen continuously.

The current evidence-based indications for hormonal therapy are summarized in Table 13.6. These include newly diagnosed metastatic disease, adjuvant therapy of node-positive disease discovered at prostatectomy, and in combination with radiotherapy in patients with intermediate/high-risk disease. In practice, ADT is employed much more widely, and its use in the setting of biochemical progression alone is controversial. Because men with PSA-only disease with a PSA-DT of less than 6 months have a more aggressive disease course, the use of ADT in this subset of patients is under intense investigation. This is based on the notion that in addition to the adjuvant setting for high-risk disease, ADT may also confer a survival benefit in rapidly progressive micrometastatic disease. In the metastatic setting, ADT is palliative and not curative; hence there has been debate

Table 13.6 ADT: Indications.

– Newly diagnosed metastatic disease

– Adjuvant therapy of node-positive disease discovered at prostatectomy

– Combined with radiotherapy in patients with intermediate/high-risk disease

Note. Use of ADT in patients with biochemical progression is controversial.

about the optimal timing of its use. Randomized placebo-controlled studies of estrogen therapy (diethylstilbestrol) in men with newly diagnosed advanced prostate cancer were done in the early 1970s. These studies clearly showed that immediate hormonal therapy delayed disease progression, but the excessive risk of cardiovascular toxic effects associated with diethylstilbestrol confounded any survival advantage. Hence hormonal treatment was reserved for symptomatic disease. The availability of GnRH agonists and nonsteroidal antiandrogens from the 1980s has led to the earlier use of hormonal therapy. The Medical Research Council of the United Kingdom conducted a randomized trial in over 900 men of early versus late ADT in patients with locally advanced disease or asymptomatic metastatic disease: 71 percent of 465 patients in the deferred-treatment arm died of prostate cancer versus 62 percent of 469 patients in the immediate-treatment arm ($p = .001$). Furthermore, when comparing the deferred arm versus the immediate-treatment arm, extraskeletal metastases occurred in 11.8 percent versus 7.9 percent of patients; the incidence of spinal cord compression was 4.9 percent versus 1.9 percent; and the frequency of ureteral obstruction was 11.8 percent versus 7.0 percent, respectively.[35] Thus, in the setting of advanced prostate cancer, ADT confers important quality-of-life benefits. However, a survival benefit exclusively in the subset of patients with metastatic disease remains to be proven.

The median duration of response to first-line ADT in metastatic prostate cancer can range from 12 to 30 months, being dependent on the Gleason score of the tumor. Patients are considered to be castrate-resistant if they have a rising PSA

Table 13.7 Side effects of ADT.

"Big three"	Body image: "What you see"	Metabolic: "What you don't see"	CNS and psyche: "What you feel"
Loss of libido	Weight gain	Loss of BMD	Fatigue
Erectile dysfunction	Gynecomastia	Anemia	Lack of energy, lack of initiative
Hot flashes	Loss in muscle mass, strength	Onset/worsening of lipids, HTN, diabetes, CVD	Depression
	Decreased penis size and testes		Emotional lability
	Hair changes		Cognitive function

Note. BMD = bone mineral density; HTN = hypertension; CVD = cardiovascular disease; adapted from Higano.[52]

and/or progressive metastatic disease, despite castrate testosterone levels. The continuation of ADT in the setting of castrate-resistant disease is currently recommended given that some of the tumor clones continue to be androgen-dependent. Thus continuous androgen suppression with the duration of treatment with secondary hormonal therapies and chemotherapy is standard practice. It is also a necessary prerequisite for patients to enter protocol therapy for progressive castrate-resistant prostate cancer (CRPC).

ADT has a wide variety of side effects (Table 13.7), all of which increase with time.[36–37] The most common ones include hot flashes, decreased libido, erectile dysfunction, weight gain, and insomnia. Hot flashes occur in over 90 percent of men on ADT, and a variety of medications have been tried with variable success to alleviate these. The more effective of these medications include low-dose megestrol acetate, selective serotonin uptake inhibitors like venlafaxine and paroxetine, gabapentin, and transdermal estrogens. The sexual side effects can be mitigated somewhat with the use of antiandrogen monotherapy (as testosterone levels are maintained). However, antiandrogens can be associated with hepatic dysfunction, painful gynecomastia, and gastrointestinal effects, including nausea, diarrhea, and constipation. Furthermore, in multiple settings, antiandrogen monotherapy has been associated with worse disease-related outcomes when compared with ADT.

Osteopenia and/or osteoporosis is invariably associated with prolonged ADT within 6–9 months of initiation as ADT increases bone turnover and decreases bone mineral density (BMD). The average bone loss is 2–3 percent per year, and osteoporotic skeletal fractures occur in up to 20 percent of men within 5 years of starting

ADT. Other aggravating factors in the elderly include reduced intake of calcium, low vitamin D levels, alcohol abuse, smoking, and chronic use of corticosteroids. All men on ADT should have baseline dual-energy X-ray absorptiometry scans and should be on measures to mitigate osteopenia (Table 13.8). Recent reports show that weekly oral bisphosphanates can increase BMD by 2 to 3 percent every year and that the more potent intravenous amino bisphosphanates every 6–12 months can increase BMD by 5–6 percent every year, as opposed to a 2–3 percent loss in BMD on the placebo arms.[38]

Diabetes and cardiovascular diseases (coronary artery disease and myocardial infarction) are also more commonly associated with ADT. In a population-based cohort of over 73,000 Medicare enrollees aged 66 years or older, the overall incidence of cardiovascular complications was

Table 13.8 Osteoporosis: Prevention.

Prevention
Vitamin D: 800–1,000 IU/d
Calcium: 1,200 mg/d
Weight-bearing exercise
Smoking and alcohol use moderation

Bisphosphonates and SERMs
    FDA approved only for established osteoporosis
    Awaiting randomized results for fracture end points

Denosumab
    Monoclonal antibody targeting RANKL
    Ongoing randomized, double-blind, placebo-controlled phase III trial

Note. FDA = U.S. Food and Drug Administration; RANKL = receptor activator of nuclear factor kappa B ligand; SERM = Selective estrogen receptor modulator; Adapted from Greenspan.[53]

36 percent in men on an LHRH analog and 7 percent in men who had undergone a bilateral orchiectomy.[39] In the latter group, the only significant association was with diabetes. Several other complications, including cognitive deficits, depression, anemia, and decrease in lean body mass and increase in fat mass, are also receiving increased attention. Exercise, counseling, and a healthy diet form the basis of treating most of these complications.

Intermittent androgen deprivation has been advocated to decrease side effects from ADT and also to potentially increase the time to androgen independence.[40] With this strategy, patients are cycled on and off hormonal therapy based on PSA response. Once patients achieve a PSA nadir in response to ADT, they are taken off therapy and monitored; treatment is reinitiated based on absolute PSA value and/or PSA doubling time. Although intermittent ADT is now widely used and in most cases decreases the side effects attributable to ADT, its long-term efficacy is currently being addressed by two large, randomized intergroup trials with survival and quality of life as primary end points. Interim results from these trials have reported that the intermittent approach is not inferior to continuous ADT.

Antiandrogen monotherapy either with bicalutamide 50 mg once daily or with 150 mg once daily remains controversial. Compared to ADT, both doses are inferior with respect to disease control and survival. Because antiandrogen monotherapy preserves testosterone levels and mitigates some of the side effects associated with ADT, its use may be considered, under careful monitoring, in men who are intolerant of LHRH analog therapy.

H.2. Second-line hormonal therapy

There are several potential second- (and third-) line hormonal treatments for patients who fail first-line therapy. If the patient is receiving combined androgen blockage, the first treatment modality is antiandrogen withdrawal. The median duration of response is approximately 4–6 months, but very rarely the benefit may extend for 1–2 years. Some patients also benefit from the addition of a second antiandrogen. Ketoconazole, which decreases the production of adrenal androgens, has also been widely studied, has PSA response rates in the 40–50 percent range, but has not been associated with a survival benefit. However, all trials with ketoconazole are confounded by

the concomitant use of hydrocortisone (to prevent adrenal insufficiency) as it is known that steroids alone can produce a 10 percent PSA response.

The decision to pursue secondary hormonal manipulations will likely depend on several factors. Available data suggest that patients with a significant and prolonged response to initial hormonal therapy or a significant antiandrogen withdrawal response may be good candidates for a trial of secondary hormonal therapy. Patients with a good performance status and rapid PSA doubling times may receive more benefit from upfront chemotherapy.

H.3. Castrate-resistant prostate cancer

Eventually, all patients with metastatic prostate cancer on ADT develop androgen independence, with the mean time to progression being 12–30 months and primarily driven by disease biology. Thus androgen independence or hormone resistance or castrate resistance is defined as evidence of disease progression (PSA or measurable disease or both) in the face of castrate serum testosterone levels. Recent data suggest that the intratumoral levels of androgens are persistently high, and hence the appropriate term for this disease state is *castrate-resistant prostate cancer* (CRPC).[41–42]

Multiple potential mechanisms foster CRPC: upregulated enzymes of steroidogenesis within the tumor (primary and metastatic), increased tissue production of androgens, persistent AR signaling despite low serum androgens, AR mutations, AR signaling via alternate ligands. The end result of all these phenomena is persistent AR-dependent signaling in the tumor. Until recently, in the appropriate patient, chemotherapy was the mainstay for the treatment of CRPC. However, elucidation of the preceding mechanisms of CRPC has led to the development of new agents that are currently in trial: a new generation of AR blockers (MDV 3100) and agents that block intratumoral steroidogenesis (abiraterone).[43]

Chemotherapy

CRPC was once labeled "chemotherapy-resistant." However, new agents have been demonstrated to positively impact both palliative and survival end points. Mitoxantrone with prednisone was the first combination to be approved for the treatment of CRPC, for providing a palliative benefit in patients with painful bone metastases. Docetaxel is the first chemotherapeutic agent with demonstrated survival benefit in prostate cancer and has become standard of care for first-line therapy in CRPC. In two phase III clinical trials, docetaxel in combination with prednisone improved median survival from 16 to 18.5 months (24% increase) when compared with mitoxantrone and prednisone.[44] Currently a number of trials are ongoing both in first- and second-line CRPC, combining these cytotoxics with agents targeting the vasculature. Also under investigation are dendritic cell–based vaccine therapies targeting prostate-specific proteins, a new generation of highly avid AR blockers, and agents that block intratumoral androgen production.

I. Supportive care

The majority of men with prostate cancer eventually develop bone metastasis, which may be associated with (1) pain, (2) cord compression or pathological fractures, and (3) reduced marrow reserve. Thus pain control, intravenous bisphosphanates,[45] palliative radiation, radioisotopes, and blood product support are an integral part of caring for the patient with prostate cancer. Visceral disease with urinary obstruction may require either a stent or a nephrostomy tube. Bleeding from the bladder, secondary to prior radiation (radiation cystitis), can be a vexing problem and may eventually require an indwelling catheter.

J. Conclusions

Prostate cancer is primarily a disease of older men. At every stage of the disease – screening to treatment – there is controversy regarding the most optimal approach in the elderly. Given the heterogeneity of the elderly, the trade-off between efficacy and side effects needs to be evaluated constantly, and treatment needs to be individualized. Screening is not currently recommended for patients over 75 years or with a life expectancy of under 10 years. For the large group of patients diagnosed with apparently localized prostate cancer of low to intermediate risk, active monitoring and delayed treatment with curative intent are emerging as the option of choice. Aggressive prostate cancer will need some form of immediate therapy – most likely radiation based. In the setting of metastatic disease, the early use of ADT is likely to be beneficial. Older men with CRPC should receive chemotherapy when indicated, with particular attention to appropriate supportive care. Promising new agents and therapies for CRPC are currently under investigation and are eagerly awaited.

References

1. Jemal A, Siegel R, Ward E, et al. Cancer statistics. *CA Cancer J Clin.* 2008;58:71–96.

2. Damber JE, Aus G. Prostate cancer. *Lancet.* 2008;371:1710–1721.

3. National Cancer Institute, Surveillance Epidemiology and End Results (SEER). *Cancer Stat Fact Sheets: Cancer of the Prostate.* Rockville, MD, 2008.

4. Abate-Shen C, Shen MM. Molecular genetics of prostate cancer. *Genes Dev.* 2000;14:2410–2434.

5. Gelmann EP. Complexities of prostate-cancer risk. *N Engl J Med.* 2008;358:961–963.

6. Tomlins SA, Bjartell A, Chinnaiyan AM, et al. ETS gene fusions in prostate cancer: from discovery to daily clinical practice. *Eur Urol.* 2009;56:275–286.

7. Ross RK, Bernstein L, Lobo RA, et al. 5-alpha-reductase activity and risk of prostate cancer among Japanese and US white and black males. *Lancet.* 1992;339:887–889.

8. Paris PL, Kupelian PA, Hall JM, et al. Association between a CYP3A4 genetic variant and clinical presentation in African-American prostate cancer patients. *Cancer Epidemiol Biomarkers Prev.* 1999;8:901–905.

9. Palapattu GS, Sutcliffe S, Bastian PJ, et al. Prostate carcinogenesis and inflammation: emerging insights. *Carcinogenesis.* 2005;26:1170–1181.

10. Ma J, Li H, Mucci L. Prediagnostic body mass index (BMI) and prostate cancer mortality: a 21-year survival analysis in the Physicians' Health Study. Presented at: Multidisciplinary Prostate Cancer Symposium (ed). Orlando, FL, 2005.

11. Lippman SM, Klein EA, Goodman PJ, et al. Effect of selenium and vitamin E on risk of prostate cancer and other cancers: the Selenium and Vitamin E Cancer Prevention Trial (SELECT). *JAMA.* 2009;301:39–51.

12. Thompson IM, Goodman PJ, Tangen CM, et al. The influence of finasteride on the development of prostate cancer. *N Engl J Med.* 2003;349:215–224.

13. Oesterling JE, Jacobsen SJ, Chute CG, et al. Serum prostate-specific antigen in a community-based population of healthy men. Establishment of age-specific reference ranges. *Jama.* 1993;270:860–864.

14. Barry MJ. Screening for prostate cancer–the controversy that refuses to die. *N Engl J Med.* 2009;360:1351–1354.

15. Screening for Prostate Cancer: U.S. Preventive Services Task Force Recommendation Statement. *Ann Intern Med.* 2008;149:185–191.

16. *Prostate cancer.* Available at: http://www.cdc.gov/cancer/prostate.

17. Bill-Axelson A, Holmberg L, Ruutu M, et al. Radical Prostatectomy versus Watchful Waiting in Early Prostate Cancer. *N Engl J Med.* 2005;352:1977–1984.

18. Partin AW, Kattan MW, Subong EN, et al. Combination of prostate-specific antigen, clinical stage, and Gleason score to predict pathological stage of localized prostate cancer. A multi-institutional update. *JAMA.* 1997;277:1445–1451.

19. Cooperberg MR, Broering JM, Litwin MS, et al. The contemporary management of prostate cancer in the United States: lessons from the cancer of the prostate strategic urologic research endeavor (CapSURE), a national disease registry. *J Urol.* 2004;171:1393–1401.

20. Sun L, Gancarczyk K, Paquette EL, et al. Introduction to Department of Defense Center for Prostate Disease Research Multicenter National Prostate Cancer Database, and analysis of changes in the PSA-era. *Urologic Oncology.* 2001;6:203–209.

21. D'Amico AV, Chen MH, Roehl KA, et al. Preoperative PSA velocity and the risk of death from prostate cancer after radical prostatectomy. *N Engl J Med.* 2004;351:125–135.

22. D'Amico AV, Moul JW, Carroll PR, et al. Surrogate end point for prostate cancer-specific mortality after radical prostatectomy or radiation therapy. *J Natl Cancer Inst.* 2003;95:1376–1383.

23. Freedland SJ, Moul JW. Prostate specific antigen recurrence after definitive therapy. *J Urol.* 2007;177:1985–1991.

24. Albertsen PC, Hanley JA, Fine J. 20-year outcomes following conservative management of clinically localized prostate cancer. *JAMA.* 2005;293:2095–2101.

25. Speight JL, Roach M, 3rd. Radiotherapy in the management of clinically localized prostate cancer: evolving standards, consensus, controversies and new directions. *J Clin Oncol.* 2005;23:8176–8185.

26. Klotz L. Active Surveillance for Prostate Cancer: For Whom? *J Clin Oncol.* 2005;23:8165–8169.

27. Wei JT, Dunn RL, Sandler HM, et al. Comprehensive comparison of health-related quality of life after contemporary therapies for localized prostate cancer. *J Clin Oncol.* 2002;20:557–566.

28. Bolla M, de Reijke TM, Zurlo A, Collette L. Adjuvant hormone therapy in locally advanced and localized prostate cancer: three EORTC trials. *Front Radiat Ther Oncol.* 2002;36:81–86.

29. Messing EM, Manola J, Yao J, et al. Immediate versus deferred androgen deprivation treatment in patients with node-positive prostate cancer

after radical prostatectomy and pelvic lymphadenectomy. *Lancet Oncol.* 2006;7:472–479.

30. Pilepich MV, Winter K, John MJ, et al. Phase III radiation therapy oncology group (RTOG) trial 86-10 of androgen deprivation adjuvant to definitive radiotherapy in locally advanced carcinoma of the prostate. *Int J Radiat Oncol Biol Phys.* 2001;50:1243–1252.

31. D'Amico AV, Manola J, Loffredo M, et al. 6-month androgen suppression plus radiation therapy vs radiation therapy alone for patients with clinically localized prostate cancer: a randomized controlled trial. *JAMA.* 2004;292: 821–827.

32. Stephenson AJ, Shariat SF, Zelefsky MJ, et al. Salvage radiotherapy for recurrent prostate cancer after radical prostatectomy. *JAMA.* 2004;291: 1325–1332.

33. Loblaw DA, Virgo KS, Nam R, et al. Initial hormonal management of androgen-sensitive metastatic, recurrent, or progressive prostate cancer: 2006 update of an American Society of Clinical Oncology practice guideline. *J Clin Oncol.* 2007;25:1596–1605.

34. Mohler JL, Gregory CW, Ford OH, 3rd, et al. The androgen axis in recurrent prostate cancer. *Clin Cancer Res.* 2004;10:440–448.

35. Immediate versus deferred treatment for advanced prostatic cancer: initial results of the Medical Research Council Trial. The Medical Research Council Prostate Cancer Working Party Investigators Group. *Br J Urol.* 1997;79:235–246.

36. Harle LK, Maggio M, Shahani S, et al. Endocrine complications of androgen-deprivation therapy in men with prostate cancer. *Clin Adv Hematol Oncol.* 2006;4:687–696.

37. Michaelson MD, Cotter SE, Gargollo PC, et al. Management of complications of prostate cancer treatment. *CA Cancer J Clin.* 2008;58:196–213.

38. Smith MR, McGovern FJ, Zietman AL, et al. Pamidronate to prevent bone loss during androgen-deprivation therapy for prostate cancer. *N Engl J Med.* 2001;345:948–955.

39. Keating NL, O'Malley AJ, Smith MR. Diabetes and cardiovascular disease during androgen deprivation therapy for prostate cancer. *J Clin Oncol.* 2006;24:4448–4456.

40. Boccon-Gibod L, Hammerer P, Madersbacher S, et al. The role of intermittent androgen deprivation in prostate cancer. *BJU Int.* 2007;100: 738–743.

41. Feldman BJ, Feldman D. The development of androgen-independent prostate cancer. *Nat Rev Cancer.* 2001;1:34–45.

42. Montgomery RB, Mostaghel EA, Vessella R, et al. Maintenance of intratumoral androgens in metastatic prostate cancer: a mechanism for castration-resistant tumor growth. *Cancer Res.* 2008;68:4447–4454.

43. Attard G, Reid AHM, Yap TA, et al. Phase I Clinical Trial of a Selective Inhibitor of CYP17, Abiraterone Acetate, Confirms That Castration-Resistant Prostate Cancer Commonly Remains Hormone Driven. *J Clin Oncol.* 2008;26:4563–4571.

44. Tannock IF, de Wit R, Berry WR, et al. Docetaxel plus prednisone or mitoxantrone plus prednisone for advanced prostate cancer. *N Engl J Med.* 2004;351:1502–1512.

45. Saad F, Gleason DM, Murray R, et al. Long-term efficacy of zoledronic acid for the prevention of skeletal complications in patients with metastatic hormone-refractory prostate cancer. *J Natl Cancer Inst.* 2004;96:879–882.

46. Ries L, Harris R. 2001–2005 NCI SEER cancer statistics review. *Ann Intern Med.* 2002;13:917.

47. Kattan M, Eastham J, Stapleton A, et al. A preoperative nomogram for disease recurrence following radical prostatectomy for prostate cancer. *J. Natl Cancer Inst.* 1998;90: 766–771.

48. Bolla M, Collette L, Blank L, et al. Long-term results with immediate androgen suppression and external irradiation in patients with locally advanced prostate cancer (an EORTC study): a phase III randomised trial. *Lancet.* 2002;360: 103–106.

49. Shipley WU, Kaufman DS, Tester WJ, et al. Overview of bladder cancer trials in the Radiation Therapy Oncology Group. *Cancer.* 2003;97: 2115–2119.

50. Messing EM, Manola J, Sarosdy M, et al. Immediate hormonal therapy compared with observation after radical prostatectomy and pelvic lymphadenectomy in men with node-positive prostate cancer. *N Engl J Med.* 1999;341: 1781–1788.

51. Sharifi N, Gulley JL, Dahut WL. Androgen Deprivation Therapy for Prostate Cancer. *JAMA.* 2005;294:238–244.

52. Higano CS. Side effects of androgen deprivation therapy: monitoring and minimizing toxicity. *Urology.* 2003;61:32–38.

53. Greenspan SL. Approach to the prostate cancer patient with bone disease. *J Clin Endocrinol Metab.* 2008;93:2–7.

54. Scher HI, Halabi S, Tannock I, et al. Design and End Points of Clinical Trials for Patients With Progressive Prostate Cancer and Castrate Levels of Testosterone: Recommendations of the Prostate Cancer Clinical Trials Working Group. *J Clin Oncol.* 2008;26:1148–1159.

Management of ovarian and endometrial cancer in older adults

William P. Tew and Vivian von Gruenigen

A. Introduction

Global improvements in health care and an increased life expectancy have led to a significant increase in the number of elderly women worldwide. In developed countries, a woman's life expectancy was 81.1 years in 1991 and is expected to rise to 90.4 years by 2020. In fact, over the next decades, approximately 20 percent of the world population is estimated to be over age 65 years. As more women age, there will be a steep increase in the incidence of diagnosed malignancies, including gynecologic cancers.[1,2]

B. Ovarian cancer

Advancing age is considered a risk factor for survival in ovarian cancer. Several groups reported at least a twofold increased risk of death in women older than 65 years of age.[3,4] In the United States, the age-specific mortality rate for ovarian cancer increases with age, reaching 37 out of 100,000 for women aged 65–74 years and 53 out of 100,000 for women aged 75 years and over.[1] There have been various theories proposed to account for this survival disparity in older women, including (1) more aggressive cancer with advanced age, (2) inherent resistance to chemotherapy, (3) individual patient factors such as multiple concurrent medical problems, and (4) physician and health care biases toward the elderly that lead to inadequate surgery, less than optimal chemotherapy, and poor enrollment in clinical trials.[5]

B.1. Risk factors

In 2008, an estimated 21,650 new cases of ovarian cancer were diagnosed in the United States and, despite being less common than cancers of the uterus and cervix, will result in more deaths than both of those combined.[6] Ovarian cancer is primarily a disease of postmenopausal women and has an age-related increase in incidence. Between 2001 and 2005, the average age of a patient with ovarian cancer was 63 years (20% between 65 and

74 years old, 19.2% between 75 and 84 years old, and 7.4% over 85 years of age).[7]

Risks to the development of epithelial ovarian cancer are linked to factors that produce incessant ovulation during one's lifetime such as null or low parity and possibly fertility drug use. Family history remains a strong risk factor, particularly among those with a breast-ovarian cancer syndrome (BRCA-1 or -2) and hereditary nonpolyposis colorectal syndrome (HNPCC, Lynch II syndrome). In those with hereditary mutations, onset of diagnosis is typically at a younger age.[8] However, in women with BRCA mutations, the associated risk of ovarian, fallopian tube, or peritoneal cancer can occur at any age, including over 70.[9] Bilateral prophylactic oophorectomy is reported to cut the risk of ovarian cancer by 96 percent and the risk of breast cancer by 53 percent among BRCA carriers.[10,11] Given their significant prognostic and potential risk-reducing options for patients and their families, a detailed family history is vital in all patients with ovarian cancer.

B.2. Diagnosis

Epithelial ovarian cancer is rarely diagnosed at an early stage because the disease causes few specific symptoms, particularly when it is localized to the ovary. Unlike breast and colon cancer, there is no currently accepted screening tool to detect ovarian cancer at an early stage. For example, CA125, a tumor-associated antigen that is elevated in 80 percent of women with advanced ovarian cancer, is elevated in fewer than 50 percent of early-stage cases.[12]

Therefore, outside families with high genetic risk syndromes, most women are diagnosed following several months of nonspecific abdominal symptoms. Thus more than 70 percent of patients will present with disease beyond the confines of the ovary at initial diagnosis. With tumor spread into the pelvis and abdominal cavity, patients often complain of abdominal or pelvic pain, pressure, distension, and early satiety.[13] Elderly women with nonspecific abdominal symptoms may be at even higher risk of a misdiagnosis given increased comorbidities and polypharmacy.[14] One retrospective study examined the types of symptoms and diagnostic procedures reported in Medicare claims of 3,250 women aged 65 years and older 12 months before diagnosis for women with ovarian cancer.[15] Over 80 percent of women with ovarian cancer had at least one target sign or symptom 12 months before diagnosis. Gastrointestinal symptoms, such as nausea, vomiting, and constipation, diarrhea, or other digestive disorders, were associated with later-stage cancer. Among those with at least one symptom, women with gynecologic symptoms were operated on earlier and with higher frequency. Awareness of the potential for unresolved gastrointestinal symptoms to be indicators for ovarian cancer is vital.

B.3. Prognostic factors

The initial stage, grade, histology type, and number of residual tumors at the beginning of adjuvant chemotherapy in advanced stages of ovarian cancer are the most significant prognostic factors for survival. Stage III–IV, high-grade tumors, clear-cell histology, and surgical debulking with greater than 1 cm of residual tumor (suboptimal) are well established as poor risk features.[16]

Age of the patient has been consistently described as a poor prognostic factor, but the etiology is debated.[3,16–22] A large retrospective review was conducted through the Gynecologic Oncology Group (GOG) of 1,895 patients with stage III epithelial ovarian cancer who had undergone primary surgery followed by six cycles of intravenous platinum and paclitaxel. Increasing age was associated with increased risks for disease progression.[16]

Extracted from the Surveillance, Epidemiology, and End Results (SEER) database (1988–2001), 400 patients were aged less than 30 years (very young), 11,601 patients were aged 30–60 years (young), and 16,164 were aged over 60 years (older). Of the very young, young, and older patients, 261 (65.3%), 4,664 (40.2%), and 3,643 (22.5%) had stage I–II disease, respectively. Across all stages, very young women had a significant survival advantage over the young and older groups, with 5-year disease-specific survival estimates at 78.8 percent versus 58.8 and 35.3 percent, respectively. This survival difference between the age groups persists even after adjusting for race, stage, grade, and surgical treatment.[18]

Using the Geneva Cancer Registry, 736 women diagnosed with primary ovarian cancer were studied with respect to tumor characteristics, treatment patterns, and age: young (70 years or younger) versus older (over 70 years) by logistic regression. Older women presented at more advanced stages and were less often treated by optimal surgery and chemotherapy. The 5-year disease-free survival was 53 percent in younger women in comparison to 18 percent in older women, an absolute difference of 35 percent. Five-year disease-specific survival was 18 percent among old versus young women. After adjustment for tumor characteristics and treatment, older women still had a 1.8-fold increased risk of dying of ovarian cancer compared to younger women.[20]

B.4. Surgery

In most patients, the initial diagnosis of ovarian cancer is made at an exploratory laparotomy. The standard surgical procedure for a patient suspected of having ovarian cancer requires that the entire abdominal cavity be adequately visualized. If ovarian cancer is confirmed on frozen-section pathologic examination, the completion operation should include a total abdominal hysterectomy, bilateral salpingo-oophorectomy, omentectomy, retroperitoneal lymph node sampling, inspection under the diaphragms, random biopsies, and peritoneal cavity washes. After cytoreduction surgery, patients whose largest residual unresectable nodule measures 1 cm or less are defined as having *optimal* debulking, and those with larger nodules are termed *suboptimal*. Success of cytoreduction surgery is significantly related to prognosis.[23]

Less aggressive surgical procedures (i.e., less optimal debulking or less radical surgery) contribute to poorer outcome in elderly patients with advanced ovarian cancer.[24,25] Wright and colleagues showed a similar rate of optimal cytoreduction and postoperative complications for patients younger or older than age 70 with all stages of ovarian cancer.[26] Aggressive optimal cytoreduction can be achieved in the majority of patients with multiple surgical risk factors and is associated with a low complication rate.[27] Elderly patients with advanced disease had an equivalent rate of optimal cytoreduction as well as the proportion cytoreduced to no visible disease.[28] Bruchim and colleagues demonstrated that patients aged 70 years or older were less likely to undergo primary cytoreduction and more likely to receive neoadjuvant chemotherapy.[29]

Elderly patients with ovarian cancer and their surgeons are often faced with questions of how aggressive their surgery should be. For women older than 80, approximately 40 percent are not offered a definitive surgical cytoreduction, and most are not referred to a gynecologic oncology specialist.[5] In one series, patients older than 80 were mostly cared for by general surgeons (31%) and obstetrician-gynecologists (29%).[4] For the oldest patients (over 80 years of age), the decision is often less aggressive treatment. In a SEER review, older patients underwent fewer operations compared to younger patients, with optimal cytoreduction decreasing with age: 43.7 percent (under 60 years old), 29.5 percent (60–79 years old), and 21.7 percent (over 80 years old).[5] Is this disparity due to older patients being less willing to undergo surgery? Likely not. As Nordin and colleagues showed in a cohort of 189 women with ovarian cancer, patients over age 75 years had the same desire for a curative surgical attempt as younger patients.[30]

Serious medical comorbidities are common in the elderly, and the concern for high surgical morbidity/mortality can affect decision making of both the surgeon and the patient. In one study, 83 percent of women older than 80 years had serious comorbidities such as stroke, heart disease, or hypertension. Although cytoreduction was attempted in 88 percent in this cohort, only 25 percent of patients achieved optimal debulking and developed high rates of serious morbidity (38%), postoperative mortality (13%), and intensive-care monitoring (75%).[31]

However, with improvements in surgical technique and postoperative care, surgical morbidity in the elderly has improved over the past decades, as was shown by Susini's group. In fact, in his retrospective review, women older than 70 had significantly shorter hospital stays as well as lower transfusion rates, morbidity, and perioperative mortality (2%) in comparison to patients at the same hospital 1 decade earlier.[32] Since the mean age was only 73 in this retrospective review and multidimensional factors such as functional status or comorbidities were not taken into account, the study does not clarify the concern for operative risk in the frail or very old (aged over 80 years). Primary surgical care for ovarian cancer in women aged over 80 years is associated with utilization of significant health care resources and worse short-term outcomes compared to younger women.[33] Clearly prospective trials in this high-risk population are needed.

B.5. Chemotherapy

First line

Ovarian cancer is one of the most chemotherapy-sensitive malignancies, and treatment has a strong impact on survival in the postoperative (first-line) settings. For newly diagnosed stage III and IV patients, the superior chemotherapy regimen has evolved over the past decades from cyclophosphamide-based regimens to a current standard: intravenous carboplatin (area under the curve [AUC] of 5–7.5) and paclitaxel (175 mg/m^2).[34,35] On the basis of a variety of phase III trials employing this regimen following maximal cytoreduction, the expected progression-free survival (PFS) and overall survival (OS) is as follows: stage III optimal (PFS 21–28 months, OS 52–57 months) and stage III suboptimal (PFS 18 months, OS 38 months).

The poor prognosis of many older women with ovarian cancer is partly because of the reduced use of standard chemotherapy. Reports have suggested that only half of women over age 65 receive standard first-line platinum-based therapy, and the likelihood of receiving it decreased with age, independent of comorbidity.[36] In one population-based study, Hershman's group found that only about half of women with advanced ovarian cancer over age 65 were treated with platinum-based chemotherapy; however, survival improved by 38 percent in the treated women, similar to the benefits described in randomized controlled trials among younger patients. The greatest benefit was seen when platinum was combined with paclitaxel.[37]

In a SEER review, Sundararajan and colleagues found that older patients treated with any chemotherapy had actually increased in the years of 1992–1996, with 83 percent of patients receiving any chemotherapy treatment (single-agent or combination regimens) within 4 months of diagnosis.[38] However, as age increased, the odds ratio (OR) of patients receiving chemotherapy dropped significantly. With 65–69 years as a reference, OR was 0.96 for ages 70–74, 0.65 for ages 75–79, 0.24 for ages 80–84, and 0.12 for ages 85 and over. The disparities for the oldest patients were also observed in the nonwhite subgroup. Although not specified in their report, fear of excessive toxicity, patient preference, and unequal access to care were felt to be the major contributors.

Several strategies have been described to improve the tolerability of the first-line treatment, including single-agent carboplatin, low-dose weekly schedules, and dose reductions.[39–42] In a series of twenty-six ovarian cancer patients older than 70 years (median 77), weekly carboplatin (AUC 2) and paclitaxel (60 mg/m^2) on day 1, 8, and 15 every 4 weeks demonstrated a favorable toxicity profile.[40] Patients had a high incidence of comorbidity (54% with two or more) and dependence (31% activities of daily living [ADLs], 50% instrumental ADLs). Despite these barriers, only 11 percent had high-grade toxicity: grade 3 heart rhythm, grade 3 increase of liver transaminases, and prolonged hematological toxicity. Grade 1 neuropathy was reported in four cases. RECIST (Response Evaluation Criteria in Solid Tumors) response rate was 38.5 percent, and median overall survival was 32 months, which appears lower than expected with this regimen and diagnosis.

A second retrospective study compared two cohorts older than 70 years who received either standard or reduced-dose carboplatin-paclitaxel.[42] A reduced dose consisted of carboplatin AUC 4–5 and paclitaxel 135 mg/m^2. A standard dose consisted of carboplatin AUC 5–6 and paclitaxel 175 mg/m^2. Patients who received a reduced dose ($n = 26$) were significantly older than patients who received a standard dose ($n = 74$; median age 77.0 vs. 74.7, respectively, $p = .014$). There were no differences in stage, comorbidity scores, cytoreductive status, or growth factor administration between cohorts. Patients receiving a standard dose were more likely to experience grade 3–4 neutropenia (54.1% vs. 19.2%, $p = .002$) and cumulative toxicity and to require treatment delays. Although PFS was poorer in patients who received a standard dose ($p = .02$), on multivariate analysis, only the administration of the standard-dose regimen predicted toxicity ($p = .008$). There were no differences in progression-free or overall survival between cohorts, although on multivariate analysis, these data suggest that reduced-dose carboplatin-paclitaxel may be better tolerated but equally effective as the standard regimen in elderly ovarian cancer patients.

Others have argued to use single-agent carboplatin particularly in frail or the oldest patients (greater than 80 years), given the lack of reliable toxicity and efficacy data in the elderly population.[39] The results from the ICON 3 study are cited as a rationale; single-agent carboplatin was shown to have high efficacy, and with attention to the subgroup analysis of those over 65 years (30% of patients), carboplatin-paclitaxel

did not significantly improve efficacy.[43] In addition, other studies have illustrated that paclitaxel significantly increases neutropenia, thrombocytopenia, infection, alopecia, and sensory neuropathy without clear efficacy advantages to carboplatin alone.[41]

However, despite these thoughtful treatment modifications, several retrospective studies have suggested that elderly women who can tolerate cytoreductive surgery should receive combination standard doses of platinum-taxane chemotherapy.[28,44,45] We recently reported a cohort study of all 292 patients with stages IIIC–IV ovarian cancer who had their primary surgery at Memorial Sloan-Kettering Cancer Center from 1998 to 2004 and subsequently began a platinum-taxane chemotherapy regimen. Of these, 108 (37%) were older than 65 years, and 184 (63%) were younger than 65. Stage of disease, optimal cytoreduction rate, number of chemotherapy cycles, and chemotherapy regimen alterations were similar between groups. However, the older cohort had a lower median carboplatin (AUC) dose. Older patients achieved a clinical complete response with a similar frequency to those aged under 65 years (70% vs. 79%), similar rates of platinum sensitivity at 6 months (61% vs. 65%), and similar overall median survival (52 vs. 55 months). However, selection bias in this fit population, who can tolerate surgery and seek out a tertiary center, can limit the results generalizability.[28]

A second study from Italy reported on 148 consecutive women with gynecologic malignancies over the age of 70 who were treated with chemotherapy between 1999 and 2000.[45] The median age was 73 years (range 70–84, 37% over 75 years). Most patients had ovarian cancer (70%) and comorbid conditions (80%). Standard schedules were administered to 97 percent of cases with 1,046 cycles of therapy administered (median 6, range 1–35 per patient). Most received platinum-combination chemotherapy regimens (72%) rather than single-agent regimens (28%). Toxicity was primarily hematologic (grade 3–4, 38%), and only 7 percent required discontinuation and delay over 7 days was required in 17 percent of cases, although from a subgroup analysis, those older than 75 years required more drug delays and dose reductions. In addition, the number of patients receiving several lines of chemotherapy diminished: one regimen (57%), two (33%), three (6%), and four (4%). However, from these results, chronological age did not adversely influence the ability to receive aggressive treatment.

B.6. Intraperitoneal chemotherapy

Cisplatin-based intraperitoneal (IP) chemother-apy has a demonstrated survival benefit in opti-mally cytoreduced patients with advanced ovar-ian cancer and is gradually becoming a standard of care.[46–48] The survival advantages have been observed across all age groups. In the most recent IP study (GOG 172) reported by Armstrong and colleagues, 39 percent of the 205 women who received IP cisplatin-paclitaxel were elderly: 26 percent (61–70 years), 12 percent (71–80 years), and 1 percent (over age 80).[48] Their functional sta-tus was good (92%, GOG performance status 0–1).

Despite growing acceptance of its superior survival advantages, several concerns remain: technical difficulties (IP catheter placement and complications) and increased toxicities (renal dys-function, neuropathy). In GOG 172, fewer than 50 percent of all patients were able to complete four or more cycles of the IP regimen because of toxicity, regardless of age. In a quality-of-life (QOL) assessment, physical and functional well-being and ovarian cancer symptoms were signif-icantly worse in the IP arm, particularly before cycle 4.[49] Patients in the IP arm also reported sig-nificantly worse abdominal discomfort and neuro-toxicity 3–6 weeks and 12 months after complet-ing IP treatment. However, the QOL of both the IV and IP groups improved over time.

How does an oncologist apply these results to their older population? First, the major limitation to the study was that patients received IP cisplatin. By the age of 70, renal function may have declined by 40 percent, and this reduction in glomerular fil-tration rate may lead to enhanced toxicity of drugs, particularly those with significant renal excretion such as cisplatin.[50–52] On GOG 172, patients were required to have a serum creatinine less than 1.2 mg/dL; however, creatinine clearance is a more sensitive marker for renal dysfunction and should be used.[53] The second limitation was the use of paclitaxel as its drug clearance declines with age and its toxicities, such as neuropathy and cytope-nias, heighten.[54] To improve tolerability, future tri-als will need to consider elimination of the day 8 IP paclitaxel, substitution of IP carboplatin, sub-stitution of IV paclitaxel with IV docetaxel to reduce neurotoxicity, and the use of more aggres-sive IV hydration. Clearly we need prospective tri-als designed specifically for older patients with an emphasis of pharmacokinetics and toxicity to bet-ter screen this vulnerable patient group.[55] Until that time, IP chemotherapy should still be offered as an option to older women, particularly those with good functional status, as long as kidney function is carefully assessed and drugs are dosed accordingly.

Second line

Treatment for recurrent ovarian cancer is divided into relapse at under 6 months as platinum-resistant and at more than 6 months as platinum-sensitive. For platinum-sensitive patients, trials show survival advantage to a doublet combina-tion with carboplatin and either paclitaxel or gem-citabine.[56,57] Choice is often based on the toxic-ity profile, and in older patients, gemcitabine may offer less neuropathy, but cytopenias may be more significant.

For platinum-resistant disease, chemotherapy is typically given as a single agent, and responses range from 10 to 25 percent with a median dura-tion from 4 to 8 months. Common options include liposomal doxorubicin, topotecan, gemcitabine, weekly paclitaxel, and Navelbine.[58] Unfortunately, few retrospective studies have been reported in older ovarian cancer patients. However, on the basis of extensive studies from lung and breast cancer in older patients, most of these single-agent drugs are well tolerated.[59,60] With platinum-resistant ovarian cancer, Gronlund and colleagues described their experience with topotecan (1 mg/m^2 over 5 days) in 57 elderly patients and found no significant differences in toxicity profile or response between an older (over 65 years) and younger (under 65 years) cohort. Performance sta-tus was a better predictor of response and survival in both cohorts.[61] Currently most oncologists use liposomal doxorubicin or weekly topotecan for older patients with platinum resistance given an improved toxicity profile.[62,63]

Recent data show support for antivascular strategies such as bevacizumab. Hypertension and arterial thrombosis risk may be heightened in an elder with more comorbidity.[64] Moreover, in the ovarian cancer population, high bowel perforation rates (up to 11%) are worrisome.[65]

Finally, because these chemotherapy options only offer palliation, many argue to focus on better supportive measures rather than more chemother-apy. In one study, there was a significant cost differ-ence with no appreciable improvement in survival between ovarian cancer patients treated aggres-sively with chemotherapy versus those enrolled in hospice at the final months of their life. The authors suggest that earlier hospice enrollment is beneficial, particularly in the older frail patients.[66]

B.7. Geriatric assessment

Future studies may benefit from the inclusion of a comprehensive geriatric assessment (CGA) to better identify areas of vulnerability and potentially predict tolerability and response to cancer treatments. This evaluation would include a patient's functional status (i.e., ability to live independently at home and in the community), comorbid medical conditions, cognition, psychological status, social functioning support, and nutritional status.[67] We have taken a lead part in a multi-institutional prospective study (NCT00477958, national principal investigator [PI], Arti Hurria, MD; Memorial Sloan-Kettering PI, William Tew, MD) with 600 cancer patients (including patients with gynecologic malignancies) to evaluate the utility of a geriatric assessment to predict toxicity to chemotherapy. Each patient undergoes a CGA before initiation of a new chemotherapy regimen and on completion of the regimen. The study is expected to conclude by 2010.

A study was performed in 83 patients with advanced ovarian cancer who were aged 70 years and older and who received carboplatin (AUC 5) and cyclophosphamide (600 mg/m^2) on day 1 of six 28-day cycles. Comorbidities, medications, cognitive functions (mini-mental test), nutritional status, and autonomy were collected prospectively. Sixty patients (72%) received six chemotherapy cycles without severe toxicity or tumor progression. Multivariate analysis revealed three factors as independent predictors of significant toxicity: symptoms of depression at baseline, dependence (defined as living at home with assistance or living in a specialized institution with medical assistance), and performance status of 2 or less. Independent prognostic factors identified for overall survival (Cox model) were depression, FIGO (International Federation of Gynecology and Obstetrics) stage IV, and more than six different comedications per day. These data show the potential for a CGA to predict toxicity and overall survival of elderly advanced ovarian carcinoma patients.[68]

B.8. Quality of life and survivorship

Along with a geriatric assessment, QOL is an important component of assessing the effects of cancer, therapy, and survivorship. While the traditional use is for comparisons of treatment groups, QOL can also be utilized for descriptive aspects and generate a global number from individual QOL tools. In addition, relationships can be explored between physical, functional, emotional, and social domains, along with specific line questions.[69]

Elderly women with cancer have larger impacts on physical and functional domains compared to emotional aspects of QOL. Using the Iowa Women's Health Registry, over 25,000 elderly female cancer survivors reported functional limitations.[70] Women closer to diagnosis reported more limitations in functioning than those farther from treatment. In addition, 54 percent of patients with ovarian cancer reported at least one limitation, and many two. These limitations included problems with housework, walking, and meal preparation.

QOL is altered by surgery in elderly women with ovarian cancer. In one series, women undergoing surgery for the possibility of ovarian cancer were followed preoperatively until 6 months after chemotherapy.[71,72] Surgery made a large impact on QOL, especially in regard to the physical and functional domains. Results from other surgical studies in the elderly undergoing gynecologic surgery are quite varied as they are without controls, use different definitions of *elderly*, and do not address QOL.[25–27]

After surgery, ovarian cancer patients undergo adjuvant chemotherapy; however, research on QOL of patients during treatment has included heterogeneous populations. Schink and colleagues assessed QOL in 59 ovarian cancer patients before, during, and 1 year after chemotherapy.[73] Patients ranged in age from 34 to 84 years, with a median age of 64 years. Global QOL and physical well-being scores improved throughout chemotherapy. A larger series assessed QOL in 152 ovarian cancer patients after surgical debulking and at regular intervals during chemotherapy with two different treatment arms.[74] Patients ranged in age from 22 to 85 years, with a median age of 58 years. There was deterioration seen in QOL during chemotherapy, followed by clinical improvements compared with baseline over time. These improvements persisted for the duration of follow-up at 2 years.

Factors other than cancer and its treatment may have significant effects on QOL and affect assessment of treatments. Wan and colleagues examined the relationship between demographic variables (including age), clinical factors, and social characteristics and measures on the four subscales in cancer patients.[75] They found lower QOL scores among those with poorer performance status, younger patients, and lower socioeconomic status. Movsas and colleagues speculated that the observation of decreased QOL in younger patients may be due to the devastating impact of a cancer diagnosis at a younger age.[76]

QOL is affected by clinical factors, including age. In one study of women with endometrial or ovarian cancer, age and educational level were positively correlated with physical well-being, while increasing patient weight was negatively correlated.[77] Social well-being was positively correlated with the global mental score and negatively correlated with patient weight and educational level. Age was positively correlated with physical and emotional well-being.

In an ancillary data analysis the GOG measured demographic variables, QOL domains, and line items to determine relationships in women actively receiving chemotherapy for ovarian cancer.[71] Patients ranged in age from 45 to 72, with a median age of 60 years. The ovarian cancer patients had global QOL scores similar to the U.S. female adult population. However, the reported subscale scores were significantly lower in physical, functional, and emotional well-being and higher in social well-being subscales. In the physical domain, significant differences were observed in symptoms (nausea, pain, feeling ill, and being bothered by the side effects of treatment) as well as more general effects (lack of energy, meeting needs of family, forced to spend time in bed). In the functional subscale, a significantly higher proportion of women selected the worst categories of sleeping well. In the emotional domain, there were significant differences in feeling nervous and worrying about dying. In regard to the elevated social domain, it may be that patients with cancer receive more social support during adjuvant therapy. As the elderly have a tendency to have a poor performance status, those with a compromised performance status of more than 1 reported lower QOL. With respect to the elderly, age was positively correlated with positive emotions.

End of life

The majority of women with ovarian cancer present with advanced-stage disease, and the majority recur and die of cancer. Therefore, as death may be a part of the trajectory of disease, QOL at the end of life is a natural study point. A prospective, longitudinal cohort study of patients with advanced cancer found that EOL discussions were associated with less aggressive medical care near death and earlier hospice referrals.[78] These discussions did not increase in the elderly as there were no associations between discussions and age. However, others have found the elderly with cancer less likely to receive aggressive care.[24]

Aggressive medical care at the end of life is associated with worse QOL near death.[26,78] Unfortunately, patients with ovarian cancer frequently receive aggressive medical care at the end of life.[79] A retrospective study measured the aggressiveness of cancer care within the last month of life. Significant clinical events (SCE) specific to patients with ovarian cancer were defined as ascites, bowel obstruction, and pleural effusion. Mean age at death was 63, with a range of 21–89. Patients had significantly increased hospitalizations and SCE as they approached the end of life. There was no difference in the pattern of hospitalizations and SCE between the top and bottom survival quartiles. Therefore, if patients lived short or long after diagnosis, they died in a similar pattern. Patients with a shorter survival time had a trend toward increased chemotherapy during their last 3 months of life and had increased overall aggressiveness of care. Those who received aggressive care did not have improvement in survival. Increasing hospitalizations with SCE should be indicators of the appropriateness of reducing cure-oriented therapies and increasing palliative interventions. By recognizing the end of life, physicians and patients can focus on pain and symptom management to improve QOL.

C. Endometrial cancer

Endometrial carcinoma (EMC) is the most common gynecologic malignancy in the United States, with 40,100 woman diagnosed and 7,470 dying of this disease in 2008.[6] EMC is a disease of postmenopausal woman with a median age of 63 at time of diagnosis.[6] Advanced age has been found to be an independent predictor for survival and poor outcomes. Several theories have been suggested: (1) EMC in older women tends to have more aggressive histologic features such as deep myometrial invasion, poor differentiation, higher stage, and extrauterine spread; (2) less aggressive surgical approaches or postoperative treatments are used; and/or (3) higher comorbidities, particularly associated with both older age and EMC (obesity, hypertension, and diabetes), are found. In this section, we will review the prognostic implications of advanced age as well as the experience with surgical, radiation, and chemotherapeutic approaches in older patients with EMC.

C.1. Diagnosis and prognostic features

EMC is typically found at early stages (80% confined to uterus) because of early onset of symptoms, notably abnormal vaginal bleeding. This often leads to a clinical workup, including a pelvic ultrasound to access the endometrial stripe and ultimately an endometrial biopsy.[80] The risk of EMC increases with age and time from menopause.[81,82] Therefore the gold standard test, dilation and curettage, must be performed to completely rule out EMC in an older woman. Risk factors such as diabetes, hypertension, obesity, and prior hormonal therapy (i.e., tamoxifen) increase the pretest probability of cancer. Family history of cancer has not been a good indictor of personal risk to endometrial cancer in postmenopausal women because HNPCC is typically diagnosed in younger women.[83] Prognosis is based on stage, histology, tumor grade, lymphovascular invasion, ethnicity (i.e., African American), and advanced age.[84-86]

Older patients with endometrial cancer are often at risk for comorbidities, with obesity being prominent among them. Though endometrial cancer is most commonly diagnosed at an early stage, patients are at significant risk from premature death from these other comorbid conditions.[87] Survival decreases significantly in patients older than 50, and this decreased survival associated with age is unrelated to surgical stage or grade of the adenocarcinoma.[84] However, the poor prognosis associated with advanced age may be in part associated with the decreased frequency of surgical treatment.[88] In addition, obesity in endometrial cancer patients does not significantly differ based on age as obesity is associated with higher mortality from causes other than endometrial cancer.[89] A recent study examined if rates of disease recurrence, treatment-related adverse effects, and survival differ between obese or morbidly obese and nonobese patients. Of importance, body mass index (BMI) was not significantly different based on age. In this GOG study, obesity was associated with higher mortality from causes other than endometrial cancer but not disease recurrence.

C.2. Surgery

Treatment of endometrial cancer involves primary surgical staging (hysterectomy, bilateral salpingo-oophorectomy, washing, and lymph node sampling) followed in some cases with adjuvant radiotherapy and/or chemotherapy.[90] The poor prognosis associated with advanced age may be in part associated with the decreased frequency of proper surgery.[88] Because over 70 percent of women are obese, and many are elderly, they are likely to have medical comorbidities and increased risk for perioperative morbidity.

Vaginal hysterectomy for endometrial cancer is an option in patients who are unable to undergo general anesthesia secondary to their comorbidities.[91] Because most elderly patients with endometrial cancer have early-stage disease, a simple vaginal hysterectomy performed with regional anesthesia, such as an epidural or a spinal, may be a reasonable option without compromising survival.[92] Another option in the frail elderly with endometrial cancer is to treat primarily with radiation therapy.[93] Several studies have shown that minimally invasive surgical (MIS) staging for endometrial cancer is associated with overall excellent surgical outcomes, shorter hospitalization, and less postoperative pain.

In terms of the optimal surgical approach, in a retrospective review of MIS approaches performed in 100 EMC patients, Fader and colleagues demonstrated that total laparoscopic hysterectomy may be more feasible to perform (in terms of operative time and blood loss) than laparoscopic-assisted vaginal hysterectomy in obese women.[94] Furthermore, Gehrig and colleagues recently queried what the optimal minimally invasive surgical approach in morbidly obese EMC patients was and concluded that robotic surgery was superior to conventional laparoscopy, with shorter operative time, less blood loss, increased lymph node retrieval, and shorter hospital stay.[95]

The advantages of robotic-assisted MIS include three-dimensional vision, wristed instrumentation, ergonomic positioning, magnification, telestration, and the ability to offer more MIS to obese patients.[95-97] Disadvantages include financial burden, as the da Vinci unit presently costs over $1 million (http://www.intuitivesurgical.com/). In addition, lack of tactile feedback, the learning curve, training of residents, and docking are barriers that need to be addressed.

Once the decision is made to take the elderly with endometrial cancer to the operating room, the intraoperative procedure does not change. However, these patients may have increased postoperative morbidity. One retrospective review evaluated the effect of age on surgical morbidity and outcomes in patients with endometrial cancer.[98] Intraoperatively, there are no differences in the percentage of patients with lymph node sampling, operative time, blood loss, or complications. Postoperatively, older patients had more wound infections, more cardiac events, and more episodes of bowel ileus.

C.3. Radiation

Adjuvant therapy recommendations for elderly endometrial cancer patients may be hampered by comorbidity. A retrospective study analyzing postoperative radiotherapy for early-stage elderly endometrial cancer patients revealed that associated pelvic-vaginal relapse rates were higher in elderly patients not treated with radiotherapy.[99] In two other large series, older patients had a far worse prognosis, independent of other high-risk features (lymphovascular invasion, serous histology).[100,101] Moreover, the rate of complications was found to be similar in both older and younger age groups (3% grade 3 or higher, CTCAEv3).[100] Therefore advanced age is often considered crucial in determining whether to offer radiation and which type (intravaginal or pelvic).[102–106]

C.4. Chemotherapy

Chemotherapy is being used with much higher frequency in endometrial cancer. In the past, chemotherapy was reserved only for patients who relapsed, which accounts for only 10–20 percent of all EMC patients. The most active agents include platinum, anthracyclines, taxanes, and hormonal blockade agents, as outlined in a recent review.[107] As discussed earlier in this chapter, these agents present challenges for an older patient, particularly when given as combination therapy such as a three-drug regimen of paclitaxel, doxorubicin, and cisplatin (TAP). Unfortunately, dedicated trials with older women are lacking. Over the past 2 years, chemotherapy has also been incorporated into the adjuvant treatment of patients with stage III or IV and early-stage cancer with high-risk features such as serous histology.[108–110] Clearly, given the older demographics associated with EMC, geriatric assessment and QOL measurements will be vital components to determine the feasibility of these newer standard treatments.

C.5. Quality of life and survivorship

The most common problem endometrial cancer survivors confront is obesity and related morbidi-

ties. Unfortunately, obesity continues to rise in the United States, including among the elderly. It is estimated that the prevalence of obesity in adults aged 60 years and older will increase from 32 percent in 2000 to 37 percent in 2010.[111] A recent prospective study reported that nearly 70 percent of women with early endometrial cancer were obese, which is a markedly increased number compared to older reports.[112] When assessing obesity-associated cancers, it appears that patients with endometrial cancer are the most morbid as most have stage I disease yet are at significant risk for premature death.[87] While the impact of weight on cancer recurrence does not appear to be a factor in endometrial cancer, obese endometrial cancer survivors have a higher mortality from causes not related to cancer.[89] Endometrial cancer survivors have numerous comorbidities related to their obesity, including hypertension, diabetes mellitus, cardiovascular disease, osteoarthritis, and pulmonary disease.[113] Improving medical comorbidities through weight management in survivors may lead to improved overall QOL and survival.

QOL is an important component of assessing cancer survivorship. It is imperative to measure and understand alterations in specific cancer populations to assess unmet needs and develop strategies for improvement. As mentioned previously in this chapter, different aspects of QOL are altered in ovarian cancer patients as scores are lower in physical and emotional well-being subscales. However, patients with endometrial cancer have significant decreases in the physical and functional domains based on increasing weight.

Among endometrial cancer survivors, obesity and increasing age affect QOL. The elderly are a heterogeneous population with regard to QOL. As patients age, certain aspects of their QOL decline, including global physical health. However, with advancing age, an improvement in mental health is perceived.[114] QOL is related to performance status and comorbidity and less to chronological age. As weight increases, comorbidities increase also, affecting QOL. In a prospective examination of QOL, general health status, and obesity in women with early-stage endometrial cancer, women with a BMI more than 30 (obese) had decreased physical QOL scores.[115] There was also an inverse relationship between the global physical health composite score and BMI. A recent cross-sectional survey of Canadian endometrial cancer survivors revealed that those patients with morbid obesity had a QOL score 3 times lower than women with a normal

BMI.[116] This suggests that if weight is decreased, survivors' QOL may be improved.

Obesity influences all domains of QOL but particularly the physical component. Obese women rated their QOL lower on all domains of the SF-36, a general health measure, compared to normal-weight women.[116–117] Apovian and colleagues conducted a prospective study assessing the physical domain in obese elderly women and ascertained that a higher BMI is significantly associated with poor upper- and lower-body function.[118] Most studies conclude that obesity has a greater impact on physical versus mental health.[116,119] Others have concurred with these findings but question a confounding effect because of the presence of accompanying chronic illness.[119] Multiple studies have found that obese individuals who are following a healthy diet and engage in regular exercise have a higher QOL compared to those who do not.[120–122]

There have been limited studies specifically assessing QOL in women with endometrial cancer. Limitations of prior research have included heterogeneous gynecologic populations, receiving different adjuvant therapies.[123–125] Klee and colleagues assessed 49 women with endometrial cancer who received adjuvant radiation therapy and concluded that most patients experience physical side effects and had overall lower QOL compared to a matched population of healthy women.[126] Li and colleagues evaluated 61 women with clinical stage I–III endometrial cancer 5–7 years after primary treatment.[127] All patients received surgery; however, the adjuvant treatments received were diverse and included observation, radiation, and/or chemotherapy. The study did not use a standard QOL measurement tool, and it is unclear whether the questionnaires consisted of specific domains with the ability for comparisons. A more recent larger study compared QOL among 5- to 10-year survivors of stage I–II endometrial cancer treated with surgery alone or surgery with external-beam pelvic adjuvant therapy.[128] Using an adapted version of the Charlson score, comorbidity appeared to be the only variable that was negatively and independently associated with all subscales. On multivariate analyses, adjuvant radiation therapy was independently and negatively associated with vitality and physical and social well-being scale scores. Unfortunately, BMI was not a controlled variable. In addition, other investigators believe that adjuvant treatment for endometrial cancer patients at intermediate risk for recurrence is vaginal radiation, not pelvic radiation.

C.6. Lifestyle

Cancer survivors do not always engage in healthy lifestyle behaviors. Few cancer survivors are meeting physical activity levels or five servings of fruits and vegetables a day, as recommended by many medical societies.[129] Blanchard and colleagues' trend analyses have shown a positive association between the numbers of lifestyle behavior recommendations being met and QOL for breast, prostate, colorectal, bladder, uterine, and skin melanoma cancer survivors. In addition, the association between current lifestyle recommendations and QOL in cancer survivors appears to be cumulative.

A recent ancillary analysis of two prospective endometrial cancer QOL trials revealed that scores were similar to normative data in age-matched women without cancer.[94] Although summary patient scores were similar to normative scores, when considering increasing BMI, analysis revealed a significant decrease in the physical component and the functional domains based on increasing weight. BMI was inversely correlated with functional, physical, and social well-being and with several decreases in line items within the functional domain, including ability at work and being content. BMI also had an inverse relationship with the "lack of energy" item in the physical domain. Fatigue was present in nearly 30 percent of survivors, which increased as weight increased.

It is imperative to implement lifestyle interventions to improve survivorship of endometrial cancer patients who are at increased risk for poor QOL and premature death. A recent randomized controlled study of an interventional lifestyle program in 45 endometrial cancer survivors demonstrated that patients can lose weight and improve their exercise for 6 months following the intervention. The trial focused on improving walking, nutritional quality, and behavioral modification. Even though the average age in the study was 54 years, with five patients over the age of 65 years, there was no difference between weight loss and physical activity based on age.

D. Conclusion

To improve the benefit and tolerability of cancer treatment, we must develop new geriatric-specific trials and encourage enrollment of older patients in current clinical trials. Age appears to be an important factor influencing treatment selection among patients with gynecologic cancers, and elderly patients may be inappropriately denied participation in research.[130] In addition, standard treatment options, such as a gynecologic oncology surgical referral and postoperative chemotherapy and/or radiation, should be discussed. To be mindful and respectful, one must define the goals of treatment for patients and their families (palliative vs. curative) as well as treatment toxicities. As the field of geriatric oncology evolves, guidelines will ultimately assist in these difficult decisions.

References

1. Edwards BK, Howe HL, Ries LA, et al. Annual report to the nation on the status of cancer, 1973–1999, featuring implications of age and aging on U.S. cancer burden. *Cancer.* 2002;94:2766–2792.

2. Yancik R, Ries LA. Cancer in older persons: an international issue in an aging world. *Semin Oncol.* 2004;31:128–136.

3. Thigpen T, Brady MF, Omura GA, et al. Age as a prognostic factor in ovarian carcinoma. The Gynecologic Oncology Group experience. *Cancer.* 1993;71:606–614.

4. Hightower RD, Nguyen HN, Averette HE, et al. National survey of ovarian carcinoma. IV: Patterns of care and related survival for older patients. *Cancer.* 1994;73:377–383.

5. Pignata S, Vermorken JB. Ovarian cancer in the elderly. *Crit Rev Oncol Hematol.* 2004;49: 77–86.

6. Jemal A, Siegel R, Ward E, et al. Cancer statistics, 2008. *CA Cancer J Clin.* 2008;58:71–96.

7. Ries LA, Melbert D, Krapcho M, et al. *SEER Cancer Statistics Review, 1975–2005.* Bethesda, MD: National Cancer Institute; 2008.

8. Watson P, Butzow R, Lynch HT, et al. The clinical features of ovarian cancer in hereditary nonpolyposis colorectal cancer. *Gynecol Oncol.* 2001;82:223–228.

9. Chen S, Iversen ES, Friebel T, et al. Characterization of BRCA1 and BRCA2 mutations in a large United States sample. *J Clin Oncol.* 2006;24:863–871.

10. Haber D. Prophylactic oophorectomy to reduce the risk of ovarian and breast cancer in carriers of BRCA mutations. *N Engl J Med.* 2002;346: 1660–1662.

11. Kauff ND, Domchek SM, Friebel TM, et al. Risk-reducing salpingo-oophorectomy for the prevention of BRCA1- and BRCA2-associated breast and gynecologic cancer: a multicenter, prospective study. *J Clin Oncol.* 2008;26: 1331–1337.

12. Chi DS, Sabbatini P. Advanced ovarian cancer. *Curr Treat Options Oncol.* 2000;1:139–146.

13. Mirhashemi R, Nieves-Neira W, Averette HE. Gynecologic malignancies in older women. *Oncology.* 2001;15:580–586; discussion 592–594, 597–598.

14. Lambrou NC, Bristow RE. Ovarian cancer in elderly women. *Oncology.* 2003;17:1075–1081; discussion 1081, 1085–1086, 1091.

15. Ryerson AB, Eheman C, Burton J, et al. Symptoms, diagnoses, and time to key diagnostic procedures among older U.S. women with ovarian cancer. *Obstet Gynecol.* 2007;109:1053–1061.

16. Winter III WE, Maxwell GL, Tian C, et al. Prognostic factors for stage III epithelial ovarian cancer: a Gynecologic Oncology Group Study. *J Clin Oncol.* 2007;25:3621–3627.

17. Chan JK, Loizzi V, Lin YG, et al. Stages III and IV invasive epithelial ovarian carcinoma in younger versus older women: what prognostic factors are important? *Obstet Gynecol.* 2003;102:156–161.

18. Chan JK, Urban R, Cheung MK, et al. Ovarian cancer in younger vs older women: a population-based analysis. *Br J Cancer.* 2006;95: 1314–1320.

19. Markman M, Lewis Jr JL, Saigo P, et al. Impact of age on survival of patients with ovarian cancer. *Gynecol Oncol.* 1993;49:236–239.

20. Petignat P, Fioretta G, Verkooijen HM, et al. Poorer survival of elderly patients with ovarian cancer: a population-based study. *Surg Oncol.* 2004;13:181–186.

21. Du XL, Sun CC, Milam MR, et al. Ethnic differences in socioeconomic status, diagnosis, treatment, and survival among older women with epithelial ovarian cancer. *Int J Gynecol Cancer.* 2008; 18(4):660–669.

22. Pectasides D, Fountzilas G, Aravantinos G, et al. Epithelial ovarian carcinoma in younger vs older women: is age an independent prognostic factor? The Hellenic Oncology Cooperative Group experience. *Int J Gynecol Cancer.* 2007;17: 1003–1010.

23. Bristow RE, Tomacruz RS, Armstrong DK, et al. Survival effect of maximal cytoreductive surgery for advanced ovarian carcinoma during the platinum era: a meta-analysis. *J Clin Oncol.* 2002;20:1248–1259.

24. Wimberger P, Lehmann N, Kimmig R, et al. Impact of age on outcome in patients with advanced ovarian cancer treated within a prospectively randomized phase III study of the Arbeitsgemeinschaft Gynaekologische Onkologie Ovarian Cancer Study Group (AGO-OVAR). *Gynecol Oncol.* 2006;100:300–307.

25. Uyar D, Frasure HE, Markman M, et al. Treatment patterns by decade of life in elderly women (> or = 70 years of age) with ovarian cancer. *Gynecol Oncol.* 2005;98:403–408.

26. Wright JD, Herzog TJ, Powell MA. Morbidity of cytoreductive surgery in the elderly. *Am J Obstet Gynecol.* 2004;190:1398–1400.

27. Sharma S, Driscoll D, Odunsi K, et al. Safety and efficacy of cytoreductive surgery for epithelial ovarian cancer in elderly and high-risk surgical patients. *Am J Obstet Gynecol.* 2005;193: 2077–2082.

28. Eisenhauer EL, Tew WP, Levine DA, et al. Response and outcomes in elderly patients with stages IIIC–IV ovarian cancer receiving

platinum-taxane chemotherapy. *Gynecol Oncol.* 2007;106:381–387.

29. Bruchim I, Altaras M, Fishman A. Age contrasts in clinical characteristics and pattern of care in patients with epithelial ovarian cancer. *Gynecol Oncol.* 2002;86:274–278.

30. Nordin AJ, Chinn DJ, Moloney I, et al. Do elderly cancer patients care about cure? Attitudes to radical gynecologic oncology surgery in the elderly. *Gynecol Oncol.* 2001;81:447–455.

31. Cloven NG, Manetta A, Berman ML, et al. Management of ovarian cancer in patients older than 80 years of Age. *Gynecol Oncol.* 1999;73: 137–139.

32. Susini T, Scambia G, Margariti PA, et al. Gynecologic oncologic surgery in the elderly: a retrospective analysis of 213 patients. *Gynecol Oncol.* 1999;75:437–443.

33. Diaz-Montes TP, Zahurak ML, Giuntoli II RL, et al. Surgical care of elderly women with ovarian cancer: a population-based perspective. *Gynecol Oncol.* 2005;99:352–357.

34. McGuire WP, Hoskins WJ, Brady MF, et al. Cyclophosphamide and cisplatin compared with paclitaxel and cisplatin in patients with stage III and stage IV ovarian cancer. *N Engl J Med.* 1996;334:1–6.

35. Ozols RF, Bundy BN, Greer BE, et al. Phase III trial of carboplatin and paclitaxel compared with cisplatin and paclitaxel in patients with optimally resected stage III ovarian cancer: a Gynecologic Oncology Group study. *J Clin Oncol.* 2003;21: 3194–3200.

36. Maas HA, Kruitwagen RF, Lemmens VE, et al. The influence of age and co-morbidity on treatment and prognosis of ovarian cancer: a population-based study. *Gynecol Oncol.* 2005;97:104–109.

37. Hershman D, Jacobson JS, McBride R, et al. Effectiveness of platinum-based chemotherapy among elderly patients with advanced ovarian cancer. *Gynecol Oncol.* 2004;94:540–549.

38. Sundararajan V, Hershman D, Grann VR, et al. Variations in the use of chemotherapy for elderly patients with advanced ovarian cancer: a population-based study. *J Clin Oncol.* 2002;20:173–178.

39. Pignata S, Monfardini S. Single agents should be administered in preference to combination chemotherapy for the treatment of patients over 70 years of age with advanced ovarian carcinoma. *Eur J Cancer.* 2000;36:817–820.

40. Pignata S, Breda E, Scambia G, et al. A phase II study of weekly carboplatin and paclitaxel as first-line treatment of elderly patients with advanced ovarian cancer. A Multicentre Italian Trial in Ovarian cancer (MITO-5) study. *Crit Rev Oncol Hematol.* 2008:66(3):229–236.

41. Tredan O, Geay JF, Touzet S, et al. Carboplatin/ cyclophosphamide or carboplatin/paclitaxel in elderly patients with advanced ovarian cancer? Analysis of two consecutive trials from the Groupe d'Investigateurs Nationaux pour l'Etude des Cancers Ovariens. *Ann Oncol.* 2007;18: 256–262.

42. Fader AN, Gruenigen VV, Gibbons H, et al. Improved tolerance of primary chemotherapy with reduced-dose carboplatin and paclitaxel in elderly ovarian cancer patients. *Gynecol Oncol.* 2008.

43. Group ICON: Paclitaxel plus carboplatin versus standard chemotherapy with either single-agent carboplatin or cyclophosphamide, doxorubicin, and cisplatin in women with ovarian cancer: the ICON3 randomised trial. *Lancet.* 2002;360: 505–515.

44. Villella JA, Chaudhry T, Pearl ML, et al. Comparison of tolerance of combination carboplatin and paclitaxel chemotherapy by age in women with ovarian cancer. *Gynecol Oncol.* 2002;86:316–322.

45. Ceccaroni M, D'Agostino G, Ferrandina G, et al. Gynecological malignancies in elderly patients: is age 70 a limit to standard-dose chemotherapy? An Italian retrospective toxicity multicentric study. *Gynecol Oncol.* 2002;85:445–450.

46. Alberts DS, Liu PY, Hannigan EV, et al. Intraperitoneal cisplatin plus intravenous cyclophosphamide versus intravenous cisplatin plus intravenous cyclophosphamide for stage III ovarian cancer. *N Engl J Med.* 1996;335: 1950–1955.

47. Markman M, Bundy BN, Alberts DS, et al. Phase III trial of standard-dose intravenous cisplatin plus paclitaxel versus moderately high-dose carboplatin followed by intravenous paclitaxel and intraperitoneal cisplatin in small-volume stage III ovarian carcinoma: an intergroup study of the Gynecologic Oncology Group, Southwestern Oncology Group, and Eastern Cooperative Oncology Group. *J Clin Oncol.* 2001;19: 1001–1007.

48. Armstrong DK, Bundy B, Wenzel L, et al. Intraperitoneal cisplatin and paclitaxel in ovarian cancer. *N Engl J Med.* 2006;354:34–43.

49. Wenzel LB, Huang HQ, Armstrong DK, et al. Health-related quality of life during and after intraperitoneal versus intravenous chemotherapy for optimally debulked ovarian cancer: a Gynecologic Oncology Group Study. *J Clin Oncol.* 2007;25:437–443.

50. Brenner BM, Meyer TW, Hostetter TH. Dietary protein intake and the progressive nature of kidney disease: the role of hemodynamically mediated glomerular injury in the pathogenesis of progressive glomerular sclerosis in aging, renal

ablation, and intrinsic renal disease. *N Engl J Med.* 1982;307:652–659.

51. Launay-Vacher V, Chatelut E, Lichtman SM, et al. Renal insufficiency in elderly cancer patients: International Society of Geriatric Oncology clinical practice recommendations. *Ann Oncol.* 2007;18:1314–1321.

52. Launay-Vacher V, Oudard S, Janus N, et al. Prevalence of renal insufficiency in cancer patients and implications for anticancer drug management: the renal insufficiency and anticancer medications (IRMA) study. *Cancer.* 2007;110:1376–1384.

53. Lichtman SM, Wildiers H, Launay-Vacher V, et al. International Society of Geriatric Oncology (SIOG) recommendations for the adjustment of dosing in elderly cancer patients with renal insufficiency. *Eur J Cancer.* 2007;43:14–34.

54. Lichtman SM, Hollis D, Miller AA, et al. Prospective evaluation of the relationship of patient age and paclitaxel clinical pharmacology: Cancer and Leukemia Group B (CALGB 9762). *J Clin Oncol.* 2006;24:1846–1851.

55. Lichtman SM, Wildiers H, Chatelut E, et al. International Society of Geriatric Oncology Chemotherapy Taskforce: evaluation of chemotherapy in older patients – an analysis of the medical literature. *J Clin Oncol.* 2007;25:1832–1843.

56. Parmar MK, Ledermann JA, Colombo N, et al. Paclitaxel plus platinum-based chemotherapy versus conventional platinum-based chemotherapy in women with relapsed ovarian cancer: the ICON4/AGO-OVAR-2.2 trial. *Lancet.* 2003;361:2099–2106.

57. Pfisterer J, Plante M, Vergote I, et al. Gemcitabine plus carboplatin compared with carboplatin in patients with platinum-sensitive recurrent ovarian cancer: an intergroup trial of the AGO-OVAR, the NCIC CTG, and the EORTC GCG. *J Clin Oncol.* 2006;24:4699–4707.

58. Bukowski RM, Ozols RF, Markman M. The management of recurrent ovarian cancer. *Semin Oncol.* 2007;34:S1–S15.

59. Gridelli C, Langer C, Maione P, et al. Lung cancer in the elderly. *J Clin Oncol.* 2007;25:1898–1907.

60. Wildiers H, Kunkler I, Biganzoli L, et al. Management of breast cancer in elderly individuals: recommendations of the International Society of Geriatric Oncology. *Lancet Oncol.* 2007;8:1101–1115.

61. Gronlund B, Hogdall C, Hansen HH, et al. Performance status rather than age is the key prognostic factor in second-line treatment of elderly patients with epithelial ovarian carcinoma. *Cancer.* 2002;94:1961–1967.

62. Gordon AN, Tonda M, Sun S, et al. Long-term survival advantage for women treated with pegylated liposomal doxorubicin compared with topotecan in a phase 3 randomized study of recurrent and refractory epithelial ovarian cancer. *Gynecol Oncol.* 2004;95:1–8.

63. Morris RT. Weekly topotecan in the management of ovarian cancer. *Gynecol Oncol.* 2003;90: S34–S38.

64. Kabbinavar FF, Hurwitz HI, Yi J, et al. Addition of bevacizumab to fluorouracil-based first-line treatment of metastatic colorectal cancer: pooled analysis of cohorts of older patients from two randomized clinical trials. *J Clin Oncol.* 2009;27:199–205.

65. Burger RA. Experience with bevacizumab in the management of epithelial ovarian cancer. *J Clin Oncol.* 2007;25:2902–2908.

66. Lewin SN, Buttin BM, Powell MA, et al. Resource utilization for ovarian cancer patients at the end of life: how much is too much? *Gynecol Oncol.* 2005;99:261–266.

67. Hurria A, Lichtman SM, Gardes J, et al. Identifying vulnerable older adults with cancer: integrating geriatric assessment into oncology practice. *J Am Geriatr Soc.* 2007;55:1604–1608.

68. Freyer G, Geay JF, Touzet S, et al. Comprehensive geriatric assessment predicts tolerance to chemotherapy and survival in elderly patients with advanced ovarian carcinoma: a GINECO study. *Ann Oncol.* 2005;16:1795–1800.

69. Cella DF, Tulsky DS, Gray G, et al. The Functional Assessment of Cancer Therapy (FACT) Scale: development and validation of the general measure. *J Clin Oncol.* 1993;11:570–579.

70. Sweeney C, Schmitz KH, Lazovich D, et al. Functional limitations in elderly female cancer survivors. *J Natl Cancer Inst.* 2006;98:521–529.

71. von Gruenigen VE, Gil K, Huang H, et al. Quality of life in ovarian cancer patients during chemotherapy: a Gynecologic Oncology Group study. *Gynecol Oncol.* 2008;108:S28–S29.

72. von Gruenigen VE, Frasure HE, Grandon M, et al. Longitudinal assessment of quality of life and lifestyle in newly diagnosed ovarian cancer patients: the roles of surgery and chemotherapy. *Gynecol Oncol.* 2006;103:120–126.

73. Schink JC, Weller E, Harris LS, et al. Outpatient taxol and carboplatin chemotherapy for suboptimally debulked epithelial carcinoma of the ovary results in improved quality of life: an Eastern Cooperative Oncology Group phase II study (E2E93). *J Cancer.* 2001;7:155–164.

74. Bezjak A, Tu P, Bacon M, et al. Quality of life in ovarian cancer patients: comparison of paclitaxel plus cisplatin, with cyclophosphamide plus

cisplatin in a randomized study. *J Clin Oncol.* 2004;22:4595–4603.

75. Wan GJ, Counte MA, Cella DF, et al. An analysis of the impact of demographic, clinical and social factors on health related quality of life. *Value Health.* 1999;2:308–318.

76. Movsas B, Scott C, Watkins-Bruner D. Pretreatment factors significantly influence quality of life in cancer patients: a Radiation Therapy Oncology Group (RTOG) analysis. *Int J Radiat Oncol Biol Phys.* 2006;65: 830–835.

77. Gil KM, Gibbons HE, Hopkins MP, et al. Baseline characteristics influencing quality of life in gynecologic cancer. *Health Qual Life Outcomes.* 2007;5:25–32.

78. Earle CC, Landrum MB, Souza JM, et al. Aggressiveness of cancer care near the end of life: is it a quality-of-care issue? *J Clin Oncol.* 2008;26:3860–3866.

79. von Gruenigen VE, Daly B, Gibbons HE, et al. Indicators of survival duration in ovarian cancer and implications for aggressiveness of care. *Cancer.* 2008;112(10):2221–2227.

80. Bruchim I, Biron-Shental T, Altaras MM, et al. Combination of endometrial thickness and time since menopause in predicting endometrial cancer in women with postmenopausal bleeding. *J Clin Ultrasound.* 2004;32(5):219–224.

81. van Doorn HC, Opmeer BC, Jitze Duk M, et al. The relation between age, time since menopause, and endometrial cancer in women with postmenopausal bleeding. *Int J Gynecol Cancer.* 2007;17(5):1118–1123.

82. Somoye G, Olaitan A, Mocroft A, et al. Age related trends in the incidence of endometrial cancer in South East England 1962–1997. *J Obstet Gynaecol.* 2005;25(1):35–38.

83. Olson JE, Sellers TA, Anderson KE, et al. Does a family history of cancer increase the risk for postmenopausal endometrial carcinoma? A prospective cohort study and a nested case-control family study of older women. *Cancer.* 1999;85(11):2444–2449.

84. Farley JH, Nycum LR, Birrer MJ, et al. Age-specific survival of women with endometrioid adenocarcinoma of the uterus. *Gynecol Oncol.* 2000;79(1):86–89.

85. Ueda SM, Kapp DS, Cheung MK. Trends in the demographics and clinical characteristics in women diagnosed with corpus cancer and their potential impact on the increasing number of deaths. *Am J Obstet Gynecol.* 2008;198(218): E1–E6.

86. Chan JK, Tian C, Monk BJ, et al. Gynecologic Oncology Group. Prognostic factors for high-risk early-stage epithelial ovarian cancer: a Gynecologic Oncology Group study. *Cancer.* 2008;112(10):2202–2210.

87. Calle EE, Rodriguez C, Walker-Thurmond K, et al. Overweight, obesity, and mortality from cancer in a prospectively studied cohort of U.S. adults. *N Engl J Med.* 2003;348:1625–1638.

88. Ahmed A, Zamba G, DeGeest K, et al. The impact of surgery on survival of elderly women with endometrial cancer in the SEER program from 1992–2002. *Gynecol Oncol.* 2008;111(1):35–40.

89. von Gruenigen VE, Tian C, Frasure H, et al. Treatment toxicity, disease recurrence and survival as related to obesity in women with early endometrial carcinoma: a Gynecologic Oncology Group study. *Cancer.* 2006;107:2786–2791.

90. Trimble EL, Kosary C, Park RC. Lymph node sampling and survival in endometrial cancer. *Gynecol Oncol.* 1998;71(3):340–343.

91. Chan JK, Lin YG, Monk BJ, et al. Vaginal hysterectomy as primary treatment of endometrial cancer in medically compromised women. *Obstet Gynecol.* 2001;97(5 Pt 1):707–711.

92. Susini T, Massi G, Amunni G, et al. Vaginal hysterectomy and abdominal hysterectomy for treatment of endometrial cancer in the elderly. *Gynecol Oncol.* 2005;96(2):362–367.

93. Nag S, Erickson B, Parikh S. The American Brachytherapy Society recommendations for high-dose-rate brachytherapy for carcinoma of the endometrium. *Int J Radiat Oncol Biol Phys.* 2000;48(3):779–790.

94. Fader AN, Michener CM, Giannios N, et al. Total laparoscopic hysterectomy versus laparoscopic-assisted vaginal hysterectomy in endometrial cancer: surgical and survival outcomes. *J Min Inv Gynecol.* 2009;16(3):333–339.

95. Gehrig PA, Cantrell LA, Shafer A, et al. What is the optimal minimally invasive surgical procedure for endometrial cancer staging in the obese and morbidly obese woman? *Gynecol Oncol.* 2008;111(1):41–45.

96. Boggess JF, Gehrig PA, Cantrell L, et al. A comparative study of 3 surgical methods for hysterectomy with staging for endometrial cancer: robotic assistance, laparoscopy, laparotomy. *Am J Obstet Gynecol.* 2008;199:360–362.

97. Seamon LG, Cohn DE, Richardson DL, et al. Robotic hysterectomy and pelvic-aortic lymphadenectomy for endometrial cancer. *Obstet Gynecol.* 2008;112:1207–1213.

98. Lachance JA, Everett EN, Greer B, et al. The effect of age on clinical/pathologic features, surgical morbidity, and outcome in patients with endometrial cancer. *Gynecol Oncol.* 2006;101(3): 470–475.

99. Truong PT, Kader HA, Lacy B, et al. The effects of age and comorbidity on treatment and outcomes

in women with endometrial cancer. *Am J Clin Oncol.* 2005;28(2):157–164.

100. Alektiar KM, Venkatraman E, Abu-Rustum, et al. Is endometrial carcinoma intrinsically more aggressive in elderly patients? *Cancer.* 2003;98(11):2368–2377.

101. Jolly S, Vargas CE, Kumar T, et al. The impact of age on long-term outcome in patients with endometrial cancer treated with postoperative radiation. *Gynecol Oncol.* 2006;103(1):87–93.

102. Creutzberg CL, van Putten WL, Warlam-Rodenhuis CC, et al. Outcome of high-risk stage IC, grade 3, compared with stage I endometrial carcinoma patients: the Postoperative Radiation Therapy in Endometrial Carcinoma Trial. *J Clin Oncol.* 2004;22(7):1234–1241.

103. Creutzberg CL, van Putten WL, Koper PC, et al. Surgery and postoperative radiotherapy versus surgery alone for patients with stage-1 endometrial carcinoma: multicentre randomised trial. PORTEC Study Group. Post Operative Radiation Therapy in Endometrial Carcinoma. *Lancet.* 2000;355(9213):1404–1411.

104. Keys HM, Roberts JA, Brunetto VL, et al. A phase III trial of surgery with or without adjunctive external pelvic radiation therapy in intermediate risk endometrial adenocarcinoma: a Gynecologic Oncology Group study. *Gynecol Oncol.* 2004;92(3):744–751.

105. Citron JR, Sutton H, Yamada SD, et al. Pathologic stage I-II endometrial carcinoma in the elderly: radiotherapy indications and outcome. *Int J Radiat Oncol Biol Phys.* 2004;59(5):1432–1438.

106. Alektiar KM, Venkatraman E, Chi DS, et al. Intravaginal brachytherapy alone for intermediate-risk endometrial cancer. *Int J Radiat Oncol Biol Phys.* 2005;62(1):111–117.

107. Fleming GF. Systemic chemotherapy for uterine carcinoma: metastatic and adjuvant. *J Clin Oncol.* 2007;25(20):2983–2990.

108. Alvarez Secord A, Havrilesky LJ, Bae-Jump V, et al. The role of multi-modality adjuvant chemotherapy and radiation in women with advanced stage endometrial cancer. *Gynecol Oncol.* 2007;107(2):285–291.

109. Goldberg H, Miller RC, Abdah-Bortnyak R, et al. Rare Cancer Network. Outcome after combined modality treatment for uterine papillary serous carcinoma: a study by the Rare Cancer Network (RCN). *Gynecol Oncol.* 2008;108(2):298–305.

110. Randall ME, Filiaci VL, Muss H, et al. Gynecologic Oncology Group Study. Randomized phase III trial of whole-abdominal irradiation versus doxorubicin and cisplatin chemotherapy in advanced endometrial carcinoma: a Gynecologic Oncology Group study. *J Clin Oncol.* 2006;24(1):36–44.

111. Arterburn DE, Crane PK, Sullivan SD. The coming epidemic of obesity in elderly Americans. *J Am Geriatr Soc.* 2004;52(11):1907–1912.

112. von Gruenigen VE, Frasure HE, Grandon M, et al. Impact of obesity and age on quality of life in gynecologic surgery. *Am J Obstet Gynecol.* 2005;193:1369–1375.

113. Everett E, Tamini H, Geer B, et al. The effect of body mass index on clinical/pathologic features, surgical morbidity, and outcome in patients with endometrial cancer. *Gynecol Oncol.* 2003;90:150–157.

114. Cassileth BR, Lusk EJ, Strouse TB, et al. Psychosocial status in chronic illness: a comparative analysis of six diagnostic groups. *N Engl J Med.* 1984;311(8):506–511.

115. von Gruenigen VE, Courneya K, Gibbons H, et al. Feasibility and effectiveness of a lifestyle intervention program in obese endometrial cancer patients: a randomized trial. *Gynecol Oncol.* 2008;109(1):19–26.

116. Larsson U, Karlsson J, Sullivan M. Impact of overweight and obesity on health-related quality of life: a Swedish population study. *Int J Obes Relat Metab Disord.* 2002;26(3):417–424.

117. Lopez-Garcia E, Banegas JR, Gutierrez-Fisac JL, et al. Relation between body weight and health-related quality of life among the elderly in Spain. *Int J Obes.* 2003;27:701–709.

118. Apovian CM, Frey CM, Wood GC, et al. Body mass index and physical function in older women. *Obes Res.* 2002;10:740–747.

119. Doll HA, Petersen SE, Stewart-Brown SL. Obesity and physical and emotional well-being: associations between body mass index, chronic illness and the physical and mental components of the SF-36 questionnaire. *Obes Res.* 2000;8(2):160–170.

120. Fontaine KR, Barofsk I, Andersen RE, et al. Impact of weight loss on health-related quality of life. *Qual Life Res.* 1999;8:275–277.

121. Hulens M, Vansant G, Claessens AL, et al. Health-related quality of life in physically active and sedentary obese women. *Am J Hum Biol.* 2002;14:777–785.

122. Hassan MK, Joshi AV, Madhavan SS, et al. Obesity and health-related quality of life: a cross-sectional analysis of the US population. *Int J Obes.* 2003;27:1227–1232.

123. Lutgendorf SK, Anderson B, Rothrock N, et al. Quality of life and mood in women receiving extensive chemotherapy for gynecologic cancer. *Cancer.* 2002;87:178–184.

124. Miller BE, Pittman B, Case D, et al. Quality of life after treatment for gynecologic malignancies: a pilot study in an outpatient clinic. *Gynecol Oncol.* 2002;87(2):178–184.

125. Chan YM, Ngan HY, Li BY, et al. A longitudinal study on quality of life after gynecologic cancer treatment. *Gynecol Oncol.* 2001;83(1):10–19.

126. Klee M, Machin D. Health-related quality of life of patients with endometrial cancer who are disease-free following external irradiation. *Acta Oncol.* 2001;40(7):816–824.

127. Li C, Samsioe G, Iosif C. Quality of life in endometrial cancer survivors. *Maturitas.* 1999;31(3):227–236.

128. van de Poll-Franse LV, Mols F, Essink-Bot ML, et al. Impact of external beam adjuvant radiotherapy on health-related quality of life for long-term survivors of endometrial adenocarcinoma: a population-based study. *Int J Radiat Oncol Biol Phys.* 2007;69(1):125–132.

129. Blanchard CM, Courneya KS, Stein K. Cancer survivors' adherence to lifestyle behavior recommendations and associations with health-related quality of life: results from the American Cancer Society's SCS-II. *J Clin Oncol.* 2008;26(13):2198–2204.

130. Moore DH, Kauderer JT, Bell J, et al. An assessment of age and other factors influencing protocol versus alternative treatments for patients with epithelial ovarian cancer referred to member institutions: a Gynecologic Oncology Group study. *Gynecol Oncol.* 2004;94:368–374.

Part 3 Management of hematologic malignancies in older adults

15 Management of myelodysplasia in older adults

Heidi D. Klepin and Bayard L. Powell

A. Introduction

The myelodysplastic syndromes (MDSs) encompass a heterogenous group of clonal hematopoietic disorders characterized by ineffective hematopoiesis, peripheral blood cytopenias, and typically, hypercellularity of the bone marrow. In these diseases, cells of the affected lineage are unable to undergo maturation and differentiation, resulting in cytopenias. The major clinical significance of these disorders is the morbidity associated with profound cytopenias and the potential to evolve into acute myelogenous leukemia (AML). The natural history of MDS varies widely from indolent to rapidly progressive disease. Understanding of the underlying molecular and cellular defects continues to evolve along with the availability of treatments for this complex group of disorders.

B. Epidemiology

MDSs are clearly diseases of aging patients, with a median age at diagnosis of 76 years.[1] Over 80 percent of MDS cases reported to the Surveillance, Epidemiology, and End Results (SEER) program between 2001 and 2003 were diagnosed in individuals 60 years of age or older (Figure 15.1).[1] The incidence of MDS has only recently been recorded by the SEER registry, with 10,300 incident cases diagnosed in 2003. About two-thirds of patients with MDS are elderly males. Unfortunately, survival for MDS has been poor, with a reported 3-year overall survival rate of 35 percent.[1] The incidence of these disorders is likely to rise with the aging of the U.S. population, making this an increasingly important public health concern.

The predominant risk factor associated with MDS is advanced age. The majority of patients diagnosed with MDS have no other known predisposing factor. Exposures that have been associated with subsequent development of MDS include chemotherapy, radiation, agricultural chemicals (i.e., pesticides), solvents, and tobacco smoking.[2] Of these, exposure to alkylating agent

chemotherapy (i.e., melphalan) has been most well defined. Alkylating agent–associated MDS typically presents within 5–7 years after exposure and is associated with abnormalities in chromosomes 5 and 7.[3]

C. Diagnosis

Diagnosis of MDS relies mainly on peripheral blood and bone marrow findings. The diagnosis should be suspected in individuals presenting with cytopenia. In clinical studies, the majority of patients have a hemoglobin of less than 11, a platelet count less than 100,000, and an absolute neutrophil count less than 1,000 at the time of diagnosis. However, careful attention should be paid to consistent decreases in blood counts over time in an older adult, which may signify early-developing MDS. A frequent presentation can be progressive macrocytic anemia in an older adult. Many patients are asymptomatic at the time of diagnosis. However, careful history taking should include questions regarding recurrent infections, bruising, bleeding, duration of cytopenia, and need for red cell transfusion. The differential diagnosis for suspected MDS includes AML, aplastic anemia, megaloblastic anemia (B_{12} and folate deficiency), copper deficiency, viral infections (HIV), large granular lymphocytic leukemia, paroxysmal nocturnal hemoglobinuria, and heavy-metal poisoning.

The initial serologic workup includes a complete blood count with differential, reticulocyte count, red blood cell folate, serum B12, iron studies, and review of the peripheral smear. Classic peripheral blood findings associated with MDSs include macrocytosis and hypogranular, hypolobated neutrophils (pseudo-Pelger-Huët anomaly).

A bone marrow biopsy with cytogenetic analysis is required to confirm the diagnosis. The bone marrow is typically hypercellular and demonstrates evidence of dysplasia. Morphologic analysis also provides information on the percentage

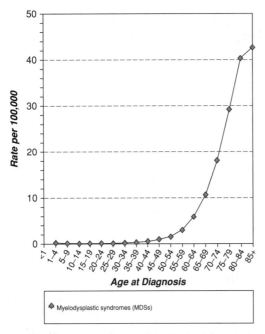

Rate per 100,000

Age at Diagnosis

◆ Myelodysplastic syndromes (MDSs)

Figure 15.1 Age-specific Surveillance, Epidemiology, and End Results incidence rate for myelodysplastic syndrome, 2001–2003 (http://seer.cancer.gov/).

of myeloblasts in the marrow. Cytogenetic abnormalities play a critical role in the diagnosis and prognosis of MDS. Clonal chromosomal abnormalities can be detected in approximately 50 percent of patients with MDS.[4,5] Common cytogenetic abnormalities involve chromosomes 5, 7, 8, or 20. Deletions of chromosomes 5 or 7 are characteristic of therapy-related MDS caused by alkylating agents or radiation exposure. Diagnosis of certain MDS subtypes (such as the 5q– syndrome) is entirely dependent on detection of specific cytogenetic abnormalities. Cytogenetic testing, therefore, should be performed as part of bone marrow evaluation in all patients with suspected MDS to enhance diagnosis and inform treatment options as well as prognosis.

D. Classification

The classification of MDS has evolved over the past 10 years. In 1982, the French-American-British (FAB) Cooperative Group established a classification system with five diagnostic categories based on peripheral blood and bone marrow characteristics. These include refractory anemia (RA), RA with ring sideroblasts (RARS), RA with excess blasts (RAEB), RAEB in transformation (RAEBT), and chronic myelomonocytic leukemia (CMML).

A more recent classification scheme was proposed and updated by the World Health Organi-

zation (WHO) that incorporates evolving knowledge of the biology of disease, including the significance of cytogenetic abnormalities. This classification scheme is presented in Table 15.1 and better reflects the heterogeneity of MDS. There are several important differences between the FAB and WHO classifications. The WHO classification defines over 20 percent blasts (RAEBT) as AML; defines CMML as a myelodysplastic/myeloproliferative disease; and adds new categories of MDS such as the 5q– syndrome.

E. Prognosis

The natural history of patients with MDS is quite variable and can range from a chronic relatively indolent disease to an acute fulminant and progressive process. It is well established that mutagen-induced MDS is associated with a poor prognosis and that increased age is also a negative prognostic factor. However, the heterogeneity of this disease has complicated accurate prognostication in de novo MDS.

The International Prognostic Scoring System (IPSS) (Table 15.2) was developed to risk-stratify patients at the time of diagnosis based on cytogenetic, morphologic, and clinical data. The IPSS for MDS was developed based on an analysis of 816 patients that demonstrated that specific cytogenetic abnormalities, the percentage of blasts in the bone marrow, and the number of hematopoietic lineages involved in the cytopenia were the most important variables in disease outcome.[6] Risk scores are determined based on these variables, and a categorization of low risk, intermediate-1, intermediate-2, and high risk is assigned (Table 15.3). The IPSS has demonstrated improved prognostic discrimination over earlier classification schemes and has been incorporated into clinical practice and subsequent trial design.[7]

There are multiple known prognostic factors not included in the IPSS classification. For example, chronologic age is not incorporated into the IPSS score. The prognostic impact of increasing age, however, differs by IPSS risk group (Table 15.4). In the analysis by Greenberg and colleagues reported on earlier, survival for high-risk patients was independent of age. This suggests that survival was driven primarily by tumor biology in these patients.[6] Survival for low-risk patients was strongly dependent on age, with median survival of 9.0 years versus 3.9 years for age groups under 70 and 70 and older, respectively. These findings

Table 15.1 World Health Organization classification of peripheral blood and bone marrow findings in myelodysplastic syndromes.

Disease	Blood findings	Bone marrow findings
Refractory cytopenias with unilineage dysplasia (RCUD) Refractory anemia Refractory neutropenia Refractory thrombocytopenia	Unicytopenia or bicytopenia No or rare blasts	Dysplasia in ≤10% of cells in one myeloid lineage <5% blasts <15% ringed sideroblasts
Refractory anemia with ringed sideroblasts (RARS)	Anemia No blasts	≥15% ringed sideroblasts Erythroid dysplasia only <5% blasts
Refractory cytopenia with multilineage dysplasia (RCMD)	Cytopenias No or rare blasts (<1%) No Auer rods <1 × 10^9/L monocytes	Dysplasia in ≥10% of the cells of two or more myeloid cell lines <5% blasts in marrow No Auer rods ±15% ringed sideroblasts
Refractory anemia with excess blasts-1 (RAEB-1)	Cytopenias <5% blasts No Auer rods <1 × 10^9/L monocytes	Unilineage or multilineage dysplasia 5–9% blasts No Auer rods
Refractory anemia with excess blasts-2 (RAEB-2)	Cytopenias 5–19% blasts Auer rods ± <1 × 10^9/L monocytes	Unilineage or multilineage dysplasia 10–19% blasts Auer rods ±
Myelodysplastic syndrome-unclassified (MDS-U)	Cytopenias ≤1% blasts	Dysplasia <10% of cells in one or more myeloid cell lines accompanied by a cytogenetic abnormality that is characteristic for MDS <5% blasts
MDS associated with isolated del (5q)	Anemia Usually normal or increased platelet count <1% blasts	Normal to increased megakaryocytes with hypolobated nuclei <5% blasts Isolated del (5q) cytogenetic abnormality No Auer rods

Note. Adapted from Brunning et al.[34]

suggest that additional factors such as comorbid disease may influence survival in the setting of more indolent MDS.

There are several limitations to the IPSS classification system: (1) it does not account for duration of disease, (2) subjects who received prior therapy or had secondary MDS were excluded, and (3) it does not account for performance status or comorbid disease. Additional classification schemes are being developed that include

Table 15.2 International Prognostic Scoring System (IPSS) for myelodysplastic syndromes (MDSs).

Prognostic variable	Score value				
	0	0.5	1.0	1.5	2.0
Bone marrow blasts (%)	<5	5–10	–	11–20	21–30
Karyotype[a]	Good	Intermediate	Poor	–	–
Cytopenias	0/1	2/3	–	–	–

Note. This research was originally published by Greenberg et al.[6]
[a]Karyotype definitions are as follows: good risk – normal, –Y, del (5q), del (20q); poor risk – ≥ 3 abnormalities, abnormal chromosome 7; intermediate risk – all other abnormalities.

Table 15.3 Median survival by IPSS category for MDS.

IPSS risk category	Overall score	Median survival (years)
Low	0	5.7
Intermediate-1	0.5–1.0	3.5
Intermediate-2	1.5–2.0	1.2
High	≥2.5	0.4

Note. This research was originally published by Greenberg et al.[6]

prognostic factors such as poor performance status, older age, prior transfusions, and time elapsed from diagnosis.[8-10]

F. Treatment

There are few effective therapies for MDS. However, treatment strategies have been evolving in recent years to target higher-risk MDS and subgroups defined by specific cytogenetic abnormalities. Treatment goals for MDS therapy include managing cytopenias, improving quality of life, decreasing progression to AML, and improving overall survival. In 2000, the International Working Group (IWG) developed standardized response criteria to be used in clinical trials with a focus on each of these goals.[11,12] These response criteria provided specific definitions of multiple outcomes such as remission, relapse, survival, cytogenetic response, and hematologic improvement. Adaptation of these measures in clinical trials provides a mechanism for comparison of investigational treatments.

Current treatment recommendations for MDS involve a risk-adapted therapeutic approach and continue to evolve. In general, the National Comprehensive Cancer Center (NCCN) guidelines recommend classifying patients into relatively low risk (IPSS low or intermediate-1 categories) and higher risk (IPSS intermediate-2 and high)

Table 15.4 Age-related median survival in years within IPSS group.

	Age < 70 years	Age ≥ 70 years
IPSS risk category		
Low	9.0	3.9
Intermediate-1	4.4	2.4
Intermediate-2	1.3	1.2
High	0.4	0.4

Note. This research was originally published by Greenberg et al.[6]

categories.[7] Supportive care aimed at controlling symptoms related to cytopenias is the mainstay of treatment for low-risk patients.

F.1. Supportive care

Supportive care with red cell and platelet transfusions and antibiotics for infection has long been considered standard therapy for most patients with MDS. Hematopoietic growth factors such as recombinant erythropoietin (epoetin alpha) are also used to try to minimize transfusion requirements in responding patients. Patients with symptomatic anemia, normal cytogenetics, and a serum erythropoietin level under 500 U/L may benefit from epoetin alpha or a longer-acting darbepoetin alfa. Response rates in studies using the IWG criteria are approximately 50 percent (major response is defined by a hemoglobin increase over 2 g/dL or transfusion independence; minor response is defined by a hemoglobin increase of 1–2 g/dL or 50% reduction for transfusion-dependent patients).[13] Overall response rates appear similar for both agents.[13] Small studies have suggested that granulocyte colony stimulating factor (G-CSF) has a synergistic effect in combination with epoetin for treatment of anemia.[14-16] Low-dose G-CSF dosed three times per week can be added to erythropoietin if response is inadequate to epoetin alone.[17] Responses in hemoglobin levels are typically evident within 6–8 weeks of treatment. Ongoing treatment is not indicated if no response is detected during this time period.

Overall, in selected patients, use of growth factors for symptomatic anemia has been associated with improved quality of life and decreased transfusion requirement without increased risk of progression to AML.[15,18,19] Patients most likely to respond to use of erythropoietin are those with IPSS scores of low/intermediate-1, serum erythropoietin levels less than 500, and transfusion requirements of less than 2 units of red cells per month.[18] The NCCN recommends a target hemoglobin of 12 g/dL or less. To date, there are no randomized clinical trial data to support a survival benefit with use of these agents in MDS, so the rationale for treatment is symptom management and quality of life.

Over time, most patients become transfusion-dependent, increasing the risk of iron overload. Secondary iron overload negatively affects survival in transfusion-dependent patients.[20] The mechanism linking transfusional iron overload and decreased survival in MDS is not yet clear.

However, iron overload has been associated with damage to the heart, liver, and endocrine glands.[21] Current consensus guidelines recommend iron chelation therapy for those patients most likely to suffer negative consequences from chronic iron overload.[22,23] At-risk patients include those with lower-risk MDS, ongoing transfusion dependence, and anticipated survival of greater than 1 year. Presence of cardiac or hepatic dysfunction should also be considered. In this setting, the NCCN recommends initiation of iron chelation therapy after 20–30 units of red cells have been transfused or the serum ferritin is over 2,500 mcg/L. Serum ferritin can be used to monitor efficacy of chelation with goal ferritin under 1,000 mcg/L on treatment. Chelation agents include deferoxamine or the oral agent deferasirox.[24]

F.2. Chemotherapy

Patients in the higher-risk IPSS categories are more likely to experience morbidity related to cytopenias and to progress to acute leukemia in a shorter time interval from diagnosis. For patients who present with high-risk disease or show evidence of progression to high-risk disease during follow-up, treatment with low-intensity chemotherapy should be considered. The low-intensity chemotherapeutic agents that have demonstrated efficacy in the treatment of MDS are the hypomethylating agents 5-azacytidine and decitabine.

The first chemotherapy agent to demonstrate efficacy in treatment of MDS was 5-azacytidine. A randomized controlled trial of 191 patients conducted by the national cooperative group Cancer and Leukemia Group B (CALGB) comparing treatment with 5-azacytidine to supportive care alone for high-risk MDS demonstrated significant improvements in response time to AML progression, and survival.[25] Patients included in this trial had higher-risk MDS. Eligible patients (median age 68 years) met FAB classification criteria for MDS; patients with RA or RARS met additional criteria of significant marrow dysfunction. The 5-azacitidine was administered at a dose of 75 mg/m^2 for 7 consecutive days on a 28-day cycle. The response rate (complete and partial) was 23 percent in the treatment arm, with median time to leukemic progression of 21 versus 13 months for supportive care ($p = .007$). There was no significant overall survival benefit seen in this study, although this analysis was complicated by the fact

that patients receiving supportive care were permitted to cross over to active treatment during the study. In an effort to eliminate the confounding effect of treatment crossover, a survival analysis was performed from a 6-month landmark date. The three subgroups evaluated included patients receiving supportive care who either never crossed over or crossed over after 6 months, patients receiving supportive care who crossed over before 6 months, and patients initially randomized to 5-azacitidine. The median survival (after the 6-month landmark date) for the three groups was 11, 14, and 18 months, respectively.

Of importance, this study also evaluated quality-of-life outcomes.[26] Treatment with 5-azacitidine in this population was associated with statistically significant improvement in fatigue, dyspnea, self-reported physical functioning, and psychological distress. Quality-of-life differences were maintained after controlling for the number of transfusions received. The improvements in both disease-related outcomes and quality of life established the use of 5-azacitidine as a standard of care for treatment of high-risk MDS. Another randomized controlled international trial of 358 patients confirmed an overall survival benefit favoring 5-azacitidine over physician-directed conventional care (supportive care, 58.7%; low-dose cytarabine, 27.3%; or intensive chemotherapy, 14%).[27]

On the basis of treatment experience from these randomized studies, it is generally recommended to treat for approximately four to six cycles, if tolerated, to determine response for individual patients. In the CALGB study, treatment was continued for three cycles after achieving complete remission or for as long as a treatment benefit persisted in patients with a lesser response.

The U.S. Food and Drug Administration has also approved decitabine, a second pyrimidine nucleoside analog of cytidine that inhibits DNA methylation for the treatment of higher-risk MDS. A randomized study of 170 patients (median age 70 years) compared decitabine versus supportive care for patients who met FAB classification for MDS and had an IPSS score of 0.5 or higher.[28] The dose schedule was 15 mg/m^2 given intravenously every 8 hours for 3 days on a 6-week cycle. Patients treated with decitabine had a 17 percent overall response rate (complete and partial) with an additional 13 percent demonstrating hematologic improvement. Patients with intermediate-2 or high-risk disease by IPSS classification demonstrated improvement in progression to AML (12 vs. 6.8 months). In this study, the median number of treatment cycles administered was three (range 0–9) with responding patients receiving a median of six cycles (range 2–8). Temporary dose reduction or delay was required in 35 percent of patients on treatment. Evaluation of quality of life demonstrated improvements in global health status, fatigue, and dyspnea, favoring active treatment.

A follow-up randomized study evaluated different treatment dosing schedules of decitabine.[29] In this study, 95 patients were randomized to one of three schedules given every 4 weeks: (1) 20 mg/m^2 intravenously daily for 5 days; (2) 20 mg/m^2 subcutaneously daily for 5 days; or (3) 10 mg/m^2 intravenously daily for 10 days. The 5-day intravenous schedule that had the highest dose intensity was determined to be optimal with a response rate of 39 percent compared with 21 percent and 24 percent, respectively ($p < .05$). This dosing schedule is convenient for outpatient treatment and has become an acceptable option in clinical practice. At the present time, there are no randomized clinical trial data that compare decitabine directly to 5-azacitidine. These agents are generally considered to be similar in efficacy. Current evidence would suggest that the patients most likely to benefit from these agents are those with intermediate-2 or high-risk classification by IPSS.

Though these medications are associated with toxicity, they represent the mainstay of treatment for older adults with higher-risk MDS who have a good performance status. The primary toxicity seen is myelosuppression. Often cytopenias will worsen in the first few months of treatment prior to demonstrating evidence of response.[25] Consequences of myelosuppression can be managed in older adults with temporary increased use of transfusion support, growth factor support, and prophylactic antibiotics for neutropenia. Higher-intensity therapy such as standard allogeneic transplantation, to date the only curative therapy for MDS, is generally restricted to younger adults with acceptable donors because of the high morbidity and mortality associated with the therapy itself.

F.3. Biologic therapy

Treatment options have expanded for patients with MDS associated with chromosome 5q deletion. The 5q– syndrome is a specific MDS subset defined by deletion of the long arm of chromosome 5 as the sole abnormality without excess bone marrow blasts. The 5q– syndrome typically manifests as refractory anemia, often with normal or even increased platelet counts, and is considered a more favorable MDS subset because a large percentage of patients do not progress to acute leukemia.[30] Lenalidomide, an oral immunomodulatory drug, has demonstrated efficacy in this setting. In a phase II clinical trial of 148 patients, significant decrease in transfusion requirements and reversal of cytogenetic abnormalities were demonstrated.[31] Eligible patients met FAB criteria for MDS, had a chromosome 5q31 deletion that was either in isolation or combined with additional cytogenetic abnormalities, low or intermediate-1 IPSS score, and transfusion-dependent anemia. The majority of patients (64%) had isolated 5q deletion. Lenalidomide was dosed 10 mg daily orally for 21 days of a 4-week cycle. Transfusion independence was achieved in 67 percent of participants. Median time to response was rapid at 4.6 weeks. A substantial proportion of evaluable patients also had cytogenetic improvement, including complete cytogenetic remission. The primary toxicity in this study was myelosuppression with neutropenia and thrombocytopenia. This typically occurred within the first 8 weeks of treatment. Dose adjustment was required in 84 percent of patients. This drug has become the standard of care for treatment of transfusion-dependent, lower-risk patients with chromosome 5q deletion and reinforces the clinical and therapeutic importance of cytogenetic evaluation in MDS.

G. Unresolved issues for the aging patient

Despite recent advances in pharmacologic treatment options, there are unresolved clinical questions related to the treatment of older adults with MDS. One major issue is patient selection. Clinical trials in MDS have included a substantial number of older adults. However, most studies included only patients with Eastern Cooperative Oncology Group (ECOG) performance scores of 0–2.[25,28] Many older adults with MDS in clinical practice present with impaired performance status. It is unclear if the beneficial results seen in clinical trials can be extrapolated to older adults with impaired performance status. This results in a substantial proportion of older adults for whom there is no evidence-based treatment recommendation.

Clinical experience suggests that some older adults with poor performance status may benefit from low-intensity chemotherapy, particularly those whose functional decline was related to disease progression. Alternatively, some older adults with impaired functional status may experience increased morbidity with active treatment. The interaction between the presence of specific comorbidities and treatment benefit has also been understudied and remains a concern during treatment decision-making for this population. Clinical trials are needed that target older adults with impaired performance status with a focus on both disease-specific outcomes and quality of life. In addition, patient-selection algorithms specific to the older adult need to be tested to help identify which patient-specific factors are the most important determinants of treatment benefit and morbidity.

Another issue for treatment of MDS in older adults is the balance between ongoing maintenance therapy for disease control and quality of life. Optimal duration of treatment for high-risk patients who respond to hypomethylating agents is unclear. Studies would suggest continuing treatment until intolerance or progression. Over time, many older adults can develop increased toxicity and decline in functional status because of ongoing treatment. The impact of continuous treatment versus sequential treatment strategies on disease control and quality of life is unclear. Planned sequential treatment strategies might offer the benefit of disease control with intermittent time off therapy to maximize quality of life.

H. Future directions

There are multiple new therapeutic approaches for MDS under investigation. There is an increasing focus on development of targeted therapies that is informed by improved understanding of biologic mechanisms underlying the heterogeneity of MDS. Future treatment algorithms will likely differentiate specific disease subtypes, such as the 5q− syndrome, that are susceptible to targeted therapeutic approaches. Combining novel agents with hypomethylating agents to improve efficacy is another investigational approach. Finally, improved patient-assessment strategies will help identify which older patients with high-risk MDS may benefit from more aggressive treatment approaches such as reduced-intensity allogeneic transplantation.[32,33]

I. Conclusions

MDS represents a heterogeneous group of disorders of variable natural history. Older adults represent the majority of patients diagnosed with MDS and will continue to increase in number with the aging of the population. Treatment goals include managing cytopenias, improving quality of life, decreasing progression to AML, and improving overall survival. Current treatment recommendations involve a risk-adapted approach ranging from supportive care in lower-risk patients to low-intensity therapy with hypomethylating agents in higher-risk disease. Current risk-stratification tools, such as the IPSS classification, are useful for prognostication. However, additional patient-specific characteristics, such as comorbidity and functional status, need to be studied in the context of active treatment to guide decision making for many older adults with MDS. Future trials will attempt to identify additional targets for directed therapies as well as combination therapy that will improve both survival and quality of life for older adults.

References

1. Ma X, Does M, Raza A, et al. Myelodysplastic syndromes: incidence and survival in the United States. *Cancer.* 2007;109:1536–1542.

2. Strom SS, Gu Y, Gruschkus SK, et al. Risk factors of myelodysplastic syndromes: a case-control study. *Leukemia.* 2005;19:1912–1918.

3. Kantarjian HM, Keating MJ, Walters RS, et al. Therapy-related leukemia and myelodysplastic syndrome: clinical, cytogenetic, and prognostic features. *J Clin Oncol.* 1986;4:1748–1757.

4. Haase D, Germing U, Schanz J, et al. New insights into the prognostic impact of the karyotype in MDS and correlation with subtypes: evidence from a core dataset of 2124 patients. *Blood.* 2007;110:4385–4395.

5. Pozdnyakova O, Miron PM, Tang G, et al. Cytogenetic abnormalities in a series of 1,029 patients with primary myelodysplastic syndromes: a report from the US with a focus on some undefined single chromosomal abnormalities. *Cancer.* 2008;113:3331–3340.

6. Greenberg P, Cox C, LeBeau MM, et al. International scoring system for evaluating prognosis in myelodysplastic syndromes. *Blood.* 1997;89:2079–2088.

7. Greenberg PL, Baer MR, Bennett JM, et al. Myelodysplastic syndromes clinical practice guidelines in oncology. *J Natl Compr Canc Netw.* 2006;4:58–77.

8. Bernasconi P, Klersy C, Boni M, et al. World Health Organization classification in combination with cytogenetic markers improves the prognostic stratification of patients with de novo primary myelodysplastic syndromes. *Br J Haematol.* 2007;137:193–205.

9. Kantarjian H, O'Brien S, Ravandi F, et al. Proposal for a new risk model in myelodysplastic syndrome that accounts for events not considered in the original International Prognostic Scoring System. *Cancer.* 2008;113:1351–1361.

10. Malcovati L, Germing U, Kuendgen A, et al. Time-dependent prognostic scoring system for predicting survival and leukemic evolution in myelodysplastic syndromes. *J Clin Oncol.* 2007;25:3503–3510.

11. Cheson BD, Bennett JM, Kantarjian H, et al. Report of an international working group to standardize response criteria for myelodysplastic syndromes. *Blood.* 2000;96:3671–3674.

12. Cheson BD, Greenberg PL, Bennett JM, et al. Clinical application and proposal for modification of the International Working Group (IWG) response criteria in myelodysplasia. *Blood.* 2006;108:419–425.

13. Moyo V, Lefebvre P, Duh MS, et al. Erythropoiesis-stimulating agents in the treatment of anemia in myelodysplastic syndromes: a meta-analysis. *Ann Hematol.* 2008;87:527–536.

14. Balleari E, Rossi E, Clavio M, et al. Erythropoietin plus granulocyte colony-stimulating factor is better than erythropoietin alone to treat anemia in low-risk myelodysplastic syndromes: results from a randomized single-centre study. *Ann Hematol.* 2006;85:174–180.

15. Jadersten M, Malcovati L, Dybedal I, et al. Erythropoietin and granulocyte-colony stimulating factor treatment associated with improved survival in myelodysplastic syndrome. *J Clin Oncol.* 2008;26:3607–3613.

16. Negrin RS, Stein R, Doherty K, et al. Maintenance treatment of the anemia of myelodysplastic syndromes with recombinant human granulocyte colony-stimulating factor and erythropoietin: evidence for in vivo synergy. *Blood.* 1996;87:4076–4081.

17. Casadevall N, Durieux P, Dubois S, et al. Health, economic, and quality-of-life effects of erythropoietin and granulocyte colony-stimulating factor for the treatment of myelodysplastic syndromes: a randomized, controlled trial. *Blood.* 2004;104:321–327.

18. Hellstrom-Lindberg E, Gulbrandsen N, Lindberg G, et al. A validated decision model for treating the anaemia of myelodysplastic syndromes with erythropoietin + granulocyte colony-stimulating factor: significant effects on quality of life. *Br J Haematol.* 2003;120:1037–1046.

19. Jadersten M, Montgomery SM, Dybedal I, et al. Long-term outcome of treatment of anemia in MDS with erythropoietin and G-CSF. *Blood.* 2005;106:803–811.

20. Malcovati L, Porta MG, Pascutto C, et al. Prognostic factors and life expectancy in myelodysplastic syndromes classified according to WHO criteria: a basis for clinical decision making. *J Clin Oncol.* 2005;23:7594–7603.

21. Andrews NC. Disorders of iron metabolism. *N Engl J Med.* 1999;341:1986–1995.

22. Bennett JM. Consensus statement on iron overload in myelodysplastic syndromes. *Am J Hematol.* 2008;83:858–861.

23. Gattermann N. Overview of guidelines on iron chelation therapy in patients with myelodysplastic syndromes and transfusional iron overload. *Int J Hematol.* 2008;88:24–29.

24. Metzgeroth G, Dinter D, Schultheis B, et al. Deferasirox in MDS patients with transfusion-caused iron overload – a phase-II study. *Ann Hematol.* 2009;88:301–310.

25. Silverman LR, Demakos EP, Peterson BL, et al. Randomized controlled trial of azacitidine in patients with the myelodysplastic syndrome: a study of the cancer and leukemia group B. *J Clin Oncol.* 2002;20:2429–2440.

26. Kornblith AB, Herndon JE, Silverman LR, et al. Impact of azacytidine on the quality of life of patients with myelodysplastic syndrome treated in a randomized phase III trial: a Cancer and Leukemia Group B study. *J Clin Oncol.* 2002;20:2441–2452.

27. Fenaux P, Mufti GJ, Hellstrom-Lindberg E, et al. Efficacy of azacitidine compared with that of conventional care regimens in the treatment of higher-risk myelodysplastic syndromes: a randomised, open-label, phase III study. *Lancet Oncol.* 2009;10:223–232.

28. Kantarjian H, Issa JP, Rosenfeld CS, et al. Decitabine improves patient outcomes in myelodysplastic syndromes: results of a phase III randomized study. *Cancer.* 2006;106:1794–1803.

29. Kantarjian H, Oki Y, Garcia-Manero G, et al. Results of a randomized study of 3 schedules of low-dose decitabine in higher-risk myelodysplastic syndrome and chronic myelomonocytic leukemia. *Blood.* 2007; 109:52–57.

30. Kelaidi C, Eclache V, Fenaux P. The role of lenalidomide in the management of myelodysplasia with del 5q. *Br J Haematol.* 2008;140:267–278.

31. List A, Dewald G, Bennett J, et al. Lenalidomide in the myelodysplastic syndrome with chromosome 5q deletion. *N Engl J Med.* 2006;355:1456–1465.

32. Estey E, de Lima M, Tibes R, et al. Prospective feasibility analysis of reduced-intensity conditioning (RIC) regimens for hematopoietic stem cell transplantation (HSCT) in elderly patients with acute myeloid leukemia (AML) and high-risk myelodysplastic syndrome (MDS). *Blood.* 2007;109:1395–1400.

33. Lubbert M, Bertz H, Ruter B, et al. Non-intensive treatment with low-dose 5-aza-2′-deoxycytidine (DAC) prior to allogeneic blood SCT of older MDS/AML patients. *Bone Marrow Transplant.* 2009;44(9):585–588.

34. Brunning R, et al. *Tumours of Hematopoietic and Lymphoid Tissues.* Geneva: World Health Organization; 2008.

Management of chronic leukemia in older adults

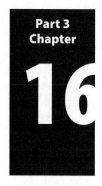

Martha Wadleigh and Richard Maury Stone

The approach to the older patient with chronic leukemia in many ways is no different from that of the younger patient. Treatment options are tailored to the goals of therapy as well as to the functional capacity of the patient. In recent years, there has been an expansion of treatment options with targeted therapy, antibody therapy, and reduced-intensity stem cell transplant that improves the balance between efficacy and tolerability. This chapter will focus on the more common disorders of chronic myelogenous leukemia (CML) and chronic lymphocytic leukemia (CLL) and the management of these disorders as it relates to the older patient.

A. Chronic myelogenous leukemia

A.1. Clinical features and epidemiology

CML is a clonal hematopoietic neoplasm originating in the pluripotent stem cell of the bone marrow and characterized by the Philadelphia chromosome. CML has a worldwide annual incidence of one to two cases per 100,000 people. It occurs in all age groups with a median age of diagnosis in the fifth and sixth decades of life and with a slight male predominance. Of note, patients over age 60 years account for a total of 60 percent of all cases.[1] The majority of patients are diagnosed while in the chronic phase, and almost half of patients will be asymptomatic at the time of diagnosis. Common signs and symptoms at presentation include fatigue, weight loss, night sweats, splenomegaly, and anemia.

Morphologically, CML is characterized by leukocytosis and/or thrombocytosis in the peripheral blood, often with basophilia and eosinophilia. Granulocytes are typically mature, though there is a spectrum of immaturity in the peripheral blood with usually less than 5 percent blasts. An absolute monocytosis may be present, but the overall percentage is usually less than 3 percent. At diagnosis, the bone marrow is hypercellular with an increased myeloid-to-erythroid ratio. In chronic

phase, blasts account for less than 5 percent of the marrow cellularity. Megakaryocytes may be increased and morphologically are smaller than normal and have hypolobated nuclei. Reticulin fibrosis is found in one-third of newly diagnosed patients and correlates with increased megakaryocytes and a larger spleen.[2,3]

Historically (preimatinib era) after a median of 5 years or so, CML typically progresses from chronic phase (CP) to an accelerated phase (AP) and eventually to blast crisis (BC), which can be either myeloid or lymphoid in lineage.[4] There are different definitions and criteria for AP. The World Health Organization (WHO)[5] defines AP by the presence of any one of the following: (1) persistent or increasing white blood cell count ($>10 \times 10$/L) and/or persistent or increasing splenomegaly unresponsive to therapy, (2) persistent thrombocytosis ($>1000 \times 10^9$/L) uncontrolled by therapy, (3) persistent thrombocytopenia ($<100 \times 10^9$/L) unrelated to therapy, (4) clonal cytogenetic evolution occurring after the initial diagnostic karyotype, (5) 20 percent or more basophils in the peripheral blood, and (6) 10–19 percent myeloblasts in the blood or bone marrow. Blast phase is diagnosed when blasts are 20 percent or more in the blood and/or bone marrow or when there is an extramedullary blast population or granulocytic sarcoma.

A.2. Molecular biology

Although initially described in the middle of the nineteenth century, CML was not well understood until 1960, when Nowell and Hungerford detected the recurrent chromosomal abnormality, later called the Philadelphia chromosome, that is the hallmark of this disease. It was later recognized that the Philadelphia chromosome resulted from the t(9;22) translocation,[6] involving the breakpoint cluster region (BCR) on chromosome 22 and the ABL kinase on chromosome 9, leading to the BCR-ABL fusion gene.[7] Critical experiments using murine models have demonstrated the oncogenic potential of the BCR-ABL gene.[8,9] Of importance, BCR-ABL is a constitutively active cytoplasmic tyrosine kinase that activates downstream kinases that prevent apoptosis among other functions. Understanding how this gene works has been key to the development of targeted therapy in this disease.

A.3. Diagnosis

The presence of the Philadelphia chromosome by cytogenetic analysis or the BCR-ABL by fluorescent in situ hybridization (FISH) or polymerase chain reaction (PCR) on the peripheral blood can establish the diagnosis of CML. Although not necessary to establish the diagnosis of CML, a bone marrow biopsy and aspirate done at the time of diagnosis is useful and recommended to determine phase of disease at presentation (which has treatment implications) as well as to assess for other cytogenetic abnormalities that may have prognostic implications.

A.4. Treatment

Treatment options for patients aged over 60 years have greatly expanded over the past decade with the advent of reduced-intensity stem cell transplantation and the orally available tyrosine kinase inhibitors imatinib, dasatinib, and nilotinib, which target the BCR-ABL gene. Historically, treatment for CML was not targeted to BCR-ABL. Initially, radiotherapy was used, followed by cytoreductive agents such as busulfan and hydroxyurea, which controlled blood counts but did little to target the molecular pathogenesis of the disease or affect overall survival. Interferon alpha, introduced in the 1980s, was the first agent to eradicate the Philadelphia chromosome, at least in a subset of patients. With imatinib mesylate and the second-generation tyrosine kinase inhibitors, the treatment paradigm has shifted to one of targeted therapy.

A.5. Imatinib mesylate in chronic phase disease

Imatinib mesylate is an orally available tyrosine kinase inhibitor that has relative selectivity for the BCR-ABL tyrosine kinase. Phase I[10] and II[11] trials using this drug in patients intolerant or resistant to interferon therapy demonstrated hematologic responses in 95 percent of patients, with complete cytogenetic responses in more than 40 percent of patients in CP at doses of 400 mg/d. No maximum tolerated dose was determined in the dose-escalation study; however, most responses and inhibition of BCR-ABL were seen at doses of over 300 mg, so 400 mg/d was chosen as the standard starting dose. Of importance, imatinib demonstrated a low toxicity profile in these early studies.

The International Randomized Study of Interferon (IRIS) plus Ara-C vs. STI571 in Chronic Myeloid Leukemia trial,[12] a prospective randomized phase III trial comparing imatinib 400 mg daily to the combination of interferon alpha and cytarabine in previously untreated chronic phase, established imatinib as the best initial treatment for newly diagnosed CML. After a median follow-up of 19 months, the estimated hematologic, major cytogenetic remission, and complete cytogenetic remission were superior in the imatinib-treated group compared to the combination-therapy arm (Table 16.1). At 18 months, the estimated rate of freedom from progression to accelerated-phase or blast crisis CML was 96.7 percent for the imatinib group compared to 91.5 percent for the combination therapy ($p < .001$). Furthermore, imatinib was better tolerated than the combination therapy, with only 12 patients discontinuing imatinib therapy secondary to an adverse event compared to 33 patients in the combination arm.

The results of this study have been updated and published now with a median follow-up of 5 years.[13] At the time of this analysis, 368 of the original 553 (68%) patients randomized to imatinib were still on study, taking imatinib and in

Table 16.1 Results of the IRIS trial at 19 months' and 60 months' follow-up.

Response	Initial treatment: 19 months' follow-up[12]		60 months' follow-up[13]
	Imatinib ($n = 553$)	IFN-α + ara-C ($n = 553$)	Continued imatinib ($n = 382$)
Median age (range)	50 (18–70)	51 (18–70)	
Complete hematologic	95.3	55.5	98
Major cytogenetic	85.2	22.1	92
Complete cytogenetic	73.8	8.5	87
Partial cytogenetic	11.4	13.6	–

complete cytogenetic remission. The cumulative best rate of complete cytogenetic response was 87 percent by 60 months, and only 7 percent of patients had progressive disease on imatinib therapy. Of importance, molecular response has prognostic significance. Those patients who achieved a complete cytogenetic remission by 18 months and a 3-log reduction of the BCR-ABL transcript level by PCR compared to a laboratory standard had a progression-free survival of 100 percent compared to 87 percent for those without a cytogenetic remission ($p < .001$).[13] For those patients in complete cytogenetic remission, the likelihood of achieving a major molecular response defined as a 3-log reduction of the BCR-ABL transcript improves over time. Of 124 patients from the IRIS trial who had samples available after 12 and 48 months of treatment with imatinib, the proportion of molecular responses increased from 53 to 80 percent.[13] Unfortunately, owing to allowed crossover from the interferon-cytarabine arm to imatinib, an intention-to-treat survival analysis would not be informative. However, results with imatinib compared to historical controls demonstrate the superiority of imatinib in terms of survival.[14,15]

No maximally tolerated dose was identified in the early-phase studies. This prompted investigators to evaluate if higher doses of imatinib result in a higher proportion of patients achieving complete cytogenetic and major molecular remissions at 1 year with the aim of improving progression-free survival. A nonrandomized, single-institution phase II study comparing imatinib 800 mg daily to imatinib 400 mg daily demonstrated a higher proportion of complete cytogenetic, major molecular remissions, and complete molecular remission is in the higher-dose imatinib group.[16] However, the higher doses resulted in much greater myelosuppression, requiring dose reduction in one-third of patients originally assigned to the 800-mg arm. Unfortunately, larger randomized trials evaluating the efficacy of higher initial doses of imatinib have not demonstrated meaningful differences in complete cytogenetic remissions at 1 year, and only one trial has demonstrated a statistically significant difference in the time to major molecular remission (Table 16.2).[17–20] At this time, there is no clear-cut benefit of higher doses of imatinib in newly diagnosed patients, but longer follow-up is needed.

Imatinib is well tolerated, and discontinuation of the drug secondary to adverse events or side effects is uncommon. For the most part, toxicity with imatinib is generally mild to moderate. The most common grade 1 and 2 nonhematologic toxicities are edema, nausea, muscle cramps, fatigue, and diarrhea. The treatment for these is

Table 16.2 Imatinib dosing and outcomes.

Study	Patients	Imatinib dosing	Outcomes (400 mg vs. 600 or 800 mg)
SPIRIT[20]	$n = 636$ newly diagnosed 63% intermediate- to high-risk Sokal	400 mg ($n = 159$) 600 mg ($n = 160$)	CCyR 6 months: 49% vs. 68%, $p < .01$ CCyR 12 months: 55% vs. 62%, ns MMR 6 months: 20% vs. 31%, ns MMR 12 months: 38% vs. 49%, ns Overall D/C rate: 21% vs. 23%, ns
European LeukemiaNet[17]	$n = 216$, high risk	400 mg ($n = 108$) 600 mg ($n = 108$)	CCyR 6 months: 50% vs. 52%, ns CCyR at 12 months: 58% vs. 65%, ns MMR at 6 months: 25% vs. 31%, ns MMR at 12 months: 33% vs. 40%, ns Projected 4-year OS: 84% vs. 91%, ns
TOPS[18]	$n = 476$ 61% intermediate- to high-risk Sokal (400 mg) 58% intermediate- to high-risk Sokal (800 mg)	400 mg ($n = 157$) 800 mg ($n = 319$)	CCyR 6 months: 45% vs. 57%, $p = .0146$ CCyR 12 months: 66% vs. 70%, ns Time to MMR: 13.6 vs. 8.4 months, $p = .0038$ On treatment at 1 year: 92% vs. 90%, ns
German CML Study IV[19]	$n = 1,242$	400 mg ($n = 312$) 800 mg ($n = 303$, (100% high risk)	Responses comparable, data not reported

Note. CCyR, complete cytogenetic response; DC, discontinuation; MMR, major molecular response; OS, overall survival; SPIRIT, randomized comparison of imatinib vs. imatinib combination therapies in newly diagnosed CML; TOPS, tyrosine kinase inhibitor optimization and selectivity.

often supportive, and decreasing the dose of imatinib is not recommended. Elevated liver enzymes can occur, and it is recommended to monitor liver function tests periodically as liver failure has been described. Oftentimes, discontinuation of the imatinib results in resolution of liver abnormalities, and rechallenge with imatinib with or without concomitant steroids can be undertaken.

A certain degree of myelosuppression is common with imatinib at doses of 400 mg, and the frequency increases with higher doses.[16] The etiology of the myelosuppression is not well understood. Patients with gastrointestinal tumors treated with imatinib do not get the same degree of myelosuppression with comparable doses.[21] It is postulated that the myelosuppression seen with the initiation of treatment may be a result of eradiation of the malignant clone and delayed recovery of the normal progenitor cells.[21,22] The recommendation is to interrupt imatinib dosing in the setting of severe pancytopenia and to restart when the cytopenia has resolved. Dose reductions are not recommended out of concern for the development of resistance. Small studies support the use of granulocyte colony-stimulating factor to treat neutropenia[23] and erythropoietin-stimulating factors to treat the anemia.[24]

The literature regarding the tolerability and efficacy of imatinib in the elderly is scarce. In the IRIS trial, 20 percent of patients were older than 60 years of age. There is no indication that they had more difficulty in terms of side effects. In this study, baseline Sokol risk score, which includes age, was predictive of response. Two series have been published that specifically address the use of imatinib in elderly patients.[25,26] The general conclusions from these series is that older patients have similar cytogenetic response rates and survival compared to younger patients and that age may not be an independent poor prognostic factor as originally thought.

A.6. Imatinib in advanced disease

Rarely, patients present with advanced-phase disease. In the early trials of imatinib in advanced disease, many of the patients had demonstrated interferon resistance, and these patients do worse than those who are merely intolerant to interferon. Results of these early trials indicate that hematologic and cytogenetic responses to imatinib can be seen, but the duration of response is much shorter than what is seen in chronic phase.[27,28] Cytogenetic remission is more frequent in accelerated phase than blast crisis. Furthermore, the appropriate starting dose for patients with advanced-phase disease is 600 mg/d or more.

A.7. Resistance and second-generation tyrosine kinase inhibitors

Despite imatinib's impressive efficacy, resistance is a real clinical problem. After initiation of treatment, it is important to actively monitor patients with a series of tests to ensure that they are responding appropriately (Tables 16.3 and 16.4) and not developing resistance. If a patient does not achieve the important benchmarks of hematologic remission or cytogenetic remission at the appropriate times, then the patient has primary resistance. Secondary resistance can develop in patients who initially respond to imatinib but then lose their response and is often first manifested by a rise in the quantitative PCR. Imatinib resistance is seen in all phases of the disease, but is

Table 16.3 Definitions of response.[90]

Response	Definition
Complete hematologic remission	Normal white count with a normal differential and platelets <450 × 10^9/L No extramedullary disease
Cytogenetic response	
Minor cytogenetic remission	35–90% Ph-positive metaphases
Major cytogenetic remission	<35% Ph-positive metaphases
Complete cytogenetic remission	0% Ph-positive metaphases
Molecular response	
Major molecular response	≥3-log reduction of BCR-ABL mRNA compared with a standardized baseline
Complete molecular response	No detectable BCR-ABL transcript by nested real-time quantitative PCR assays

Note. BCR, breakpoint cluster region; PCR, polymerase chain reaction; Ph, Philadelphia chromosome.

Table 16.4 Optimization of response by NCCN guidelines.[91]

Response	Time of response			
	3 months	6 months	12 months	18 months
Optimal	CHR	CCR	CCR	CCR
Suboptimal			No CCR	No CCR
Failure	No CHR	No CyR	No MCR or cytogenetic relapse	No MCR or cytogenetic relapse

Note. CHR, complete hematologic remission; CCR, complete cytogenetic remission; MCR, major cytogenetic remission; CyR, cytogenetic response.

more frequent in advanced-phase disease. Factors including compliance, bioavailability, pharmacodynamics, BCR-ABL kinase domain mutations, or a combination have been identified as contributing to the development of resistance. When a patient demonstrates resistance, mutation testing of the BCR-ABL kinase is appropriate. These mutations frequently occur at specific locations within the gene such that they prevent imatinib binding in the active site or create a conformational change in the protein that prevents imatinib binding. Newer, second-generation tyrosine kinase inhibitors have been developed to help combat resistance and are currently available.

A.8. Dasatinib

Dasatinib is an orally available dual ABL and Src kinase inhibitor with specificity for C-Kit, EPHA2, and PDGFRB. It is over 300 times more potent against BCR-ABL than imatinib and binds to both the active and inactive conformations of the kinase.[29] It inhibits 18 of the 19 BCR-ABL imatinib-resistant mutations but importantly has no efficacy in the T315I mutation, which is resistant to imatinib, dasatinib, and nilotinib.[30] It is currently approved by the U.S. Food and Drug Administration for the treatment of CML in chronic phase, accelerated phase, or blast crisis, with resistance or intolerance to imatinib. The recommended starting dose for chronic phase is 100 mg daily and 140 mg daily for CML in accelerated phase or blast crisis. Dasatinib is generally well tolerated. The most common nonhematologic toxicities seen were diarrhea, headache, hemorrhage, musculoskeletal pain, fatigue, and rash. Fluid retention is also common. In particular, pleural effusions have been demonstrated in 22 percent of patients, but only 5 percent of cases were grade 3 or 4.[31] Myelosuppression is also common, occurring with all phases of disease but most commonly in advanced-stage disease. Studies are ongoing to determine its efficacy compared to imatinib in newly diagnosed chronic phase.

A.9. Nilotinib

Nilotinib is an analog of imatinib and was developed as a second-generation tyrosine kinase inhibitor with specificity for the BCR-ABL, KIT, PDGFR, and Ephrin receptor kinases. It is 30 times more potent than imatinib against BCR-ABL and can overcome imatinib resistance in 32 of 33 imatinib-resistant BCR-ABL mutations.[29,32–35] Similar to dasatinib, it is not effective against the T315I mutation. It is approved for use in imatinib-resistant or intolerant CML in chronic phase or accelerated phase, but not blast crisis. Responses were greater in patients who are intolerant to imatinib versus those who were resistant. The starting dose is 400 mg twice daily. The most common nonhematologic toxicities include elevated bilirubin, hypophosphatemia, elevated lipase, and hyperglycemia. Of importance, given the risk of QT prolongation, there is a black-box warning regarding sudden cardiac death. QT needs to be monitored with the initiation of therapy, and the drug should not be used in patients with hypokalemia, hypomagnesaemia, or prolonged QT. Nilotinib is metabolized by the CYP3A4 hepatic enzymes. Concomitant use of medications that prolong the QT interval as well as CYP3A4 inhibitors should be avoided. There is also a food effect such that if taken with food, the drug levels can increase; therefore the medication should be taken on an empty stomach. Phase II and III studies are ongoing evaluating the use of nilotinib in newly diagnosed patients, and preliminary results indicate that it does lead to impressive molecular remissions by 12 months in low-risk patients.[36,37]

A.10. Interferons

Before the availability of imatinib, interferon was considered the first-line treatment for patients not eligible for allogeneic stem cell transplantation, but now its role in the treatment of CML is largely historical. Several randomized studies demonstrated that interferon alpha induced cytogenetic responses that correlated with improved survival compared to chemotherapy.[38–41] A meta-analysis of seven randomized clinical trials comparing interferon alpha to chemotherapy in CML reported a 5-year survival rate of 57 percent with interferon alpha and 42 percent with chemotherapy.[42] These studies verified the use of complete cytogenetic remission as a surrogate end point for survival in CML. Randomized studies evaluating the benefit of the addition of low-dose cytarabine to interferon alpha have demonstrated higher rates of major cytogenetic responses (defined as less than 35% metaphases of a 20-metaphase spread with the Philadelphia chromosome) with the combination, which translated into a survival benefit in one study[43] but not another.[44] Lower doses of interferon (3 MIU five times a week) are as effective and better tolerated than higher doses (5 MIU/m^2 body surface area/d).[45]

Long-term results of 317 patients who achieved complete cytogenetic remission with interferon treatment found that 53 percent of patients were still alive in chronic phase. Of note, 18 percent (56 patients) in this series were more than 60 years of age at the time of diagnosis. In this analysis, the 10-year overall survival from first complete cytogenetic response was dependent on Sokal risk score at presentation, with 89 percent 10-year survival for the low-risk group versus 70 percent for the intermediate-risk group.[46]

Overall, interferon results in 10–30 percent major cytogenetic response rate and 10 percent complete cytogenetic response. The median time to complete cytogenetic response is approximately 19 months, with just over 60 percent of cases in complete cytogenetic remission after 2 years.[46] Elderly patients are as likely to respond to interferon treatment as younger patients.[47] Unfortunately, interferon is not well tolerated, often requiring dose reduction in elderly patients.[47–49] In a retrospective review of two large randomized trials of interferon versus chemotherapy, patients older than 60 had a statistically significant lower median daily dose of interferon administered compared to younger patients.[47] Frequent side effects include flulike symptoms, fevers, rigors, myalgias, weight loss, granulocytopenia, thrombocytopenia, and central nervous system side effects, which occurred with similar frequency in older patients as they did in younger patients.[47] Severe central nervous system side effects, including lethargy, fatigue, depression, insomnia, reduced attention span, and memory deficits, have been reported in up to 24 percent of patients receiving therapy.[50] Patients with a preexisting neurologic or psychiatric diagnosis are at increased risk of developing such side effects. Age was not identified as a risk factor for central nervous toxicity; however, in the analysis of the Cancer and Leukemia Group B (CALGB) study using interferon alpha 2b and low-dose ara-C, of the 22 patients who developed severe neurophysiatric toxicity, 10 were aged 55 years or older.[50]

A.11. Reduced-intensity stem cell transplantation

To date, the only potential curative option for CML remains allogeneic stem cell transplantation. However, a conventional myeloablative approach is not an option for patients older than 60 years of age because of the high mortality and morbidity associated with such a procedure. In an effort to expand the benefits of stem cell transplantation to older patients or those with comorbidities, reduced-intensity conditioning (RIC) regimens were introduced. The rationale behind this approach was to lessen the toxicity of the preparative conditioning regimen, which in turn would lead to decreased treatment-related mortality but still allow for the immunologic graft-versus-leukemia (GVL) effect to occur. Several studies have demonstrated that donor lymphocyte infusions result in molecular remissions following relapse after a stem cell transplant in patients with CML,[51,52] providing strong evidence for a GVL effect in this disease.

To date, several series have now been published evaluating the efficacy of this treatment modality for CML. In a small German series, 35 patients aged 45–62 underwent RIC from either a matched sibling donor or an unrelated matched donor. The majority of these patients were in first chronic phase. After a median follow-up of 30 months, 63 percent of the patients were alive. Treatment-related mortality at day +100 was 11 percent; all patients had a cytogenetic remission. Relapse occurred in 5 (14%) patients.[53] Patients in first chronic phase fared the best. In another small series of patients from Israel, 24 patients aged 3–63 years with CML were conditioned with fludarabine, low-dose busulfan, and anti-T-lymphocyte globulin (ATG). All patients had rapid engraftment. After a median follow-up of 42 months, 21 of 24 patients were alive without disease.[54]

At the M. D. Anderson, 64 patients with advanced CML underwent nonmyeloablative transplantation.[55] Patients received one of four nonablative conditioning regimens. These were older patients with a median age of 52 (range of 17–72). Only 20 percent of patients were in first chronic phase; the rest had more advanced disease and were heavily pretreated, with 10 patients having undergone prior allogeneic or autologous stem cell transplantation. With a median follow-up of 7 years, overall survival and progression-free survival at 5 years were 33 percent and 20 percent, respectively. Treatment-related mortality increased over time and was 33 percent, 39 percent, and 48 percent at +100 days, 2 years, and 5 years, respectively. Again, stage of disease was predictive of overall and progression-free survival.

The European Group for Blood and Marrow Transplantation evaluated the outcomes of RIC transplantation in 186 patients with CML.[56] Median age was 50 years (range was 17–65); 64 percent were in the first chronic phase; 13 percent second chronic phase; 17 percent accelerated phase and 6 percent blast crisis. The day +100 transplantation-related mortality was 6.1 percent but rose to 23 percent at 2 years. Conditioning with fludarabine, busulfan, and ATG had the lowest treatment-related mortality at 1 year. Acute graft-versus-host disease (GVHD) occurred in 32 percent and chronic GVHD in 43 percent, of which 24 percent was extensive. At 3 years, the overall survival and progression-free survival was 58 percent and 37 percent, respectively. Advanced-phase disease was associated with inferior outcomes.

Taken together, these data indicate that for the selected older patient who fails imatinib or second-generation tyrosine kinase inhibitor therapy, RIC stem cell transplantation is an option that provides a reasonable long-term survival but does have substantial treatment-related mortality over time, likely related to complications of chronic GVHD. Few studies to date address the feasibility of this approach in older patients alone. This modality of treatment is really for those patients with an excellent performance status and adequate organ function (normal kidney and liver function) and seems to benefit those in chronic phase over those with more advanced disease.

A.12. Conclusions

1. Diagnosis of CML should include bone marrow biopsy, cytogenetics, FISH, and quantitative PCR.
2. Initial treatment with imatinib at a starting dose of 400 mg/d is recommended with careful monitoring to ensure that patients achieve benchmarks of remission at specified time points.
3. BCR-ABL mutation analysis should be performed at the appearance of disease resistance.
4. Second-generation tyrosine kinase inhibitors have excellent response rates in those who are imatinib resistant or intolerant and have acceptable toxicity profiles.
5. Reduced-intensity allogeneic stem cell transplant is an option of last resort for the fit elderly patient with a suitable match who has failed oral tyrosine kinase inhibition.

B. Chronic lymphocytic leukemia in older adults

B.1. Introduction

CLL, best considered an indolent B cell lymphoproliferative neoplasm, is probably the most common of the leukemias.[57] This disease, like acute myeloid leukemia, is a disease of older adults with a median age being in the upper end of the seventh decade of life. However, unlike acute myeloid leukemia, distinct treatment algorithms based on age are not generally employed, nor is prognosis grossly affected by the patient's age. Patients who present with similar disease features may have highly variable natural histories. Recent advances in the therapeutic management of chronic lymphocytic leukemia both in the setting of initial therapy and management of recurrent disease have been applicable to patients of all age cohorts. However, age-specific issues could play a factor in deciding which of the available therapeutic options to choose.

B.2. Diagnosis

The diagnosis of chronic lymphocytic leukemia is usually straightforward. Patients present with lymphocytosis; greater than 5,000 lymphocytes/μL should prompt strong consideration of this diagnosis (and such elevation for 3 or more months represents the minimum diagnostic criteria).[58–60] CLL lymphocytes are mature appearing on smear but may have smudged nuclei. Immunophenotypic analysis yields a characteristic pattern of CD5 and CD23 expression on B lymphocytes, which are generally CD19 and dimly CD20 positive and CD10 negative. Weak surface immunoglobulin staining is present. Patients with CLL may also present with lymphadenopathy and/or splenomegly as well as anemia and thrombocytopenia. Small lymphocytic lymphoma (SLL), a low-grade non-Hodgkin's lymphoma, is a lymph node tropic variant of CLL. Cells from pathologic nodes from SLL patients appear to be identical to the circulating cells in CLL from a morphological and biological standpoint. A more aggressive variant of CLL, prolymphocytic leukemia, is characterized by a relative low level of CD5 expression, a higher level of surface immunoglobulin expression, and a morphological metamorphosis to activated-appearing lymphocytes with young-appearing nuclei, often containing multiple nucleoli.[61] Once a diagnosis of CLL is established, generally by a review of the peripheral blood smear with appropriate immunophenotypic studies, an additional staging workup includes a computerized tomography scan of the chest, abdomen, and pelvis (positron emission tomography scans are not particularly helpful because of the lack of the avidity of CLL lymphocytes)[62] and routine biochemical evaluation of liver function tests, including serum lactate dehydrogenase (LDH) and quantitation of serum immunoglobulins (patients with these B-cell neoplasms often present with compensatory hypogammaglobulinemia, which could lead to infection with encapsulated micro-organisms such as *H. flu* and *S. pneumococcus*). The nature of infectious complications in CLL is important, particularly in the elderly, for whom awareness and treatment of incipient pneumonias or other upper respiratory infections could be lifesaving. The value of a bone marrow examination in CLL is somewhat controversial because all patients have bone marrow involvement; whether the bone marrow involvement is nodular or diffuse may have some prognostic significance.[63]

B.3. Staging and prognosis

Classic staging for CLL patients relies on notation of lymphadenopathy (number of nodal groups and location), the presence or absence of splenomegly, and the presence or absence of anemia and thrombocytopenia. Note that age does not enter into the prognostic model of the Rai classification system, which divides patients into five subgroups, or the Binet system,[64] which classifies patients into three subgroups (Table 16.5). In Rai[65] stage III or IV patients, the thrombocytopenia or anemia should not be related to autoimmune destruction, which yields a much better prognosis. The prognosis of Rai stage 0 patients (elevated lymphocytic count without lymphadenopathy, splenomegly, anemia, or thrombocytopenia) is equivalent to that of age-matched controls. Recently, a CLL precursor disease, monoclonal B-cell lymphocytosis (MBL), has been defined as an entity wherein under $500/\mu L$ monoclonal B cells with CLL immunophenotype are present without other CLL disease features.[66] MBL is detectable in 5.1 percent of individuals between the ages of 62 and 80 years. About 1 percent of such people annually develop CLL that requires treatment.[66]

Given the heterogeneity within the Rai and Binet subgroups, a number of refinements have been made which take into account karyotypic and genetic characteristics of the malignant

Table 16.5 Rai[65] and Binet[64] staging of chronic lymphocytic leukemia (CLL).

Binet system			Rai system	
Stage	Description	Risk status	Stage	Description
0	Lymphocytosis, lymphocytes in blood >15,000/mcL, and >40% lymphocytes in the bone marrow	Good	A	Hemoglobin ≥10 g/dL and platelets ≥100,000 mm³ and <3 enlarged areas
I	Stage 0 with enlarged node(s)	Intermediate	B	Hemoglobin ≥10 g/dL and platelets ≥100,000 mm³ and ≥3 enlarged areas
II	Stage 0–1 with splenomegaly, hepatomegaly, or both	Intermediate		
III	Stage 0–II with hemoglobin <11.0 g/dL or hematocrit <33%	High	C	Hemoglobin <10 g/dL and/or platelets <100,000 mm³ and any number of enlarged areas
IV	Stage III with platelets <100,000/mcL	High		

Table 16.6 Karyotype and CLL.[80,92]

Karyotype-based prognosis in CLL	
Favorable	13q– (if sole)
Intermediate	Normal or trisomy12
Unfavorable	T (11q;v)
	17p–
	11q–

lymphocytes. Standard karyotypic analysis relies on cells in cycle that can generate metaphases, which does not always occur in CLL cells with low proliferative thrust. The advent of FISH has made possible the characterization of chromosomal abnormalities in a large percentage of CLL patients. Single-nucleotide polymorphism analysis promises even more refined prognosis based on genetic abnormalities. Patients with a 17p deletion (involving loss of p53 tumor suppressor gene) have a remarkably inferior prognosis, whereas those with deletion of the long arm of chromosome 13 have a superior prognosis (Table 16.6).

Analysis of certain genetic and immunophenotypic features have further refined prognosis in CLL. Expression of the ZAP 70 protein is clearly associated with an adverse prognosis.[67,68] Corresponding to the stage of differentiation at which the malignant cell arises, B cells that have yet to undergo mutation in their immunoglobulin heavy chain region are more immature; CLL patients whose cells have unmutated heavy chains have an adverse prognosis compared to patients whose CLL cells have already undergone rearrangement of their immunoglobulin heavy chain genes.[69] While of important prognostic significance, this test is not widely available. The use of CD38 expression may be a surrogate marker for patients with unmutated (poor prognosis) CLL.[69] A prognostic scoring system that takes into account clinical, cytogenetic, and genetic features has been proposed.

B.4. Treatment Considerations

Decision regarding treatment initiation

Many patients with CLL can be managed without therapy. It does not appear that early initiation of therapy, at least for the average patient with low-stage CLL, is advantageous.[70] First, many patients with very low stage CLL will never have any clinical problems, and therefore early treatment would make little sense. Second, initia-

tion of treatment in the presymptomatic phase has not been shown to prolong overall survival. Criteria for initiation of treatment in CLL have been established. Such criteria generally require the presence of constitutional symptoms (fatigue, night sweats, weight loss, and fever without infection), symptomatic lymphadenopathy, and/or splenomegaly or cytopenias. Treatment for patients whose peripheral blood leukocyte counts double in less than 6 months is also reasonable. It is important to distinguish cytopenias that arise from a high degree of bone marrow involvement as opposed to those due to autoimmune anemia or thrombocytopenia. Though it can sometimes be difficult to distinguish autoimmune cytopenia from lack of platelet production, the presence of a warm auto antibody against red cells and an elevated reticulocyte count should prompt the use of steroids.[71] Though initiation of therapy is not based on patient age, even older patients who have symptomatic lymphadenopathy, splenomegaly, or cytopenias should be treated in a similar fashion as those with younger patients with the same disease.

A major issue that has emerged recently with the advent of the cytogenetic and genetically based prognostic factors is whether patients with a known adverse prognosis should be treated in the presymptomatic stage. The current best answer to this question is that treatment should be initiated only on the basis of clinical features. An important intergroup CALGB-led trial will, it is hoped, answer this question. Patients with adverse genetic prognostic factors will be randomized to early treatment or observation until standard treatment criteria are met. The primary end point is not overall survival but rather time to require second treatment.

Initial treatment

For patients whose only clinical problems are bulky nodes, localized radiation can be helpful. When systemic treatment is required, there are a number of therapeutic choices available. The most important choices include the alkylating agents chlorambucil, bendamustine, or fludarabine (a nucleoside analog) alone or in combination with rituximab and/or cyclophosphamide, and pentostatin (nucleoside analog)-containing regimens. Rituximab, an anti-CD20 monoclonal antibody, though effective in low-grade lymphomas, is not greatly effective as a single agent in CLL, perhaps because of the relative low level of surface CD20 expression. Randomized trials do not provide the answer to the optimal therapy. However, a large randomized trial comparing fludarabine to chlorambucil showed that fludarabine produced a much higher likelihood of complete (20% vs. 4%) or partial remission (43% vs. 33%) and a superior disease-free survival without an overall survival benefit.[72] Nonetheless, this large CALGB study prompted the common use of fludarabine-based regimens for symptomatic patients with CLL. Fludarabine has some important side effects that could be potentially devastating, particularly in an older person, including immunosuppression and occasional generation of autoimmune hemolysis or thrombocytopenia. CALGB 9712[73] showed that fludarabine plus rituximab (at least in the context of a phase II trial) was associated with a high response rate, probably higher than historical controls who received fludarabine alone.[74] Rituximab is an immunosuppressive agent and is associated with reactivation of hepatitis infection; pretreatment screening is mandated.

Both alemtuzumab[75] (anti-CD52 monoclonal antibody) and bendamustine[76] as single agents have been shown to be better than chlorambucil as initial treatment. On the other hand, a large amount of phase II data with the regimen consisting of fludarabine, cyclophosphamide, and rituximab (FCR) suggest an impressively high complete remission rate and likelihood of long-term survival.[77,78] However, the FCR regimen is quite myelosuppressive, so caution is in order for older adults. The Eastern Cooperative Oncology Group led an intergroup study that showed that cyclophosphomide plus fludarabine was superior to fludarabine alone.[79,80] Pentostatin-containing regimens (rather than using fludarabine) have similar activity.[81–83]

Treatment of relapsed disease

Because none of the upfront regimens can be considered curative, patients will generally have recurrent CLL within 5 years of initiation of initial treatment. The duration of the initial disease-free period is an important prognostic factor for response to subsequent therapy. An approved therapy for relapsed CLL, alemtuzumab (trade name Campath), a monoclonal antibody to the ubiquitously expressed CD52 epitope, is associated with a significant response rate.[84,85] Side effects include profound immunosuppression and should be used with caution (requires obligatory pneumocytis carinii [PCP] and cytomegalovirus [CMV] prophylaxis)[86] in most patients, including older adults, with this disease. Patients with relapsed CLL who can be shown to have respon-

sive disease may be candidates for allogeneic stem cell transplantation. In a small series from Seattle,[87] 64 patients with advanced CLL underwent reduced-intensity allogeneic stem cell transplant. The median age of this study was 56 years (range 44–69 years), and overall survival and disease-free survival were 60 percent and 52 percent, respectively. Older adults with aggressive yet responsive disease who have a reasonable performance status could be considered for reduced-intensity allogeneic stem cell transplantation, but long-term results are difficult to discern given the selection bias inherent in small studies.[87]

Rather than basing the treatment decision solely on patient age (owing to the lack of easily discernible intrinsic biologic differences), most recommend a performance status or frailty-based algorithm for therapeutic choice. For example, frail patients with significant degrees of comorbidity might not be able to tolerate a nucleoside analog and could be better candidates for chlorambucil with or without prednisone. In patients over age 70, the National Comprehensive Cancer Network (NCCN) guidelines[88] recommend considering alkylating agent–based approaches before those involving fludarabine. FCR in treatment-naive patients should be more strongly considered for younger patients or those with relapsed CLL of any age. For the older adult with a 17p deletion, the prognosis is so poor that more aggressive treatment (e.g., with chemoimmunotherapy including a nucleoside analog) can be considered for upfront use. A discussion of new approaches[89] including novel monoclonal antibodies (e.g., lumiliximab [anti-CD23] and ofatumumab [anti-CD20]) and agents useful in other lymphomas (lenalidomide, flavopiridol, or oblimersen) may be applicable in older adults with advanced disease.

B.5. Conclusions

1. Diagnosis is based on the presence of an absolute lymphocytosis over 5,000 lymphocytes/μL for 3 or more months with the immunophenotype CD19, CD20 (dim), CD5, and CD23 positive, CD10 negative.

2. Interphase FISH at diagnosis provides important prognostic information.

3. Other molecular tests to define prognosis, including immunoglobulin heavy chain mutational status and ZAP70, are not commercially available. CD38 is a surrogate marker for patients with unmutated

immunoglobulin heavy chain, which confers a poor prognosis.

4. Early treatment of asymptomatic disease has not been shown to improve overall survival. Indications for treatment include the presence of nonautoimmune cytopenias, symptomatic lymphadenopathy, or hepatosplenomegaly; disease-related B symptoms; extreme lymphocytosis and autoimmune hemolytic anemia; or thrombocytopenia nonresponsive to therapy.

5. Initial treatment for patients aged 70 years or older includes chlorambucil and steroids prior to initiating treatment with fludarabine.

6. Combination therapy such as fludarabine, cyclophosphamide, and rituximab should be considered for younger, treatment-naive patients or those with relapse CLL of any age.

References

1. National Cancer Institute. *SEER Survival Monograph: Cancer Survival among Adults: U.S. SEER Program, 1988–2001, Patient and Tumor Characteristics*. Bethesda, MD: National Cancer Institute; 2007.

2. Dekmezian R, Kantarjian HM, Keating MJ, et al. The relevance of reticulin stain-measured fibrosis at diagnosis in chronic myelogenous leukemia. *Cancer*. 1987;59(10):1739–1743.

3. Buesche G, Hehlmann R, Hecker H, et al. Marrow fibrosis, indicator of therapy failure in chronic myeloid leukemia – prospective long-term results from a randomized-controlled trial. *Leukemia*. 2003;17(12):2444–2453.

4. Kantarjian HM, Dixon D, Keating MJ, et al. Characteristics of accelerated disease in chronic myelogenous leukemia. *Cancer*. 1988;61(7):1441–1446.

5. Swerdlow SH, Campo E, Harris NL, et al. *WHO Classification of Tumours of Haematopoietic and Lymphoid Tissues*. 4th ed. Lyon, France: International Agency for Research on Cancer; 2008.

6. Rowley JD. Letter: A new consistent chromosomal abnormality in chronic myelogenous leukaemia identified by quinacrine fluorescence and Giemsa staining. *Nature*. 1973;243(5405):290–293.

7. Shtivelman E, Lifshitz B, Gale RP, et al. Fused transcript of Abl and Bcr genes in chronic myelogenous leukaemia. *Nature*. 1985;315(6020):550–554.

8. Daley GQ, Van Etten RA, Baltimore D. Induction of chronic myelogenous leukemia in mice by the P210Bcr/Abl gene of the Philadelphia chromosome. *Science*. 1990;247(4944):824–830.

9. Li S, Ilaria Jr RL, Million RP, et al. The P190, P210, and P230 forms of the BCR/ABL oncogene induce a similar chronic myeloid leukemia-like syndrome in mice but have different lymphoid leukemogenic activity. *J Exp Med*. 1999;189(9):1399–1412.

10. Druker BJ, Talpaz M, Resta DJ, et al. Efficacy and safety of a specific inhibitor of the BCR-ABL tyrosine kinase in chronic myeloid leukemia. *N Engl J Med*. 2001;344(14):1031–1037.

11. Kantarjian H, Sawyers C, Hochhaus A, et al. Hematologic and cytogenetic responses to imatinib mesylate in chronic myelogenous leukemia. *N Engl J Med*. 2002;346(9):645–652.

12. O'Brien SG, Guilhot F, Larson RA, et al. Imatinib compared with interferon and low-dose cytarabine for newly diagnosed chronic-phase chronic myeloid leukemia. *N Engl J Med*. 2003;348(11):994–1004.

13. Druker BJ, Guilhot F, O'Brien SG, et al. Five-year follow-up of patients receiving imatinib for chronic myeloid leukemia. *N Engl J Med*. 2006;355(23):2408–2417.

14. Roy L, Guilhot J, Krahnke T, et al. Survival advantage from imatinib compared with the combination interferon-alpha plus cytarabine in chronic-phase chronic myelogenous leukemia: historical comparison between two phase 3 trials. *Blood*. 2006;108(5):1478–1484.

15. Kantarjian HM, Talpaz M, O'Brien S, et al. Survival benefit with imatinib mesylate versus interferon-alpha-based regimens in newly diagnosed chronic-phase chronic myelogenous leukemia. *Blood*. 2006;108(6):1835–1840.

16. Kantarjian H, Cortes J, O'Brien S, et al. High rates of early major and complete cytogenetic responses with imatinib mesylate therapy given at 400 mg or 800 mg orally daily in patients with newly diagnosed Philadelphia chromosome positive chronic myeloid leukemia in chronic phase [abstract]. *Proc Am Soc Clin Oncol*. 2002;21:261a.

17. Baccarani M, Rosti G, Castagnetti F, et al. A comparison of imatinib 400 mg and 800 mg daily in the front-line treatment of patients with high risk, Philadelphia-positive, chronic myeloid leukaemia: a European LeukemiaNet study. *Blood*. 2009;113(19):4497–4504.

18. Cortes J, Baccarani M, Guilhot F, et al. A phase III, randomized, open-label study of 400 mg versus 800 mg of imatinib mesylate (IM) in patients with newly diagnosed, previously untreated chronic myeloid leukemia in chronic phase (CML-CP) using molecular endpoints: Tyrosine Kinase Inhibitor Optimization and Selectivity Study. *Journal of Clinical Oncology*. 2010;28(3):424–430.

19. Hehlmann R, Sausselle S, Lauseker M, et al. Randomized comparison of imatinib 400 mg vs. imatinib + INF vs. imatinib + ARAC v. imatinib after INF vs. imatinib 800 mg: optimized treatment and survival. Designed First Interim Analysis of the German CML Study IV. *ASH Annu Meet Abstr*. 2008;112(11):75.

20. Guilhot F, Mahon FX, Guilhot J, et al. Randomized comparison of imatinib versus imatinib combination therapies in newly diagnosed chronic myeloid leukaemia (CML) patients in chronic phase (CP): first results of the phase III (SPIRIT) trial from the French CML group (F1 LMC). *ASH Annu Meet Abstr*. 2008;112(11):74.

21. Demetri GD, von Mehren M, Blanke CD, et al. Efficacy and safety of imatinib mesylate in advanced gastrointestinal stromal tumors. *N Engl J Med*. 2002;347(7):472–480.

22. Cortes J, Ault P, Koller C, et al. Efficacy of imatinib mesylate in the treatment of idiopathic hypereosinophilic syndrome. *Blood*. 2003;101(12):4714–4716.

23. Quintas-Cardama A, Kantarjian H, O'Brien S, et al. Granulocyte-colony-stimulating factor (filgrastim) may overcome imatinib-induced neutropenia in patients with chronic-phase chronic myelogenous leukemia. *Cancer*. 2004;100(12):2592–2597.

24. Cortes J, O'Brien S, Quintas A, et al. Erythropoietin is effective in improving the anemia induced by imatinib mesylate therapy in patients with chronic myeloid leukemia in chronic phase. *Cancer*. 2004;100(11):2396–2402.

25. Cortes J, Talpaz M, O'Brien S, et al. Effects of age on prognosis with imatinib mesylate therapy for patients with Philadelphia chromosome-positive chronic myelogenous leukemia. *Cancer*. 2003;98(6):1105–1113.

26. Latagliata R, Breccia M, Carmosino I, et al. Elderly patients with Ph+ chronic myelogenous leukemia (CML): results of imatinib mesylate treatment. *Leuk Res*. 2005;29(3):287–291.

27. Talpaz M, Silver RT, Druker BJ, et al. Imatinib induces durable hematologic and cytogenetic responses in patients with accelerated phase chronic myeloid leukemia: results of a phase 2 study. *Blood*. 2002;99(6):1928–1937.

28. Sawyers CL, Hochhaus A, Feldman E, et al. Imatinib induces hematologic and cytogenetic responses in patients with chronic myelogenous leukemia in myeloid blast crisis: results of a phase II study. *Blood*. 2002;99(10):3530–3539.

29. O'Hare T, Walters DK, Stoffregen EP, et al. In vitro activity of Bcr-Abl inhibitors AMN107 and BMS-354825 against clinically relevant imatinib-resistant Abl kinase domain mutants. *Cancer Res*. 2005;65(11):4500–4505.

30. Bradeen HA, Eide CA, O'Hare T, et al. Comparison of imatinib mesylate, dasatinib (BMS-354825), and nilotinib (AMN107) in an n-ethyl-n-nitrosourea (ENU)-based mutagenesis screen: high efficacy of drug combinations. *Blood*. 2006;108(7):2332–2338.

31. McFarland KL, Wetzstein GA. Chronic myeloid leukemia therapy: focus on second-generation tyrosine kinase inhibitors. *Cancer Control*. 2009;16(2):132–140.

32. Weisberg E, Manley P, Mestan J, et al. AMN107 (nilotinib): a novel and selective inhibitor of BCR-ABL. *Br J Cancer*. 2006;94(12):1765–1769.

33. Weisberg E, Manley PW, Breitenstein W, et al. Characterization of AMN107, a selective inhibitor of native and mutant Bcr-Abl. *Cancer Cell*. 2005;7(2):129–141.

34. Golemovic M, Verstovsek S, Giles F, et al. AMN107, a novel aminopyrimidine inhibitor of Bcr-Abl, has in vitro activity against imatinib-resistant chronic myeloid leukemia. *Clin Cancer Res*. 2005;11(13):4941–4947.

35. Verstovsek S, Golemovic M, Kantarjian H, et al. AMN107, a novel aminopyrimidine inhibitor of p190 Bcr-Abl activation and of in vitro proliferation of Philadelphia-positive acute lymphoblastic leukemia cells. *Cancer*. 2005;104(6):1230–1236.

36. Rosti G, Castagnetti F, Poerio A, et al. High and early rates of cytogenetic and molecular response with nilotinib 800 mg daily as first line treatment of Ph-positive chronic myeloid leukemia in chronic phase: results of a phase 2 trial of the GIMEMA CML Working Party [abstract]. *ASH Annu Meet Abstr*. 2008;112(11):181.

37. Cortes J, O'Brien S, Jones D, et al. Efficacy of nilotinib (formerly AMN107) in patients (Pts) with newly diagnosed, previously untreated Philadelphia chromosome (Ph)-positive chronic myelogenous leukemia in early chronic phase (CML-CP) [abstract]. *ASH Annu Meet Abstr*. 2008;112(11):446.

38. Interferon alfa-2a as compared with conventional chemotherapy for the treatment of chronic myeloid leukemia. The Italian Cooperative Study Group on Chronic Myeloid Leukemia. *N Engl J Med*. 1994;330(12):820–825.

39. Hehlmann R, Heimpel H, Hasford J, et al. Randomized comparison of interferon-alpha with busulfan and hydroxyurea in chronic myelogenous leukemia. The German CML Study Group. *Blood*. 1994;84(12):4064–4077.

40. Allan NC, Richards SM, Shepherd PC. UK Medical Research Council randomised, multicentre trial of interferon-alpha n1 for chronic myeloid leukaemia: improved survival irrespective of cytogenetic response. The UK Medical Research Council's Working Parties for Therapeutic Trials in Adult Leukaemia. *Lancet*. 1995;345(8962):1392–1397.

41. Ohnishi K, Ohno R, Tomonaga M, et al. A randomized trial comparing interferon-alpha with busulfan for newly diagnosed chronic myelogenous leukemia in chronic phase. *Blood*. 1995;86(3):906–916.

42. Randomized study on hydroxyurea alone versus hydroxyurea combined with low-dose interferon-alpha 2b for chronic myeloid leukemia. The Benelux CML Study Group. *Blood*. 1998;91(8):2713–2721.

43. Guilhot F, Chastang C, Michallet M, et al. Interferon alfa-2b combined with cytarabine versus interferon alone in chronic myelogenous leukemia. French Chronic Myeloid Leukemia Study Group. *N Engl J Med*. 1997;337(4):223–229.

44. Baccarani M, Rosti G, de Vivo A, et al. A randomized study of interferon-alpha versus interferon-alpha and low-dose arabinosyl cytosine in chronic myeloid leukemia. *Blood*. 2002;99(5):1527–1535.

45. Kluin-Nelemans HC, Buck G, le Cessie S, et al. Randomized comparison of low-dose versus high-dose interferon-alfa in chronic myeloid leukemia: prospective collaboration of 3 joint trials by the MRC and HOVON groups. *Blood.* 2004;103(12):4408–4415.

46. Bonifazi F, de Vivo A, Rosti G, et al. Chronic myeloid leukemia and interferon-alpha: a study of complete cytogenetic responders. *Blood.* 2001;98(10):3074–3081.

47. Berger U, Engelich G, Maywald O, et al. Chronic myeloid leukemia in the elderly: long-term results from randomized trials with interferon alpha. *Leukemia.* 2003;17(9):1820–1826.

48. Cortes J, Kantarjian H, O'Brien S, et al. Result of interferon-alpha therapy in patients with chronic myelogenous leukemia 60 years of age and older. *Am J Med.* 1996;100(4):452–455.

49. Hilbe W, Apfelbeck U, Fridrik M, et al. Interferon-alpha for the treatment of elderly patients with chronic myeloid leukaemia. *Leuk Res.* 1998;22(10):881–886.

50. Hensley ML, Peterson B, Silver RT, et al. Risk factors for severe neuropsychiatric toxicity in patients receiving interferon alfa-2b and low-dose cytarabine for chronic myelogenous leukemia: analysis of Cancer and Leukemia Group B 9013. *J Clin Oncol.* 2000;18(6):1301–1308.

51. Horowitz MM, Gale RP, Sondel PM, et al. Graft-versus-leukemia reactions after bone marrow transplantation. *Blood.* 1990;75(3):555–562.

52. Kolb HJ, Schattenberg A, Goldman JM, et al. Graft-versus-leukemia effect of donor lymphocyte transfusions in marrow grafted patients. *Blood.* 1995;86(5):2041–2050.

53. Weisser M, Schleuning M, Ledderose G, et al. Reduced-intensity conditioning using TBI (8 Gy), fludarabine, cyclophosphamide and ATG in elderly CML patients provides excellent results especially when performed in the early course of the disease. *Bone Marrow Transplant.* 2004;34(12):1083–1088.

54. Or R, Shapira MY, Resnick I, et al. Nonmyeloablative allogeneic stem cell transplantation for the treatment of chronic myeloid leukemia in first chronic phase. *Blood.* 2003;101(2):441–445.

55. Kebriaei P, Detry MA, Giralt S, et al. Long-term follow-up of allogeneic hematopoietic stem-cell transplantation with reduced-intensity conditioning for patients with chronic myeloid leukemia. *Blood.* 2007;110(9):3456–3462.

56. Crawley C, Szydlo R, Lalancette M, et al. Outcomes of reduced-intensity transplantation for chronic myeloid leukemia: an analysis of prognostic factors from the Chronic Leukemia Working Party of the EBMT. *Blood.* 2005;106(9):2969–2976.

57. Jemal A, Siegel R, Ward E, et al. Cancer statistics, 2008. *CA Cancer J Clin.* 2008;58(2):71–96.

58. Cheson BD, Bennett JM, Grever M, et al. National Cancer Institute–sponsored Working Group guidelines for chronic lymphocytic leukemia: revised guidelines for diagnosis and treatment. *Blood.* 1996;87(12):4990–4997.

59. Eichhorst B, Hallek M. Revision of the guidelines for diagnosis and therapy of chronic lymphocytic leukemia (CLL). *Best Pract Res Clin Haematol.* 2007;20(3):469–477.

60. Hallek M, Cheson BD, Catovsky D, et al. Guidelines for the diagnosis and treatment of chronic lymphocytic leukemia: a report from the International Workshop on Chronic Lymphocytic Leukemia updating the National Cancer Institute–Working Group 1996 guidelines. *Blood.* 2008;111(12):5446–5456.

61. Hercher C, Robain M, Davi F, et al. A multicentric study of 41 cases of B-prolymphocytic leukemia: two evolutive forms. *Leuk Lymphoma.* 2001;42(5):981–987.

62. Seam P, Juweid ME, Cheson BD. The role of FDG-PET scans in patients with lymphoma. *Blood.* 2007;110(10):3507–3516.

63. Rozman C, Montserrat E, Rodriguez-Fernandez JM, et al. Bone marrow histologic pattern – the best single prognostic parameter in chronic lymphocytic leukemia: a multivariate survival analysis of 329 cases. *Blood.* 1984;64(3):642–648.

64. Binet JL, Auquier A, Dighiero G, et al. A new prognostic classification of chronic lymphocytic leukemia derived from a multivariate survival analysis. *Cancer.* 1981;48(1):198–206.

65. Rai KR, Sawitsky A, Cronkite EP, et al. Clinical staging of chronic lymphocytic leukemia. *Blood.* 1975;46(2):219–234.

66. Rawstron AC, Bennett FL, O'Connor SJ, et al. Monoclonal B-cell lymphocytosis and chronic lymphocytic leukemia. *N Engl J Med.* 2008;359(6):575–583.

67. Crespo M, Bosch F, Villamor N, et al. ZAP-70 expression as a surrogate for immunoglobulin-variable-region mutations in chronic lymphocytic leukemia. *N Engl J Med.* 2003;348(18):1764–1775.

68. Wiestner A, Rosenwald A, Barry TS, et al. ZAP-70 expression identifies a chronic lymphocytic leukemia subtype with unmutated immunoglobulin genes, inferior clinical outcome, and distinct gene expression profile. *Blood.* 2003;101(12):4944–4951.

69. Damle RN, Wasil T, Fais F, et al. Ig V gene mutation status and CD38 expression as novel prognostic indicators in chronic lymphocytic leukemia. *Blood.* 1999;94(6):1840–1847.

70. Chemotherapeutic options in chronic lymphocytic leukemia: a meta-analysis of the randomized trials. *J Natl Cancer Inst.* 1999;91:861–868.

71. Hamblin TJ. Autoimmune complications of chronic lymphocytic leukemia. *Semin Oncol.* 2006;33(2):230–239.

72. Rai KR, Peterson BL, Appelbaum FR, et al. Fludarabine compared with chlorambucil as primary therapy for chronic lymphocytic leukemia. *N Engl J Med.* 2000;343(24):1750–1757.

73. Byrd JC, Peterson BL, Morrison VA, et al. Randomized phase 2 study of fludarabine with concurrent versus sequential treatment with rituximab in symptomatic, untreated patients with B-cell chronic lymphocytic leukemia: results from Cancer and Leukemia Group B 9712 (CALGB 9712). *Blood.* 2003;101(1):6–14.

74. Byrd JC, Rai K, Peterson BL, et al. Addition of rituximab to fludarabine may prolong progression-free survival and overall survival in patients with previously untreated chronic lymphocytic leukemia: an updated retrospective comparative analysis of CALGB 9712 and CALGB 9011. *Blood.* 2005;105(1):49–53.

75. Hillmen P, Skotnicki AB, Robak T, et al. Alemtuzumab compared with chlorambucil as first-line therapy for chronic lymphocytic leukemia. *J Clin Oncol.* 2007;25(35):5616–5623.

76. Knauf WU, Lissichkov T, Aldaoud A, et al. Bendamustine versus chlorambucil in treatment-naive patients with B-cell chronic lymphocytic leukemia (B-CLL): results of an international phase III study [abstract]. *ASH Annu Meet Abstr.* 2007;110(11):2043.

77. Keating MJ, O'Brien S, Albitar M, et al. Early results of a chemoimmunotherapy regimen of fludarabine, cyclophosphamide, and rituximab as initial therapy for chronic lymphocytic leukemia. *J Clin Oncol.* 2005;23(18):4079–4088.

78. Wierda W, O'Brien S, Wen S, et al. Chemoimmunotherapy with fludarabine, cyclophosphamide, and rituximab for relapsed and refractory chronic lymphocytic leukemia. *J Clin Oncol.* 2005;23(18):4070–4078.

79. Flinn IW, Neuberg DS, Grever MR, et al. Phase III trial of fludarabine plus cyclophosphamide compared with fludarabine for patients with previously untreated chronic lymphocytic leukemia: US Intergroup Trial E2997. *J Clin Oncol.* 2007;25(7):793–798.

80. Grever MR, Lucas DM, Dewald GW, et al. Comprehensive assessment of genetic and molecular features predicting outcome in patients with chronic lymphocytic leukemia: results from the US Intergroup Phase III Trial E2997. *J Clin Oncol.* 2007;25(7):799–804.

81. Weiss MA, Maslak PG, Jurcic JG, et al. Pentostatin and cyclophosphamide: an effective new regimen in previously treated patients with chronic lymphocytic leukemia. *J Clin Oncol.* 2003;21(7):1278–1284.

82. Lamanna N, Kalaycio M, Maslak P, et al. Pentostatin, cyclophosphamide, and rituximab is an active, well-tolerated regimen for patients with previously treated chronic lymphocytic leukemia. *J Clin Oncol.* 2006;24(10):1575–1581.

83. Kay NE, Geyer SM, Call TG, et al. Combination chemoimmunotherapy with pentostatin, cyclophosphamide, and rituximab shows significant clinical activity with low accompanying toxicity in previously untreated B chronic lymphocytic leukemia. *Blood.* 2007;109(2):405–411.

84. Keating MJ, Flinn I, Jain V, et al. Therapeutic role of alemtuzumab (Campath-1H) in patients who have failed fludarabine: results of a large international study. *Blood.* 2002;99(10):3554–3561.

85. Stilgenbauer S, Dohner H. Campath-1H-induced complete remission of chronic lymphocytic leukemia despite p53 gene mutation and resistance to chemotherapy. *N Engl J Med.* 2002;347(6):452–453.

86. O'Brien SM, Keating MJ, Mocarski ES. Updated guidelines on the management of cytomegalovirus reactivation in patients with chronic lymphocytic leukemia treated with alemtuzumab. *Clin Lymphoma Myeloma.* 2006;7(2):125–130.

87. Sorror ML, Maris MB, Sandmaier BM, et al. Hematopoietic cell transplantation after nonmyeloablative conditioning for advanced chronic lymphocytic leukemia. *J Clin Oncol.* 2005;23(16):3819–3829.

88. Non Hodgkin's lymphoma. In: *National Comprehensive Cancer Network Clinical Practice Guidelines in Oncology.* http://www.nccn.org/index.asp

89. O'Brien S. New agents in the treatment of CLL. *Hematol Am Soc Hematol Educ Prog.* 2008;2008:457–464.

90. Goldman JM. How I treat chronic myeloid leukemia in the imatinib era. *Blood.* 2007;110(8):2828–2837.

91. Chronic myelogenous leukemia. In: *National Comprehensive Cancer Network Clinical Practice Guidelines in Oncology.* http://www.nccn.org/index.asp

92. Dohner H, Stilgenbauer S, Benner A, et al. Genomic aberrations and survival in chronic lymphocytic leukemia. *N Engl J Med.* 2000;343(26):1910–1916.

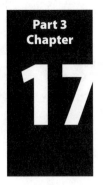

Management of acute myeloid leukemia in older adults

Arati V. Rao and Joseph O. Moore

A. Introduction

It is estimated that acute myeloid leukemia (AML) accounts for 70 percent of newly diagnosed acute leukemias. In the United States, approximately 13,000 individuals were diagnosed with AML in 2008, and nearly 9,000 died of the disease.[1] Notably, 35 percent of patients with newly diagnosed AML are 75 years of age or older, and the median age at diagnosis is 67 years. The incidence of AML will likely increase over time, as the number of individuals over 65 years of age in the United States – estimated to be 37.3 million in 2006 – is expected to double by year 2030 and represent 20 percent of the population.[2] Elderly patients, defined in the AML literature as those aged 60 years or older, historically have lower complete remission (CR) and relapse-free survival (RFS) rates when compared to their younger counterparts. In elderly patients with AML, CR rates vary between 30 and 50 percent, with the lowest value reported for patients aged 70–75 years (CR rate about 38%) and for those over 75 years (CR rate about 22%).[3,4] In contrast, in patients aged up to 50–55 years, CR rates vary between 70 and 80 percent. More important, most studies have shown that median RFS in AML patients older than 60 years is significantly lower, that is, less than 12 months, as opposed to younger adults (i.e., up to 50 years of age), who tend to have longer RFS of almost 24 months. The reason for these poor CR rates and survival includes a combination of host-related factors and the underlying biology of AML.[5] The cost of treating elderly AML patients is also a burgeoning problem, as was demonstrated in a retrospective analysis of Medicare payments among 2,657 adults 65 years and older with AML.[6] The mean standard error (SE) in total Medicare payments was $41,594 ± $870 (in 1998 U.S. dollars), 84 percent of which was attributed to inpatient payments. In the 2 years after the AML diagnosis, 790 patients (30%) underwent chemotherapy. These patients had costs almost 3 times higher than those of other patients, and their median survival was 6 months longer. The use of hospice care was rare and utilized only by 17 percent of patients. Oldest patients also had the highest average payments per month of follow-up ($26,272 for patients over 85 years of age compared to $8,922 for patients aged 65–74 years).

However, the past 10 years have seen the emergence of multiple chemotherapeutic and targeted agents that have provided the treating oncologist with many new therapeutic strategies to better treat the elderly patient with AML. In this chapter, we will review the underlying causes for the aggressive biology of AML in the elderly, quality-of-life (QOL) issues, various therapeutic options for induction therapy, the role of hematopoietic growth factors, newer targeted agents being utilized in AML, and future directions.

B. Host-related factors and biological features of acute myeloid leukemia (AML) in the elderly

There is considerable evidence to suggest that AML is a very different disease in older patients and that the underlying biology is fairly aggressive (Table 17.1).[7] Some of the biological features include multilineage involvement and trilineage dysplasia.[8] This leads to higher incidence of clonal remissions and higher relapse rates. The combination of impaired hematopoiesis and persistence of the leukemic clone may explain the impaired marrow-repopulating efficiency and reduced tolerance to induction and consolidation chemotherapy. This is also seen in myelodysplastic syndromes (MDSs), a condition that often precedes the development of AML. Data from a number of multicenter studies indicate that a small number of older patients with de novo AML may have actually suffered from a previous occult preleukemic/MDS phase. Moreover, some patients affected by AML with trilineage dysplasia may relapse as MDS after initial induction chemotherapy, further suggesting that their supposed de novo AML actually represented an evolution of a preceding occult MDS.[9,10] It has also been

245

Table 17.1 Characteristics of acute myeloid leukemia (AML) biology in elderly versus younger individuals.[1,16,18,94]

Characteristic	Elderly AML	Younger AML
Population incidence/100,000	17.6	1.8
Secondary AML	24–56%	8%
TRM with induction therapy	25–30%	5–10%
Complete remission	38–62%	65–73%
FLT3 mutation	34%	20%
MDR1 expression	71%	35%
Favorable cytogenetics		
t(8;21)	2%	9%
inv 16 or t(16;16)	1–3%	10%
t(15;17)	4%	6–12%
Intermediate-risk cytogenetics		
+8	6–10%	4%
Normal karyotype	31%	34–45%
Unfavorable cytogenetics		
−7, −5, inv 3 or t(3;3)	8–9%	3%
Complex	18%	7%

Note. TRM = treatment-related mortality; FLT3 = FMS-like tyrosine kinase-3; MDR1 = multidrug resistance 1; inv = inversion; t = translocation.

demonstrated that leukemic blasts derived from elderly AML patients are less likely to undergo apoptosis following treatment with cytarabine and daunorubicin.[11]

One reason for the varying nature of the biology of elderly AML is thought to be the aging of the hematopoietic stem cell (HSC), which is a result of several processes that include DNA damage, telomere shortening, and oxidative stress.[12] It is also important to point out that homing of primitive stem/progenitor cells to the bone marrow represents the crucial first step to successful engraftment after transplantation. One elegant study has quantitatively determined that recipient age has a dramatic influence on HSC homing, and the seeding efficiency of young HSCs in the bone marrow of old mice is only one-third to one-half that measured in young mice.[13] This striking difference points to a decline in the capacity of the marrow stroma to capture or retain – or both – stem cells in old age. In an attempt to better understand the mechanisms underlying hematopoietic aging gene expression, profiling revealed that HSC aging is accompanied by the systemic down-regulation of genes mediating lymphoid specification and function and up-regulation of genes involved in specifying myeloid fate and function.[14] In this study, HSCs from old mice expressed elevated levels of many genes involved in leukemic transformation. These data support a model in which age-dependent alterations in gene expression at the stem cell level presage downstream developmental

potential and thereby contribute to age-dependent immune decline, and perhaps also to the increased incidence of leukemia in the elderly.

More recently, immunophenotyping has yielded some valuable results in elderly AML patients.[15] In one study, the authors investigated expression of the membrane antigens CD13, CD15, CD33, and CD34 by flow cytometry in 273 elderly patients (median age 69 years) with newly diagnosed AML and demonstrated that CD13 was expressed in 73 percent of patients, CD15 was expressed in 43 percent of patients, CD33 was expressed in 64 percent of patients, and CD34 was expressed in 66 percent of patients. Three risk groups were defined based on CD34 and CD33 antigen expression: the poor-risk group included patients with CD34-positive/CD33-positive or CD34-negative/CD33-negative disease, the intermediate-risk group included patients with CD34-positive/CD33-negative disease, and the favorable-risk group included patients with CD34-negative/CD33-positive disease. After cytogenetic analyses, immunophenotype was the most significant prognostic factor in terms of survival in a multivariate analysis ($p = .03$ and $p < .0001$, respectively).

Several studies have confirmed that karyotypic abnormalities carrying an adverse prognostic significance are more frequently detected in elderly than younger AML patients. These include −7, 7q−, −5, and 5q−; abnormalities of 11q and 17p; and +8 and several complex or multiple

Table 17.2 Genetic alterations and their impact on clinical outcome in AML.[15,19,26,28,95]

Mutation	Characteristic
FLT3-ITD	Higher white blood cell counts, higher peripheral blasts, lower percentage CD34+ cells, normal karyotype, yet worse CR and survival
RAS	Lower percentage of peripheral and marrow blasts, N-ras mutation likely associated with M4, worse CR and survival
BAALC	Overexpression leads to worse CR, DFS, and OS
MLL-PTD	Shorter CR duration and worse overall survival
TP53	Elderly patients, unfavorable cytogenetics, worse CR and survival
CEBPA	If mutation + longer CR duration and OS than wild-type gene
NPM1	Younger, higher white blood cell counts, normal karyotype, not seen with M0 AML; mutation if + lends to better CR and survival, especially in normal karyotype patients who are also FLT3 –

Note. FLT3 = FMS-like tyrosine kinase-3; CR = complete response; BAALC = brain and acute leukemia, cytoplasmic; DFS = disease-free survival; OS = overall survival; MLL-PTD = mixed lineage leukemia and partial tandem duplication; TP53 = tumor protein 53; CEBPA = CCAAT/enhancer binding protein; NPM1 = nucleophosmin; M0 = French American British AML Subtype M0.

abnormalities involving two, three, or more chromosomes. As in younger patients with AML, cytogenetic abnormalities predict response to induction therapy in the elderly.[16] This was confirmed by assessment of the cytogenetic findings and clinical outcome of 1,065 elderly individuals who had enrolled in the MRC AML11 trial.[17] More recently, a study of 635 elderly AML patients (excluding M3) led to the conclusion that pretreatment cytogenetics along with white blood cell count (WBC), marrow blast percentage, sex, and age have prognostic significance in elderly patients with AML. Patients with five or more chromosomal aberrations appear to benefit minimally from current treatment and are better suited for investigational therapy or supportive care.[18]

Another factor that contributes to poor prognosis in the elderly is the higher expression by leukemic cells of multidrug resistance gene (MDR1) compared to younger patients.[19,20] MDR1, located on chromosome 7, encodes for a membrane transporter protein, P-glycoprotein (P-gp), and is responsible for drug efflux and subsequent drug resistance. Apart from its role as a drug-efflux pump, P-gp has been implicated as an inhibitor of apoptosis in leukemic cells.[21] Other genes involved in drug resistance include MRP1 and its various homologues. Lung resistance protein (LRP), breast cancer resistance protein (BRCP), and glutathione S-transferases have also been implicated in drug resistance mechanisms in AML.[19,20] About 20–30 percent of newly diagnosed AML cases express the MDR1 gene compared to 70–75 percent of patients with refractory, relapsed, and secondary AML. Accordingly, lower CR rates and shorter remission durations have been reported in adult patients with MDR1+ disease as compared with those with a MDR1– phenotype. Recently, MDR status has been incorporated into prognostic models for AML, and efforts to modulate multidrug resistance with pharmacologic agents are ongoing. Several trials have utilized the first-generation P-gp inhibitors quinine and cyclosporine-A in combination with chemotherapy for treatment of relapsed AML.[22-25] While two of these studies found no difference in CR rate, disease-free survival (DFS), or overall survival (OS) between patients who received a P-gp inhibitor as part of induction and those who did not, one trial that included cyclosporine as part of induction therapy did demonstrate improvement in RFS and OS.[24] The addition of cyclosporine did not increase toxicity associated with induction therapy, and the survival benefit conferred by the addition of cyclosporine to induction occurred in patients with higher levels of P-gp expression.

A number of genetic alterations also affect clinical outcome in AML (Table 17.2). The prevalence and potential biological role of these mutations in the elderly have been investigated in several studies. In one study of 140 elderly AML patients, for example, FLT3, RAS, and TP53 mutations were found in 34 percent, 19 percent, and 9 percent of patients, respectively.[26] A meta-analysis of four studies that evaluated the prognostic significance of FLT3 mutations was able to demonstrate that FLT3 mutations have an adverse effect on the outcome for AML.[27] Also seen are nucleophosmin (*NPM1*) gene mutations that occur frequently in younger patients and are typically associated with normal karyotype. However, one study has evaluated the correlation between mutations in *NPM1* and *FLT3* genes and outcome in 99 elderly patients (median age 71 years, range 60–85 years) with newly diagnosed for AML.[28] In this study, primary treatment approach was curative in 54 patients, palliative in 38 patients, and supportive only in the remaining 7 patients. In patients who were *FLT3* negative, presence of the *NPM1* mutation was associated with a higher CR rate (40.5% in *NPM1*– vs. 80.0% in *NPM1*+, $p = .03$) but not with a significant difference in DFS or OS. Meanwhile, presence of the *FLT3* mutation was associated with a decrease in OS regardless of *NPM1* status (210 days in *FLT3*+ vs. 634 days in *FLT3*–, $p = .03$). One recent study utilized clinically annotated microarray data from 425 patients with newly diagnosed de novo AML and conducted gene expression analysis by applying previously defined and tested signature profiles reflecting deregulation of oncogenic signaling pathways, altered tumor environment, and signatures of chemotherapy sensitivity. As expected elderly patients had very poor survival when compared to their younger counterparts and were more resistant to an anthracycline, and this may be explained by the finding that elderly AML patients were noted to have a higher probability of RAS, Src, and TNF (tumor necrosis factor) pathway activation. When patients were stratified by their molecular mutation status, it was noted that elderly AML patients, irrespective of their *FLT3* and *NPM1* status had higher RAS, Src, and TNF pathway activation compared to the younger AML patients.[28a]

The previously mentioned biological factors act along with the usual host-related factors in elderly AML patients. These include an age-associated decline in kidney and liver functions and an increase in comorbid conditions among the elderly such as heart disease, renal insufficiency, vascular disease, and coexisting hematologic conditions that all impact the metabolism of chemotherapeutic agents and the ability to withstand intensive therapy. Elderly patients are also more likely than younger patients to develop severe, life-threatening infections during the course of treatment.[29] Also, as might be expected, some older individuals with AML tend to have poor performance status (PS) at diagnosis in comparison to younger individuals, and multiple studies have now demonstrated a correlation between poor performance status and unfavorable response to therapy. One retrospective analysis of 968 adults with AML on five Southwest Oncology Group trials was able to demonstrate that not only do elderly patients with AML present with worse PS but also patients who were younger (56 years of age and younger) with PS of 2 had a 2 percent chance of dying within 30 days of induction therapy compared to 31 percent in patients 66–75 years and 50 percent in those aged over 75 years with the same PS.[30]

C. Decision making and quality of life in elderly AML patients

Older patients with AML and advanced MDS are often left with the difficult task of making the decision between receiving intensive induction chemotherapy or nonintensive chemotherapy and best supportive care. When this was evaluated prospectively in 43 patients, it was noted that the choice for intensive therapy was associated with younger age (66 vs. 76 years, $p = .01$) but not with performance status, comorbidities, or QOL.[31] In all, 63 percent of patients reported not being offered other treatment options despite physician documentation of alternatives. Patient and physician estimates of cure differed significantly: 74 percent of patients estimated their chance of cure to be 50 percent or greater, yet for 89 percent of patients, physician estimates of cure were 10 percent or less. Patients who received intensive therapy experienced decreased QOL at 2 weeks but rebounded to baseline and to nonintensive chemotherapy levels by 6 weeks.

This has also been corroborated by another study that evaluated the effect of intensive induction therapy on the QOL and functional status of 60 elderly AML patients. The authors monitored QOL before, during, and after therapy and concluded that receiving intensive chemotherapy does not appear to lead to worse QOL or functional status than more palliative approaches.[32] They noted that basic activities of daily living (ADL) scores did not change over time, whereas instrumental ADL scores declined slightly regardless of treatment. One interesting study has also been able to demonstrate that elderly patients with AML and MDS are highly symptomatic and experience cognitive impairment and fatigue before the initiation of their treatment.[33] This is thought to be due to increased levels of circulating cytokines (IL-6, TNF-α), providing some support to the hypothesis that cancer-related symptoms are related at least in part to cytokine-immunologic activation. This has also been demonstrated in another study of 65 elderly AML patients, where it was noted that fatigue was the most universal symptom in AML patients irrespective of the type of treatment, that is, intensive versus nonintensive therapy.[34] There was a correlation between fatigue scores and both WBC counts and lactate dehydrogenase level (LDH) levels, and one possible explanation is that WBC count and LDH level may reflect the burden of rapid cell turnover or breakdown, with resultant leakage of intracellular contents and alterations in cytokine levels. Future studies need to focus on exploring relationships between fatigue and depression, cytokines, and other factors to identify potential intervention targets.

D. Therapeutic options for elderly AML patients

The most appropriate management of AML in elderly patients is still a highly controversial issue because of the clinical and biological heterogeneity of these patients. However, at least three different approaches are currently used: palliative treatment, attenuated chemotherapy, and standard intensive chemotherapy. It is noteworthy that the therapeutic choice for an individual patient should be based on objective criteria and not solely on chronological age and the physician's attitude. As indicated earlier, elderly AML patients generally want to be treated with induction therapy and retain their QOL and functional status with both intensive and nonintensive therapy.

D.1. Palliative therapy and best supportive care

A landmark study has evaluated the value of intensive induction compared to palliative care in elderly (aged 65 years or older) AML patients.[35] Thirty-one patients received one or two courses of daunorubicin, vincristine, and cytarabine for remission induction, followed by one additional cycle for consolidation, compared to 29 patients who were randomized to "wait and see" and supportive care plus mild cytoreductive chemotherapy only for relief of progressive AML-related symptoms. As expected, OS was significantly longer in patients who received intensive treatment, and surprisingly, hospitalization rates were no different between

the two arms. Thus palliation should be limited to patients with unfavorable prognostic factors, very poor performance status, or severe comorbid diseases in whom chemotherapy may result in unacceptable toxicity without any meaningful advantage in survival.

D.2. Attenuated chemotherapy

Attenuated chemotherapy uses the principle of combining one or more chemotherapeutic agents (e.g., oral etoposide, hydroxyurea, cytarabine, etc.) given orally or at lower doses parenterally to achieve a CR.[36] One randomized study in 51 elderly AML patients compared the use of etoposide, thioguanine, idarubicin (ETI) to thioguanine, ara-C, daunorubicin (TAD).[37] The CR rate was 60 percent in the ETI group and 23 percent in the TAD group ($p = .007$). In another study of 217 elderly AML patients who were deemed unfit for intensive chemotherapy and were randomized to receive low-dose ara-C (20 mg by subcutaneous injection twice daily for 10 days) or oral hydroxyurea with or without all-trans retinoic acid (ATRA),[38] patients in the low-dose ara-C arm had better CR rate (18% vs. 1%, $p = .00006$) and better OS. Of note, patients who had adverse cytogenetics did not benefit from ATRA. Toxicity scores or supportive care requirements did not differ between the treatment arms. More recently, hypomethylating agents like 5-aza-2-deoxycytidine (decitabine) and 5-azacytidine (azacytidine) have been successfully used in some trials to treat AML in the elderly and have been described in more detail later in this chapter.

D.3. Standard intensive induction therapy and role of postremission therapy

Since the 1970s, intensive chemotherapy with the "7 + 3" regimen (cytarabine [for 7 days] and an anthracycline such as daunorubicin or idarubicin, or the anthracenedione mitoxantrone [for 3 days]) has been standard therapy for AML.[39,40] There have been no studies using the 7 + 3 regimen specifically in elderly AML patients, and CR rates in various studies range from 30 to 50 percent in elderly patients. In addition to intensive induction chemotherapy, most treatment regimens for older patients with AML include postremission chemotherapy or consolidation therapy to prevent relapse. The benefit of such an approach is less clear in older patients, for whom median

DFS is approximately 1 year, whether or not they receive consolidation therapy. This has been demonstrated in a landmark CALGB trial, where high-dose cytarabine was superior to lower doses of cytarabine, with a 4-year DFS of 44 percent and a 4-year OS of 46 percent in AML patients aged less than 60 years.[41] However, in patients aged 60 years or older, among whom only 29 percent were able to complete all four cycles of high-dose cytarabine, the 4-year DFS was 16 percent or less, and 4-year OS was only 9 percent. Cerebellar toxicity occurred in over 30 percent of elderly patients who received high-dose cytarabine (HiDAC). Poor tolerance of HiDAC thus presumably accounted for the inferior outcome observed in elderly patients treated with HiDAC as compared to younger patients who received such therapy. In another recent study of 40 elderly AML patients treated with standard 7 + 3 induction therapy, patients who achieved a CR were treated with consolidation therapy with cytarabine at 400 mg/m^2.[42] However, it was noted that there was no difference in DFS or OS whether or not patients received postremission therapy. Thus the role of postremission therapy continues to be controversial, and the decision to do so should be made jointly by the patient and treating oncologist.

D.4. Role of gemtuzumab ozogamicin (Mylotarg)

Gemtuzumab ozogamicin (GO) is a humanized anti-CD33 monoclonal antibody conjugated to a derivative of the cytotoxic antibiotic calicheamicin.[43] The agent selectively targets CD33 antigen, which is expressed on 90 percent of myeloid blast cells. Binding of the antibody to CD33 results in internalization and release of calicheamicin, leading to cell death. GO received U.S. Food and Drug Administration approval in May 2000 for monotherapy in patients 60 years of age or older with relapsed, CD33-positive AML who are not considered candidates for cytotoxic chemotherapy. In 2005, the Mylotarg Study Group reported updated results from three multicenter, open-label, single-arm, phase II studies in 277 patients with CD33-positive AML at first recurrence, in which patients received two intravenous doses of GO 9 mg/m^2.[44] Among individuals 60 years or older, the overall response rate (ORR) was 24 percent, the CR rate 12 percent, and complete remission with incomplete platelet recovery rate (CRp) was 12 percent. Patients in whom a CR after initial therapy persisted longer than 12 months

prior to relapse experienced the best response to GO, with an ORR of 35 percent. Infusion-related events included chills, fever, nausea, hypotension, and hypertension, all of which occurred in 8 percent of cases or less. Grade 3 or 4 neutropenia and thrombocytopenia developed in 98–99 percent of patients. Other important, though less frequent, therapy-related toxicities included hyperbilirubinemia, elevations in liver transaminases, and hepatic veno-occlusive disease (VOD). The higher incidence of VOD after stem cell transplantation was seen in patients who received GO within 6 months of the procedure.[45] GO has also been studied as part of first-line therapy in older patients with AML. In a phase II trial involving 12 individuals aged 65 or older with newly diagnosed AML, patients were scheduled to receive GO 9 mg/m^2 on days 1 and 14.[46] Those who recovered bone marrow function received consolidation therapy with GO 6 mg/m^2 45–60 days after induction, followed by maintenance GO 3 mg/m^2 every 4 weeks. CR was attained in 25 percent of patients, and only one patient was taken off study due to unsatisfactory bone marrow recovery. One phase I study tested intensive, dose-dense therapy with HiDAC and GO as the sole induction and consolidation therapy in nine newly diagnosed patients with AML aged 60 years or older. In this small study, the ORR was high at 88 percent, with 66 percent CR, and two patients continue to be alive (DFS 50 and 59 months). All patients had significant hematologic toxicity with grade 4 pancytopenia, and two patients developed dose-limiting reversible neurotoxicity.[47]

D.5. Role of hematopoietic stem cell transplantation

Elderly patients with AML are often poor candidates for hematopoietic stem cell transplantation (HSCT) because of comorbid medical conditions, and most of the randomized trials are conducted in patients aged over 50 years. More recently, however, the development of reduced-intensity conditioning (RIC) regimens has challenged convention regarding patient age and HSCT.[48,49] There is increasing evidence derived from clinical trials that appropriately selected individuals may benefit from allogeneic SCT following RIC. In one phase II trial, for instance, 19 older patients (median age 64 years) with AML or high-risk MDS who received a RIC regimen consisting of fludarabine, melphalan, and carmustine followed by allogeneic SCT achieved a CR of 89 percent

CR and 1-year survival rate of 68 percent.[48,49] The feasibility and efficacy of autologous SCT have also been studied. In a phase II study involving 160 elderly patients with AML (median age 69 years), patients were treated with intensive induction chemotherapy and, if CR was achieved, one cycle of consolidation therapy followed by autologous SCT for selected patients under 70 years of age.[50] While autologous SCT was feasible in this population, it did not prevent early relapse and thus did not translate into longer DFS or OS. Thus enrolling elderly AML patients on HSCT clinical trials should be a priority with better selection criteria (other than chronological age), better tolerated preparative regimens, and supportive care measures.

E. New and emerging therapeutic modalities for treatment of AML in the elderly

Given the poor response rates and high toxicity from traditional 7 + 3 induction therapy in elderly AML patients, there is an impetus to develop induction therapy that includes more targeted agents that might perhaps lead to better CR rates at the cost of much less toxicity. Drugs or treatment modalities discussed in this chapter include (1) novel chemotherapeutic agents (e.g., cloretazine, clofarabine, and troxacitabine), (2) farnesyltransferase inhibitors (e.g., tipifarnib), (3) *FLT3* inhibitors, (4) differentiation therapy using hypomethylating agents or histone deacetylase inhibitors, and (5) other agents.

E.1. Novel chemotherapeutic agents

There have been many new chemotherapeutic agents tested in elderly AML patients. Cloretazine (VNP40101M) is a member of the novel sulfonylhydrazine class of alkylating agents that causes DNA damage by releasing the DNA chloroethylating agent 90CE after entering the blood. In a multicenter phase II study, 104 older patients with previously untreated AML or high-risk MDS received cloretazine 600 mg/m^2 as a single intravenous infusion.[51] Notably, patients enrolled in this trial included those with Eastern Cooperative Oncology Group (ECOG) 2 performance status (30%), preexisting cardiac disease (45%), and preexisting hepatic disease (24%). Despite this, an ORR of 32 percent with 28 percent CR was achieved, and ORR in patients with de novo AML was

50 percent. Grade 3 or 4 myelosuppression was seen in 100 percent of patients, while severe infection with febrile neutropenia occurred in 21 percent of patients and 1-year survival was 14 percent. In a confirmatory phase II trial of single-agent cloretazine administered as a 600 mg/m^2 infusion to 85 elderly patients (median age 73) with poor-risk de novo AML, an ORR of 35 percent was achieved with 28 percent CR, and the response rate was 34 percent in patients over age 70.[52] Cloretazine has also been combined with cytarabine in the treatment of AML. Results from a double-blind, placebo-controlled, randomized phase III study using high-dose continuous-infusion cytarabine (1.5 g/m^2 d1–3) with or without cloretazine (600 mg/m^2 d1) for the treatment of AML patients in first relapse have been recently reported. Although the ORR in the combination arm was nearly twice that in the cytarabine alone arm (37% vs. 19%), the death rate was significantly higher in the combination arm (39% vs. 8.6%).[53] The majority of deaths in patients who received combination therapy occurred as a result of infection, sepsis, or pneumonia. The study has now been placed on hold, pending further investigation of the excess mortality observed when the two agents were used in combination.

In recent years, research has sought to refine the use of nucleoside analogs in AML patients in whom cytarabine forms the cornerstone of induction therapy. These efforts have focused primarily on two new agents: clofarabine and troxacitabine. Clofarabine is a next-generation nucleoside analog designed to combine the most favorable pharmacokinetic properties of fludarabine and cladribine and, at the same, time to avoid the dose-limiting neurotoxicity of other deoxynucleoside analogs. Initial phase I and II trials of clofarabine monotherapy in the setting of relapsed or refractory AML yielded encouraging results, with significant response rates and a favorable toxicity profile featuring minimal neurotoxicity.[54] More recently, preliminary results were reported from a single-arm phase II trial involving previously untreated elderly patients (median age 71) with one or more adverse prognostic factors who received clofarabine monotherapy.[55] Clofarabine was administered as a 30 mg/m^2 (induction) or 20 mg/m^2 (reinduction/consolidation) infusion days 1–5 of each cycle to a maximum of six cycles. Treatment-related toxicity, primarily hematologic, was manageable, and the ORR was 43 percent, with 40 percent CR. A phase II study in 32 relapsed and refractory AML patients (median age 59 years) using clofarabine 40 mg/m^2 intravenously for 5 days along with cytarabine 1,000 mg/m^2 intravenously for 5 days led to ORR of 38 percent, with 22 percent CR.[56] This approach was extended to the treatment of 60 newly diagnosed AML patients aged 50 years or older with doses of clofarabine and cytarabine similar to upfront induction therapy and produced higher ORR of 60 percent with 52 percent CR.[57] Myelosuppression was common, and four patients died during induction. Adverse events included diarrhea, nausea, vomiting, mucositis, skin reactions, liver test abnormalities, and infusion-related facial flushing and headaches. Thus the combination of clofarabine and cytarabine does lead to good response rates, but it does not appear to improve survival in comparison to other regimens.

Troxacitabine is an L-nucleoside analog (most nucleoside analogs are in D-configuration) that has been studied in phase I/II studies as monotherapy in patients with relapsed or refractory AML.[58] The dose-limiting toxicity of the drug included mucositis and hand-foot syndrome. This drug has shown promise in younger AML patients but has yet to be studied specifically in the elderly.[59]

Sapacitabine is a deoxycytidine nucleoside analog that causes single-strand DNA breaks. In a phase I trial, sapacitabine was given in a dose-escalation pattern from 75 to 375 mg orally twice a day for 7 days every 3–4 weeks to 29 patients. It led to a decrease in bone marrow blasts by 50 percent, and the dose-limiting toxicity was delayed myelosuppression.[60] Currently phase II studies using 325 mg orally twice a day for 7 days every 3 weeks in AML patients are ongoing.

E.2. Farnesyltransferase inhibitors

This class of agents targets the enzyme farnesyltransferase, which catalyzes the transfer of a farnesyl moiety to the C-terminus cysteine residue of Ras and other proteins.[61] This posttranslational modification directs proteins to the plasma membrane, where they carry out their specific cellular, or in the case of mutated Ras, oncogenic function. Thus disruption of these events theoretically interrupts the oncogenic activity of mutated Ras.

In one phase II trial, the oral farnesyltransferase inhibitor tipifarnib was evaluated in poor-risk elderly patients with previously untreated AML.[62] Patients were treated with tipifarnib 600 mg orally twice daily for 21 days, followed by a 42-day rest period. Up to four cycles of therapy

were given to patients who experienced a clinical response. There was an ORR of 23 percent with 14 percent CR, and among individuals who experienced a CR, the median duration of survival was 18 months. Serious drug-related toxicity occurred in 47 percent of patients. Eleven patients (7%) died within 30 days of the final dose of tipifarnib from causes other than progressive disease. A majority of patients (60%) required hospitalization during treatment with tipifarnib for a median duration of 14 days. Tipifarnib was then evaluated in a second trial involving individuals with relapsed or refractory AML, where patients received tipifarnib 600 mg orally twice daily for 21 days of each 4-week cycle until disease progression. Though the drug was well tolerated, only 4 percent of patients achieved any response.[62] Finally, tipifarnib was compared to best supportive care in the management of elderly patients in a study that enrolled 457 AML patients over the age of 70 who did not wish to undergo combination chemotherapy. At the time of interim analysis, there was no survival difference between patients who received tipifarnib and those who received best supportive care, and final results from this interesting study are pending.[63]

E.3. *FLT3* inhibitors

A member of the class III receptor tyrosine kinase family, the FMS-like tyrosine kinase-3 (*FLT3*) receptor, plays an important regulatory role in normal hematopoiesis.[64] Mutations of *FLT3* in AML were first described over 10 years ago and are now known to occur in a substantial percentage of patients with the disease. An internal tandem duplication (ITD) involving the juxtamembrane of *FLT3* occurs in 15–35 percent of patients with AML, while a mutation in the tyrosine kinase domain occurs in 5–10 percent and the presence of the *FLT3*-ITD mutation confers a poor prognosis.[27] Several phase I and phase II trials have assessed the activity of *FLT3* inhibitors in patients with relapsed/refractory AML or in older patients with disease not amenable to therapy with conventional chemotherapy.[65] Recently, a phase I–II trial employed the oral *FLT3* inhibitor lestaurtinib (CEP701) as first-line therapy in previously untreated older patients with AML who were not candidates for intensive chemotherapy.[66] Patients were treated regardless of their FLT mutation status and received lestaurtinib 60 mg orally twice daily initially with dose escalation to 80 mg twice daily, as tolerated. There were no complete or partial remissions, though a bone marrow response occurred in 19 percent of patients with an 11 percent hematologic response. The most common therapy-related high-grade toxicities of nausea and diarrhea occurred in fewer than 10 percent of patients. Further clinical trials are necessary to define the role of *FLT3* inhibition in treatment of AML, but the mutated receptor remains an attractive target given its prevalence and biological function within hematopoietic cells.

E.4. Differentiation therapy

DNA methylation, nucleosome remodeling, and histone modifications play a role in gene silencing, and when these processes are usurped, it leads to inappropriate silencing and contributes to carcinogenesis. Drugs that lead to reexpression of silenced genes through DNA hypomethylation and protein/histone acetylation have shown promise in AML.[67,68] The histone deacetylase inhibitors include drugs like vorinostat, MS-275, valproic acid, and depsipeptide. The hypomethylating agents include 5-azacytidine and decitabine. A phase I study of the histone deacetylase inhibitor MS-275 in patients with relapsed, refractory, or newly diagnosed poor-risk AML confirmed the agent's biologic activity, as reflected by increases in H3/H4 acetylation and p21 expression, but failed to show clinical responsiveness based on standard response criteria, and further studies are ongoing.[69] Valproic acid has also shown synergistic activity with ara-C, and this combination has been tested in 31 frail elderly AML patients. Eleven of 31 patients (35%) had hematological improvement, including 7 CR (22%) with clearing of blasts in the marrow and normalization of blood counts, and there was minimal toxicity. The authors concluded that this combination was a feasible option for frail elderly patients who were not candidates for intensive therapy.[70]

The hypomethylating agent 5-azacytidine at a dose of 75 mg/m^2 subcutaneously has been evaluated in 55 elderly AML patients, and this led to an ORR of 35 percent with 16 percent CR. The authors also concluded that 5-azacytidine is more effective in de novo AML patients as compared to pretreated (refractory and/or relapsed) disease, and AML patients responding to the drug have a significant survival advantage compared to nonresponders.[71] Similarly, decitabine (20 mg/m^2 IV over 1 hour for 5 days every 4 weeks) has been evaluated in 55 elderly AML patients (median age

74 years) where the ORR was 26 percent with 24 percent CR. The 30-day mortality rate on this trial was 4 percent, which compares favorably to the approximately 20 percent mortality rate typically seen in this population treated with standard induction therapy.[72] A large phase III study utilizing decitabine is currently ongoing in this patient population.

E.5. Other agents

There has been a deluge of clinical trials recently utilizing several novel agents in AML. Some of these have yet to be studied specifically in elderly AML patients. Bcl-2, a potent inhibitor of apoptosis, is overexpressed in various hematologic malignancies, including AML, and has been explored as a therapeutic target. Phase I and II studies of the Bcl-2 antisense oligonucleotide G3139 as part of induction therapy in AML patients with relapsed, refractory, and previously untreated disease demonstrated biological activity with a decrease in Bcl-2 expression following therapy, significant clinical responses, and minimal toxicity.[73] However, a randomized phase III trial involving untreated older individuals with AML who received cytarabine and daunorubicin with or without Bcl-2 antisense oligonucleotide showed no difference in CR rate or OS between the two treatment groups.[74] Interestingly, in one phase II study, 48 elderly AML patients in first relapse were treated with oblimersen 7 mg/kg/d given as a continuous intravenous infusion on days 1–7 and 15–21, along with GO 9 mg/m^2 given intravenously on days 4 and 18. Twelve of 48 patients (25%) achieved a major response (five complete response and seven complete response without platelet recovery). Ten of the 12 patients who achieved a major response survived more than 6 months compared with six of 36 nonresponders.[75]

Another area of research includes the potential role of vascular endothelial growth factor (VEGF) and its receptor, VEGFR2, which are overexpressed in the bone marrow of patients with AML.[76] In vitro studies suggest VEGF inhibits apoptosis and promotes survival in AML by inducing expression of Bcl-2.[77] A single-arm phase II trial of bevacizumab in combination with cytarabine and mitoxantrone yielded an ORR of 48 percent and a CR rate of 33 percent with a favorable toxicity profile.[78] Also, c-Kit, a class III receptor tyrosine kinase, is expressed on AML blasts in 63–80 percent of patients. One study randomized 34 elderly AML patients to low-dose ara-C versus low-dose ara-C plus imatinib and found no superiority in ORR in the combination arm.[79] Finally, there are emerging data on the role the PI3-kinase and AKT/m TOR pathways in the pathogenesis of AML, and these may serve as therapeutic targets for drug development in AML.[80] All these agents warrant further evaluation of their role in the treatment of elderly AML.

F. Hematopoietic growth factors in elderly AML

The major causes of death from induction therapy in elderly AML patients include infections (mainly fungal and bacterial) and hemorrhage.[81] Improvements in supportive care may decrease treatment-associated mortality among elderly adults with AML, thereby increasing the likelihood of complete remission. The use of hematopoietic growth factors was previously controversial because it was thought that leukemia cells possess receptors for hematopoietic growth factors such as granulocyte-macrophage colony-stimulating factor (GM-CSF), which stimulates the cells to proliferate and worsen the disease.[82–84] There have been several landmark studies with respectable numbers of patients that have studied this question and randomized patients to receiving standard induction therapy with cytarabine plus an anthracycline with or without a CSF. Briefly, four studies have studied GM-CSF, and though all four showed a statistically significant decrease in the number of neutropenia days, only one study demonstrated an improvement in CR rates, decrease in early deaths, and improvement in DFS or OS in these patients.[85–89] One study utilized G-CSF and showed statistically significant improvement in CR rates and neutropenia, but again, early death, DFS, and OS were not affected.[90]

The AML-13 trial studied recombinant G-CSF, lenograstim, in 722 patients with median age 68 years and newly diagnosed AML who were randomized into four treatment arms: (1) no G-CSF, (2) G-CSF during chemotherapy, (3) G-CSF after chemotherapy until day 28 or recovery of polymorphonuclear leukocytes, and (4) G-CSF during and after chemotherapy.[91] The CR rate was significantly higher in patients who received G-CSF during chemotherapy (groups B and D), but there was no difference in OS between the four groups. Patients who received G-CSF after chemotherapy had a shorter time to neutrophil recovery and a shorter hospitalization. The authors concluded

that although priming with G-CSF can improve the CR rate, the use of G-CSF during and/or after chemotherapy has no effect on the long-term outcome of AML in older patients.

In summary, studies utilizing GM-CSF have shown a decrease in the median duration of neutropenia without any effect on CR rates and overall mortality. Studies utilizing G-CSF have also shown a decrease in the median duration of neutropenia and actual improvement in CR rates but no effect on mortality.

G. Summary and conclusions for future directions

There has been a concerted effort to better understand the biology of AML in the elderly. Over the past few years, there has been an increase in the number of clinical trials in this patient population and the number of publications to help guide the treating oncologist. The importance of understanding tumor biology to select patients likely to respond to a given therapy has been previously illustrated by the example of trastuzumab in breast cancer.[92] More recently, gene expression profiling was utilized to improve risk classification and outcome prediction in 170 older AML patients whose median age was 65 years, and it was demonstrated that gene expression signatures provide insight into novel groups of AML not predicted by traditional studies that impact prognosis and potential therapy.[93] A critical step in translating these findings to real-time clinical practice is to prospectively validate the approach in the setting of a clinical trial. However, this has not been studied in a prospective fashion, and at the present time, we are unable to predict (other than for acute promyelocytic leukemia) if patients should receive (1) traditional 7 + 3 induction chemotherapy; (2) induction therapy with other chemotherapeutic agents, for example, gemcitabine or cloretazine; or (3) targeted agents based on oncogenic pathway predictors (e.g., Src inhibitors) or molecular mutations (e.g., FLT3 inhibitors), alone or in combination with chemotherapeutic agents. The ultimate aim should be to improve the response rates and survival rates in elderly AML patients without increasing toxicity from induction therapy. The data in this chapter provide evidence of emerging treatment options in all aspects of care for older adults with AML and highlight the need for further studies in this patient population.

References

1. Jemal A, Siegel R, Ward E, et al. Cancer statistics, 2008. *CA Cancer J Clin.* 2008;58:71–96.

2. Yancik R. Population aging and cancer: a cross-national concern. *Cancer J.* 2005;11:437–441.

3. Baudard M, Marie JP, Cadiou M, et al. Acute myelogenous leukaemia in the elderly: retrospective study of 235 consecutive patients. *Br J Haematol.* 1994;86:82–91.

4. Taylor PR, Reid MM, Stark AN, et al. De novo acute myeloid leukaemia in patients over 55-years-old: a population-based study of incidence, treatment and outcome. Northern Region Haematology Group. *Leukemia.* 1995;9:231–237.

5. Pinto A, Zagonel V, Ferrara F. Acute myeloid leukemia in the elderly: biology and therapeutic strategies. *Crit Rev Oncol Hematol.* 2001;39:275–287.

6. Menzin J, Lang K, Earle CC, et al. The outcomes and costs of acute myeloid leukemia among the elderly. *Arch Int Med.* 2002;162:1597–1603.

7. Bowen DT. Etiology of acute myeloid leukemia in the elderly. *Semin Hematol.* 2006;43:82–88.

8. Fialkow PJ, Singer JW, Raskind WH, et al. Clonal development, stem-cell differentiation, and clinical remissions in acute nonlymphocytic leukemia. *N Engl J Med.* 1987;317:468–473.

9. Goasguen JE, Matsuo T, Cox C, et al. Evaluation of the dysmyelopoiesis in 336 patients with de novo acute myeloid leukemia: major importance of dysgranulopoiesis for remission and survival. *Leukemia.* 1992;6:520–525.

10. Larson RA. Treatment of acute myeloid leukemia with antecedent myelodysplastic syndrome. *Leukemia.* 1996;10(suppl 1):23–25.

11. Garrido SM, Cooper JJ, Appelbaum FR, et al. Blasts from elderly acute myeloid leukemia patients are characterized by low levels of culture- and drug-induced apoptosis. *Leuk Res.* 2001;25:23–32.

12. Kamminga LM, de Haan G. Cellular memory and hematopoietic stem cell aging. *Stem Cells.* 2006;24:1143–1149.

13. Liang Y, Van Zant G, Szilvassy SJ. Effects of aging on the homing and engraftment of murine hematopoietic stem and progenitor cells. *Blood.* 2005;106:1479–1487.

14. Rossi DJ, Bryder D, Zahn JM, et al. Cell intrinsic alterations underlie hematopoietic stem cell aging. *Proc Natl Acad Sci USA.* 2005;102:9194–9199.

15. Plesa C, Chelghoum Y, Plesa A, et al. Prognostic value of immunophenotyping in elderly patients with acute myeloid leukemia: a single-institution experience. *Cancer.* 2008;112:572–580.

16. Grimwade D, Walker H, Oliver F, et al. The importance of diagnostic cytogenetics on outcome in AML: analysis of 1,612 patients entered into the MRC AML 10 trial. The Medical Research Council Adult and Children's Leukaemia Working Parties. *Blood.* 1998;92:2322–2333.

17. Grimwade D, Walker H, Harrison G, et al. The predictive value of hierarchical cytogenetic classification in older adults with acute myeloid leukemia (AML): analysis of 1065 patients entered into the United Kingdom Medical Research Council AML11 trial. *Blood.* 2001;98:1312–1320.

18. Cancer and Leukemia Group B, Farag SS, Archer KJ, et al. Pretreatment cytogenetics add to other prognostic factors predicting complete remission and long-term outcome in patients 60 years of age or older with acute myeloid leukemia: results from Cancer and Leukemia Group B 8461. *Blood.* 2006;108:63–73.

19. Drenou B, Fardel O, Amiot L, et al. Detection of P glycoprotein activity on normal and leukemic CD34+ cells. *Leuk Res.* 1993;17:1031–1035.

20. Leith CP, Kopecky KJ, Chen IM, et al. Frequency and clinical significance of the expression of the multidrug resistance proteins MDR1/P-glycoprotein, MRP1, and LRP in acute myeloid leukemia: a Southwest Oncology Group Study. *Blood.* 1999;94:1086–1099.

21. Smyth MJ, Krasovskis E, Sutton VR, et al. The drug efflux protein, P-glycoprotein, additionally protects drug-resistant tumor cells from multiple forms of caspase-dependent apoptosis. *Proc Natl Acad Sci USA.* 1998;95:7024–7029.

22. Baer MR, George SL, Dodge RK, et al. Phase 3 study of the multidrug resistance modulator PSC-833 in previously untreated patients 60 years of age and older with acute myeloid leukemia: Cancer and Leukemia Group B Study 9720. *Blood.* 2002;100:1224–1232.

23. Daenen S, Van Der Holt B, Verhoef GEG, et al. Addition of cyclosporin A to the combination of mitoxantrone and etoposide to overcome resistance to chemotherapy in refractory or relapsing acute myeloid leukaemia: a randomised phase II trial from HOVON, the Dutch-Belgian Haemato-Oncology Working Group for adults. *Leuk Res.* 2004;28:1057–1067.

24. List AF, Kopecky KJ, Willman CL, et al. Benefit of cyclosporine modulation of drug resistance in patients with poor-risk acute myeloid leukemia: a Southwest Oncology Group study. *Blood.* 2001;98:3212–3220.

25. Solary E, Drenou B, Campos L, et al. Quinine as a multidrug resistance inhibitor: a phase 3 multicentric randomized study in adult de novo acute myelogenous leukemia. *Blood.* 2003;102:1202–1210.

26. Stirewalt DL, Kopecky KJ, Meshinchi S, et al. FLT3, RAS, and TP53 mutations in elderly patients with acute myeloid leukemia. *Blood*. 2001;97:3589–3595.

27. Yanada M, Matsuo K, Suzuki T, et al. Prognostic significance of FLT3 internal tandem duplication and tyrosine kinase domain mutations for acute myeloid leukemia: a meta-analysis. *Leukemia*. 2005;19:1345–1349.

28. Scholl S, Theuer C, Scheble V, et al. Clinical impact of nucleophosmin mutations and Flt3 internal tandem duplications in patients older than 60 yr with acute myeloid leukaemia. *Eur J Haematol*. 2008;80:208–215.

28a. Rao AV, Valk PJM, Metzeler KH, et al. Age-specific differences in oncogenic pathway dysregulation and anthracycline sensitivity in patients with acute myeloid leukemia. *Journal of Clinical Oncology* 2009;27:5580–5586.

29. Fanci R, Leoni F, Longo G. Nosocomial infections in acute leukemia: comparison between younger and elderly patients. *New Microbiol*. 2008;31:89–96.

30. Appelbaum FR, Gundacker H, Head DR, et al. Age and acute myeloid leukemia. *Blood*. 2006;107:3481–3485.

31. Sekeres MA, Stone RM, Zahrieh D, et al. Decision-making and quality of life in older adults with acute myeloid leukemia or advanced myelodysplastic syndrome. *Leukemia*. 2004;18:809–816.

32. Alibhai SMH, Leach M, Kermalli H, et al. The impact of acute myeloid leukemia and its treatment on quality of life and functional status in older adults. *Crit Rev Oncol Hematol*. 2007;64:19–30.

33. Meyers CA, Albitar M, Estey E. Cognitive impairment, fatigue, and cytokine levels in patients with acute myelogenous leukemia or myelodysplastic syndrome. *Cancer*. 2005;104:788–793.

34. Alibhai SMH, Leach M, Kowgier ME, et al. Fatigue in older adults with acute myeloid leukemia: predictors and associations with quality of life and functional status. *Leukemia*. 2007;21:845–848.

35. Lowenberg B, Zittoun R, Kerkhofs H, et al. On the value of intensive remission-induction chemotherapy in elderly patients of 65+ years with acute myeloid leukemia: a randomized phase III study of the European Organization for Research and Treatment of Cancer Leukemia Group. *J Clin Oncol*. 1989;7:1268–1274.

36. Bouabdallah R, Lefrere F, Rose C, et al. A phase II trial of induction and consolidation therapy of acute myeloid leukemia with weekly oral idarubicin alone in poor risk elderly patients. *Leukemia*. 1999;13:1491–1496.

37. Ruutu T, Almqvist A, Hallman H, et al. Oral induction and consolidation of acute myeloid leukemia with etoposide, 6-thioguanine, and idarubicin (ETI) in elderly patients: a randomized comparison with 5-day TAD. Finnish Leukemia Group. *Leukemia*. 1994;8:11–15.

38. Burnett AK, Milligan D, Prentice AG, et al. A comparison of low-dose cytarabine and hydroxyurea with or without all-trans retinoic acid for acute myeloid leukemia and high-risk myelodysplastic syndrome in patients not considered fit for intensive treatment. *Cancer*. 2007;109:1114–1124.

39. Yates J, Glidewell O, Wiernik P, et al. Cytosine arabinoside with daunorubicin or adriamycin for therapy of acute myelocytic leukemia: a CALGB study. *Blood*. 1982;60:454–462.

40. Rai KR, Holland JF, Glidewell OJ, et al. Treatment of acute myelocytic leukemia: a study by cancer and leukemia group B. *Blood*. 1981;58:1203–1212.

41. Mayer RJ, Davis RB, Schiffer CA, et al. Intensive postremission chemotherapy in adults with acute myeloid leukemia. Cancer and Leukemia Group B. *N Engl J Med*. 1994;331:896–903.

42. Abou-Jawde RM, Sobecks R, Pohlman B, et al. The role of post-remission chemotherapy for older patients with acute myelogenous leukemia [see comment]. *Leuk Lymphoma*. 2006;47:689–695.

43. Dowell JA, Korth-Bradley J, Liu H, et al. Pharmacokinetics of gemtuzumab ozogamicin, an antibody-targeted chemotherapy agent for the treatment of patients with acute myeloid leukemia in first relapse. *J Clin Pharmacol*. 2001;41:1206–1214

44. Larson RA, Sievers EL, Stadtmauer EA, et al. Final report of the efficacy and safety of gemtuzumab ozogamicin (Mylotarg) in patients with CD33-positive acute myeloid leukemia in first recurrence. *Cancer*. 2005;104:1442–1452.

45. Wadleigh M, Richardson PG, Zahrieh D, et al. Prior gemtuzumab ozogamicin exposure significantly increases the risk of veno-occlusive disease in patients who undergo myeloablative allogeneic stem cell transplantation [see comment]. *Blood*. 2003;102:1578–1582.

46. Nabhan C, Rundhaugen LM, Riley MB, et al. Phase II pilot trial of gemtuzumab ozogamicin (GO) as first line therapy in acute myeloid leukemia patients age 65 or older. *Leuk Res*. 2005;29:53–57.

47. Rao AV, Rizzieri DA, Gockerman JP, et al. Dose dense, high intensity therapy in newly diagnosed elderly patients with acute myeloid leukemia using gemtuzumab ozogamicin (Mylotarg^{TM}) and high dose cytarabine (Hi-DAC). Paper presented at: American Society of Hematology Annual Meeting; December 10–13, 2005; Atlanta, GA.

48. Bertz H, Potthoff K, Finke J. Allogeneic stem-cell transplantation from related and unrelated donors in older patients with myeloid leukemia. *J Clin Oncol*. 2003;21:1480–1484.

49. Scott BL, Sandmaier BM, Storer B, et al. Myeloablative vs nonmyeloablative allogeneic transplantation for patients with myelodysplastic syndrome or acute myelogenous leukemia with multilineage dysplasia: a retrospective analysis. *Leukemia*. 2006;20:128–135.

50. Archimbaud E, Jehn U, Thomas X, et al. Multicenter randomized phase II trial of idarubicin vs mitoxantrone, combined with VP-16 and cytarabine for induction/consolidation therapy, followed by a feasibility study of autologous peripheral blood stem cell transplantation in elderly patients with acute myeloid leukemia. *Leukemia*. 1999;13:843–849.

51. Giles F, Rizzieri D, Karp J, et al. Cloretazine (VNP40101M), a novel sulfonylhydrazine alkylating agent, in patients age 60 years or older with previously untreated acute myeloid leukemia. *J Clin Oncol*. 2007;25:25–31.

52. Schiller GJ, DeAngelo D, Vey N, et al. A phase II study of VNP40101M in elderly patients (pts) with de novo poor risk acute myelogenous leukemia (AML) [abstract 7026]. Paper presented at: American Society of Clinical Oncology Annual Meeting; May 30–June 3, 2008; Chicago, IL.

53. DeAngelo DOBS, Vey N, et al. A double blind placebo-controlled randomized phase III study of high dose continuous infusion cytosine arabinoside (araC) with or without VNP40101M in patients (pts) with first relapse of acute myeloid leukemia (AML). Paper presented at: American Society of Clinical Oncology Annual Meeting; May 30–June 3, 2008; Chicago, IL.

54. Kantarjian HM, Gandhi V, Kozuch P, et al. Phase I clinical and pharmacology study of clofarabine in patients with solid and hematologic cancers. *J Clin Oncol*. 2003;21:1167–1173.

55. Erba HP, Kantarjian D,KH, Claxton D, et al. Phase II study of single agent clofarabine in previously untreated older adult patients with acute myelogenous leukemia (AML) unlikely to benefit from standard induction chemotherapy. Paper presented at: American Society of Clinical Oncology Annual Meeting; May 30–June 3, 2008; Chicago, IL.

56. Faderl S, Verstovsek S, Cortes J, et al. Clofarabine and cytarabine combination as induction therapy for acute myeloid leukemia (AML) in patients 50 years of age or older. *Blood*. 2006;108:45–51.

57. Faderl S, Ferrajoli A, Wierda W, et al. Clofarabine combinations as acute myeloid leukemia salvage therapy [see comment]. *Cancer*. 2008;113:2090–2096.

58. Giles FJ, Cortes JE, Baker SD, et al. Troxacitabine, a novel dioxolane nucleoside analog, has activity in patients with advanced leukemia. *J Clin Oncol*. 2001;19:762–771.

59. Giles FJ, Faderl S, Thomas DA, et al. Randomized phase I/II study of troxacitabine combined with cytarabine, idarubicin, or topotecan in patients with refractory myeloid leukemias. *J Clin Oncol*. 2003;21:1050–1056.

60. Plunkett W, Faderl S, Cortes J, et al. Phase I study of sapacitabine, an oral nucleoside analogue, in patients with advanced leukemias or myelodysplastic syndromes. *J Clin Oncol*. 2007;25(18 suppl):7063.

61. End DW, Smets G, Todd AV, et al. Characterization of the antitumor effects of the selective farnesyl protein transferase inhibitor R115777 in vivo and in vitro. *Cancer Res*. 2001;61:131–137.

62. Harousseau J-L, Lancet JE, Reiffers J, et al. A phase 2 study of the oral farnesyltransferase inhibitor tipifarnib in patients with refractory or relapsed acute myeloid leukemia. *Blood*. 2007;109:5151–5156.

63. Harousseau J-L, Jedrzejczak WW, Martinelli G, et al. A randomized phase 3 study of tipifarnib compared to best supportive care (including hydroxyurea) in the treatment of newly diagnosed acute myeloid leukemia (AML) in patients 70 years or older. Paper presented at: American Society of Hematology Annual Meeting; December 8–11, 2007; Atlanta, GA.

64. Nakao M, Yokota S, Iwai T, et al. Internal tandem duplication of the flt3 gene found in acute myeloid leukemia. *Leukemia*. 1996;10:1911–1918.

65. Smith BD, Levis M, Beran M, et al. Single-agent CEP-701, a novel FLT3 inhibitor, shows biologic and clinical activity in patients with relapsed or refractory acute myeloid leukemia. *Blood*. 2004;103:3669–3676.

66. Knapper S, Burnett AK, Littlewood T, et al. A phase 2 trial of the FLT3 inhibitor lestaurtinib (CEP701) as first-line treatment for older patients with acute myeloid leukemia not considered fit for intensive chemotherapy. *Blood*. 2006;108:3262–3270.

67. Altucci L, Clarke N, Nebbioso A, et al. Acute myeloid leukemia: therapeutic impact of epigenetic drugs. *Int J Biochem Cell Biol*. 2005;37:1752–1762.

68. Kosugi H, Towatari M, Hatano S, et al. Histone deacetylase inhibitors are the potent inducer/enhancer of differentiation in acute myeloid leukemia: a new approach to anti-leukemia therapy. *Leukemia*. 1999;13:1316–1324.

69. Gojo I, Jiemjit A, Trepel JB, et al. Phase 1 and pharmacologic study of MS-275, a histone deacetylase inhibitor, in adults with refractory and relapsed acute leukemias. *Blood.* 2007;109:2781–2790.

70. Braiteh F, Soriano AO, Garcia-Manero G, et al. Phase I study of epigenetic modulation with 5-azacytidine and valproic acid in patients with advanced cancers. *Clin Cancer Res.* 2008;14:6296–6301.

71. Luca Maurillo AS, Genuardi M, Spagnoli A, et al. 5-Azacytidine for the treatment of acute myeloid leukemia: a retrospective, multicenter study of 55 patients [abstract 1947]. Paper presented at: Annual Meeting of the American Society of Hematology; Nov. 16, 2008; San Francisco, CA.

72. Cashen AF, O'Donnell MR, Larsen JS, et al. Preliminary results of a multicenter phase II trial of 5-day decitabine as front-line therapy for elderly patients with acute myeloid leukemia (AML) [abstract 560]. Paper presented at: Annual Meeting of the American Society of Hematology; Nov. 16, 2008; San Francisco, CA.

73. Marcucci G, Stock W, Dai G, et al. Phase I study of oblimersen sodium, an antisense to Bcl-2, in untreated older patients with acute myeloid leukemia: pharmacokinetics, pharmacodynamics, and clinical activity. *J Clin Oncol.* 2005;23:3404–3411.

74. Marcucci G, Moser B, Blum W, et al. A phase III randomized trial of intensive induction and consolidation chemotherapy +/– oblimersen, a proapoptotic Bcl-2 antisense oligonucleotide in untreated acute myeloid leukemia patients > 60 years old. Paper presented at: American Society of Clinical Oncology Annual Meeting; June 1–5, 2007; Chicago, IL.

75. Moore J, Seiter K, Kolitz J, et al. A phase II study of Bcl-2 antisense (oblimersen sodium) combined with gemtuzumab ozogamicin in older patients with acute myeloid leukemia in first relapse. *Leuk Res.* 2006;30:777–783.

76. Padro T, Bieker R, Ruiz S, et al. Overexpression of vascular endothelial growth factor (VEGF) and its cellular receptor KDR (VEGFR-2) in the bone marrow of patients with acute myeloid leukemia. *Leukemia.* 2002;16:1302–1310.

77. Dias S, Shmelkov SV, Lam G, et al. VEGF(165) promotes survival of leukemic cells by Hsp90-mediated induction of Bcl-2 expression and apoptosis inhibition. *Blood.* 2002;99:2532–2540.

78. Karp JE, Gojo I, Pili R, et al. Targeting vascular endothelial growth factor for relapsed and refractory adult acute myelogenous leukemias: therapy with sequential 1-beta-d-arabinofuranosylcytosine, mitoxantrone, and bevacizumab. *Clin Cancer Res.* 2004;10: 3577–3585.

79. Heidel F, Cortes J, Rucker FG, et al. Results of a multicenter phase II trial for older patients with c-Kit-positive acute myeloid leukemia (AML) and high-risk myelodysplastic syndrome (HR-MDS) using low-dose Ara-C and imatinib. *Cancer.* 2007;109:907–914.

80. Park S, Chapuis N, Bardet V, et al. PI-103, a dual inhibitor of class IA phosphatidylinositide 3-kinase and mTOR, has antileukemic activity in AML. *Leukemia.* 2008;22:1698–1706.

81. Kantarjian H, O'Brien S, Cortes J, et al. Results of intensive chemotherapy in 998 patients age 65 years or older with acute myeloid leukemia or high-risk myelodysplastic syndrome: predictive prognostic models for outcome. *Cancer.* 2006;106:1090–1098.

82. Budel LM, Dong F, Lowenberg B, et al. Hematopoietic growth factor receptors: structure variations and alternatives of receptor complex formation in normal hematopoiesis and in hematopoietic disorders. *Leukemia.* 1995;9:553–561.

83. Lowenberg B, Touw IP. Hematopoietic growth factors and their receptors in acute leukemia. *Blood.* 1993;81:281–292.

84. Lowenberg B, Delwel R, Touw I. Hematopoietic growth factors and in vitro growth of human acute myeloblastic leukemia. *Crit Rev Oncol Hematol.* 1990;10:1–8.

85. Lowenberg B, Suciu S, Archimbaud E, et al. Use of recombinant GM-CSF during and after remission induction chemotherapy in patients aged 61 years and older with acute myeloid leukemia: final report of AML-11, a phase III randomized study of the Leukemia Cooperative Group of European Organisation for the Research and Treatment of Cancer and the Dutch Belgian Hemato-Oncology Cooperative Group. *Blood.* 1997;90:2952–2961.

86. Rowe JM, Andersen JW, Mazza JJ, et al. A randomized placebo-controlled phase III study of granulocyte-macrophage colony-stimulating factor in adult patients (>55 to 70 years of age) with acute myelogenous leukemia: a study of the Eastern Cooperative Oncology Group (E1490). *Blood.* 1995;86:457–462.

87. Rowe JM, Neuberg D, Friedenberg W, et al. A phase 3 study of three induction regimens and of priming with GM-CSF in older adults with acute myeloid leukemia: a trial by the Eastern Cooperative Oncology Group. *Blood.* 2004;103:479–485.

88. Stone RM, Berg DT, George SL, et al. Granulocyte-macrophage colony-stimulating factor after initial chemotherapy for elderly patients with primary acute myelogenous

leukemia. Cancer and Leukemia Group B. *N Engl J Med*. 1995;332:1671–1677.

89. Witz F, Sadoun A, Perrin MC, et al. A placebo-controlled study of recombinant human granulocyte-macrophage colony-stimulating factor administered during and after induction treatment for de novo acute myelogenous leukemia in elderly patients. Groupe Ouest Est Leucemies Aigues Myeloblastiques (GOELAM). *Blood*. 1998;91:2722–2730.

90. Dombret H, Chastang C, Fenaux P, et al. A controlled study of recombinant human granulocyte colony-stimulating factor in elderly patients after treatment for acute myelogenous leukemia. AML Cooperative Study Group. *N Engl J Med*. 1995;332:1678–1683.

91. Amadori S, Suciu S, Jehn U, et al. Use of glycosylated recombinant human G-CSF (lenograstim) during and/or after induction chemotherapy in patients 61 years of age and older with acute myeloid leukemia: final results of

AML-13, a randomized phase-3 study. *Blood*. 2005;106:27–34.

92. Bedard PL, Piccart-Gebhart MJ. Current paradigms for the use of HER2-targeted therapy in early-stage breast cancer. *Clin Breast Cancer*. 2008;4(suppl):S157–S165.

93. Wilson CS, Davidson GS, Martin SB, et al. Gene expression profiling of adult acute myeloid leukemia identifies novel biologic clusters for risk classification and outcome prediction. *Blood*. 2006;108:685–696.

94. Grimwade D, Moorman A, Hills R, et al. Impact of karyotype on treatment outcome in acute myeloid leukemia. *Ann Hematol*. 2004;83(suppl 1):S45–S48.

95. Van Den Heuvel-Eibrink MM, Van Der Holt B, Burnett AK, et al. CD34-related coexpression of MDR1 and BCRP indicates a clinically resistant phenotype in patients with acute myeloid leukemia (AML) of older age. *Ann Hematol*. 2007;86:329–337.

Hematopoietic cell transplantation in older adults

Andrew S. Artz and William B. Ershler

A. Introduction

Hematopoietic cell transplantation (HCT) is applied to high-risk hematologic diseases to overcome poor outcomes from non-HCT approaches. Historically, the associated morbidity and mortality limited application to adults less than 50 years of age. Many advances, including reduced-intensity conditioning for allogeneic HCT, have led to improved tolerance and removed traditional age barriers. In parallel, risk-assessment tools such as comorbidity measures have recently been applied to facilitate decisions regarding HCT eligibility and tolerance. The dismal outcome of some hematologic malignancies in older adults warrants early consideration of HCT. In this chapter, we will summarize the data and future directions for HCT in adults 50 years and older, with an emphasis on allogeneic HCT for acute myeloid leukemia (AML).

B. Epidemiology of hematologic diseases in the elderly

The incidence of leukemia rises and the prognosis declines with each decade of life.[1,2] The abysmal outcomes of older adults with present therapy for some hematologic diseases drive the need to consider alternative strategies. For example, AML, the most common indication for allogeneic HCT, has a 10-fold greater incidence in adults 65 years and over relative to young adults.[1] Estimated 5-year survival for older AML patients in registry studies hovers around 3 percent, compared to 30 percent in younger adults. Moreover, the secular trend of improved survival over time for younger adults has not been realized in the elderly. Among the relatively healthy older adults enrolled in cooperative group studies for newly diagnosed AML or acute lymphoblastic leukemia (ALL), advancing age remains tightly linked to lower remission rates as well as shorter disease-free and overall survival.[1,3] The poor prognosis of older adults relates both to reduced tolerance to treatment and adverse biologic features of the disease.[3,4] The rising num-

ber and proportion of older adults underscores a pressing need for better treatment strategies.

C. Autologous and allogeneic hematopoietic cell transplantation (HCT)

Autologous and allogeneic HCT represent two quite different approaches, with distinct disease indications, toxicity patterns, and efficacy. Autologous HCT relies on high-dose myeloablative chemotherapy to achieve disease control. Reinfusion of previously harvested cryopreserved autologous hematopoietic cells rescues the patient from chemotherapy-induced marrow aplasia. The most common indications for autologous HCT are multiple myeloma (MM) and non-Hodgkin's lymphoma (NHL), diseases more common among older adults.

Allogeneic HCT requires hematopoietic cells collected from a human leukocyte antigen (HLA) adequately matched donor. After administration of conditioning chemotherapy, cryopreserved or freshly collected donor hematopoietic cells are infused intravenously. Advantages of allogeneic HCT include a tumor-free graft and the benefit of an immune response of the donor cells against the recipient malignancy (i.e., graft vs. leukemia). Unique problems related to an allograft include a risk of immune-based graft rejection; graft-versus-host disease (GVHD), in which the donor cells recognize the recipient as foreign; and profound immune suppression. The wider-ranging toxicities as well as the tremendous resources in planning and managing an allogeneic HCT mandate an even more thorough pretransplant evaluation. For this reason, we devote more time to decisions related to allogeneic HCT.

D. The current era: Increased utilization of HCT in older adults

The past decade has witnessed major advances in HCT that have led to a rising number of older

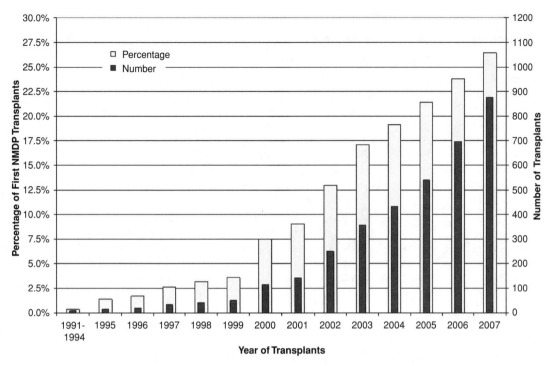

Figure 18.1 National Marrow Donor Registry recipients over 55 years of age.

adults undergoing HCT who were previously excluded. As recently as the 1980s, autologous HCT studies generally enrolled adults under 60 years of age,[5,6] and allogeneic HCT studies were usually restricted to adults 50 years or younger.[7] However, older adults represent an increasingly larger absolute number and proportion of patients receiving a transplant in the modern era. The Center for International Blood and Marrow Transplantation (CIBMTR) now reports that 53 percent and 20 percent of autografts are for patients over 50 and 60 years of age, respectively. In a recent CIBMTR analysis of NHL patients, only 20.7 percent of patients receiving autografts were 55 years or older between the years 1990 and 1994. In contrast, between 1999 and 2000, 40.4 percent fell into the older age category.[8] For allograft recipients for malignant disease from 2001 to 2007, over 20 percent were performed for those 51 – 60 years of age, and a remarkable 10 percent were over 60 years of age (https://campus.mcw.edu/AngelUploads/Content/CS_IBMTR2/_assoc/ECCBED0AF0A4492BB667FB6227DC7C06/summary05_Pt1_files/frame.htm) Figure 18.1 depicts the rapid rise for patients 55 years and older among unrelated donor allogeneic transplants facilitated by the National Marrow Donor Registry (NMDP). Nevertheless, only a small fraction of older adults with stan-

dard transplant indications actually proceed to HCT.

E. Applying HCT to older adults

The presence of hematologic disease whereby long-term disease control is unlikely after standard treatment prompts consideration of HCT, either autologous, allogeneic, or both. As with most of geriatric oncology, the lack of randomized or prospective trials among older adults comparing HCT to non-HCT therapy presents a formidable obstacle. Disease-based indications for HCT are derived primarily from studies conducted on adults less than 50 years of age (http://www.marrow.org/PHYSICIAN/Tx_Indications_Timing_Referral/Recommended_Timing_for_Tx_Cons/index.html). To the extent that hematologic diseases have even worse outcomes in older adults than in younger adults (e.g., lymphoma, AML, ALL, myelodysplastic syndromes), disease-based HCT indications seem reasonable. MM and NHL are the main indications for an autograft, whereas leukemias account for over three-fourths of allogeneic HCT.[9]

F. Transplant tolerability

Reduced tolerance to HCT complications has been the major reservation in applying HCT,

Table 18.1 Trends promoting hematopoietic cell transplant (HCT) for older adults.

Characteristic	Example
Reduced-intensity conditioning[a]	Fewer acute regimen–related toxicities
Peripheral blood stem cells	Reduces time to neutrophil engraftment
	Easier collection of hematopoietic cells for patients and donors
Supportive care	Better infectious monitoring (e.g., CMV prophylaxis and early identification)
Infectious disease	Better infectious disease monitoring (e.g., CMV detection) and better treatments for opportunistic infections
Growth factors	Facilitate stem cell collection and reduce neutropenia phase post-HCT
Immunosuppression[a]	More tolerable immunosuppression-reducing toxicity
Human leukocyte antigen (HLA) matching[a]	Better HLA matching reduces post-HCT complications
Donor registries[a]	Merging of registry databases electronically facilitates unrelated donor identification; cord blood banks provide resource for unrelated cord blood
Patient health	Older adults have fewer disabilities and longer life expectancy, allowing for more intensive treatment
Societal attitudes	Patient and physician attitudes have shifted to expect life-prolonging treatment for older adults

[a]Restricted to allogeneic HCT. CMV = Cytomegalovirus

and for that matter other intensive therapies, to older adults. Traditional myeloablative conditioning regimens (e.g., total body irradiation) can provoke serious organ complications and infections, resulting in substantial morbidity and mortality irrespective of age. Over the past two decades, a confluence of transplant and societal factors has pushed HCT to an increasingly older population (Table 18.1).

F.1. Reduced-intensity conditioning

Reduced-intensity conditioning (RIC) regimens for allogeneic HCT have been the factor most frequently credited with improved tolerance, at least for allogeneic recipients. RIC incorporates fewer myeloablative drugs or doses but retains adequate immunosuppression to achieve donor hematopoietic cell engraftment.[10,11] A transient state of mixed chimerism may occur whereby the donor and recipient cells coexist posttransplant. The European Group for Blood and Marrow Transplantation Registry (EBMTR) reports that 31 percent of allogeneic transplants now incorporate RIC,[9] rarely used before 2000, and this trend is growing. RIC regimens vary in the degree of immunosuppression and myeloablation. Transplant-related mortality ranges from 3 to 55 percent and may be less than myeloablative approaches. Randomized studies are lacking, and patients undergoing RIC are often considered ineligible for standard myeloablative regimens. RIC comes at a cost; reducing the conditioning regimen

intensity and possibly the greater use of immunosuppression may subject patients to higher relapse rates.[12–15]

F.2. Nonconditioning factors

A host of factors other than RIC may play an essential albeit less well recognized role in expanding HCT eligibility (Table 18.1). For example, the myeloablative conditioning employed in autologous HCT has changed little over the past decade; nevertheless, increases in autologous HCT among older adults have paralleled the increase for allogeneic HCT. In addition, the majority of allogeneic HCT recipients over the age of 50 years still receive myeloablative conditioning regimens. A major non-regimen-related advance has been better diagnosis and management of opportunistic infections such as cytomegalovirus and aspergillosis.[16–18] Although more difficult to quantify, nontransplant factors cannot be underestimated. Secular trends are such that an older person today has fewer comorbid conditions or disabilities than in prior generations,[19] increasing tolerability to intensive therapy. Prolonged life expectancy and/or shifts in societal attitudes about older adults are likely to influence patients' and physicians' decisions.

F.3. Donors

Finding the optimal HLA-compatible donor represents a major obstacle and modifiable factor for allogeneic HCT. An HLA-matched sibling at HLA-A, HLA-B, HLA-C, HLA-DRB1 (i.e., 8/8 match), and possibly other loci continues to be the gold standard. Donor selection for older recipients has important nuances. On average, HLA-matched siblings will also be older, raising issues about the upper age or health limitations for donor collection. Older donor age slightly diminishes hematopoietic cell yields.[20] In our own data, among 106 granulocyte colony-stimulating factor (G-CSF) mobilized peripheral blood stem cell related sibling donors 50 years of age, only 6.4 percent had an inadequate mobilization, defined by a peripheral blood CD34 of under 20 cells/uL on day 5 after G-CSF mobilization.[20a]

An expanding number of volunteer unrelated donors and electronic integration of worldwide donor registries increases the probability of identifying a well-matched unrelated donor. Most important, better HLA matching using molecular techniques has reduced the traditional outcome disparity for unrelated donors to the point that HLA-matched related and unrelated donors have converged, at least for AML.[21,22]

Debate continues about whether one should select younger over older unrelated donors, independent of patient age. Kollman and colleagues evaluated unrelated donor bone marrow transplants and found that donor age 45 years and older increased the risk of GVHD and mortality.[23] However, in a recent analysis of registry data better adjusted for HLA mismatches, Lee and colleagues did not appreciate an impact of older donor age.[24] Another smaller study raised the possibility that older donor age among related donor HCT might lead to worse outcomes.[25] Whether a younger unrelated donor would be preferred over an older sibling donor remains to be established. Schetelig and colleagues suggested a trend toward better outcomes with unrelated allografts compared to sibling donors among AML patients 50 years and over after an allogeneic HCT.[26] However, the limited availability and the 2- to 4-month delay in procuring a fully matched unrelated donor suggest that healthy, HLA-compatible siblings should be preferred when available. Cord blood units (CBU) have emerged as a promising alternative donor source for those lacking HLA-compatible sibling donors. CBU can be procured quickly, are more permissive for HLA mismatches, and may have a reduced risk of chronic GVHD.[27] However, the low cell doses in CBU lead to very slow engraftment, leaving patients vulnerable to prolonged neutropenia. Several recent series suggest favorable outcomes for adults over 50 years of age after CBU.[28–30] Thus unrelated adult donors and CBUs have become viable donor sources for older allogeneic HCT recipients.

G. Outcomes

G.1. Autologous hematopoietic cell transplantation

To the extent that autologous HCT relies on high-dose chemotherapy, any improvements in outcomes over time relate to either better patient selection or advances in supportive care. The most obvious advance has been the use of peripheral blood stem cells harvested after chemotherapy and/or cytokine mobilization instead of bone marrow harvests. Early studies indicated suboptimal outcomes and high transplant-related mortality (TRM) of older adults after autologous bone marrow transplantation.[31–33] More recent data, primarily using peripheral blood stem cell products, suggest improved outcomes. Among 26 elderly MM patients over 70 years of age who were treated with melphalan, there were no deaths by day 100.[34] The EBMTR reviewed results for diffuse large B-cell lymphoma after auto-HCT. Adults 60 years and over comprised 18 percent of patients, were more likely to have active disease at the time of transplant, and were more likely to have slightly higher TRM. Three-year overall survival was 60 percent in the older adults compared to 70 percent in those less than 60 years ($p < .001$).[35] A CIBMTR analysis of NHL patients showed for patients age 55 years or greater inferior overall survival (RR = 1.5, 1.33–1.69) for both aggressive histology and (RR = 1.33, 95% confidence interval [CI] 1.04–1.71) for follicular grades 1 and 2.[8] Among the subjects 65 years and older, the TRM at 1 year was 11 percent between 1990 and 2000, and the 5-year overall survival was 29 percent; outcomes improved over time. The data for autologous HCT among older adults appear promising in light of the high risk and relapsed diseases undergoing transplant and the fact that auto-HCT outcomes are continually improving. The value of autologous HCT for AML in first remission remains controversial.[36,37] Because AML tends to have highly unfavorable disease characteristics among older adults and the toxicity of autologous HCT for older adults has been high, an allogeneic HCT is usually favored.

263

Table 18.2 Clinical studies of allogeneic transplant for adults 50 years and over.

Author/year	Age Median	Age Range	Donor	N	Regimen	Disease	TRM Day (D)/year
Konuma, 2009[30a]	52	50–55	Cord	19	TBI + cy	AML + ALL	1 year, 5%
Uchida, 2008[28]	61	55–79	Cord	70	Flu/TBI/mel	Heme malig	100 D, 43%
Majhail, 2008[29]	58	55–70	Sib	47	TBI + Flu/cy, Flu/bu, Cla/Bu	Heme malig	180 D, 23%
	59	55–69	Cord	43	180 D, 28%		
Falda, 2007[83]	62	60–70	Sib	32	Flu/TBI	Heme malig	100 D, 6% 1 year, 13%
Ditschkowski, 2006[42a]	57	50–67	Sib and MUD	214	Flu/cy/TBI Bu/cy Flu/cy/treo	Heme malig	100 D, 13–30%, 1 year, 21–46%
Kroger, 2006[84]	60	44–70	Sib and MUD	26	Flu/treo/ATG	MDS, AML	100 D, 28%
Tsirigotis, 2006[85]	60	55–69	Sib and MUD	37	Flu/Bu/ATG	Heme malig	100 D, 22% 1 year, 32%
Wallen, 2005[86a]	63	60–68	Sib	52	Ablative regimens	Heme malig MDS 67%	100 D, 27% 3 year, 43%
Gupta, 2005[87]	64	61–70	Sib	24	Flu/TBI	MDS, AML	100 D, 8% 2 year, 25%
Corradino, 2005[88]	59	55–69	Sib	160	Flu/thio/cy	Heme malig	5 year, 19%
Shimoni, 2005[89]	58	56–66	MUD	36	Flu/bu/treo OR Mel/ATG or Camp	Heme malig	1 year, 39%
Allyea, 2005[13]	58	51–70	Sib-MUD	71	Flu/bu	Heme malig	100 D, 6%
Allyea, 2005[13a]	54	51–66	Sib MUD	81	TBI/cy Bu/cy	Heme malig	100 D, 30%
Weisser, 2004[90]	51	45–62	Sib and MUD	35	Flu/cy/TBI/ATG	CML	100 D, 11% 1 year, 29%
Shapira, 2004[91]	63	60–67	Sib MUD	17	Flu/bu Flu/TBI, Bu alone	Heme malig	100 D, 33%
Bertz, 2003[92]	64	60–70	Sib MUD	19	Flu/mel/carmustine +/- ATG	Myeloid	1 year, 22%
Wong, 2003[43]	59	55–69	Sib MUD	29	Flu/mel, Flu/bu +/− ATG for MUD	Myeloid	1 year, 55%
de la Camara, 2002[93a]	53	50–59	Sib	32	Bu/cy TBI/cy	Myeloid	100 D, 9%
Deeg, 2000[94a]	59	55–66	Sib	50	Bu/cy TBI/cy Bu/TBI	MDS	2 year, 39%
Du, 1998[95a]	53.7	50–62	Sib	59	Bu/cy TBI/cy	Heme malig	100 D, 24% 1 year, 36%

Table 18.2 *(cont.)*

Author/year	Age Median	Age Range	Donor	N	Regimen	Disease	TRM Day (D)/year
Aggregate data							
Schetelig, 2008[26]	57	57–72	Sib and MUD	368	Various	AML	2 year, 23–37%
Aoudjhane, 2005[40]	57	50–73	Sib	315	Various	AML	2 year, 18%
Aoudjhane, 2005[40a]	54	50–64	Sib	407	Various	AML	2 year, 32%
Yanada, 2004[39a]	52	50–67	Sib and MUD	398	Various		100 D, 17% 1 year, 35%

Note. TRM = transplant-related mortality; Sib = sibling donor; MUD = matched-unrelated donor; Treo = treosulfan; Flu = fludarabine; Bu = busulfan; Cla = cladribine; Cy = cyclophosphamide; TBI = total body irradiation; ATG = antithymocyte globulin; Camp = alemtuzumab (Campath); Heme malig = hematologic malignancies; AML = acute myeloid leukemia; ALL = acute lymphoblastic leukemia.
[a] Ablative regimens.

H. Allogeneic hematopoietic cell transplantation

Allogeneic HCT data from the 1980s suggested that age 50 years and older was associated with worse outcomes.[38] In the modern era, many groups have reexamined allogeneic HCT among older adults (Table 18.2). Common features include a less intensive preparative regimen incorporating fludarabine and AML/MDS as the most frequent indications. The varied diseases, eligibility, and conditioning regimens limit insight into disease control or survival; nevertheless, estimates of toxicity can be determined based on TRM (i.e., death without disease relapse). Studies pooling data across centers, such as registry studies, indicate TRM of around 20–35 percent at 1–2 years.[26,39,40] Comparative studies suggest that RIC regimens among older adults lead to reduced TRM.[13,40] Nevertheless, the 30 percent TRM found in myeloablative regimens may not necessarily be prohibitive, depending on the nontransplant prognosis. GVHD may be more common among older adults[41,42] and increase the risk of TRM.

Registry data reveal that 1-year survival for all diseases transplanted is over 40 percent for those 60 years and over receiving an allogeneic HCT (Figure 18.2). Overall survival for AML and MDS, the most common indications for allogeneic HCT, is around 30–50 percent for adults 50 years and older.[26,40,43] For older adults with AML achieving first complete remission and treated on a chemotherapy consolidation protocol, overall survival is less than 20 percent at 5 years.[44] In light of the dismal outcomes among older AML patients, the results appear encouraging. Important differences may exist in comparing HCT recipients to data derived from other studies. It is well appreciated how patient selection can influence allogeneic HCT outcomes.[45] Patients undergoing allogeneic HCT typically have very adverse disease features; however, they also have reasonably good or excellent health, insurance coverage, and disease kinetics that allow proceeding to allogeneic HCT in remission. In addition, older age for allogeneic HCT is usually defined as greater than 50 years of age. Very few patients over the age of 70 years have received an allogeneic HCT, and 75 years is a frequent upper age limit for allogeneic HCT protocols. Estey and colleagues followed all adults 50 years and older diagnosed with AML at the M. D. Anderson Cancer Center.[46] Among those achieving first complete remission, the presence of an HLA-matched donor was associated with better outcomes. The few long-term survivors had undergone allogeneic HCT. The data

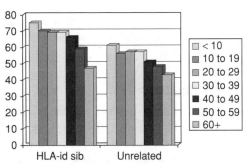

Figure 18.2 One-year survival after hematopoietic cell transplant by recipient age.

provide additional support that allogeneic HCT may extend survival for select older adults.

I. Tolerance to HCT

Absent randomized studies in older adults addressing the benefits of HCT compared to non-HCT approaches, individualized decisions must be made. After recognizing adverse disease features that represent an indication for HCT, estimates of HCT tolerance will drive transplant recommendations for older adults. Tolerance is objectively captured by TRM, which includes all deaths not related to relapse. Organ toxicity, quality of life, infections, length of hospitalization stay, and GVHD all represent important tolerance measures but are not uniformly reported.

I.1. Age

The influence of older age on HCT outcome remains highly controversial and probably overemphasized. Most of the debate revolves around patients aged 50–75 years. Studies using myeloablative conditioning for allogeneic HCT performed 1–2 decades ago showed that older age leads to greater TRM from regimen toxicities and GVHD.[47–49] Recent studies for allogeneic HCT suggest that older age imparts a small or minimal influence on outcome after RIC regimens. The younger age comparison group in studies of RIC may be problematic because they tend to have comorbid conditions or health problems that prompt enrollment on RIC protocols. In contrast, older adults are often enrolled on RIC protocols based on age alone. For example, we found that among 105 patients with hematologic malignancies given an RIC regimen, older age was marginally associated with increased TRM ($p = .05$).[50] After adjusting for comorbidity, performance status, and disease features, older age correlated more strongly with TRM (HR = 3.2, $p = .01$). Unfortunately, age by itself lacks adequate precision to predict outcomes and thus determine HCT eligibility, at least between the ages of 50 and 75 years.

I.2. Comorbidity

Although comorbidity tools are quite familiar to geriatricians, transplant physicians have only recently explored the value of comorbidity indices. For HCT, comorbid conditions are typically summarized as a composite index of medical diagnoses, excluding the primary malignancy.[51,52] In addition to helping estimate HCT tolerance, comorbidity may provide important prognostic information independent of the cancer and treatment and may also influence treatment decisions about the HCT regimen (i.e., autologous vs. allogeneic or type of conditioning). HCT recipients routinely undergo extensive testing prior to HCT, including pulmonary function tests, cardiac evaluation, and chemistry assessment of liver and renal function. Published guidelines on acceptable ranges are lacking, although many centers will consider using an RIC regimen if baseline abnormalities are outside of prespecified normal ranges (e.g., PFTs below normal or serum creatinine above the upper limit of normal). Nevertheless, single abnormalities on these routine objective tests have shown limited value in predicting HCT outcome,[53] in part because testing excludes some patients. This testing remains critical to assessing baseline function and to selecting a regimen and supportive care plan that minimizes toxicity.

As one of the most widely used comorbidity tools, the Charlson Comorbidity Index (CCI)[54,55] was an early candidate for comorbidity testing among HCT recipients. The Seattle group evaluated the non-age-adjusted CCI in the context of related and unrelated allografts.[56,57] Not surprisingly, over half of the patients receiving the less intensive conditioning regimens had comorbidity by the CCI. Among patients undergoing myeloablative conditioning, abnormalities by the CCI were infrequent. CCI scores of 3 or greater predicted more toxicity and TRM. However, only 8–18 percent of those receiving less intensive conditioning fell into the high comorbidity category. A subsequent series from the same institution revealed an even lower prevalence and predictive value for high CCI scores.[58] Others have also shown the limited predictive value of the CCI.[50] In the autologous setting, a CCI score of 1 or more showed a marginal trend toward decreased autologous HCT tolerance,[59] again with few patients categorized as a CCI of 3 or more. The Kaplan-Feinstein Scale (KF)[60] has also been evaluated and revealed slightly greater sensitivity in that 47 percent showed some abnormality by KF compared to only 26 percent by CCI[50] among adults undergoing an RIC allogeneic HCT. In multivariable analysis, neither the CCI nor the KF predicted increased TRM. Thus the CCI and KF have limited sensitivity in the setting of HCT. Not surprisingly, older adults undergoing HCT tend to have greater comorbidity.[50,61]

Sorror and colleagues pioneered the development of the Hematopoietic Cell Transplantation-Specific Co-morbidity Index (HCT-CI), a more sensitive comorbidity tool derived specifically from patients who received an allogeneic HCT. As expected, the HCT-CI shows much greater sensitivity than the CCI.[58,61] For example, 62 percent showed an abnormality by HCT-CI compared to only 12 percent using the CCI. At 2 years, the HCT-CI predicted for increased TRM (HR = 3.5, 95% CI 2.0–6.3) and inferior overall survival (HR = 2.7, 95% CI 1.8–4.1). In the autologous setting, the HCT-CI also more strongly predicts toxicity than the CCI.[59] However, confirmatory studies among allogeneic HCT recipients in other centers have shown the HCT-CI to be less predictive of TRM than originally reported.[61–63] Interestingly, after RIC using T-cell depletion to minimize GVHD, comorbidity by the HCT-CI did not predict TRM.[64,65] These data suggest that less intensive regimens that minimize GVHD might attenuate the impact of higher comorbidity, at least with respect to TRM. Whether more sensitive measures of comorbidity, such as the cumulative illness rating scale, will hold additional value requires testing. Comorbidity tools such as the HCT-CI represent a significant advance in providing more accurate estimates of HCT tolerance and comparing study populations.[61] However, comorbidity alone also lacks discriminative capacity to alter HCT decision making for the majority of subjects. Ironically, the call to measure comorbidity stems from application of HCT in older adults; nevertheless, these studies typically do not address the influence of comorbidity among older adults alone, and older age is almost always restricted to 75 years or younger.

One might expect comorbidity to specifically predict for TRM, the standard measure of transplant tolerance. Interestingly, higher comorbidity more reliably predicts worse overall survival rather than TRM,[50,64,66] in part because higher comorbidity tracks with more advanced disease at HCT.[67] Thus comorbidity may also be a surrogate for disease and death because of disease relapse and represents another limitation in assessing HCT tolerance. Other instruments other than comorbidity tools are necessary to accurately gauge transplant tolerance.

I.3. Functional assessment

Functional assessment has long been recognized as a strong gauge of health status.[68] The simplest functional status measures, performance status (PS) either by Karnofsky Performance score (KPS) or the Eastern Cooperative Oncology Group Performance score (ECOG PS), considerably impact transplant outcomes.[69–71] Most patients undergoing HCT have an ECOG PS of 0–1 or a KPS of 90–100 percent. ECOG PS of 2 strongly predicts for poor outcome but is infrequent, found in fewer than 10 percent of patients undergoing RIC allogeneic HCT.[50,72]

Other measures of functional status (e.g., disability, mobility limitations) widely used by geriatricians are of great interest but remain untested among HCT recipients. For example, in one study, 37 percent of cancer patients with a KPS less than 2 had limitations in their instrumental activities of daily living.[73] Among older adults in general, functional impairments are frequent[52] and are strongly associated with worse outcome, independent of comorbid conditions.[68,74] Functional status, independent of comorbidity, can predict toxicity and survival in older cancer patients.[73,75,76]

A combined measure of performance status and comorbidity appears to hold value for approximating HCT tolerance. Among 105 allogeneic HCT recipients, we found that a combined score of KPS and comorbidity better estimated TRM than either tool alone.[50] Patients harboring an ECOG PS of 1 and mild comorbidity were at the same heightened risk of TRM as patients with severe comorbidity or a KPS of 2. These patients overall had a 50 percent risk of TRM at 6 months compared to only 15 percent for those without these features. Using this combined measure also retained predictive value among adults 50 years and over. Sorror and colleagues have also shown a combining measure of HCT-CI, and KPS allowed for excellent risk stratification.[67]

I.4. Biomarkers

Proinflammatory cytokines, such as C-reactive protein (CRP) or interleukin 6, predict important outcomes among older adults such as functional decline, increased cardiac events, and increased mortality.[77–79] We have recently demonstrated that elevated CRP above the median of 18.5 mg/L among allogeneic HCT recipients prior to conditioning predicts for increased toxicity and TRM but not disease relapse, independent of comorbidity and KPS.[64] In addition, a rise in CRP after conditioning may also predict for increased toxicity.[80,81] As reproducible and objective measures, biomarkers could be instrumental in delineating HCT tolerance.

Numerous other geriatric domains, such as nutrition, caregiver support, and cognitive assessment, have not been evaluated in the setting of HCT. For example, delirium occurs in up to 50 percent of allogeneic HCT recipients[82] and likely more often among older adults. There is a tremendous opportunity for geriatricians to improve the care of transplant patients. Well-established methods to reduce delirium, disability, and deconditioning are poorly recognized and underutilized among HCT recipients. For example, pre-HCT cognitive evaluation would be of considerable interest.

J. Recommendations

Whereas data for autologous and allogeneic HCT remain restricted to observational studies of select older individuals, clinicians must make the best recommendation from the available studies. Enrolling older adults on HCT clinical trials remains the highest priority. For older adults between 50 and 75 years of age with disease indications for HCT, transplant should be considered if they are in good health such as an ECOG PS of 0–1 and controlled comorbid conditions. Because

of the proclivity for relapse and the delays in proceeding to HCT, particularly for allogeneic HCT, early referral to an HCT center is necessary.

K. Conclusion

Historical age restrictions are now counterbalanced by an increasing number of adults 50 years and over undergoing autologous and allogeneic HCT. Although tolerance may be less for some older adults, overall outcomes appear favorable relative to non-HCT approaches. As such, age alone should not be a contraindication to HCT. Select older adults can undergo autologous and allogeneic HCT with reasonable tolerance and reasonably good success. Assessing comorbidity and performance status may be useful in estimating HCT tolerance, although precise thresholds for eligibility remain undefined. Future risk assessment tools will be needed to determine not if but which older adults most benefit from HCT. Transplant investigators are challenged with developing better-tolerated regimens and supportive care measures, whereas geriatricians are tasked with determining which pretransplant assessment measures are most predictive of successful treatment outcomes. Ultimately, collaboration between these two fields is necessary to accomplish these goals.

References

1. Xie Y, Davies SM, Xiang Y, et al. Trends in leukemia incidence and survival in the United States (1973–1998). *Cancer.* 2003;97:2229–2235.

2. Jemal A, Siegel R, Ward E, et al. Cancer statistics, 2006. *CA Cancer J Clin.* 2006;56:106–130.

3. Appelbaum FR, Gundacker H, Head DR, et al. Age and acute myeloid leukemia. *Blood.* 2006;107:3481–3485.

4. Leith CP, Kopecky KJ, Godwin J, et al. Acute myeloid leukemia in the elderly: assessment of multidrug resistance (MDR1) and cytogenetics distinguishes biologic subgroups with remarkably distinct responses to standard chemotherapy. A Southwest Oncology Group study. *Blood.* 1997;89:3323–3329.

5. Fermand JP, Levy Y, Gerota J, et al. Treatment of aggressive multiple myeloma by high-dose chemotherapy and total body irradiation followed by blood stem cells autologous graft. *Blood.* 1989;73:20–23.

6. Barlogie B, Alexanian R, Dicke KA, et al. High-dose chemoradiotherapy and autologous bone marrow transplantation for resistant multiple myeloma. *Blood.* 1987;70:869–872.

7. Clift RA, Buckner CD, Appelbaum FR, et al. Allogeneic marrow transplantation in patients with acute myeloid leukemia in first remission: a randomized trial of two irradiation regimens. *Blood.* 1990;76:1867–1871.

8. Lazarus HM, Carreras J, Boudreau C, et al. Influence of age and histology on outcome in adult non-Hodgkin lymphoma patients undergoing autologous hematopoietic cell transplantation (HCT): a report from the Center for International Blood and Marrow Transplant Research (CIBMTR). *Biol Blood Marrow Transplant.* 2008;14:1323–1333.

9. Gratwohl A, Baldomero H, Frauendorfer K, et al. EBMT activity survey 2004 and changes in disease indication over the past 15 years. *Bone Marrow Transplant.* 2006;37:1069–1085.

10. Giralt S, Estey E, Albitar M, et al. Engraftment of allogeneic hematopoietic progenitor cells with purine analog-containing chemotherapy: harnessing graft-versus-leukemia without myeloablative therapy. *Blood.* 1997;89:4531–4536.

11. Slavin S, Nagler A, Naparstek E, et al. Nonmyeloablative stem cell transplantation and cell therapy as an alternative to conventional bone marrow transplantation with lethal cytoreduction for the treatment of malignant and nonmalignant hematologic diseases. *Blood.* 1998;91:756–763.

12. Martino R, Iacobelli S, Brand R, et al. Retrospective comparison of reduced intensity conditioning and conventional high dose conditioning for allogeneic hematopoietic stem cell transplantation using HLA identical sibling donors in myelodysplastic syndromes. *Blood.* 2006;108:836–846.

13. Alyea EP, Kim HT, Ho V, et al. Comparative outcome of nonmyeloablative and myeloablative allogeneic hematopoietic cell transplantation for patients older than 50 years of age. *Blood.* 2005;105:1810–1814.

14. de Lima M, Couriel D, Thall PF, et al. Once-daily intravenous busulfan and fludarabine: clinical and pharmacokinetic results of a myeloablative, reduced-toxicity conditioning regimen for allogeneic stem cell transplantation in AML and MDS. *Blood.* 2004;104:857–864.

15. Slattery JT, Clift RA, Buckner CD, et al. Marrow transplantation for chronic myeloid leukemia: the influence of plasma busulfan levels on the outcome of transplantation. *Blood.* 1997;89:3055–3060.

16. Herbrecht R, Denning DW, Patterson TF, et al. Voriconazole versus amphotericin B for primary therapy of invasive aspergillosis. *N Engl J Med.* 2002;347:408–415.

17. Nichols WG, Corey L, Gooley T, et al. Rising pp65 antigenemia during preemptive anticytomegalovirus therapy after allogeneic hematopoietic stem cell transplantation: risk factors, correlation with DNA load, and outcomes. *Blood.* 2001;97:867–874.

18. Kline J, Pollyea DA, Stock W, et al. Pre-transplant ganciclovir and post transplant high-dose valacyclovir reduce CMV infections after alemtuzumab-based conditioning. *Bone Marrow Transplant.* 2006;37:307–310.

19. Manton KG, Corder L, Stallard E. Chronic disability trends in elderly United States populations: 1982–1994. *Proc Natl Acad Sci USA.* 1997;94:2593–2598.

20. Vasu S, Leitman SF, Tisdale JF, et al. Donor demographic and laboratory predictors of allogeneic peripheral blood stem cell mobilization in an ethnically diverse population. *Blood.* 2008;112:2092–2100.

20a. Richa E, Papari M, Allen J, et al. Older age but not donor health impairs allogeneic granulocyte colony-stimulating factor (G-CSF) peripheral blood stem cell mobilization. Biology of blood and marrow transplantation. *Biol Blood Marrow Transplant.* 2009;11:1394–1399. Epub 2009 Sep 8.

21. Kiehl MG, Kraut L, Schwerdtfeger R, et al. Outcome of allogeneic hematopoietic stem-cell transplantation in adult patients with acute lymphoblastic leukemia: no difference in related compared with unrelated transplant in first complete remission. *J Clin Oncol.* 2004;22:2816–2825.

22. Weisdorf DJ, Anasetti C, Antin JH, et al. Allogeneic bone marrow transplantation for

chronic myelogenous leukemia: comparative analysis of unrelated versus matched sibling donor transplantation. *Blood*. 2002;99:1971–1977.

23. Kollman C, Howe CW, Anasetti C, et al. Donor characteristics as risk factors in recipients after transplantation of bone marrow from unrelated donors: the effect of donor age. *Blood*. 2001;98:2043–2051.

24. Lee SJ, Klein J, Haagenson M, et al. High-resolution donor-recipient HLA matching contributes to the success of unrelated donor marrow transplantation. *Blood*. 2007;110:4576–4583.

25. Mehta J, Gordon LI, Tallman MS, et al. Does younger donor age affect the outcome of reduced-intensity allogeneic hematopoietic stem cell transplantation for hematologic malignancies beneficially? *Bone Marrow Transplant*. 2006;38:95–100.

26. Schetelig J, Bornhauser M, Schmid C, et al. Matched unrelated or matched sibling donors result in comparable survival after allogeneic stem-cell transplantation in elderly patients with acute myeloid leukemia: a report from the cooperative German Transplant Study Group. *J Clin Oncol*. 2008;26:5183–5191.

27. Narimatsu H, Miyakoshi S, Yamaguchi T, et al. Chronic graft-versus-host disease following umbilical cord blood transplantation: retrospective survey involving 1072 patients in Japan. *Blood*. 2008;112:2579–2582.

28. Uchida N, Wake A, Takagi S, et al. Umbilical cord blood transplantation after reduced-intensity conditioning for elderly patients with hematologic diseases. *Biol Blood Marrow Transplant*. 2008;14:583–590.

29. Majhail NS, Brunstein CG, Tomblyn M, et al. Reduced-intensity allogeneic transplant in patients older than 55 years: unrelated umbilical cord blood is safe and effective for patients without a matched related donor. *Biol Blood Marrow Transplant*. 2008;14:282–289.

30. Konuma T, Takahashi S, Ooi J, et al. Myeloablative unrelated cord blood transplantation for acute leukemia patients between 50 and 55 years of age: single institutional retrospective comparison with patients younger than 50 years of age. *Ann Hematol*. 2009;88:581–588.

31. Kusnierz-Glaz CR, Schlegel PG, Wong RM, et al. Influence of age on the outcome of 500 autologous bone marrow transplant procedures for hematologic malignancies. *J Clin Oncol*. 1997;15:18–25.

32. Miller CB, Piantadosi S, Vogelsang GB, et al. Impact of age on outcome of patients with cancer undergoing autologous bone marrow transplant. *J Clin Oncol*. 1996;14:1327–1332.

33. Gopal AK, Gooley TA, Golden JB, et al. Efficacy of high-dose therapy and autologous hematopoietic stem cell transplantation for non-Hodgkin's lymphoma in adults 60 years of age and older. *Bone Marrow Transplant*. 2001;27:593–599.

34. Qazilbash MH, Saliba RM, Hosing C, et al. Autologous stem cell transplantation is safe and feasible in elderly patients with multiple myeloma. *Bone Marrow Transplant*. 2007;39:279–283.

35. Jantunen E, Canals C, Rambaldi A, et al. Autologous stem cell transplantation in elderly patients (>= 60 years) with diffuse large B-cell lymphoma: an analysis based on data in the European Blood and Marrow Transplantation registry. *Haematologica*. 2008;93:1837–1842.

36. Levi I, Grotto I, Yerushalmi R, et al. Meta-analysis of autologous bone marrow transplantation versus chemotherapy in adult patients with acute myeloid leukemia in first remission. *Leuk Res*. 2004;28:605–612.

37. Nathan PC, Sung L, Crump M, et al. Consolidation therapy with autologous bone marrow transplantation in adults with acute myeloid leukemia: a meta-analysis. *J Natl Cancer Inst*. 2004;96:38–45.

38. Ringden O, Horowitz MM, Gale RP, et al. Outcome after allogeneic bone marrow transplant for leukemia in older adults. *J Am Med Assoc*. 1993;270:57–60.

39. Yanada M, Emi N, Naoe T, et al. Allogeneic myeloablative transplantation for patients aged 50 years and over. *Bone Marrow Transplant*. 2004;34:29–35.

40. Aoudjhane M, Labopin M, Gorin NC, et al. Comparative outcome of reduced intensity and myeloablative conditioning regimen in HLA identical sibling allogeneic haematopoietic stem cell transplantation for patients older than 50 years of age with acute myeloblastic leukaemia: a retrospective survey from the Acute Leukemia Working Party (ALWP) of the European group for Blood and Marrow Transplantation (EBMT). *Leukemia*. 2005;19:2304–2312.

41. Carlens S, Ringden O, Remberger M, et al. Risk factors for chronic graft-versus-host disease after bone marrow transplantation: a retrospective single centre analysis. *Bone Marrow Transplant*. 1998;22:755–761.

42. Ditschkowski M, Elmaagacli AH, Trenschel R, et al. Myeloablative allogeneic hematopoietic stem cell transplantation in elderly patients. *Clin Transplant*. 2006;20:127–131.

43. Wong R, Giralt SA, Martin T, et al. Reduced-intensity conditioning for unrelated donor hematopoietic stem cell transplantation as treatment for myeloid malignancies in patients older than 55 years. *Blood*. 2003;102:3052–3059.

44. Stone RM, Berg DT, George SL, et al. Postremission therapy in older patients with de novo acute myeloid leukemia: a randomized trial comparing mitoxantrone and intermediate-dose cytarabine with standard-dose cytarabine. *Blood.* 2001;98:548–553.

45. Artz AS, Van Besien K, Zimmerman T, et al. Long-term follow-up of nonmyeloablative allogeneic stem cell transplantation for renal cell carcinoma: the University of Chicago experience. *Bone Marrow Transplant.* 2005;35:253–260.

46. Estey E, de Lima M, Tibes R, et al. Prospective feasibility analysis of reduced-intensity conditioning (RIC) regimens for hematopoietic stem cell transplantation (HSCT) in elderly patients with acute myeloid leukemia (AML) and high-risk myelodysplastic syndrome (MDS). *Blood.* 2007;109:1395–1400.

47. Cahn JY, Labopin M, Schattenberg A, et al. Allogeneic bone marrow transplantation for acute leukemia in patients over the age of 40 years. Acute Leukemia Working Party of the European Group for Bone Marrow Transplantation (EBMT). *Leukemia.* 1997;11:416–419.

48. Klingemann HG, Storb R, Fefer A, et al. Bone marrow transplantation in patients aged 45 years and older. *Blood.* 1986;67:770–776.

49. Przepiorka D, Smith TL, Folloder J, et al. Risk factors for acute graft-versus-host disease after allogeneic blood stem cell transplantation. *Blood.* 1999;94:1465–1470.

50. Artz AS, Pollyea DA, Kocherginsky M, et al. Performance status and comorbidity predict transplant-related mortality after allogeneic hematopoietic cell transplantation. *Biol Blood Marrow Transplant.* 2006;12:954–964.

51. Yancik R, Ganz PA, Varricchio CG, et al. Perspectives on comorbidity and cancer in older patients: approaches to expand the knowledge base. *J Clin Oncol.* 2001;19:1147–1151.

52. Yancik R, Havlik RJ, Wesley MN, et al. Cancer and comorbidity in older patients: a descriptive profile. *Ann Epidemiol.* 1996;6:399–412.

53. Alamo J, Shahjahan M, Lazarus HM, et al. Comorbidity indices in hematopoietic stem cell transplantation: a new report card. *Bone Marrow Transplant.* 2005;36:475–479.

54. Charlson M, Szatrowski TP, Peterson J, et al. Validation of a combined comorbidity index. *J Clin Epidemiol.* 1994;47:1245–1251.

55. Charlson ME, Pompei P, Ales KL, et al. A new method of classifying prognostic comorbidity in longitudinal studies: development and validation. *J Chronic Dis.* 1987;40:373–383.

56. Diaconescu R, Flowers CR, Storer B, et al. Morbidity and mortality with nonmyeloablative compared with myeloablative conditioning before hematopoietic cell transplantation from HLA-matched related donors. *Blood.* 2004;104:1550–1558.

57. Sorror ML, Maris MB, Storer B, et al. Comparing morbidity and mortality of HLA-matched unrelated donor hematopoietic cell transplantation after nonmyeloablative and myeloablative conditioning: influence of pretransplantation comorbidities. *Blood.* 2004;104:961–968.

58. Sorror ML, Maris MB, Storb R, et al. Hematopoietic cell transplantation (HCT)-specific comorbidity index: a new tool for risk assessment before allogeneic HCT. *Blood.* 2005;106:2912–2919.

59. Labonte L, Iqbal T, Zaidi MA, et al. Utility of comorbidity assessment in predicting transplantation-related toxicity following autologous hematopoietic stem cell transplantation for multiple myeloma. *Biol Blood Marrow Transplant.* 2008;14:1039–1044.

60. Kaplan MH, Feinstein AR. The importance of classifying initial co-morbidity in evaluating the outcome of diabetes mellitus. *J Chronic Dis.* 1974;27:387–404.

61. Sorror ML, Giralt S, Sandmaier BM, et al. Hematopoietic cell transplantation specific comorbidity index as an outcome predictor for patients with acute myeloid leukemia in first remission: combined FHCRC and MDACC experiences. *Blood.* 2007;110:4606–4613.

62. Guilfoyle R, Demers A, Bredeson C, et al. Performance status, but not the Hematopoietic Cell Transplantation Comorbidity Index (HCT-CI), predicts mortality at a Canadian transplant center. *Bone Marrow Transplant.* 2009;43:133–139.

63. Majhail NS, Brunstein CG, McAvoy S, et al. Does the hematopoietic cell transplantation specific comorbidity index predict transplant outcomes? A validation study in a large cohort of umbilical cord blood and matched related donor transplants. *Biol Blood Marrow Transplant.* 2008;14:985–992.

64. Artz AS, Wickrema A, Dinner S, et al. Pretreatment C-reactive protein is a predictor for outcomes after reduced-intensity allogeneic hematopoietic cell transplantation. *Biol Blood Marrow Transplant.* 2008;14:1209–1216.

65. Lim ZY, Ho AY, Ingram W, et al. Outcomes of alemtuzumab-based reduced intensity conditioning stem cell transplantation using unrelated donors for myelodysplastic syndromes. *Br J Haematol.* 2006;135:201–209.

66. Sorror ML, Maris MB, Sandmaier BM, et al. Hematopoietic cell transplantation after nonmyeloablative conditioning for advanced chronic lymphocytic leukemia. *J Clin Oncol.* 2005;23:3819–3829.

67. Sorror M, Storer B, Sandmaier BM, et al. Hematopoietic cell transplantation-comorbidity index and Karnofsky performance status are independent predictors of morbidity and mortality after allogeneic nonmyeloablative hematopoietic cell transplantation. *Cancer.* 2008;112:1992–2001.

68. Inouye SK, Peduzzi PN, Robison JT, et al. Importance of functional measures in predicting mortality among older hospitalized patients. *J Am Med Assoc.* 1998;279:1187–1193.

69. Giralt S, Thall PF, Khouri I, et al. Melphalan and purine analog-containing preparative regimens: reduced-intensity conditioning for patients with hematologic malignancies undergoing allogeneic progenitor cell transplantation. *Blood.* 2001;97:631–637.

70. Sayer HG, Kroger M, Beyer J, et al. Reduced intensity conditioning for allogeneic hematopoietic stem cell transplantation in patients with acute myeloid leukemia: disease status by marrow blasts is the strongest prognostic factor. *Bone Marrow Transplant.* 2003;31:1089–1095.

71. van Besien K, Artz A, Smith S, et al. Fludarabine, melphalan, and alemtuzumab conditioning in adults with standard-risk advanced acute myeloid leukemia and myelodysplastic syndrome. *J Clin Oncol.* 2005;23:5728–5738.

72. Gómez-Núñez M, Martino R, Caballero MD, et al. Elderly age and prior autologous transplantation have a deleterious effect on survival following allogeneic peripheral blood stem cell transplantation with reduced-intensity conditioning: results from the Spanish multicenter prospective trial. *Bone Marrow Transplant.* 2004;33:477–482.

73. Repetto L, Fratino L, Audisio RA, et al. Comprehensive geriatric assessment adds information to Eastern Cooperative Oncology Group performance status in elderly cancer patients: an Italian Group for Geriatric Oncology Study. *J Clin Oncol.* 2002;20:494–502.

74. Lee SJ, Lindquist K, Segal MR, et al. Development and validation of a prognostic index for 4-year mortality in older adults. *J Am Med Assoc.* 2006;295:801–808.

75. Extermann M, Overcash J, Lyman GH, et al. Comorbidity and functional status are independent in older cancer patients. *J Clin Oncol.* 1998;16:1582–1587.

76. Firat S, Bousamra M, Gore E, et al. Comorbidity and KPS are independent prognostic factors in stage I non-small-cell lung cancer. *Int J Radiat Oncol Biol Phys.* 2002;52:1047–1057.

77. Harris TB, Ferrucci L, Tracy RP, et al. Associations of elevated interleukin-6 and C-reactive protein levels with mortality in the elderly. *Am J Med.* 1999;106:506–512.

78. Masotti L, Ceccarelli E, Forconi S, et al. Prognostic role of C-reactive protein in very old patients with acute ischaemic stroke. *J Intern Med.* 2005;258:145–152.

79. Penninx BW, Kritchevsky SB, Newman AB, et al. Inflammatory markers and incident mobility limitation in the elderly. *J Am Geriatr Soc.* 2004;52:1105–1113.

80. Min CK, Kim SY, Eom KS, et al. Patterns of C-reactive protein release following allogeneic stem cell transplantation are correlated with leukemic relapse. *Bone Marrow Transplant.* 2006;37:493–498.

81. Schots R, Kaufman L, Van Riet I, et al. Proinflammatory cytokines and their role in the development of major transplant-related complications in the early phase after allogeneic bone marrow transplantation. *Leukemia.* 2003;17:1150–1156.

82. Fann JR, Alfano CM, Burington BE, et al. Clinical presentation of delirium in patients undergoing hematopoietic stem cell transplantation. *Cancer.* 2005;103:810–820.

83. Falda M, Busca A, Baldi I, et al. Nonmyeloablative allogeneic stem cell transplantation in elderly patients with hematological malignancies: results from the GITMO (Gruppo Italiano Trapianto Midollo Osseo) multicenter prospective clinical trial. *Am J Hematol.* 2007;82:863–866.

84. Kroger N, Shimoni A, Zabelina T, et al. Reduced-toxicity conditioning with treosulfan, fludarabine and ATG as preparative regimen for allogeneic stem cell transplantation (alloSCT) in elderly patients with secondary acute myeloid leukemia (sAML) or myelodysplastic syndrome (MDS). *Bone Marrow Transplant.* 2006;37:339–344.

85. Tsirigotis P, Bitan RO, Resnick IB, et al. A non-myeloablative conditioning regimen in allogeneic stem cell transplantation from related and unrelated donors in elderly patients. *Haematologica.* 2006;91:852–855.

86. Wallen H, Gooley TA, Deeg HJ, et al. Ablative allogeneic hematopoietic cell transplantation in adults 60 years of age and older. *J Clin Oncol.* 2005;23:3439–3446.

87. Gupta V, Daly A, Lipton JH, et al. Nonmyeloablative stem cell transplantation for myelodysplastic syndrome or acute myeloid leukemia in patients 60 years or older. *Biol Blood Marrow Transplant.* 2005;11:764–772.

88. Corradini P, Zallio F, Mariotti J, et al. Effect of age and previous autologous transplantation on nonrelapse mortality and survival in patients treated with reduced-intensity conditioning and

allografting for advanced hematologic malignancies. *J Clin Oncol.* 2005;23:6690–6698.

89. Shimoni A, Kroger N, Zabelina T, et al. Hematopoietic stem-cell transplantation from unrelated donors in elderly patients (age >55 years) with hematologic malignancies: older age is no longer a contraindication when using reduced intensity conditioning. *Leukemia.* 2005;19:7–12.

90. Weisser M, Schleuning M, Ledderose G, et al. Reduced-intensity conditioning using TBI (8 Gy), fludarabine, cyclophosphamide and ATG in elderly CML patients provides excellent results especially when performed in the early course of the disease. *Bone Marrow Transplant.* 2004;34:1083–1088.

91. Shapira MY, Resnick IB, Bitan M, et al. Low transplant-related mortality with allogeneic stem cell transplantation in elderly patients. *Bone Marrow Transplant.* 2004;34:155–159.

92. Bertz H, Potthoff K, Finke J. Allogeneic stem-cell transplantation from related and unrelated donors in older patients with myeloid leukemia. *J Clin Oncol.* 2003;21:1480–1484.

93. de la Camara R, Alonso A, Steegmann JL, et al. Allogeneic hematopoietic stem cell transplantation in patients 50 years of age and older. *Haematologica.* 2002;87:965–972.

94. Deeg HJ, Shulman HM, Anderson JE, et al. Allogeneic and syngeneic marrow transplantation for myelodysplastic syndrome in patients 55 to 66 years of age. *Blood.* 2000;95:1188–1194.

95. Du W, Dansey R, Abella EM, et al. Successful allogeneic bone marrow transplantation in selected patients over 50 years of age – a single institution's experience. *Bone Marrow Transplant.* 1998;21:1043–1047.

19

Management of non-Hodgkin's lymphoma in older adults

Anne H. Blaes and Vicki A. Morrison

A. Incidence

Non-Hodgkin's lymphoma (NHL) is currently the fifth most common malignancy in women and the sixth most common in men in the United States.[1] It is estimated that approximately 35,450 men and 30,670 women will be diagnosed with NHL in 2008, and 19,160 patients will die from this disease in 2008.[2] Over the last 2 decades, the incidence of NHL has been increasing across all adult age groups, rising by as much as 8–10 percent per year.[3-6] Specifically, the incidence is rising in patients aged over 60 years.[7-9] Among U.S. men, the incidence of NHL ranged from 13.1 per 100,000 in people aged 40–44 years to 51.2 per 100,000 in people aged 60–64 years and 133 per 100,000 in people aged 80–84 years.[10] This increasing incidence is relevant in the elderly population; though patients aged over 65 years represent 13 percent of the population, 53 percent of all new cases occur in this age group. The median age of patients at diagnosis of NHL is 67 years. With the population over 75 years and 85 years tripling and doubling, respectively, by 2030, the occurrence of NHL in this older patient population will pose an increasing problem.[6,11]

B. Impact of aging

Though overall progress in the management of cancer, and specifically NHL, has been made in the last few decades, cancer-specific mortality continues to increase as a function of age. In general, older patients have a number of factors, including concomitant medical conditions (comorbidities) and physiologic and functional changes, that can affect prognosis, treatment, and outcomes (Table 19.1).[12,13] Kidney and liver function also decline as a natural part of aging. Ultimately, these factors may lead to modifications in treatment as well as changes in treatment outcomes.[14] For example, though anthracyclines are known to improve survival in NHL patients, physicians may be reluctant to give chemotherapy to the elderly, and only 42 percent of 4,000 patients aged over 65 years

with diffuse large B-cell lymphoma received doxorubicin in a recent report.[15] In terms of cognitive function, it is essential to consent patients for chemotherapy, yet up to 30 percent of the elderly have cognitive impairment.[14] Depression remains a problem in the elderly, which can impair outlook on cancer care and treatment. Nutritionally, 40 percent of hospitalized cancer patients are at risk for or already have developed malnutrition. The social environment and access to care may also be a barrier. These issues can be challenges in the care of elderly patients with NHL.

Finally, the presence of comorbidities and polypharmacy may also influence a patient's care.[14] In one study, 35 percent of patients between the ages of 65 and 79 years in the United States had at least two chronic diseases. This number, however, increased to 70 percent in patients over 80 years of age.[16] The presence of comorbidities can lead to polypharmacy and potential drug interactions with chemotherapy. The presence of comorbidities may also lead to alterations in cancer outcome. Common comorbidities such as diabetes have been shown in one study to be associated with a worse cancer outcome.[17] All these issues related to functional status, cognitive abilities, emotional conditions, comorbidities, nutritional status, polypharmacy, and the patient's social and environmental situation need to be considered in the care of these patients, leading to a multidisciplinary approach in treating the elderly with NHL.

Age is also a barrier to enrollment in clinical trials.[18] Despite a high incidence of cancer in the elderly, older patients make up only 20 percent of those in phase II clinical trials. Although clinical trials remain the main approach for evaluating the safety and efficacy of cancer treatment, few elderly are actually enrolled in these trials.

While a number of factors influence the care of elderly patients with NHL, the question arises as to why older patients have a poorer outcome and whether the disease is biologically different in elderly patients. In clinical trials, however,

Table 19.1 Factors influencing cancer care in the elderly.

Functional status
Cognitive abilities
Emotional conditions
Comorbid conditions
Nutritional status
Polypharmacy
Alterations in pharmacokinetics
Social and environmental situation

it has been demonstrated that if older patients with diffuse aggressive NHL receive full-dose chemotherapy, their outcome is comparable to that of younger patients.[19–22] There is no difference in disease stage by age in patients with follicular, Burkitt's, or lymphoblastic lymphoma. Though not completely understood, elderly patients with diffuse aggressive NHL appear to have more advanced-stage disease.

C. Epidemiology and classification of non-Hodgkin's lymphoma (NHL) in the elderly

Risk factors for the development of NHL have been identified and are not specific for age. These risk factors include occupational exposures to agricultural herbicides, pesticides, or industrial solvents; alterations in the immune system, including autoimmune disorders and congenital and acquired immunodeficiencies; and the adminis-

tration of chronic immunosuppressive therapy as well as infectious etiologies. The latter include infections with HIV, human T-lymphotropic virus types I/II, Epstein Barr virus, *Helicobacter pylori*, *Borellia burgdorferi*, and *Chlamydia psittaci*.[23,24]

Over the years, there have been a number of different classification systems used to differentiate the subtypes of NHL. In 2001, the World Health Organization incorporated a classification scheme that included morphologic, immunophenotypic, and genetic features as well as clinical aspects. Within the previously recognized Revised European American Lymphoma (REAL) classification schema that was developed in 1994,[25] all lymphoma subtypes may be observed in elderly patients.[26,27] However, there tends to be a higher percentage of patients with aggressive lymphoma,[26] with elderly patients having a slightly higher tendency for developing lymphocytic/lymphoplasmocytic lymphoma, diffuse large B-cell lymphoma, and peripheral T-cell lymphoma (Table 19.2). Anaplastic large-cell lymphoma, lymphoblastic lymphoma, and Burkitt's lymphoma are less commonly seen in the elderly. It is unclear whether specific chromosomal or genetic abnormalities are associated with the development of NHL in the elderly, with few studies in this area. Additionally, extranodal sites of involvement are more common in older than in younger patients. Specifically, extranodal sites that commonly occur in patients over 60 years of age include primary lymphomas of the testes, epidural space, and skin (B cells).[28–30]

Table 19.2 Frequency of different lymphoma reports in the REAL classification of patients according to age (n = 1,283).

Lymphoma subtype	No. pts	Patients in each age category (%)				
		≤30–35	35–49	50–59	60–69	≥70
Small lymphocytic	98	1	14	18	33	34
Mucosa-associated lymphoid tissue	108	9	14	24	26	27
Marginal zone (splenic and nodal)	32	6	22	22	34	16
Follicular	317	8	22	22	26	22
Mantle cell	72	–	11	31	33	25
Diffuse large B cell	448	16	15	16	21	32
Peripheral T cell	93	11	18	17	26	28
Anaplastic large T/null cell	32	53	19	6	13	9
Burkitt's	9	78	–	11	11	–
Lymphoblastic	28	68	14	14	4	–
Unclassified	46	6	22	20	22	30
All patients	1,283	13	17	19	24	27

Note. REAL = Revised European-American Lymphoma. Adapted from Thieblemont and Coiffier.[26]

D. Staging and prognostic factors

The Ann Arbor staging system has been traditionally used to stage NHL.[31] This staging system divides NHL into limited (stages I, II) and advanced (stages III, IV) disease. A staging evaluation should typically include a physical examination; a computerized tomography scan of the chest, abdomen, and pelvis and other sites as indicated; a bilateral bone marrow biopsy and aspiration; and laboratory tests. The bone marrow sample should be evaluated for standard histology, in addition to flow cytometry, immunohistochemistry, and cytogenetic analysis. Laboratory testing should include blood counts, lactate dehydrogenase (LDH), B2-microglobulin, and serologies for HIV and hepatitis B and C. The evaluation of baseline kidney and liver function should also be taken into consideration as alterations in these values may lead to a change in therapy.

E. Prognostic information

The International NHL Prognostic Factors Project (IPI) identified prognostic factors for patients with aggressive NHL treated with doxorubicin-based regimens (Table 19.3). Age, specifically over 60 years, was the most important factor independently associated with outcome. An advanced age resulted in a lower response rate and decreases in disease-free and overall survival (OS). This has subsequently been confirmed in other studies as well.[19,20] The other poor prognostic factors identified by the IPI include an elevated LDH, poor performance status (PS 2–4), advanced-stage disease, and more than one site of extranodal involvement. Subsequent studies have identified the absence of cell surface expression of HLA-DR and beta-2 microglobulin with a poor response to treatment.[32–34]

For patients with follicular lymphoma, a similar prognostic scheme, known as the FLIPI index,

Table 19.3 International Prognostic Index (IPI) and Follicular Lymphoma International Prognostic Index (FLIPI).

IPI	FLIPI
Age > 60 years	Age > 60 years
Stage III, IV	Stage III, IV
Lactate dehydrogenase > normal	Hemoglobin <12 g/dL
No. extranodal sites ≥ 2	No. extranodal sites > 4
Performance status ≥ 2	Lactate dehydrogenase > normal

was developed. The five prognostic indicators include age (less than or more than 60 years), Ann Arbor stage, hemoglobin (over or under 12 g/dL), number of involved nodal areas (more than or less than 4), and LDH. With these five indicators, three risk factor groups have been identified with low- (no or one adverse factors), intermediate- (two factors), and poor-risk (three or more adverse factors) disease associated with 10-year overall survival of 71 percent, 51 percent, and 36 percent, respectively.

F. Therapy of diffuse large B-cell lymphoma in the elderly

For decades, the standard approach to diffuse large B-cell lymphoma in the elderly consisted of cyclophosphamide, adriamycin, vincristine, and prednisone (CHOP) chemotherapy.[35] In patients aged 65–75 years, CHOP chemotherapy resulted in complete remission rates of 50 percent. In patients under 75 years of age, complete remission rates were 40 percent with a median remission duration of 16 months. The basis for the CHOP regimen resulted from an intergroup trial in which CHOP was compared to other combination chemotherapy regimens (m-BACOD [methotrexate, bleomycin, adriamycin, cyclophosphamide, vincristine, dexamethasone], Pro-MACE-CytaBOM, MACOP-B), with no significant difference in efficacy (complete remission [CR], overall response [OR], progression-free survival [PFS]) being found but fewer adverse events seen with CHOP therapy.[36]

Over the last decade, the introduction of the monoclonal antibody targeting CD20, rituximab, has led to a new standard of care (Table 19.3). Initially, rituximab therapy was studied in 40 patients with low-grade B-cell NHL.[37–39] This study demonstrated a prolonged remission duration and a favorable safety profile. Subsequently, rituximab has been studied in combination with CHOP chemotherapy (R-CHOP). An initial phase II trial examined 33 patients with aggressive lymphoma who received six cycles of chemotherapy with R-CHOP.[40] Rituximab, 375 mg/m^2, was given 2 days before CHOP. Ten of these 33 patients were over 60 years of age. The overall response rate was 94 percent (61% CR, 33% partial remission [PR]) at a median follow-up of 26 months. Rituximab was generally well tolerated in all ages, including the older patients.

In a subsequent phase III trial of the Groupe d'Etude des Lymphomes de l'Adulte, Coiffer and colleagues reported the results of 399 patients aged 60–80 years with untreated diffuse large B-cell lymphoma who were randomized to either R-CHOP or CHOP chemotherapy.[41] Rituximab, 375 mg/m^2, was given on day 1 of each cycle. The complete response rate, at an initial median follow-up of 2 years, was 76 percent for R-CHOP as compared with 63 percent for the CHOP arm ($p = .005$). In the most recent report with 7 years of follow-up, event-free, disease-free, and overall survival all continued to be significantly better in patients treated with R-CHOP than with CHOP.[42] The 7-year overall survival advantage was present across all age groups. Specifically, for patients aged 60–69 years, overall survival was 58 percent with R-CHOP versus 40 percent with CHOP; for ages 70–74 years, 55 percent versus 41 percent; and for ages 75–80 years, 41 percent versus 21 percent, respectively. The 7-year overall survival was also favorable in those with poor risk characteristics (age over 75 years, PS = 2, presence of B symptoms, stage IV disease, elevated LDH, and the presence of marrow involvement).

In the subsequent phase III U.S. intergroup trial,[43] 632 patients with untreated diffuse aggressive NHL were randomized to therapy with R-CHOP or CHOP for a maximum of eight cycles. Two doses of rituximab, 375 mg/m2, were given prior to cycle 1, with an additional dose of rituximab administered prior to cycles 3, 5, and 7. The 415 patients with an initial response to therapy (CR or PR) underwent a second randomization to either maintenance rituximab (375 mg/m2 weekly for 4 weeks, given every 6 months for 2 years) or observation. Of these 415 patients, 352 were considered evaluable. The overall response rate to induction chemotherapy was 77 percent with R-CHOP and 76 percent with CHOP. With a median follow-up of 5.5 years, the 6-year failure-free survival was 45 percent in those who received maintenance rituximab and 36 percent for those randomized to observation.[44] For those patients receiving CHOP induction therapy, the median time to treatment failure (TTF) was 5.2 years with maintenance rituximab and 1.6 years with maintenance observation ($p = .0004$). In contrast, in those patients who received R-CHOP induction therapy, the median TTF was comparable among the two groups (5.6 years with maintenance rituximab group and 5.4 years with observation). In a weighted analysis, the use of maintenance rituximab did not change overall survival, regardless of the type of induction therapy received. Overall, these large phase III trials led to R-CHOP becom-

ing the standard of care in the treatment of aggressive lymphoma, including both elderly and young patients.

Finally, the German Lymphoma Study Group has subsequently studied the administration of CHOP chemotherapy on an every-14-day schedule (CHOP-14) as opposed to the more traditional every-21-day schedule (CHOP-21).[45] Initially, the group randomized patients to CHOP-14 versus CHOP-21 (CR 70% vs. 60%), CHOEP-14 (cyclophosphamide, doxorubicin, etoposide, vincristine, and prednisone), or CHOEP-21 (71.6% vs. 76.1%). The addition of etoposide to CHOP, however, appeared to be more toxic in this patient population. In the subsequent RICOVER-60 study, 1,222 patients aged 61–80 years[46] were randomized to therapy with CHOP-14 or CHOP-R-14. This study included patients with stage I disease. Overall, the CR rates improved with the addition of rituximab (68% CHOP-14, 78% R-CHOP-14 after six cycles). With a median follow-up of 35 months, the 3-year event-free survival after six cycles of CHOP-R-14 chemotherapy was 67 percent compared to 47 percent with CHOP-14. Improvements were also seen in PFS (56.9% CHOP-14, 73.4% R-CHOP-14, $p = .0001$) and OS (67.7% CHOP-14, 78.1% R-CHOP-14, $p = .0181$) with the addition of rituximab. CHOP-R-14 was well tolerated in these older patients. However, Tholstrup and colleagues subsequently reported an analysis of 65 patients treated with CHOP-14, stratifying the patients into high-risk (age over 75 years with PS over 3) and standard-risk (age 60–75 years with PS less than 3 or age less than 60 years) subgroups.[47] There was a higher frequency of hospitalizations (88% vs. 68%) in the very high risk group, with most of these hospitalizations due to opportunistic infections, malnutrition, and declining performance status.

On the basis of these studies, it appears that R-CHOP therapy is well tolerated in the elderly (Table 19.4). The feasibility of delivering full-dose CHOP chemotherapy has been advocated.[48-51] Campbell and colleagues found that the subset of patients ($n = 60$) at least 65 years of age with a favorable PS (less than 2) and few comorbidities could tolerate CHOP without growth factor support.[49] Jacobson and colleagues reported that full-dose CHOP with prophylactic growth factor support could be administered to patients over the age of 60 years with a low rate of neutropenia and neutropenic fever.[51]

Though it appears that R-CHOP is both effective and tolerated, a number of approaches have

Table 19.4 The use of R-CHOP/CHOP in the elderly.

Trial (reference)	n	Age (years)	IPI (%)				DFS and OS	
GELA[41,42]	399	60–80 (median 69)						
8 cycles			0–1	2	3	4–5	(at 5 years)	
R-CHOP	202		14	32	39	15	66%	58%
CHOP	197		12	35	42	12	45%	45%
U.S. intergroup[43,44]		≥60						
Induction: 6–8 cycles	632							
			1	2	3	4–5		
R-CHOP	267	Median 69	12	35	44	9		
CHOP	279	Median 70	14	36	41	9		
Maintenance	415							
Rituximab	174							
Observation	178							
RICOVER-60[46]	1,222	61–80						
			1	2	3	4–5	(at 3.5 years)	
R-CHOP-14 X 6		Median 69	31	29	25	15	73.4%	78.1%
R-CHOP-14 X 8		Median 68	30	27	25	18	68.8%	72.5%
CHOP-14 X 6		Median 68	32	26	26	16	56.9%	67.7%
CHOP-14 X 8		Median 68	30	29	26	16	56.9%	67.7%

Note. CHOP = cyclophosphamide, vincristine, and prednisone; R-CHOP = rituximab + CHOP; GELA = Groupe d'Etude des Lymphomes de l'Adulte; IPI = International Prognostic Index; DFS = disease-free survival; OS = overall survival.

been taken to minimize therapy-related toxicity while maximizing outcome in the elderly population. The use of non-anthracycline-containing regimens has been studied. The administration of cyclophosphamide, vincristine, procarbazine, and prednisone (COPP) was found to result in a lower CR rate and shorter survival compared with anthracycline-containing regimens.[52] In a phase III trial of the Dutch Cooperative Hematology Group, 145 patients over 65 years of age were randomized to CHOP or cyclophosphamide, mitoxantrone, vincristine, and prednisone (CNOP).[53] In this trial, the CR rate for CHOP was 49 percent and CNOP was 31 percent ($p = .03$) with a statistically significant prolongation in OS in the CHOP group ($p = .029$). In this trial, toxicities were similar, except for less nausea and alopecia with CNOP. In some other studies in which mitoxantrone was used, fewer cardiac complications occurred, but there was a significant amount of myelotoxicity.[54–58] Other anthracyclines, such as idarubicin and epirubicin, have been utilized in CHOP or P-VABEC-like regimens with acceptable toxicities.[59–61] Additionally, the administration of liposomal doxorubicin has been studied in the elderly. In phase II trials, pegylated liposomal dox-

orubicin was substituted for standard doxorubicin in the CHOP regimen (CCOP).[62,63] Within one of these phase II trials, in which 33 patients over 60 years of age were treated, the overall response rate was 64 percent (49% CR, 15% PR). Sixty-four percent of patients developed grade 3 or 4 neutropenia.[63] It appears that liposomal doxorubicin may be an acceptable alternative; however, further randomized trials need to investigate whether this is well tolerated and truly less toxic. Finally, lower-intensity CHOP has been administered to patients over the age of 80 years and may prolong survival.[26] Italiano and colleagues reported the results of 24 patients over the age of 80 years treated with R-CHOP at a mean dose reduction of 30 percent. The overall response rate was 79 percent with a 2-year OS of 63 percent.[64]

For elderly patients with cardiac disease, liposomal doxorubicin can be substituted for standard doxorubicin. The combination of pegylated liposomal doxorubicin to chemotherapy with vincristine, prednisone, and cyclophosphamide has led to overall response rates of 64–74 percent with CR of 49–59 percent.[62,63] In these two phase II trials, ejection fractions appeared to be stable; however, the follow-up of these patients was limited.

In patients who specifically have an absolute contraindication to doxorubicin chemotherapy such as an ejection fraction less than 30 percent, few data exist as to how to treat these patients. In one study of 83 patients with aggressive NHL, patients were treated with cyclophosphamide, etoposide, procarbazine, and prednisone (CEPP).[65] Of 75 evaluable patients, 40 percent achieved a CR and 32 percent had a PR. Twenty-one out of 61 (34%) patients with recurrent disease achieved a CR. On the basis of these results, though the data are limited, the use of CEPP for patients with a contraindication to doxorubicin would be favored. There may also be a role for treating these patients simultaneously with an angiotensin-converting enzyme inhibitor or beta-blocker concomitantly with chemotherapy, although additional studies are warranted to clarify the role of these medications for prophylaxis.[66,67]

Approaches to improve the outcome of elderly patients with diffuse aggressive NHL have also focused on ameliorating myelotoxicity and subsequent infectious complications with myeloid growth factor support with conflicting results.[68–70] In one study of 389 patients aged 65–90 years (median 72) years with aggressive lymphoma, in which patients were randomized to CHOP or CHOP plus filgrastim administered days 2–11, the CR rates (CHOP 55%, CHOP-filgrastim 52%, $p = .63$) and OS rates were comparable, with a median follow-up of 33 months. In this study, there was no difference in the numbers of grade 3–4 infections, hospital admissions, or days in the hospital.[68] Osby and colleagues reported differing results[69] in a study of 455 patients aged 60–86 (median 71) years who were randomized to CHOP or CNOP, alone or with filgrastim support (given on day 2 to days 10–14). Patients treated with CHOP had higher OS rates than those receiving CNOP ($p < .001$). The administration of filgrastim in conjunction with chemotherapy resulted in a reduction in grade 4 neutropenia and neutropenic fever. In addition, the relative dose intensity (RDI) was over 90 percent in those who received filgrastim support. Gómez and colleagues subsequently reported results of a phase II study in which 26 patients over 60 years of age (median 67 years) received CHOP plus sargramostim (given on days 4–13).[70] No difference in response rates or median survival was found among patients aged 61–69 years as compared to those aged over 70 years. However, patients 60–69 years of age received 86/90 planned cycles of chemotherapy, and those 70–84 years of age received only 52/72

planned cycles ($p = .00008$). The rates of neutropenia (absolute neutrophil count under 500), thrombocytopenia (platelets under 20,000), and febrile neutropenia were all significantly greater in patients over 70 years old as compared to those 61–69 years of age (neutropenia 24% vs. 73% of cycles of chemo, thrombocytopenia 5% vs. 42%, and febrile neutropenia 8% vs. 42%, respectively).

To better delineate who may benefit from the administration of hematopoietic growth factors, risk factors for the development of first-cycle neutropenia with CHOP chemotherapy in the elderly have been studied. In the study by Gómez and colleagues,[71] while hypoalbuminemia (albumin less than 3.5), an elevated lactate dehydrogenase, and the presence of marrow involvement were predictive of first-cycle neutropenia, age and performance status were not. In the U.S. intergroup study, risk factors for the development of first-cycle neutropenia with the administration of CHOP or R-CHOP chemotherapy were advancing age, PS 2–3, hemoglobin less than 12 g/dL, an elevated lactate dehydrogenase, and a high or intermediate-high IPI score.[72] Other studies have also identified kidney disease as a potential risk factor. Since these studies have been performed, the American Society of Clinical Oncology has developed guidelines for the use of growth factor support during the administration of chemotherapy.[73] For chemotherapy regimens in which the rates of neutropenia are predicted to be over 20 percent (CHOP-14, BEACOPP, etc.), prophylactic growth factor support should be administered with the first cycle of chemotherapy. For regimens in which the predicted rates of neutropenia are 10–20 percent (CHOP-21), prophylactic growth factor support should be considered with the first cycle of chemotherapy, particularly in the elderly. Any patient with a prior history of neutropenia should also receive prophylactic growth factor support with subsequent chemotherapy cycles.

Within the elderly population with aggressive lymphoma, full-dose R-CHOP appears to be the most efficacious treatment regimen. Guidelines for the use of hematopoietic growth factors exist and should be utilized as needed. It was shown in the U.S. intergroup trial that maintenance rituximab does not improve overall survival in patients who have received R-CHOP. Questions that remain unanswered include the optimal number of chemotherapy cycles and whether a 14-day or 21-day cycle interval is best. Studies are currently under way to further examine these questions.

G. Therapy of follicular lymphoma in the elderly

Approximately 30–40 percent of NHL in the elderly are follicular low-grade NHL. Unlike the diffuse aggressive lymphomas, the majority of clinical trials for the therapy of follicular lymphoma include both younger and older patients. As a result, there are limited data that focus specifically on the elderly. Patients usually present with an indolent onset of symptoms, typically with lymphadenopathy, hepatosplenomegaly, and advanced-stage disease. The presence of B symptoms is rare. Compared with other NHL, the follicular lymphomas are characterized by prolonged survival.[74–76] Though a high percentage of patients will achieve an initial complete remission following treatment with single alkylating agents, combination chemotherapy, or combined-modality treatment, a continuous rate of relapse is observed.[74] Median survival in the elderly ranges from 5 to 7 years.[77]

Patients with limited-stage (stage I–II) follicular NHL are generally treated with involved field radiation therapy, which typically results in long-term remissions.[78] In a report from Stanford University of 177 patients with stage I–II follicular lymphoma treated with involved field radiation, the median survival was 13.8 years with 5-, 10-, 15-, and 20-year survival rates of 82 percent, 64 percent, 44 percent, and 35 percent, respectively.[79] Similar results have been reported from other studies.[80,81] In one series, there was no difference in the CR rate by age, and although OS was shorter in older patients, the lymphoma-specific death rate did not vary by age.[82]

The initial approach of "watch and wait" in the elderly population has also been examined.[74] Advani and colleagues reported results of 43 patients with early-stage disease for whom therapy was deferred. Although the median age of the group was 58 years, 17 percent of the patients were over 60 years of age. With a median follow-up of 86 months, 63 percent of patients had not yet received therapy. Survival was comparable to historical series of patients receiving immediate treatment. The initial approach to watchful waiting has also been studied in patients with advanced disease, particularly in the elderly.[83–85] In one study of 309 patients with stage III and IV follicular lymphoma, patients were randomized to observation or chlorambucil 10 mg continuously. At a median follow-up of 16 years, the OS was comparable between the treatment and observation groups

($p = .84$). The actuarial chance of no treatment at 10 years from diagnosis was 19 percent (40% in those over the age of 70 years).[83] These results have been supported by additional trials as well.[84,85]

In follicular lymphoma patients with advanced disease who require treatment, a variety of therapies have been utilized over the last decade, including conventional cytotoxic agents, single-agent rituximab, rituximab-containing regimens, and radiopharmaceuticals such as tositumumab or ibritumomab tiuxetan. Some studies indicate that the CR rate with single alkylating agent therapy approaches 50 percent.[86,87] When combination chemotherapy is used, the CR rate is higher (60–80%).[88–91] However, when single-agent alkylators such as cyclophosphamide and chlorambucil were compared with combination chemotherapy such as cyclophosphamide, vincristine, and prednisone (COP), significant differences in long-term outcome, including survival, were not observed. In a large trial by the Cancer and Leukemia Group, single-agent cyclophosphamide was found to result in a similar outcome to anthracycline-based combination chemotherapy in previously untreated follicular lymphoma patients.[92] In this study, 228 patients were randomized to cyclophosphamide or CHOP with bleomycin. The median age of these patients was 56 years; slightly more than one-third of the patients were over 60 years of age. With 10-year follow-up, the overall times to failure and survival were similar in both groups. Toxicities were more common in patients receiving combination therapy. Other combination conventional cytotoxic therapies have also been studied in follicular lymphoma with similar results.[93]

Rituximab has been studied both as a single agent and in combination with chemotherapy in the treatment of follicular lymphoma. Several phase II trials demonstrated the utility of single-agent rituximab as initial therapy and in the relapsed setting.[94–98] In patients with relapsed or refractory disease, single-agent rituximab was found to have activity in patients over 60 years of age.[94–96] In the study of Hainsworth and colleagues, rituximab was administered as first-line and maintenance therapy to follicular lymphoma patients with a median age of 65 years (range to 89 years), with an overall response rate of 73 percent, including 37 percent complete responses.[97] In another trial of 50 patients with stage II–IV follicular lymphoma, the overall response rate with single-agent rituximab at 50 days was 73 percent. By polymerase chain reaction (PCR) testing for the Bcl-2 rearrangement in the peripheral blood and bone marrow, 57 percent and 31 percent of the patients became negative, respectively.[99] In these studies, rituximab appears well tolerated, particularly in the elderly population.

Rituximab has also been studied in combination with chemotherapy (cyclophosphamide, vincristine, prednisone [CVP] or CHOP).[38,100,101] In a meta-analysis by Schulz and colleagues in which seven randomized controlled trials with a total of 1,943 follicular, mantle cell, or other indolent lymphomas were evaluated, therapy with rituximab in combination with chemotherapy (R-chemo) resulted in a higher OS and overall response (OR). Therapy with R-chemo resulted in prolonged OS (HR for mortality 0.65) as compared to chemotherapy alone. This overall survival benefit with R-chemo was seen in both follicular and mantle cell histologies (HR 0.63 and 0.60, respectively).[100] The German Low Grade Lymphoma Study Group also examined rituximab plus chemotherapy in 428 patients with untreated, advanced-stage follicular lymphoma who were randomized to CHOP or R-CHOP treatment.[101] The median age of patients receiving R-CHOP was 54 years (range 29–82), with 37 percent of the patients being over 60 years of age. The median age of patients treated with CHOP was 57 years (range 27–79), with 41 percent of the patients being over 60 years of age. The addition of rituximab to CHOP chemotherapy resulted in an increased time to treatment failure ($p < .001$) and an improved overall response rate (96% vs. 90%, $p = .11$). The incidence of death during treatment was 1 percent in both arms, in which death was most commonly attributable to infection or lymphoma. R-CHOP therapy was beneficial in both younger and older patients.[101]

In follicular lymphoma, other agents, such as galiximab, CD80 monoclonal antibody, interferon, and radioimmunotherapy with toxitumumab and ibritumomab, are also being further investigated in their role in the treatment of follicular lymphoma.[102–105]

H. The role of transplantation in the elderly with NHL

The majority of patients with relapsed or refractory B-cell NHL are older than 60 years of age, yet they are often denied potentially curative high-dose therapy and autologous stem cell transplantation (SCT) because of the risk of excessive treatment-related morbidity and mortality. A few studies have demonstrated that it is possible to mobilize peripheral blood progenitor cells and to successfully undertake autologous SCT in patients over 60 years of age.[106–108] Jantunen and colleagues reviewed the results of autologous SCT in 88 NHL patients over 60 years of age treated between 1994 and 2004 at six Finnish transplant centers.[109] The median patient age was 63 years, with 17 patients being over 65 years of age, with histologies including diffuse large B-cell ($n = 29$), mantle cell ($n = 27$), follicular ($n = 15$), peripheral T-cell ($n = 12$), and other ($n = 5$) lymphoma subtypes. With a median follow-up of 21 months, 57 percent of patients were still alive, and 11 percent had early treatment-related mortality defined as death before day 100. The relapse rate after autologous SCT was 36 percent. Jantunen and colleagues also reviewed the experience of the European Blood and Marrow Transplant registry, in which 463 patients over 60 years of age (median 63, range 60–74) with diffuse large B-cell lymphoma underwent autologous SCT between 2000 and 2005.[110] The outcome of these patients was compared with a younger cohort of diffuse large B-cell lymphoma patients who received autologous SCT during this same time period. When compared with younger patients, the older patients had more often received at least two prior therapies, were less commonly in first complete remission, and received their transplant at a later time after diagnosis. With 3-year follow-up, the nonrelapse mortality in the elderly cohort was 10.8 percent compared to 6.5 percent in the younger cohort ($p = .002$). Most of these deaths were attributable to infections, which occurred equally in the young and old cohorts; however, the rate of second malignancies was higher in the elderly population. The relapse rate was 38 percent versus 32 percent ($p = .006$), and OS was 60 percent versus 70 percent ($p < .001$), respectively. It appears from these studies that autologous SCT in patients over 60 years of age is feasible. Additional prospective studies need to address measures to reduce the treatment-related mortality. Myeloablative allogeneic sibling SCT has been studied to a lesser degree in patients over 60 years of age and also warrants further investigation.[111]

I. Summary

The approach to the management of elderly patients with NHL will continue to be a significant issue, with the median age of these patients being over 60 years of age and in a setting in which the proportion of elderly patients in the population is increasing. The treatment of this patient population requires a multidisciplinary approach, given that most of these patients have comorbidities that can have an impact on the therapies being offered. Though clinical trials have expanded the knowledge base of practitioners caring for patients with NHL, most of these trials have been limited to younger, healthy patients. Future prospective studies are needed not only to investigate the efficacy of therapy in older patients but also to evaluate the toxicity profiles of these treatments. Results of these studies will be crucial in defining optimal treatment approaches in these older patients.

References

1. Jemal A, Siegel R, Ward E, et al. Cancer statistics, 2008. *CA Cancer J Clin.* 2008;58:71–96.

2. American Cancer Society. Cancer facts and figures. American Cancer Society Web site. Available at: http://www.cancer.org/downloads/STT/2008CAFFfinalsecured.pdf.

3. Devesa SS, Fears T. Non-Hodgkin's lymphoma time trends: United States and international data. *Cancer Res.* 1992;52:5432s–5440s.

4. Coleman MP, Esteve J, Damiecki P, et al. Trends in cancer incidence and mortality. *IARC Sci Publ.* 1993;121:1–806.

5. Newton R, Ferlay J, Beral V, et al. The epidemiology of non-Hodgkin's lymphoma: comparison of nodal and extra-nodal sites. *Int J Cancer.* 1997;72:923–930.

6. Thieblemont C, Coiffier B. Lymphoma in older patients. *J Clin Oncol.* 2007;25:1916–1923.

7. Roche LM, Paul SM, Costa SJ. Acquired immune deficiency syndrome and the increase in non-Hodgkin lymphoma incidence in New Jersey from 1979 to 1996. *Cancer.* 2001;92:2948–2956.

8. Roche LM, Weinstein RB, Paul SM, et al. Cancer in people with AIDS in New Jersey. *N J Med.* 2001;98:27–36.

9. Zheng T, Mayne ST, Boyle P, et al. Epidemiology of non-Hodgkin lymphoma in Connecticut: 1935–1988. *Cancer.* 1992;70:840–849.

10. Ries LAG, Melbert D, Krapcho M, et al. SEER cancer statistics review, 1975–2006. National Cancer Institute Web site. Available at: http://seer.cancer.gov/csr/1975_2006/index.html.

11. Kennedy BJ. Aging and cancer. *J Clin Oncol.* 1988;6:1903–1911.

12. Satariano WA, Ragland DR. The effect of comorbidity on 3-year survival of women with primary breast cancer. *Ann Intern Med.* 1994;120:104–110.

13. Yancik R, Wesley MN, Ries LA, et al. Effect of age and comorbidity in postmenopausal breast cancer patients aged 55 years and older. *J Am Med Assoc.* 2001;285:885–892.

14. Terret C, Zulian GB, Naiem A, et al. Multidisciplinary approach to the geriatric oncology patient. *J Clin Oncol.* 2007;25:1876–1881.

15. Hershman DL, McBride RB, Eisenberger A, et al. Doxorubicin, cardiac risk factors, and cardiac toxicity in elderly patients with diffuse B-cell non-Hodgkin's lymphoma. *J Clin Oncol.* 2008;26:3159–3165.

16. Guralnik J, LaCroix A, Everett D. Ageing in the Eighties: The Prevalence of Comorbidity and Its Association with Disability. Advance Data from Vital Health Statistics. Hyattsville, MD: National Center for Health Statistics; 1989.

17. Polednak AP. Comorbid diabetes mellitus and risk of death after diagnosis of colorectal cancer: a population-based study. *Cancer Detect Prev.* 2006; 30(5):466–472.

18. Aapro MS, Kohne CH, Cohen HJ, et al. Never too old? Age should not be a barrier to enrollment in cancer clinical trials. *Oncologist.* 2005;10:198–204.

19. Dixon DO, Neilan B, Jones SE, et al. Effect of age on therapeutic outcome in advanced diffuse histiocytic lymphoma: the Southwest Oncology Group experience. *J Clin Oncol.* 1986;4:295–305.

20. Vose JM, Armitage JO, Weisenburger DD, et al. The importance of age in survival of patients treated with chemotherapy for aggressive non-Hodgkin's lymphoma. *J Clin Oncol.* 1988;6:1838–1844.

21. Maartense E, Kluin-Nelemans HC, le Cessie S, et al. Different age limits for elderly patients with indolent and aggressive non-Hodgkin lymphoma and the role of relative survival with increasing age. *Cancer.* 2000;89:2667–2676.

22. Maartense E, Kluin-Nelemans HC, Noordijk EM. Non-Hodgkin's lymphoma in the elderly: a review with emphasis on elderly patients, geriatric assessment, and future perspectives. *Ann Hematol.* 2003;82:661–670.

23. Levine PH, Hoover R. The emerging epidemic of non-Hodgkin's lymphoma: current knowledge regarding etiological factors. *Cancer Epidemiol Biomarkers Prev.* 1992;1(6):515–517.

24. Fisher SG, Fisher RI. The epidemiology of non-Hodgkin's lymphoma. *Oncogene.* 2004;23(38):6524–6534.

25. Harris NL, Jaffe ES, Stein H, et al. A revised European-American classification of lymphoid neoplasms: a proposal from the International Lymphoma Study Group. *Blood.* 1994;84:1361–1392.

26. Thieblemont C, Coiffier B. Lymphoma in older patients. *J Clin Oncol.* 2007;25:1916–1923.

27. Greiner TC, Medeiros LJ, Jaffe ES. Non-Hodgkin's lymphoma. *Cancer.* 1995;75:370–380.

28. Ballester OF, Moscinski L, Spiers A, et al. Non-Hodgkin's lymphoma in the older person: a review. *J Am Geriatr Soc.* 1993;41:1245–1254.

29. Doll DC, Weiss RB. Malignant lymphoma of the testis. *Am J Med.* 1986;81:515–524.

30. Willemze R, Ruiter DJ, Van Vloten WA, et al. Reticulum cell sarcomas (large cell lymphomas) presenting in the skin: high frequency of true histiocytic lymphoma. *Cancer.* 1982;50:1367–1379.

31. Carbone PP, Kaplan HS, Musshoff K, et al. Report of the Committee on Hodgkin's Disease staging classification. *Cancer Res.* 1971;31:1860–1861.

32. Miller TP, Lippman SM, Spier CM, et al. HLA-DR (ia) immune phenotype predicts outcome for patients with diffuse large cell lymphoma. *J Clin Invest*. 1988;82:370–372.

33. Swan F, Huh Y, Katz R, et al. Beta-2 microglobulin (B2M) and HLA-DR cellular expression in relapsing large cell lymphomas (LCL): relationship to survival and serum B2M levels. *Blood*. 1990;76:375a.

34. Bauer KD, Merkel DE, Winter JN, et al. Prognostic implications of ploidy and proliferative activity in diffuse large cell lymphomas. *Cancer Res*. 1986;46:3173–3178.

35. McKelvey EM, Gottlieb JA, Wilson HE, et al. Hydroxyldaunomycin (Adriamycin) combination chemotherapy in malignant lymphoma. *Cancer*. 1976; 38(4):1484–1493.

36. Fisher RI, Gaynor ER, Dahlberg S, et al. Comparison of a standard regimen (CHOP) with three intensive chemotherapy regimens for advanced non-Hodgkin's lymphoma. *N Engl J Med*. 1993;328:1002–1006.

37. Czuczman MS, Grillo-López AJ, White CA, et al. Treatment of patients with low-grade B-cell lymphoma with the combination of chimeric anti-CD20 monoclonal antibody and CHOP chemotherapy. *J Clin Oncol*. 1999;17:268–276.

38. Czuczman MS, Grillo-López AJ, McLaughlin P, et al. Clearing of cells bearing the bcl-2 [t(14;18)] translocation from blood and marrow of patients treated with rituximab alone or in combination with CHOP chemotherapy. *Ann Oncol*. 2001;12:109–114.

39. Czuczman MS, Weaver R, Alkuzweny B, et al. Prolonged clinical and molecular remission in patients with low-grade or follicular non-Hodgkin's lymphoma treated with rituximab plus CHOP chemotherapy: 9-year follow-up. *J Clin Oncol*. 2004;22:4711–4716.

40. Vose JM, Link BK, Grossbard ML, et al. Phase II study of rituximab in combination with CHOP chemotherapy in patients with previously untreated, aggressive non-Hodgkin's lymphoma. *J Clin Oncol*. 2001;19:389–397.

41. Coiffier B, Lepage E, Brière J, et al. CHOP chemotherapy plus rituximab compared with CHOP alone in elderly patients with diffuse large-B-cell lymphoma. *N Engl J Med*. 2002;346:235–242.

42. Coiffier B, Feugier P, Mounier N, et al. Long term results of the GELA study comparing R-CHOP and CHOP chemotherapy in older patients with diffuse large B-cell lymphoma show good survival in poor-risk patients. *J Clin Oncol*. 2007;25(suppl):8009.

43. Habermann TM, Weller EA, Morrison VA, et al. Rituximab-CHOP versus CHOP alone or with maintenance rituximab in older patients with diffuse large B-cell lymphoma. *J Clin Oncol*. 2006;24:3121–3127.

44. Morrison VA, Weller EA, Habermann TM, et al. Maintenance rituximab (MR) compared to observation (OBS) after R-CHOP or CHOP in older patients (pts) with diffuse large B-cell lymphoma (DLBCL): an intergroup E4494/C9793 update. *J Clin Oncol*. 2007;25(suppl):8011.

45. Pfreundschuh M, Trumper L, Kloess M, et al. Two-weekly or 3-weekly CHOP chemotherapy with or without etoposide for the treatment of elderly patients with aggressive lymphomas: results of the NHL-B2 trial of the DSHNHL. *Blood*. 2004;104:634–641.

46. Pfreundschuh M, Schubert J, Ziepert M, et al. German High-Grade Non-Hodgkin Lymphoma Study Group (DSHNHL): six versus eight cycles of bi-weekly CHOP-14 with or without rituximab in elderly patients with aggressive CD20+ B-cell lymphomas: a randomised controlled trial (RICOVER-60). *Lancet Oncol*. 2008;9:105–116.

47. Tholstrup D, de Nully Brown P, Jurlander J, et al. Feasibility, efficacy and safety of CHOP-14 in elderly patients with very high-risk diffuse large B-cell lymphoma. *Eur J Haematol*. 2007;79:100–106.

48. O'Connell MJ, Earle JD, Harrington DP, et al. Initial chemotherapy doses for elderly patients with malignant lymphoma. *J Clin Oncol*. 1986;4:1418.

49. Campbell C, Sawka C, Franssen E, et al. Delivery of full dose CHOP chemotherapy to elderly patients with aggressive non-Hodgkin's lymphoma without G-CSF support. *Leuk Lymphoma*. 1999;35:119–127.

50. Sonneveld P, Huijgens PC, Hagenbeek A. Dose reduction is not recommended for elderly patients undergoing chemotherapy for non-Hodgkin lymphoma. *Ned Tijdschr Geneeskd*. 1999;143:418–419.

51. Jacobson JO, Grossbard M, Shulman LN, et al. CHOP chemotherapy with preemptive granulocyte colony-stimulating factor in elderly patients with aggressive non-Hodgkin's lymphoma: a dose-intensity analysis. *Clin Lymphoma*. 2000;1:211–217; discussion 218.

52. Liang R, Todd D, Chan TK, et al. COPP chemotherapy for elderly patients with intermediate and high grade non-Hodgkin's lymphoma. *Hematol Oncol*. 1993;11:43–50.

53. Sonneveld P, de Ridder M, Van Der Lelie H, et al. Comparison of doxorubicin and mitoxantrone in the treatment of elderly patients with advanced diffuse non-Hodgkin's lymphoma using CHOP versus CNOP chemotherapy. *J Clin Oncol*. 1995;13:2530–2539.

54. Sonneveld P, Michiels JJ. Full dose chemotherapy in elderly patients with non-Hodgkin's lymphoma: a feasibility study using a mitoxantrone containing regimen. *Br J Cancer*. 1990;62:105–108.

55. Bessell EM, Coutts A, Fletcher J, et al. Non-Hodgkin's lymphoma in elderly patients: a phase II study of MCOP chemotherapy in patients aged 70 years or over with intermediate- or high-grade histology. *Eur J Cancer*. 1994;30A:1337–1341.

56. Salvagno L, Contu A, Bianco A, et al. A combination of mitoxantrone, etoposide and prednisone in elderly patients with non-Hodgkin's lymphoma. *Ann Oncol*. 1992;3:833–837.

57. Ansell SM, Falkson G. A phase II trial of a chemotherapy combination in elderly patients with aggressive lymphoma. *Ann Oncol*. 1993;4:172.

58. Tirelli U, Zagonel V, Errante D, et al. A prospective study of a new combination chemotherapy regimen in patients older than 70 years with unfavorable non-Hodgkin's lymphoma. *J Clin Oncol*. 1992;10:228–236.

59. Zagonel V, Tirelli U, Carbone A, et al. Combination chemotherapy specifically devised for elderly patients with unfavorable non-Hodgkin's lymphoma. *Cancer Invest*. 1990;8:577–582.

60. Bertini M. Therapeutic strategies in intermediate grade lymphomas in elderly patients. the Italian Multiregional Non Hodgkin's Lymphoma Study Group (IMRNHLSG). *Hematol Oncol*. 1993;11(suppl 1):52–58.

61. Morra E, Gargantini L, Nosari A, et al. Treatment of patients with high-grade non-Hodgkin's lymphoma aged over 70 years with an all-oral regimen combining idarubicin, etoposide and alkylators. *Crit Rev Oncol Hematol*. 2000;35:95–100.

62. Zaja F, Tomadini V, Zaccaria A, et al. CHOP-rituximab with pegylated liposomal doxorubicin for the treatment of elderly patients with diffuse large B-cell lymphoma. *Leuk Lymphoma*. 2006;47:2174–2180.

63. Martino R, Perea G, Caballero MD, et al. Cyclophosphamide, pegylated liposomal doxorubicin (caelyx), vincristine and prednisone (CCOP) in elderly patients with diffuse large B-cell lymphoma: results from a prospective phase II study. *Haematologica*. 2002;87:822–827.

64. Italiano A, Jardin F, Peyrade F, et al. Adapted CHOP plus rituximab in non-Hodgkin's lymphoma in patients over 80 years old. *Haematologica*. 2005;90:1281–1283.

65. Chao NJ, Rosenberg SA, Horning SJ. CEPP(B): an effective and well-tolerated regimen in poor-risk, aggressive non-Hodgkin's lymphoma. *Blood*. 1990;76(7): 1293–1298.

66. Cardinale D, Colombo A, Sandri MT, et al. Prevention of high-dose chemotherapy-induced cardiotoxicity in high-risk patients by angiotensin-converting enzyme inhibition. *Circulation*. 2006; 114:2474–2481.

67. Kalay N, Basar E, Ozdogru I, et al. Protective effects of carvedilol against anthracycline-induced cardiomyopathy. *J Am Coll Cardiol*. 2006;48(11):2258–2262.

68. Doorduijn JK, Van Der Holt B, van Imhoff GW, et al. CHOP compared with CHOP plus granulocyte colony-stimulating factor in elderly patients with aggressive non-Hodgkin's lymphoma. *J Clin Oncol*. 2003;21:3041–3050.

69. Osby E, Hagberg H, Kvaloy S, et al. CHOP is superior to CNOP in elderly patients with aggressive lymphoma while outcome is unaffected by filgrastim treatment: results of a Nordic lymphoma group randomized trial. *Blood*. 2003;101:3840–3848.

70. Gómez H, Mas L, Casanova L, et al. Elderly patients with aggressive non-Hodgkin's lymphoma treated with CHOP chemotherapy plus granulocyte-macrophage colony-stimulating factor: identification of two age subgroups with differing hematologic toxicity. *J Clin Oncol*. 1998;16:2352–2358.

71. Gómez H, Hidalgo M, Casanova L, et al. Risk factors for treatment-related death in elderly patients with aggressive non-Hodgkin's lymphoma: results of a multivariate analysis. *J Clin Oncol*. 1998;16:2065–2069.

72. Morrison VA, Weller EA, Habermann TM, et al. Patterns of growth factor usage and febrile neutropenia among older patients with diffuse large B-cell lymphoma treated with CHOP or R-CHOP: an intergroup experience (CALGB 9793, ECOG-SWOG 4494). *Proc Am Soc Hematol*. 2004;104:904a.

73. Smith TJ, Khatcheressian J, Lyman GH, et al. 2006 update of recommendations for the use of white blood cell growth factors: an evidence-based clinical practice guidelines. *J Clin Oncol*. 2006;24:3187–3285.

74. Advani R, Rosenberg SA, Horning SJ. Stage I and II follicular non-Hodgkin's lymphoma: long-term follow-up of no initial therapy. *J Clin Oncol*. 2004;22:1454–1459.

75. Horning SJ. Natural history of and therapy for the indolent non-Hodgkin's lymphomas. *Semin Oncol*. 1993;20:75–88.

76. Horning SJ, Rosenberg SA. The natural history of initially untreated low-grade non-Hodgkin's lymphomas. *N Engl J Med*. 1984;311: 1471–1475.

77. O'Reilly SE, Connors JM, Macpherson N, et al. Malignant lymphomas in the elderly. *Clin Geriatr Med*. 1997;13:251–263.

285

78. Engelhard M, Stuschke M. 3. Report on workshop: UICC workshop "therapy of NHL in early stages," part 1: follicular lymphoma. *Ann Hematol.* 2001;80(suppl 3):B13–B15.

79. Mac Manus MP, Hoppe RT. Is radiotherapy curative for stage I and II low-grade follicular lymphoma? Results of a long-term follow-up study of patients treated at Stanford University. *J Clin Oncol.* 1996;14:1282–1290.

80. Gospodarowicz MK, Bush RS, Brown TC, et al. Prognostic factors in nodular lymphomas: a multivariate analysis based on the Princess Margaret Hospital experience. *Int J Radiat Oncol Biol Phys.* 1984;10:489–497.

81. Pendlebury S, el Awadi M, Ashley S, et al. Radiotherapy results in early stage low grade nodal non-Hodgkin's lymphoma. *Radiother Oncol.* 1995;36:167–171.

82. Tezcan H, Vose JM, Bast M, et al. Limited stage I and II follicular non-Hodgkin's lymphoma: the Nebraska Lymphoma Study Group experience. *Leuk Lymphoma.* 1999;34:273–285.

83. Ardeshna KM, Smith P, Norton A, et al. Long-term effect of a watch and wait policy versus immediate systemic treatment for asymptomatic advanced-stage non-Hodgkin lymphoma: a randomised controlled trial. *Lancet.* 2003;362(9383):516–522.

84. Kelsey SM, Newland AC, Hudson GV, et al. A British National Lymphoma Investigation randomised trial of single agent chlorambucil plus radiotherapy versus radiotherapy alone in low grade, localised non-Hodgkins lymphoma. *Med Oncol.* 1994;11(1):19–25.

85. Connors JM, O'Reilly SE. Treatment considerations in the elderly patient with lymphoma. *Hematol Oncol Clin North Am.* 1997;11:949–961.

86. Jones SE, Rosenberg SA, Kaplan HS, et al. Non-Hodgkin's lymphomas. II. Single agent chemotherapy. *Cancer.* 1972;30:31–38.

87. Kennedy BJ, Bloomfield CD, Kiang DT, et al. Combination versus successive single agent chemotherapy in lymphocytic lymphoma. *Cancer.* 1978;41:23–28.

88. Anderson T, Bender RA, Fisher RI, et al. Combination chemotherapy in non-Hodgkin's lymphoma: results of long-term followup. *Cancer Treat Rep.* 1977;61:1057–1066.

89. Jones SE, Grozea PN, Miller TP, et al. Chemotherapy with cyclophosphamide, doxorubicin, vincristine, and prednisone alone or with levamisole or with levamisole plus BCG for malignant lymphoma: a Southwest Oncology Group study. *J Clin Oncol.* 1985;3:1318–1324.

90. Jones SE, Grozea PN, Metz EN, et al. Superiority of adriamycin-containing combination chemotherapy in the treatment of diffuse lymphoma: a Southwest Oncology Group study. *Cancer.* 1979;43:417–425.

91. Glick JH, Barnes JM, Ezdinli EZ, et al. Nodular mixed lymphoma: results of a randomized trial failing to confirm prolonged disease-free survival with COPP chemotherapy. *Blood.* 1981;58:920–925.

92. Peterson BA, Petroni GR, Frizzera G, et al. Prolonged single-agent versus combination chemotherapy in indolent follicular lymphomas: a study of the cancer and leukemia group B. *J Clin Oncol.* 2003;21:5–15.

93. McLaughlin P, Hagemeister FB, Romaguera JE, et al. Fludarabine, mitoxantrone, and dexamethasone: an effective new regimen for indolent lymphoma. *J Clin Oncol.* 1996;14:1262–1268.

94. Maloney DG, Grillo-López AJ, White CA, et al. IDEC-C2B8 (rituximab) anti-CD20 monoclonal antibody therapy in patients with relapsed low-grade non-Hodgkin's lymphoma. *Blood.* 1997;90:2188–2195.

95. McLaughlin P, Grillo-López AJ, Link BK, et al. Rituximab chimeric anti-CD20 monoclonal antibody therapy for relapsed indolent lymphoma: half of patients respond to a four-dose treatment program. *J Clin Oncol.* 1998;16:2825–2833.

96. Feuring-Buske M, Kneba M, Unterhalt M, et al. IDEC-C2B8 (rituximab) anti-CD20 antibody treatment in relapsed advanced-stage follicular lymphomas: results of a phase-II study of the German low-grade lymphoma study group. *Ann Hematol.* 2000;79:493–500.

97. Hainsworth JD, Litchy S, Burris III HA, et al. Rituximab as first-line and maintenance therapy for patients with indolent non-Hodgkin's lymphoma. *J Clin Oncol.* 2002;20:4261–4267.

98. Witzig TE, Vukov AM, Habermann TM, et al. Rituximab therapy for patients with newly diagnosed, advanced-stage, follicular grade I non-Hodgkin's lymphoma: a phase II trial in the North Central Cancer Treatment Group. *J Clin Oncol.* 2005;23:1103–1108.

99. Colombat P, Salles G, Brousse N, et al. Rituximab (anti-CD20 monoclonal antibody) as single first-line therapy for patients with follicular lymphoma with a low tumor burden: clinical and molecular evaluation. *Blood.* 2001;97:101–106.

100. Schulz H, Bohlius JF, Trelle S, et al. Immunochemotherapy with rituximab and overall survival in patients with indolent or mantle cell lymphoma: a systematic review and meta-analysis. *J Natl Cancer Inst.* 2007;99:706–714.

101. Hiddemann W, Kneba M, Dreyling M, et al. Frontline therapy with rituximab added to the combination of cyclophosphamide, doxorubicin,

vincristine, and prednisone (CHOP) significantly improves the outcome for patients with advanced-stage follicular lymphoma compared with therapy with CHOP alone: results of a prospective randomized study of the German Low-Grade Lymphoma Study Group. *Blood.* 2005;106:3725–3732.

102. Witzig TE, Flinn IW, Gordon LI, et al. Treatment with ibritumomab tiuxetan radioimmunotherapy in patients with rituximab-refractory follicular non-Hodgkin's lymphoma. *J Clin Oncol.* 2002;20:3262–3269.

103. Witzig TE, Gordon LI, Cabanillas F, et al. Randomized controlled trial of yttrium-90-labeled ibritumomab tiuxetan radioimmunotherapy versus rituximab immunotherapy for patients with relapsed or refractory low-grade, follicular, or transformed B-cell non-Hodgkin's lymphoma. *J Clin Oncol.* 2002;20:2453–2463.

104. Kaminski MS, Tuck M, Estes J, et al. 131I-tositumomab therapy as initial treatment for follicular lymphoma. *N Engl J Med.* 2005;352:441–449.

105. Leonard JP, Coleman M, Kostakoglu L, et al. Abbreviated chemotherapy with fludarabine followed by tositumomab and iodine I 131 tositumomab for untreated follicular lymphoma. *J Clin Oncol.* 2005;23:5696–5704.

106. Zallio F, Cuttica A, Caracciolo D, et al. Feasibility of peripheral blood progenitor cell mobilization and harvest to support chemotherapy intensification in elderly patients with poor prognosis: non-Hodgkin's lymphoma. *Ann Hematol.* 2002;81:448–453.

107. Jantunen E, Mahlamaki E, Nousiainen T. Feasibility and toxicity of high-dose chemotherapy supported by peripheral blood stem cell transplantation in elderly patients (>/=60 years) with non-Hodgkin's lymphoma: comparison with patients <60 years treated within the same protocol. *Bone Marrow Transplant.* 2000;26:737–741.

108. Jantunen E. Autologous stem cell transplantation beyond 60 years of age. *Bone Marrow Transplant.* 2006;38:715–720.

109. Jantunen E, Itala M, Juvonen E, et al. Autologous stem cell transplantation in elderly (>60 years) patients with non-Hodgkin's lymphoma: a nation-wide analysis. *Bone Marrow Transplant.* 2006;37:367–372.

110. Jantunen E, Canals C, Rambaldi A, et al. Autologous stem cell transplantation in elderly patients (>= 60 years) with diffuse large B-cell lymphoma: an analysis based on data in the European Blood and Marrow Transplantation Registry. *Haematologica.* 2008;93:1837–1842.

111. Wallen H, Gooley TA, Deeg HJ, et al. Ablative allogeneic hematopoietic cell transplantation in adults 60 years of age and older. *J Clin Oncol.* 2005;23:3439–3446.

20 Management of multiple myeloma in older adults

Amrita Y. Krishnan

A. Introduction

Multiple myeloma is a hematologic malignancy of particular relevance for elderly patients owing to the epidemiology of the disease. The incidence of myeloma increases significantly with increasing age. For example, the age-specific incidence is less than 1 per 100,000 for persons younger than 40 years but rises to over 40 per 100,000 for persons over age 80 years.[1] The median age at diagnosis is 68 years. Treatment of myeloma in older patients is guided by multiple factors: the biology of the disease, comorbidities in the older patient, and identification of patients who would benefit from and tolerate high-dose chemotherapy with autologous stem cell rescue. The treatment of patients can vary significantly. This is in part due to variation in the age at which a myeloma patient is labeled "elderly." Some studies use a lower age of 65 years, others 70 years. Similarly, there is variation in the way patients are referred for transplant or clinical trials. Some transplant trials use age 65 as a cutoff, whereas other centers offer transplant to patients up to age 70. In addition, there is often a referral bias, with only younger patients being referred to tertiary care centers for trials. This is reflected in the median age of around 60 for myeloma patients at tertiary care centers versus community-based reports of a median age of 70 years and older.[2]

A.1. Monoclonal gammopathy of undetermined significance

Monoclonal gammopathy of undetermined significance (MGUS) may often be confused with myeloma or may be the inciting factor for referral to an oncologist to rule out a diagnosis of myeloma. It affects approximately 3 percent of persons over age 70 and is characterized by the presence of a serum monoclonal protein of 3 g/dL or less. However, what distinguishes MGUS from myeloma is the absence of boney lesions, anemia, hypercalcemia, and renal insufficiency. In addition, a bone marrow biopsy will have less than 10 percent plasma cells. There are no reliable predictors of which patients will progress to frank myeloma. A large series of 1,384 patients from the Mayo clinic with 11,009 person-years of follow-up found that on average, the risk of progression from MGUS to myeloma or related disorders was 1 percent per year and that the initial concentration of the serum monoclonal protein was a predictor of the risk of progression.[3]

A separate entity from MGUS is smoldering myeloma (SMM). This entity requires a serum M protein over 3 g/dL and bone marrow plasma cells over 10 percent. However, similar to MGUS, it requires the absence of anemia, renal insufficiency, hypercalcemia, or lytic bone lesions for diagnosis. It accounts for approximately 15 percent of all newly diagnosed cases of myeloma. What is significant is that the risk of progression to active myeloma is much greater for SMM versus MGUS. The average time to progression in one study was 2–3 years.[4] There is no specific therapy for SMM; however, close follow-up of these patients is necessary, with monitoring of blood counts and renal function.

A.2. Active myeloma

After a patient has been diagnosed with active myeloma, he or she can be staged in two ways. The traditional staging system for myeloma has been the Durie Salmon system. However, a more recent system, the International Staging System (ISS), may be more accurate. This system has been studied in over 11,000 patients worldwide, and several factors predictive of survival have been found to be significant. Three stages were defined based on albumin and B2 microglobulin (Table 20.1).[5]

Of note, age was a poor prognostic factor for all stages of disease (Table 20.2).

B. Clinical presentation and biology of disease

It is unclear whether the better survival in younger patients reflects their ability to tolerate more intensive chemotherapy or the biology of the disease in

Table 20.1 The three stages of active myeloma.

Stage I: Serum B2 microglobulin < 3.5 mg/L and serum albumin ≥ 3.5 g/dL
Stage II: Neither stage I nor stage III
Stage III: Serum B2 microglobulin ≥ 5.5 mg/L

older patients. A large retrospective study of 1,689 patients with myeloma who were younger than 50 years compared with 8,860 patients 50 years of age and older suggested that it may be in part due to the nature of the disease in older patients, though not surprisingly, the older patients also had a lower performance status.[6] Overall, younger patients presented with more favorable features such as a low ISS score. Older patients tended to have high ISS stages, increased serum creatinine, and low hemoglobin. Median age-adjusted survival was significantly longer in younger patients both after conventional-dose therapy (4.5 vs. 3.3 years, $p < .001$) and after high-dose therapy (median 7.5 vs. 5.7 years, $p = .04$). However, of note, on conventional cytogenetic analysis in 522 patients, despite the worse clinical presentation of myeloma in older patients, there was no significant difference in the proportion of patients with the poor-risk cytogenetics of deletion 13 in either age cohort. This finding is in concordance with two other smaller studies that did not reveal any association between cytogenetic abnormalities and age in a cohort of 75 patients and in a group of 175 patients.[7,8]

C. Treatment

Conventional-dose therapy for myeloma uses a variety of agents in combination. Traditional options for non-transplant-eligible patients have included melphalan and prednisone. This has been a standard of care for more than 40 years and is associated with a median survival of 29–37 months.[9] Melphalan is avoided in the transplant-eligible patient because of its potential toxicity to stem cells. Newer options include the use of thalidomide. Thalidomide was originally used in

the 1950s as a sedative; however, owing to its devastating teratogenic effects, it was initially withdrawn from the market for years. However, it had several properties that are effective against myeloma cell growth such as increasing production of interleukin 10, suppressing tumor necrosis factor, and stimulating cytotoxic T cells. Subsequently, thalidomide was shown to be an effective therapy either as a single agent or in combination with dexamethasone for patients with relapsed myeloma. Response rates of up to 66 percent were reported.[10,11] Because of its effectiveness in the relapsed setting, thalidomide was then moved to the upfront setting. A randomized trial of thalidomide plus high-dose dexamethasone versus dexamethasone alone found that the thalidomide-dexamethasone combination was more effective than dexamethasone alone in a group of newly diagnosed patients with a median age of 65 years.[12] However, the combination also had greater toxicity, manifest as grade 3 or higher deep venous thrombosis (DVT), rash, bradycardia, and neuropathy. The neurologic side effects can be particularly troublesome for older patients. A study of thalidomide and high-dose dexamethasone versus melphalan and prednisone showed higher response rates but also higher toxicity (Table 20.3) in elderly patients treated on the thalidomide-dexamethasone arm.[13]

More recent approaches have been to combine thalidomide with chemotherapy agents. Two randomized phase III trials compared thalidomide plus melphalan and prednisone (MPT) versus melphalan and prednisone (MP) in elderly patients (over 65 years) with myeloma. In one trial, melphalan was given at a dose of 4 mg/m^2 days 1–7 and prednisone at 40 mg/m^2 days 1–7 repeated every 4 weeks for six cycles. In the MPT arm, thalidomide was started on day 1 at a dose of 100 mg and continued daily through the six cycles, and then as a single agent. Of note,

Table 20.2 Poor prognostic factors for all stages of active myeloma.

Stage	Median overall survival < 65 years	Median overall survival ≥ 65 years
I	69 months	47 months
II	50 months	37 months
III	33 months	24 months

Table 20.3 Higher response rates but also higher toxicity in elderly patients treated in a study of thalidomide and high-dose dexamethasone versus melphalan and prednisone.[13]

Toxicity	Thalidomide dexamethasone (n = 134)	Melphalan prednisone (n = 134)
DVT	13 (10%)	5 (4%)
Neuropathy G1 + 2	87 (65%)	43 (32%)
Constipation G1 + 2	35 (25%)	13 (10%)
Leukopenia	4 (3%)	20 (15%)

69 percent of patients in the MPT arm were over 70 years of age.[14] Median progression-free survival (PFS) was superior in the MPT arm 21.8 months versus 14.5 months for MP ($p = .004$); however, after a median follow-up of 38.1 months, median overall survival was not significantly different at 45.1 months for MPT versus 47.6 months for MP ($p = .79$). The lack of overall survival advantage may be explained by the proportion of MP patients receiving thalidomide or novel agents such as bortezomib at relapse. The French Francophone Myeloma Intergroup (IFM) conducted a similar trial of MPT versus MP versus melphalan 100 mg/m2. With a median follow-up of 32.2 months, median PFS was 27.6 months for the MPT arm and 17.1 months for the MP arm ($p < .0001$). OS was also improved in the MPT arm at 38.6 months versus 30.3 months ($p < .0001$).[15]

D. Lenalidomide

The advent of newer immunomodulatory agents such as lenalidomide broadened the options for both transplant-eligible and non-transplant candidates. Lenalidomide is an analog of thalidomide that has a more favorable side-effect profile, specifically less sedation and neuropathy than thalidomide. It down-regulates interleukin 6 and nuclear factor kappa B and activates caspase 8 in vitro. It is 50,000 times more potent than the parent compound in inhibiting tumor necrosis factor. It was initially approved for the treatment of myeloma patients who had received one prior regimen. This was on the basis of two large, randomized trials that demonstrated superior time to progression and overall survival for the combination of lenalidomide plus high-dose dexamethasone (LD) versus dexamethasone alone.[16,17] Of note, these trials included older patients. The median age in the U.S. trial was 64 years, with a range up to 86 years. The response rate of the combination was high (61%), and it was well tolerated. The side effects in the LD arm included grade 3–4 neutropenia in 41 percent of patients and thromboembolic events in 14 percent. Strikingly, the incidence of grade 3–4 neuropathy was extremely low, at 3 percent, in the LD arm.

The high response rates and side effect profile naturally led to the exploration of the drug in the upfront setting. A phase II trial of lenalidomide plus high-dose dexamethasone was conducted.[18] The median age of the patients was 64 years (range 32–78). The overall response rate was 91 percent. Grade 3 neutropenia was seen in 12 percent. No grade 3 neuropathy was seen, and 21 percent developed grade 1–2 neuropathy. This trial confirmed the feasibility and effectiveness of lenalidomide in combination with high-dose dexamethasone. However, high doses of steroids can often be poorly tolerated by the elderly and exacerbate conditions, such as hypertension and diabetes, that are common in older patients. Hence recent trials have leaned toward a more steroid-sparing approach. The Eastern Cooperative Oncology Group (ECOG) 4A03 trial evaluated lenalidomide plus decadron in the traditional high-dose schedule versus a low-dose schedule of 40 mg weekly; 445 patients were randomized, and the primary end point was response rate at 4 months. Overall survival at preplanned interim analysis was superior with lenalidomide plus low-dose dexamethasone at 96 percent versus 87 percent in the high-dose dexamethasone arm. When patients were divided by age, the survival difference was most striking in the over 65 year group at 94 percent versus 83 percent, in contrast to 97 percent versus 92 percent in younger patients.[19] Thrombotic events were significantly lower in the low-dose dexamethasone arm. These results demonstrate that this is a very feasible, well-tolerated regimen for the elderly patient, and it has the advantage of being an oral regimen. Longer follow-up will be needed to determine the remission duration and long-term impact on survival.

Other lenalidomide-based approaches build on the MPT experience by substituting lenalidomide for thalidomide. This is more challenging in that the primary toxicity of lenalidomide is hematologic and so is the main toxicity of melphalan. In an Italian phase I trial, patients 65 years and older with newly diagnosed myeloma received nine courses of lenalidomide at escalating doses up to 10 mg maximum for 21 days.[20] Ciprofloxacin was given for antimicrobial prophylaxis and aspirin for venous thromboembolism prevention. The median age of the patients was 71 years. After one cycle, 51 percent had a response. Not surprisingly, the major toxicity was hematologic, with grade 3–4 neutropenia in 58 percent and grade 3–4 thrombocytopenia in 21 percent. The other challenge with a lenalidomide-based regimen is that the primary route of excretion of lenalidomide is renal. Elderly patients may have poor renal function because of their age and also comorbidities such as diabetes,

Table 20.4 Elderly patients may have poor renal function because of their age and also comorbidities such as diabetes, in addition to the renal compromise from their myeloma, and may require dose reductions in the lenalidomide.[21]

CrCl	Lenalidomide dose
≥50 mL/min	25 mg (full dose) every 24 hours
30 < ClCr < 50	10 mg every 24 hours
<30 mL/min (not on dialysis)	15 mg every 48 hours
<30 mL/min (requiring dialysis)	15 mg three times a week following dialysis

in addition to the renal compromise from their myeloma, and may require dose reductions in the lenalidomide (Table 20.4).[21] Alternate new guidelines released recommend administering lenalidomide 5 mg daily for patients with a ClCr < 30 or who are on dialysis.

E. Bortezomib

Nonimmunomodulatory-based treatment options include the use of bortezomib either as a single agent or in combination with steroids, anthracyclines, or a melphalan prednisone backbone. Bortezomib is a proteasome inhibitor that binds reversibly to the proteasome complex in the cell. The proteasome degrades ubiquinated proteins. The inhibition of this pathway leads to disruption of cell signaling pathways, which ultimately leads to death of the cancer cell. Bortezomib was approved by the U.S. Food and Drug Administration (FDA) in 2003 for the treatment of refractory myeloma after two prior therapies on the basis of a phase III trial that demonstrated improved time to progression and overall survival with bortezomib versus high-dose dexamethasone.[22] Specifically, overall survival was 80 percent in the bortezomib arm versus 60 percent in the high-dose dexamethasone arm. Thirty-eight percent of the patients in the bortezomib arm were aged more than 65 years. The primary grade 3–4 toxicities were thrombocytopenia (30%), neutropenia (14%), fatigue (6%), diarrhea (7%), and peripheral neuropathy (8%) in the bortezomib arm. The incidence of grade 3–4 events was 64 percent in patients under 50 years and 75 percent in patients over 65 years. As one of its primary toxicities, bortezomib is neurologic, and this might be problematic in the older patient who may already suffer from comorbidities such as diabetic neuropathy. Baseline neuropathy and comorbidities

such as diabetes may predict the occurrence of bortezomib-induced peripheral neuropathy and often correlates with its severity.[23] In fact, when neurologic complications were studied, the incidence of bortezomib-related grade 3–4 neuropathy was 14 percent for patients less than 75 years and 25 percent in older patients.[24]

Bortezomib was initially approved as a single agent for patients with relapsed myeloma. However, similar to the lenalidomide experience, the drug was soon used in combination with cytotoxic agents such as melphalan or doxorubicin. This is based on preclinical findings that drug resistance in myeloma cell lines can be overcome by combining agents, and often, as is the case of dexamethasone, a synergistic effect can be seen.[25]

A phase III trial of bortezomib plus liposomal doxorubicin (Doxil) versus bortezomib alone was conducted in patients with relapsed myeloma. Bortezomib was given on the traditional schedule of days 1, 4, 8, and 11, and the liposomal doxorubicin was added on day 4. Six hundred forty-six patients were enrolled, and median age in the bortezomib arm was 62 years (range 34–88) and 61 years (range 28–85) in the combination arm. The median time to progression increased from 6.5 months for bortezomib to 9.3 months for the combination.[26] However, the doxorubicin arm had a higher incidence of grade 3–4 adverse events, with grade 3 neutropenia and thrombocytopenia predominating. The total incidence of febrile neutropenia was 3 percent in the combination arm. Hence, though this is relatively low, it suggests that the combination regimen must be used with caution and that appropriate supportive care, such as growth factors and antibiotics, especially in an older population who are at higher risk of complications, is warranted.

Given the high response rates in the relapsed refractory patients, naturally, the drug was then explored in the upfront setting. Bortezomib was combined with melphalan and prednisone per the MPT experience. In a large phase III trial of 682 patients, bortezomib plus MP was compared with MP alone.[27] Thirty percent of the patients in the study were 75 years of age or older. They received nine 6-week cycles, with the bortezomib being given days 1, 4, 8, 11, 22, 25, and 29 for cycles 1–4 and weekly for cycles 5–9. Median time duration of response was 19.9 months in the bortezomib arm versus 13.1 months in the control group. After a median follow-up of 16.3 months, 13 percent of patients in the bortezomib arm had died versus 22 percent in the control group ($p = .008$).

The efficacy of bortezomib in three poor-risk subgroups was also assessed. One of these subgroups was defined as patients 75 years of age and older. In this subgroup of 107 patients, the median time to progression was identical as compared with 237 younger patients, though the complete remission rate was slightly lower (26% vs. 32%, $p = .29$). The adverse events were consistent with previously seen side effects for the agents, including grade 3 peripheral neuropathy in 13 percent of patients in the bortezomib arm. On the basis of these results, bortezomib also received FDA approval for previously untreated myeloma.

Building on this combination in a sort of kitchen sink approach was another phase III trial that compared bortezomib, melphalan, prednisone, and thalidomide (VMPT) versus bortezomib, melphalan, and prednisone.[28] Three hundred ninety-three patients with newly diagnosed myeloma aged 65 years and older were randomized. Initially, patients were treated with nine 6-week cycles of VMPT, with bortezomib given at 1.3 mg/m^2 days 1, 4, 8, 11, 22, 25, 29, and 32. The study was later amended to 5-week cycles, with the bortezomib given weekly days 1, 8, 15, and 22. The very good partial response rates (VGPR) were higher in the VMPT arm (55% vs. 42 percent in the VMP arm, $p = .02$). After a median follow-up of 13.6 months, the 2-year PFS was 83.9 percent for VMPT and 75.7 percent for VMP ($p = .35$). The incidence of grade 3–4 peripheral neuropathy was 18 percent in the VMPT arm and 12 percent in the VMP arm. Therefore the results suggest that VMPT is an active, well-tolerated combination in elderly patients with myeloma, with potentially higher response rates; however, it is unclear whether this will translate into an overall survival benefit. Recent trials presented in abstract form use weekly bortezomib schedules in elderly patients and have demonstrated lower neuropathy.[29,30]

F. Stem cell transplantation

Other treatment options for elderly patients may still include high-dose chemotherapy and autologous stem cell transplantation. The initial randomized trials that demonstrated the benefit of high-dose chemotherapy over conventional chemotherapy only included patients up to age 65 years.[31,32] However, as transplant-associated mortality decreases because of better supportive care, it is a feasible option for select older patients. Nonetheless, there are challenges to pursuing transplantation in elderly patients. First of all, it has been established that age is a risk factor for poor stem cell mobilization. However, it is not an absolute barrier. A retrospective trial of 21 mobilizations in patients younger than 60 years compared with 33 mobilizations in patients aged over 60 years demonstrated inferior numbers of CD34+ cells mobilized in the older patients; however, older patients were still able to mobilize sufficient numbers of cells for a transplant, though it required more days of leukapheresis.[33] The group from the University of Arkansas reported on 984 patients with myeloma undergoing mobilization. This included 106 patients 70 years or older. They found an inverse correlation with increasing age and CD34+ yield.[34]

There have been several small series of reports on older patients undergoing autologous transplantation. Obviously this is a very select group of patients with good performance status and no significant comorbidities. The University of Arkansas results highlight the challenges of transplant in older patients. First is referral bias, reflected in the fact that it took approximately 7 years to accrue 159 patients over the age of 70. Second, ultimately 40 percent of patients were not eligible because of comorbidities, lack of insurance support, inadequate psychosocial support, or patient preference.[35] Reece and colleagues described a series of 110 patients over age 60 who underwent autologous transplant.[36] The day 100 transplant-related mortality was 3 percent, though this increased to 8 percent at 1 year. Of note, almost one-third of the patients received total body irradiation (TBI) as part of their conditioning, we have now come to recognize that TBI is associated with greater toxicity in patients over the age of 55–60 and is therefore usually avoided. Other investigators have reduced the melphalan dose from the standard of 200 mg/m^2 to between 100 and 140 mg/m^2. The group from the University of Arkansas reduced the melphalan dose after experiencing a transplant-related mortality of 16 percent in the first 25 elderly patients they treated with full-dose melphalan.[35]

Nonetheless, despite all these caveats, a case control analysis by the Mayo Clinic suggested comparable toxicity and outcome for elderly myeloma patients undergoing transplant.[37] A total of 93 patients were evaluated; 33 were 70 years or older (median 71.2 years) and were matched with a group of patients 65 years or younger (median 54.3 years) at the time of transplant. The groups were matched for prognostic factors. The elderly group had a slightly higher creatinine at 1.1 (range 0.7–6.5) versus 1.0 (range 0.7–4.3) in younger patients. Thirty percent of the older patients received dose-reduced melphalan compared with 5 percent of the younger patients. There was a trend toward longer hospitalization in the older patients of 8 days and a nonsignificant difference in the rate of bacteremia between the groups. However, one patient in the elderly group died of transplant-related causes that were not specified by day 100 versus none in the younger group. The overall response rate and median time to progression and overall survival were similar between the groups. Hence, in spite of the use of reduced-dose melphalan, at least in this small series of elderly patients, transplant provided similar outcomes and mortality to a matched group of younger patients. However, this again represents a select group of patients, and not only in terms of performance status – it also selects for patients who tolerated their initial induction and survived to the time of transplant.

The role of autologous transplantation needs to be addressed in the context of durability of response. It is well known that autologous transplant is not curative. Median PFS is on the order of 3 years. The impact on short-term quality of life is significant and, especially in an elderly patient, must be strongly considered. In addition, an adequate support system must be in place for post-transplant care as one can anticipate that it would take an older patient longer to return to his or her baseline level of functioning than a younger patient.

G. Approach to the care of older adults with myeloma

Our approach to the elderly patient with myeloma is to make an assessment of whether transplantation will be a downstream option. This is based on performance status, comorbidities, and psychosocial factors. For example, assessment of the patient's ability to tolerate chemotherapy plus GCSF-based mobilization of stem cells and the potential pulmonary, hepatic, and gastrointestinal toxicity of high-dose melphalan. Other practical issues, such as who will provide care after discharge from the hospital, also need to be assessed. For patients who are potential transplant candidates, we avoid melphalan-based therapy because of the toxicity of melphalan on stem cells. This then leaves the options of bortezomib- or lenalidomide-

based treatment as induction. Both the biology of disease and the patient's comorbidities further guide this decision. The VISTA trial of Velcade (bortezomib), melphalan and prednisone demonstrated high response rates even in patients with high-risk cytogenetics. Hence, for a patient with poor-risk cytogenetics, we generally use a bortezomib-based (Velcade) regimen. If a patient has significant neuropathy, a lenalidomide-based induction is favored. If transplant is being considered, stem cells are collected after three to four cycles of induction. The decision of whether to proceed to transplant after stem cell collection or continue the current induction regimen is a difficult one as there are no mature studies in the era of novel agents of transplant versus no transplant. Generally, if the patient has achieved a VGPR or complete remission, we offer him or her the option of delaying transplant until disease progression and continuing the current therapy.

The treatment of relapsed disease follows some of the same paradigms with regard to assessing comorbidities. Patients with significant neuropathy would not receive thalidomide or bortezomib and therefore would receive lenalidomide-based treatment. Potentially autologous transplant could be considered if the patient has not had a prior transplant.

In conclusion, the treatment of myeloma in the elderly remains a challenge. The older patient tends to present with more advanced disease, though high-risk cytogenetic abnormalities are not increased in older patients. The advent of new agents, such as bortezomib and lenalidomide, has expanded treatment options for patients and led to response rates similar to high-dose chemotherapy. Unfortunately, the comorbidities of the older patient may limit the use of some therapies. For instance, underlying diabetic neuropathy could potentially worsen the severity of bortezomib-induced neuropathy. On the other hand, lenalidomide-based therapy carries a thrombotic risk. However, prophylactic anticoagulation in an elderly patient with a high potential for falls may be more risky. High-dose chemotherapy also still remains an option for a small group of elderly patients. Outcomes are similar to those of younger patients, though the early morbidity may be greater in the older patient. In general, the good news for elderly patients with myeloma is that age is no longer a barrier to participation in many clinical trials.

References

1. Anagnostopoulos A, Gika D, Symeonidis A, et al. Multiple myeloma in elderly patients: prognostic factors and outcome. *Eur J Haematol.* 2005;75(5):370–375.

2. Phekoo KJ, Schey SA, Richards MA, et al. A population study to define the incidence and survival of multiple myeloma in a national health service region in UK. *Br J Haematol.* 2004;127(3):299–304.

3. Kyle R, Therneau T, Rajkumar S, et al. A long term study of prognosis in monoclonal gammopathy of undetermined significance. *N Engl J Med.* 2002;346(8):564–569.

4. Witzig TE, Kyle RA, O'Fallon W, et al. Detection of peripheral blood plasma cells as a predictor of disease course in patients with smoldering myeloma. *Br J Haematol.* 1994;87(2):266–272.

5. Greipp PR, San Miguel J, Durie BG, et al. International staging system for myeloma. *J Clin Oncol.* 2005;23(15):3412–3420.

6. Ludwig H, Durie BG, Bolejack V, et al. Myeloma in patients younger than age 50 years presents with more favorable features and shows better survival: an analysis of 10549 patients from the International Myeloma Working Group. *Blood.* 2008;111(8):4039–4047.

7. Nilsson T, Lenhoff S, Turession I, et al. Cytogenetic features of multiple myeloma: impact of gender, age, disease phase, culture time and cytokine stimulation. *Eur J Haematol.* 2002;68(6):345–353.

8. Sagaster V, Kaufman H, Odelga V, et al. Chromosomal abnormalities of young multiple myeloma patients are not different from those of other age groups and are independent of stage according to the International Staging System. *Eur J Haematol.* 2007;78(3):227–234.

9. Alexanian R, Haut A, Khan AU, et al. Treatment for myeloma; combination chemotherapy with different melphalan dose regimens. *J Am Med Assoc.* 1969;208:1680–1685.

10. Alexanian R, Weber D, Anagnostopoulos A, et al. Thalidomide with or without dexamethasone for refractory or relapsing myeloma. *Semin Hematol.* 2003;40(suppl 4):3–7.

11. Singhal S, Mehta J, Desikan R, et al. Antitumor activity of thalidomide in refractory multiple myeloma. *N Engl J Med.* 2001;341(21):1565–1571.

12. Rajkumar SV, Rosinol L, Hussein M, et al. Multicenter randomized double-blind placebo controlled study of thalidomide plus dexamethasone compared with dexamethasone as initial therapy for newly diagnosed multiple myeloma. *J Clin Oncol.* 2008;26:2171–2177.

13. Ludwig H, Hajek R, Tothova E, et al. Thalidomide dexamethasone compared to melphalan prednisolone in elderly patients with multiple myeloma. *Blood.* 2008;113(5):3435–3442.

14. Palumbo A, Bringhen S, Caravita T, et al. Oral melphalan and predinose chemotherapy plus thalidomide compared with melphalan and predisone alone in elderly patients with myeloma: randomised controlled trial. *Lancet.* 2006;367(9513):825–831.

15. Facon T, Mary JY, Hulin C, et al. Melphalan and prednisone plus thalidomide versus melphalan and prednisone alone or reduced intensity autologous stem cell transplantation in elderly patients with multiple myeloma. *Lancet.* 2007;370(9594):1209–1218.

16. Dimopoulos M, Spencer A, Attal M, et al. Lenalidomide plus dexamethasone for relapsed or refractory multiple myeloma. *New Engl J Med.* 2007;357(21):2123–2132.

17. Weber D, Chen C, Niesvizky R. Lenalidomide plus dexamethasone for relapsed multiple myeloma in North America. *New Eng J Med.* 2007;357(21):2133–2142.

18. Rajkumar SV, Hayman S, Lacy M, et al. Combination therapy with lenalidomide plus dexamethasone for newly diagnosed myeloma. *Blood.* 2005;106(13):4050–4053.

19. Rajkumar SV, Jacobus S, Callander N, et al. A randomized trial of lenalidomide plus high dose dexamethasone (RD) versus lenalidomide plus low dose dexamethasone (Rd) in newly diagnosed multiple myeloma (E4A03): a trial coordinated by the Eastern Cooperative Oncology Group [abstract]. *Blood.* 2007;110:74.

20. Palumbo A, Falco P, Benevolo G, et al. Oral lenalidomide plus melphalan and prednisone for newly diagnosed myeloma [abstract]. *J Clin Oncol.* 2006;24 Pt 1:18.

21. Chen N, Lau H, Kong L, et al. Pharmacokinetics of lenalidomide in subjects with varying degrees of renal impairment. *J Clin Pharm.* 2007;47:1466–1475.

22. Richardson P, Sonneveld P, Schuster MW, et al. Bortezomib or high dose dexamethasone for relapsed myeloma. *New Engl J Med.* 2005;353:2487–2498.

23. Richardson PG, Briemberg H, Jagannath S, et al. Frequency, characteristics and reversibility of peripheral neuropathy during treatment of advanced multiple myeloma with bortezomib. *J Clin Oncol.* 2006;24(19):3113–3120.

24. Argyrious A, Iconomou G, Kalofonos H. Bortezomib induced peripheral neuropathy in multiple myeloma, a comprehensive review of the literature. *Blood.* 2008;112:1593–1599.

25. Ma MH, Yang HH, Parker K, et al. The proteasome inhibitor PS-341 markedly enhances sensitivity of multiple myeloma tumor cells to

chemotherapeutic agents. *Clin Cancer Res.* 2003;9:1136–1144.

26. Orlowski R, Nagler A, Sonneveld P, et al. Phase III study of pegylated liposomal doxorubicin and bortezomib compared with bortezomib alone improves time to progression in relapsed or refractory myeloma: results from DOXIL-MY3001. *J Clin Oncol.* 2007;25(25):3892–3901.

27. San Miguel J, Schlag R, Khuageva N, et al. Bortezomib plus melphalan and prednisone for initial treatment of multiple myeloma. *New Engl J Med.* 2008;359(9):906–917.

28. Palumbo A, Bringhen S, Rossi D, et al. A prospective randomized phase III study of bortezomib, melphalan, prednisone (VMPT) versus bortezomib, melphalan, and prednisone in elderly newly diagnosed myeloma patients [abstract]. *Blood.* 2008;112:652.

29. Mateos M, Oriol A, Martinez J, et al. A prospective multicenter randomized trial of Bortezomib/Melphalan/Prednisone (VMP) versus Bortezomib/Thalidomide Prednisone (VTP) with Bortezomib/Thalidomide (VT) versus Bortezomib Prednisone (VP) in elderly untreated patients with multiple myeloma older than 65 years. *Blood.* 2009;114:3.

30. Gay F. Bringhen S. Genuardi M, et al. The weekly infusion of Bortezomib reduces peripheral neuropathy. *Blood.* 2009; 114: 3887.

31. Child JA, Morgan G, Davies F, et al. High dose chemotherapy with hematopoietic stem cell rescue for multiple myeloma. *New Engl J Med.* 2003;348(19):1875–1883.

32. Attal N, Harousseau J, Stoppa A, et al. A prospective randomized trial of autologous bone marrow transplantation and chemotherapy in multiple myeloma. Intergroupe Français Du Myélome. *New Engl J Med.* 1996;335(2):91–97.

33. Fietz T, Rieger K, Dimeo F, et al. Stem cell mobilization in multiple myeloma patients: do we need an age adjusted regimen for the elderly? *J Clin Apheresis.* 2004;19(4):202–207.

34. Morris C, Siegel E, Barlogie B, et al. Mobilization of CD34+ cells in elderly patients with multiple myeloma: influence of age, prior therapy, platelet count, and mobilization regimen. *Br J Hematol.* 2003;120(2):413–423.

35. Badros A, Barlogie B, Siegel E, et al. Autologous stem cell transplantation in elderly multiple myeloma patients over the age of 70 years. *Br J Hematol.* 2001;114(3):600–607.

36. Reece DE, Bredeson C, Perez WS, et al. Autologous stem cell transplantation in multiple myeloma patients <60 years versus >= 60 years. *Bone Marrow Transplant.* 2003;32(12):1135–1143.

37. Kumar S, Dingli D, Lacy M, et al. Autologous stem cell transplantation in patients of 70 years and older with multiple myeloma: results from a matched pair analysis. *Am J Hematol.* 2008;83(8):614–617.

Part 4 Symptom management and supportive care of older adults

Optimizing quality of life in older adults with cancer

Alice B. Kornblith and Mark T. Hegel

A. Introduction

The Surveillance, Epidemiology, and End Results (SEER) data from 2001–2005 document that 55.2 percent of incident cancer patients are 65 years old or older.[1] On the basis of data from 2002–2004, the probability of developing invasive cancer in those 70 years old and older is 38.96 percent in men and 26.31 percent in women.[2] Given the high prevalence of cancer in the elderly, it is important to identify the prevalence of psychosocial problems in this age group, factors that result in patients being more vulnerable to poor psychosocial adjustment, interventions tested in older cancer patients to optimize adjustment, and suggested psychosocial interventions from other age groups or patient populations that might be effective in improving adjustment in the elderly cancer patient.

B. Psychological state

An increasing number of studies have assessed the psychosocial adjustment of the older cancer patient. Many studies have found that older cancer patients have better emotional functioning than younger patients.[3–12] In Sanson-Fisher and colleagues'[9] study, cancer patients who were 31–40 years old had significantly greater unmet psychological needs than those who were 71–90 years old. In addition, these findings are consistent with the landmark National Institute of Mental Health (NIMH) Epidemiological Catchment Area study[13] and the National Comorbidity Survey Replication study[14] involving 19,640 and 9,282 persons, respectively, which assessed the prevalence of psychiatric disorders in the general population. Both studies found that older persons had rates of psychiatric disorders that were lower than rates of psychiatric disorders in younger individuals. Factors suggested as the reasons for a better emotional adjustment in the older cancer patient were more effective skills in dealing with stress because of years of experience of coping with adverse circumstances; the common experience of

physical illnesses in the older person compared to younger cancer patients; fewer responsibilities to juggle[15–17]; and feeling that life hasn't been cut as short as younger patients might feel.

Not all studies have found a difference between younger and older patients or differences between older patients with cancer and noncancer populations. In postmenopausal breast cancer patients, Browall and colleagues[18] found no significant correlations between age (55–77 years old) and any of the assessed quality of life domains, including psychological state, with the exception of dyspnea and sexual functioning. Turner and colleagues[19] also found that there were no significant differences in anxiety and depression between younger and older lung cancer patients. Similarly, there were no differences in depressive symptoms or overall quality of life between younger and older head and neck cancer patients.[20]

Conversely, several studies have documented a decrease in psychological adjustment in older cancer patients. In Ganz and colleagues'[21] study, contradictory results were found. The overall psychological adjustment and mental health of older breast cancer patients declined over 15 months while, surprisingly, cancer-specific psychological state significantly improved. Kurtz and colleagues[22] found a steady increase in depression over 1 year in older colorectal cancer patients. There were multiple indications of a decrease in older breast cancer survivors' physical and mental health compared to older women participating in an epidemiological study.[23] Robb and colleagues[23] interpret their results as indicative of a lessening of reserve capacity in survivors, defined as the ability to "return to a normal state after periods of stress, such as a surgical procedure or illness."[23]

C. Older cancer patients in need

The literature has identified a subset of older cancer patients who experience psychological problems. There are no reported results of the prevalence of psychiatric disorders in the older cancer patient population based on clinical diagnoses. On the basis of cutoff scores of measures used to suggest a psychiatric disorder, prevalence of psychiatric symptomatology indicative of a possible psychiatric disorder in older cancer patients ranges from 3.0 to 42 percent.[4,11,19,24–27]

Significant predictors of mental health in older cancer patients can generally be grouped into sociodemographic factors (gender, race), type of treatment, physical state (symptoms and functioning, comorbid illnesses), and social factors (social limitations, social support). In the older cancer patient, depression or worse psychological state has been related to being female and African American[22]; worsening physical functioning and symptoms[22,27–31]; chronic side effects in older cancer survivors[24]; greater comorbidity[22,32]; radiation therapy for older prostate cancer patients[33,34]; cancer-related health worries (e.g., fear of recurrence, fears of a second cancer)[35]; less social support[6,21,25,30,31]; lower levels of religiosity or spirituality[31,36]; and dissatisfaction with the health care team.[21] Thus there are many factors that influence whether an older cancer patient is at a higher risk for worse mental health, even if overall older cancer patients may have better psychosocial adjustment than their younger counterparts.

C.1. Geriatric interventions to optimize the adjustment of older cancer patients

Only a handful of studies report interventions specifically tested on the older cancer patient. These include support programs[37–39]; educational/informational interventions[40,41]; monitoring of physical, psychological, and social distress[26]; exercise[42]; cognitive therapy[43]; and multimodality interventions.[44–46] Most of these studies involve small sample sizes, and some are not randomized interventions, thereby weakening the certitude of the findings.

D. Support groups

There is a growing literature testing the value of professionally led support groups, with a "planned activity component involving the sharing of experiences and mutual support among the participants."[47] Many of the group support programs include multiple components such as education, cognitive-behavioral techniques, skills training, emotional support through discussion, and relaxation training. People who benefit from support groups state that "they feel less alone with their problems"[47] and that they learned different coping skills for handling their problems. In a review of professionally led group support programs, Gottlieb and Wachala[47] concluded that patients randomized to the support group "experience significant improvement in psychological functioning compared to a randomly assigned control group. These improvements were limited to the short-term."[47]

The efficacy of support groups was examined in a prostate cancer study in which patients in peer support groups ($n = 96$; 84.4% 60 years old or older) were found to have significantly better mental health than a comparison group of prostate cancer patients from a national prostate cancer registry (Cancer of the Prostate Strategic Research Endeavor, CaPSURE).[39]

Man to Man is a national self-help program for prostate cancer patients, led by prostate cancer patients, whose goals are "(1) to provide information about diagnosis and treatment options for prostate cancer, (2) to provide support, encouragement and solutions to common problems associated with prostate cancer, and (3) to promote awareness of prostate cancer as a major healthcare concern."[38] In Man to Man programs in Florida, the typical meeting involves a speaker followed by a question and answer period and personal sharing. There was minimal attention to psychosocial issues. Four hundred and five patients from 38 Man to Man groups completed a questionnaire concerning their satisfaction with the program. When asked about which aspects of the program they valued most, of 128 responding to the question, 83 percent reported that receiving information and education about prostate cancer was the most valued.

E. Education

Education about prostate cancer and its treatment was studied using an informational booklet.[40,41] Patients were randomized to either the intervention ($n = 29$) or the control group ($n = 29$) (87.3% were 61 years old or older). Significant differences between pre- and posttest knowledge of the disease and treatment, satisfaction with care, and overall quality of life (physical, emotional, functional, and social well-being) were found in the informational booklet group, while there were no significant differences between pre- and posttest scores in the control group.

Education as an important component of support groups was also found in a randomized trial of 312 breast cancer patients across age groups (mean age 48) assessed at study entry (3 months post-diagnosis) 1–2 weeks postintervention, 6 months and 3.5 years.[48,49] Patients were randomized to an educational arm consisting of lectures followed by questions and answers ($n = 79$); peer discussion of eight weekly meetings, facilitated by a social worker and nurse, focused on expression of feelings and self-disclosure ($n = 74$); a combination of education and peer discussion ($n = 82$); and a control group ($n = 77$). At 6 months, those patients in the education groups compared to the peer discussion alone and control groups had improved psychological and physical functioning largely by "enhancing self-esteem, instilling a positive body image and reducing disturbing intrusive thoughts about the illness."[48] In the long-term follow-up study, when just the educational group alone was compared to the peer discussion group alone, the education group had significantly better mental health, vitality, and social functioning.[49]

F. Screening and referral

Screening cancer patients for psychosocial distress using a "distress thermometer," with a referral to a mental health professional for further evaluation and treatment for those scoring above distress levels, has been incorporated in the National Comprehensive Cancer Network guidelines for distress management for all cancer patients.[50,51] As early as 1993, a mixed-age group of cancer patients in clinics at Johns Hopkins were screened for psychological distress using the Brief Symptom Inventory, with high-distress patients referred to a comprehensive mental health program.[52]

Following this approach, an intervention involving screening for distress was developed by Kornblith and colleagues[26] to improve psychological adjustment of the older cancer patient. In this study, monthly telephone monitoring of older breast, prostate, and colorectal cancer patients' (65 years old or older) physical, psychological, and social distress over a 6-month period was conducted using standardized questionnaires. Those who scored above cutoff scores of distress were referred to the oncology nurse, with the oncology nurse calling the patient, evaluating the situation, and making a referral to the appropriate health professional, if needed. One hundred ninety-two patients were randomized to either the telephone monitoring and educational materials

(educational materials included cancer-related psychosocial issues and available resources) group (TM + EM) or to the educational materials (EM) only group, with 131 patients assessed at both baseline and 6 months. At 6 months, patients in the TM + EM group ($n = 69$) reported significantly less anxiety and depression compared to those in the EM group ($n = 62$). When patients were asked about what was most helpful in coping with an important problem, 41 percent of those in the TM + EM arm and 26 percent of those in the EM arm reported that talking over the phone with the research assistant about their quality of life was most helpful to them. Sixty percent of those in the TM + EM arm and 61 percent in the EM arm also reported feeling cared for between office visits. Thus just talking with the research assistant about their physical, psychological, and social problems on a monthly basis may be the effective factor of the intervention rather than the referral to the oncology nurse for a problem if distressed. This issue remains to be addressed in future research.

G. Exercise

Exercise might affect overall quality of life through an improvement in physical functioning. However, exercise studies have not targeted older cancer patients.[53] Segal and colleagues'[42] study is one of the few studies to include a substantial number of older cancer patients ($n = 155$, 70% over 65 years old). In this study, Segal and colleagues[42] tested the effects of supervised resistance training on muscular fitness and quality of life in prostate cancer patients treated with androgen deprivation therapy ($n = 82$) compared to a control group ($n = 73$). There was a significant decrease in fatigue and improved quality of life and upper and lower body muscular fitness in the exercise group. Contrary results were found in Demark-Wahnefried and colleagues'[54] study of an exercise and diet program of older breast and prostate cancer patients. Patients were randomized to either the exercise and diet program, consisting of telephone counseling and printed materials of diet and exercise ($n = 89$), or a control group ($n = 93$), in which patients received general health counseling and materials. Both groups had 12 semimonthly 20- to 30-minute sessions over a 6-month period. Though patients in the exercise and diet program arm had significantly greater diet quality and reported significantly greater self-efficacy than the control group, there were no significant differences in overall quality of life or depression between the two groups. Furthermore, Courneya and colleagues[55] reported that adherence decreased with increasing age for prostate cancer patients 75 years old and older. Clearly, with so few studies of the effect of exercise on older patients' adjustment, no conclusions can be drawn regarding its efficacy in improving their physical functioning and psychological state. More studies are needed to determine the type of exercise program that is effective in improving older cancer patients' adjustment, for which type of patient, undergoing which type of treatment, and at what point in their clinical course.

H. Cognitive therapy

Bailey and colleagues[43] developed an intervention to support prostate cancer patients during the watchful waiting period. This time of uncertainty about their disease while not being treated can be stressful to patients as they may fear that their disease will progress during this time. The intervention was delivered by telephone and was designed to improve patients' ability to cognitively reframe the way in which they viewed their illness and the continued uncertainty of watchful waiting. "In cognitive reframing, patients continually examine and reexamine illness-related events and talk about them with significant others and health care providers, to restructure their beliefs and expectations about events in such a way that they can manage them."[43] Thirty-nine patients, at an average age of 75 years old, were randomized to the intervention ($n = 20$) or usual care ($n = 19$). The watchful waiting intervention involved 5 weekly calls tailored to the specific problems that the patients raised. Several treatment strategies were used in the intervention: providing information on how prostate cancer developed and treatment options; emphasizing activities that were empowering; encouraging patients that their watch-and-wait approach was medically supported as better than undergoing current treatments; and encouraging patients to chart their prostate-specific antigen (PSA) levels if they were concerned about PSA changes, with reminders that "small fluctuations in values were probably nothing to worry about."[43] At 10 weeks' postbaseline, patients in the intervention group showed a significantly more positive perception of their future and better overall quality of life than the controls. There were no significant differences

between groups in psychological state or ability to cognitively reframe watchful waiting.

I. Multimodality interventions

Several studies used multimodality interventions for older cancer patients. In Lapid and colleagues'[44] study, a group of geriatric cancer patients with mixed disease sites ($n = 33$) were randomized to either the intervention ($n = 16$) or standard care ($n = 17$) group. The intervention consisted of eight 90-minute sessions that involved the following features: "conditioning exercises, ... educational instruction on symptom management, spiritual guidance, information on financial resources and advanced directives, cognitive-behavioral training for coping with cancer, ... open discussion and support ... and relaxation exercises."[44] Those in the geriatric intervention group showed the highest overall quality of life over an 8-week period, with spiritual well-being, emotional well-being, and overall quality of life having the greatest significant differences between the two groups.

In a second multimodality randomized trial, 72 patients involving a mixed sample of cancer diagnoses, 65 years old or older, were randomized to one of three interventions: psychopharmacologic alone (alprazolam and sulpiride) ($n = 25$), psychopharmacologic and social support from volunteers ($n = 23$), and psychopharmacologic and social support from volunteers and structured psychotherapy ($n = 24$).[45] The social support from volunteers included providing practical, informative, and emotional support. The structured psychotherapy involved the discussion of individual somatic and psychic inner experiences, autogenic training (teaching the mind and body to relax through the repetition of relaxation-producing phrases on six major themes, largely related to the body), and guided imagery (positive images suggested by the health professional or the patient, through which the patient is guided using sounds, feelings, smells, visuals, and/or tastes). Results demonstrated that older patients in the multimodality intervention groups reported significantly less anxiety and depression and better quality of life compared to those receiving psychopharmacologic agents alone. The two multimodality interventions proved almost equally effective.

Increasing hope is an interventional approach for improving quality of life among older palliative care cancer patients living at home.[46] Sixty-one terminally ill cancer patients (mean age 75 years) were randomized to the intervention involving a video on hope and a choice of one of three hope activities on which to work over a 1-week period ($n = 30$) or a standard of care control group ($n = 31$). The video included families "describing their hope and how they maintain hope."[46] Intervention group patients "chose one of three hope-focused activities: write a letter to someone, begin a hope collection or begin an 'about me' collection."[46] After 1 week, patients in the intervention group had significantly higher hope and existential well-being than those in the control group.

J. Patient characteristics

Which type of patient is most significantly affected by interventions? Results from studies of mixed-age groups suggest differences in efficacy of the intervention based on how well adjusted the patient was on entry to the intervention. In Helgeson and colleagues'[56] study of support groups for a mixed-age group of 230 breast cancer survivors, those who benefited the least were those who began with the most support. In Sheard and Maguire's[57] review of psychosocial interventions for cancer patients, across age groups, four interventions that screened patients for risk of or actual distress had the most powerful impact on emotional distress[58-61] compared to other trials in which patients were not screened for distress. Whether this would be the case for older cancer patients has yet to be answered.

K. Medication

With the exception of Mantovani and colleagues'[45] intervention, no interventions were found testing the use of psychotropics on the older cancer patient in a randomized trial. However, on the basis of clinical experience, Roth and Modi[62] have specified the appropriate use of psychotropics for the treatment of anxiety, depression, and delirium in the older cancer patient. Similar to the conclusions of Mantovani and colleagues,[45] Roth and Modi[62] suggested that multimodality therapy is preferred in the treatment of depression in the older cancer patient, with "a combination of supportive psychotherapy, cognitive-behavioral techniques, as well as antidepressant medications if needed."[62] They state that older patients with anxiety may also benefit from nonpharmacologic treatments involving psychotherapy; cognitive-behavioral interventions, which would include reframing negative thoughts; and relaxation therapies.

K.1. Other psychosocial interventions tested on nonelderly cancer patients that might be effective in improving adjustment of older cancer patients

Interventions based on studies of nonelderly cancer patients or in other patient populations that have been found to be effective in that population may be promising as effective interventions for older cancer patients. Possible candidates include online support groups, supportive-expressive therapy, behavioral activation with problem-solving skills training, and relaxation therapies. Selection of these interventions was based not only on prior success of the interventions on cancer patients and noncancer populations but also because they involve social support, which has been found to be a predictor of better adjustment (e.g., online support groups and supportive-expressive therapy); cognitive-behavioral therapies (e.g., behavioral activation/problem-solving skills training), which may appeal to older patients who do not wish to participate in psychosocial interventions involving the expression of emotions or interventions; or little strenuous activity and thus are easily accomplished in older cancer patients with physical limitations (e.g., online support groups, relaxation therapies, behavioral activation/problem-solving skills training).

L. Internet cancer support groups

Although online cancer support groups have been available since the early 1980s, they have increased dramatically over the years. As of 2003, 61.8 percent of households had computers and 87.6 percent of these households used their computers to access the Internet.[63] Internet use has likely grown since 2003. Cancer patients can interact with each other on "cancer-related news-groups, listservs, chat rooms, message boards and interactive web sites."[64] Computer-based systems would allow information seeking, social support, and patient participation in health care, which might affect quality of life.[65] Furthermore, seeking support online offers 24-hour help, convenience of availing the service from one's own home, and anonymity.

In a study of online support groups, across age groups, 1,541 messages from 947 postings were categorized.[64] Information giving and seeking comprised 28.8 percent of the messages, personal experience, 20.7 percent, and encouragement and support, 17.1 percent of messages. "Information giving/seeking was ranked first by the prostate and mixed groups, while personal experience was ranked first by the breast cancer group."[64] Thus there were gender differences between the types of intervention that patients sought, suggesting that one type of intervention may not meet the needs of all cancer patients.

One study evaluated online support groups for breast cancer patients using bulletin boards ($n = 114$). At 6 months, there was an improvement in depression, personal growth because of having had cancer, and psychosocial well-being.[66]

Two randomized trials studied the Internet as an approach to improve patients' psychological state and support.[65,67] In Winzelberg and colleagues'[67] study, 72 breast cancer patients were randomized to either a 12-week Web-based peer support program, moderated by a mental health professional whose primary role was to keep the weekly theme discussion on topics involving breast cancer and related concerns ($n = 36$), or a control group ($n = 36$). The weekly sessions were based on supportive-expressive therapy[68,69] and Kreshka's text on coping with breast cancer.[70] "Participants were able to read personal stories from survivors, share their own experiences and keep a web-based personal journal. ... Participants could log on and post comments at any time, without depending on others to be online at the same time."[67] The study found that postintervention, patients in the Web-based peer support group had significantly less depression, perceived stress, and symptoms of posttraumatic stress than the control group. In Gustafson and colleagues'[65] study, 246 breast cancer patients were randomized to either the Comprehensive Health Enhancement Support System, a Web-based system involving information, health care resources, discussion groups, personal stories from others, and coping advice ($n = 147$), or a control group that involved receiving a book about breast cancer ($n = 148$). The Internet-based support group reported significantly higher competence in dealing with information, higher levels of confidence in their doctors, and greater levels of comfort in communicating with their physicians than those in the control group. How-ever, there were no significant differences between the two groups in quality of life.

While promising, the degree to which Internet peer support will be effective with older cancer patients, and which type of older cancer patient, remains to be seen. The online support group overcomes the problems that the older cancer patient may face because of problems in physical functioning and treatment side effects that may make attending face-to-face support groups more difficult. However, older patients may be less familiar with using the Internet than younger patients, and there are economic issues that might limit the availability of the Internet to older patients on restricted incomes. In a study of Internet use among newly diagnosed patients who called the National Cancer Institute's Cancer Information Service ($n = 498$), age was the strongest predictor of type of Internet use (e.g., direct use, indirect use through others, nonuse), with those over 64.5 years old more likely to say they were not Internet users compared to younger patients.[71] Nonetheless, the studies reported earlier indicate that using online support groups may be valuable as an intervention to improve older cancer patients' knowledge of their disease and treatment, emotional support, psychological state, and satisfaction with their physician. As older cancer patients increasingly become users of the Internet, these types of interventions may be more accessible to them and perhaps effective in their adjustment.

M. Supportive-expressive group therapy

Supportive-expressive therapy is a type of support group led by a professional, in which the premise is that "sympathetic and direct confrontation with life-and-death issues result[s] in mastery rather than demoralization and that the group setting provides emotional support, enhances the patients' repertoire of coping strategies, and diminishes the sense of isolation, helplessness, and worthlessness."[72] The efficacy of supportive-expressive group therapy has been tested in several studies dating back to 1981.[72–74] In Spiegel and colleagues'[72] small study followed by Goodwin and colleagues'[73] and Kissane and colleagues'[74] studies, supportive-expressive group therapy was tested in metastatic breast cancer patients randomized to either the intervention or control group[72,73] or relaxation training.[74]

In these three studies, the support group met weekly for 1.5 hours for 1 year. In Kissane and colleagues'[74] study, the intervention as well as the control condition also included three classes of progressive muscle relaxation and guided imagery.[74] The psychosocial adjustment of those in the supportive-expressive group was found to be superior to those in the control group in all three studies. While these studies found a significant benefit of a yearly program of supportive-expressive group therapy in metastatic breast cancer patients, no significant difference in distress was found in a 12-week program for primary breast cancer patients.[75] Perhaps the negative findings in Classen and colleagues'[75] study may be due to a less sick patient population needing less support, the shortened intervention of 12 weeks rather than 1 year, or that two-thirds of the patients were not highly distressed. This latter issue was consistent with Sheard and Maguire's[57] review of the literature and Helgeson and colleagues'[56] study that demonstrated greater efficacy of interventions in those reporting greater distress.

With the success of the supportive-expressive group therapy over 1 year's time in metastatic breast cancer patients,[72–74] this approach to improving adjustment might be effective in older cancer patients who are not too ill to attend weekly group sessions for a year. As this intervention was tested in metastatic breast cancer patients across age groups, it remains for future research to test whether it would be successful in older cancer patients, male patients who may prefer educational interventions, and patients with other cancer diagnoses at different stages of disease.

N. Behavioral activation and problem-solving skills training

Behavioral activation and problem solving are distinct interventions that have been found to be effective in treating depression. However, although distinct, they may have their greatest utility when used together. They have particular value for the older person with cancer.

Behavioral activation (BA) is a psychosocial intervention originally conceptualized for the treatment of depression.[76] The primary tasks of BA are to (1) identify desired behavioral goals that are consistent with the person's life values, (2) systematically plan manageable increases in the desired activities, and (3) monitor progress and outcome. By carefully arranging for successful experiences, the goals can be achieved, and adaptive functional and emotional health can be fostered. Promoting regular contact with rewarding activities is one reason BA is effective for treating depression. A number of studies, largely conducted in psychiatric patients, support the effectiveness of BA in depression through the work of Jacobson and colleagues,[77] in a randomized trial of BA versus cognitive-behavioral therapy in outpatients with major depression ($n = 150$), and by Dimidjian and colleagues,[78] in a randomized trial of BA, cognitive therapy, and antidepressant medication in the acute treatment of adults with major depression ($n = 241$). These studies have shown BA to be equally effective to more complex psychotherapies (e.g., cognitive therapy) and even pharmacotherapy. Recently, a brief version of BA has been designed[79] and tested in a small randomized controlled trial ($n = 25$) for depression in psychiatric patients[79] and a series of case studies ($n = 6$) in depressed cancer patients.[80] However, if there are barriers to accessing the valued activity, then problem solving can be considered as a complementary, adjunctive, or alternative approach.

A problem-solving treatment model (PST) for depression was developed by D'Zurilla and Nezu[81] along with a brief version of PST, developed by Hegel and colleagues.[82] Cancer patients with weak problem-solving skills report more cancer-related problems and higher levels of anxiety and depression.[83] PST focuses on teaching a person to break down problems and identify barriers to overcoming the problem and uses a step-by-step approach to develop novel solutions. PST may assist the person to access his or her valued activities, but the emphasis is on solving problems. There are six steps to PST that are taught to the patient: (1) defining the problem, (2) setting a goal, (3) brainstorming solution alternatives, (4) evaluating and choosing a solution or solutions, (5) implementing the solutions, and (6) evaluating the outcome. Thus PST is a skills education approach that targets intractable problems. Problem solving has been shown to be effective in randomized clinical trials in the treatment of older depressed medical patients ($n = 132$)[84] and the prevention of depression in older adults with macular degeneration ($n = 206$)[85] and following stroke ($n = 176$).[86] PST has also been shown to be effective in a randomized clinical trial with a heterogeneous group of depressed long-term cancer survivors ($n = 132$).[87]

Behavioral activation and problem solving may be valuable interventions for older adults with cancer, in which the disease and its treatment cause deconditioning and nagging symptoms (e.g., fatigue, neuropathies), in addition to valued activities being disrupted. Fifty-nine percent of older cancer patients have impairments related to instrumental activities of daily living (e.g., using the telephone, taking medications, driving, etc., $n = 303$).[88] As with the limitations imposed by cancer and treatment and limitations due to impairments in instrumental activities, larger role-performance issues are also at stake such as keeping up relationships with family and friends and engaging in enjoyable activities.

Thus, given the goals and procedures of behavioral activation and problem solving and the results from the cited studies, behavioral activation and problem solving would appear to be promising for improving the adjustment and functioning of the older cancer patient. There are reasons to think that they may be most effective when used in a combined or complementary fashion. These are areas in need of further study.

O. Relaxation therapies

As can be seen from Lapid and colleagues',[44] Goodwin and colleagues',[73] and Kissane and colleagues'[74] studies, relaxation therapies were part of peer support programs that were found to be effective in improving older cancer patients' adjustment. Relaxation therapies include progressive muscle relaxation, guided imagery, meditation, autogenic training, and hypnosis.[89] In a review of interventions from 1980 to 2003 designed to improve anxiety and depression in adult cancer patients, Jacobsen and colleagues[90] concluded that in randomized studies across age groups, even when used alone, relaxation techniques prevented and relieved anxiety and depression, and relaxation combined with education and skills training prevented and relieved anxiety and depression. Furthermore, in a randomized trial, progressive muscle relaxation in cancer patients ($n = 77$) was found to be equivalent in the improvement of patients' anxiety and depressive symptoms compared to alprazolam ($n = 70$).[91] However, patients receiving alprazolam showed a slightly more rapid decrease in anxiety and depressive symptoms than those receiving progressive muscle relaxation.

In addition to a significant improvement in psychological state because of relaxation techniques, research has also demonstrated improvements in cancer-related physical symptoms, in which some studies have found a parallel improvement in psychological state. Yoo and colleagues'[92] and Molassiotis and colleagues'[93] studies have demonstrated an improvement in chemotherapy-induced nausea and vomiting in breast cancer patients being treated by progressive muscle relaxation. In 60 breast cancer patients randomized to progressive muscle relaxation and guided imagery ($n = 30$) versus a control group ($n = 30$), the intervention was found to reduce anticipatory nausea and vomiting and nausea and vomiting during chemotherapy significantly more than the control group.[92] These improvements were accompanied by improvements in emotional well-being at 3 and 6 months. In Molassiotis and colleagues'[93] study ($n = 71$), breast cancer patients randomized to progressive muscle relaxation ($n = 38$) reported significantly fewer vomiting and nausea episodes in the first 4 days after chemotherapy than the control group ($n = 33$). Psychological state was also found to significantly improve after chemotherapy in the progressive muscle relaxation group than the control group. Thus relaxation therapies may have a direct and indirect effect on psychological state through improvements in physical symptoms.

P. Conclusion

Given the scant literature concerning interventions tested in older cancer patients, the field is wide open concerning the development of interventions in this patient population. From the literature, it would seem that education alone, support programs, multimodality interventions, and the frequent assessment of physical and psychological symptoms that are conveyed to the medical team are fruitful avenues to pursue in larger randomized trials that might result in significant improvements in older cancer patients' quality of life. On the basis of one small study,[45] a multimodality intervention was found to be preferable to a single-modality intervention in older cancer patients. Other than Mantovani and colleagues'[45] study that tested the efficacy of two psychotropics (alprazolam and sulpiride) compared to the multimodality treatment arms, which included psychotropics, psychotropic drugs have not been tested for efficacy in older cancer patients. With only one study finding one type of exercise to improve quality of life in a largely older patient sample,[42] the value of different exercise programs to improve adjustment in older cancer patients remains to be further tested.

Whether the findings from the geriatric interventions would be confirmed in larger, randomized trials remains for future research, as is whether there are differences in efficacy because of different sociodemographic characteristics (e.g., gender, ethnicity, age of the older patient, educational level), functional status, type of cancer treatment, the time at which it is initiated in the patient's clinical course, and initial level of distress. Pursuit of potentially effective interventions for older cancer patients based on nongeriatric or noncancer patient populations would need to be tested in randomized trials involving geriatric cancer patients, with similar testing of efficacy according to different characteristics of the population and treatment.

With the limited number of interventions tested in geriatric cancer patients, mostly consisting of small sample sizes, and the lack of testing of nongeriatric interventions in geriatric cancer patients, it is not possible to specify which interventions might be best for which older cancer patient. Instead, the recommended approach would be to rely on the types of issues older cancer patients present and their personal preferences. The provider should discuss with the patient what types of psychosocial and physical interventions might be acceptable to them to improve their adjustment to having cancer. Issues to discuss with the older patient include the following: whether the patient prefers obtaining information, rather than emotional experiences; ease of using the computer either to obtain information or to participate in online support groups; being connected with others in-person in support groups for emotional support and methods of coping; taking medications versus psychotherapy to relieve anxiety and depression for those with anxiety disorders or clinical depression; length of time the patient is willing to be in an intervention; willingness to be followed by a nurse if distress is noted based on quality of life questionnaires; interest in complementary approaches (e.g., relaxation exercises) for psychological problems and symptom management; and degree of physical activity that would be acceptable.

As indicated in Montovani and colleagues'[45] study, multimodality interventions should be considered when discussing these various preferences with the patient. Once the patient has indicated his or her preferences for the type of intervention that would be acceptable, then the oncologist could suggest a specific intervention from those described earlier. Having these discussions with the patient is vital in that the oncologist affirms that many patients have some difficulties in adjusting to or managing their illness and its treatment, with a recommendation as to a possible psychosocial or physical intervention that might help them to optimize their adjustment.

References

1. Ries LAG, Melbert D, Krpacho M, et al., eds. *SEER Cancer Statistics Review, 1975–2005.* Bethesda, MD: National Cancer Institute; 2008.

2. American Cancer Society. *Cancer Facts and Figures 2008.* Atlanta, GA: American Cancer Society; 2008.

3. Watters JM, Yau JC, O'Rourke K, et al. Functional status is well maintained in older women during adjuvant chemotherapy for breast cancer. *Ann Oncol.* 2003;14:1744–1750.

4. Mor V, Allen S, Malin M. The psychosocial impact of cancer on older versus younger patients and their families. *Cancer.* 1994;74:2118–2127.

5. Given CW, Given BA, Stommel M. The impact of age, treatment and symptoms on the physical and mental health of cancer patients: a longitudinal perspective. *Cancer.* 1994;74(suppl): 2128–2138.

6. Parker PA, Baile WF, de Moor C, et al. Psychosocial and demographic predictors of quality of life in a large sample of cancer patients. *Psycho-Oncology.* 2003;12:183–193.

7. Hann D, Baker F, Denniston M, et al. The influence of social support on depressive symptoms in cancer patients: age and gender differences. *J Psychosom Res.* 2002;52:279–283.

8. Vinokur AD, Threatt BA, Vinokur-Kaplan D, et al. The process of recovery from breast cancer for younger and older patients: changes during the first year. *Cancer.* 1990;65:1242–1254.

9. Sanson-Fisher R, Girgis A, Boyes A, et al. Supportive Care Review Group. The unmet supportive care needs of patients with cancer. *Cancer.* 2000;88:225–236.

10. Kroenke CH, Rosner B, Chen WY, et al. Functional impact of breast cancer by age at diagnosis. *J Clin Oncol.* 2004;22:1849–1856.

11. Kornblith AB, Powell M, Regan MM, et al. Long-term psychosocial adjustment of older vs. younger survivors of breast and endometrial cancer. *Psycho-Oncology.* 2007;16:895–903.

12. Rose JH, Radziewicz R, Bowman KF, et al. A coping and communication support intervention tailored to older patients diagnosed with late-stage cancer. *Clin Interv Aging.* 2008; 3(1):77–95.

13. Robins LN, Regier DA. *Psychiatric Disorders in America: The Epidemiologic Catchment Area Study.* New York: Free Press; 1991.

14. Kessler RC, Berglund P, Demier O, et al. Lifetime prevalence and age-of-onset distribution of DSM-IV disorders in the National Comorbidity Survey Replication. *Arch Gen Psychiatry.* 2005;62:593–602.

15. Cassileth BR, Lusk EJ, Strouse TB, et al. Psychosocial status in chronic illness: a comparative analysis of six diagnostic groups. *N Eng J Med.* 1984;311:506–511.

16. Gurland, B. Epidemiology of psychiatric disorders. In: Sadavoy J, Lazarus LW, Jarvik LF, eds. *Comprehensive Review of Geriatric Psychiatry.* Washington, DC: American Psychiatric Press; 1991:25–40.

17. Mages NL, Mendelsohn GA. Effects of cancer on patients' lives: a personological approach. In: Stone GC, Cohen F, Adler NE, eds. *Health Psychology – A Handbook.* San Francisco, CA: Jossey-Bass; 1980:255–284.

18. Browall MM, Ahlberg KM, Persson LO, et al. The impact of age on health-related quality of life (HRQoL) and symptoms among postmenopausal women with breast cancer receiving adjuvant chemotherapy. *Acta Oncol.* 2008;47:207–215.

19. Turner NJ, Muers MF, Haward RA, et al. Psychological distress and concerns of elderly patients treated with palliative radiotherapy for lung cancer. *Psycho-Oncology.* 2007;16:707–713.

20. Derks W, Leeuw JR, Hordijk GJ, et al. Differences in coping style and locus of control between older and younger patients with head and neck cancer. *Clin Otolaryngol.* 2005;30:186–192.

21. Ganz PA, Guadagnoli E, Landrum MB, et al. Breast cancer in older women: quality of life and psychosocial adjustment in the 15 months after diagnosis. *J Clin Oncol.* 2003;21:4027–4033.

22. Kurtz ME, Kurtz JC, Stommel M, et al. Physical functioning and depression among older persons with cancer. *Cancer Pract.* 2001;9:11–18.

23. Robb C, Haley WE, Balducci L, et al. Impact of breast cancer survivorship on quality of life in older women. *Crit Rev Oncol Hematol.* 2007;62:84–91.

24. Deimling GT, Kahana B, Bowman KF, et al. Cancer survivorship and psychological distress in later life. *Psycho-Oncology.* 2002;11:479–494.

25. Raveis VH, Karus DG. Elderly cancer patients: correlates of depressive symptomatology. *J Psychosocial Oncol.* 1999;17(2):57–77.

26. Kornblith AB, Dowell JM, Herndon II JE, et al. Telephone monitoring of distress in advanced stage cancer patients 65 or more years old: a Cancer and Leukemia Group B Study. *Cancer.* 2006;107:2706–2714.

27. Kurtz ME, Kurtz JC, Stommel M, et al. The influence of symptoms, age, comorbidity and cancer site on physical functioning and mental health of geriatric women patients. *Women Health.* 1999;29(3):1–12.

28. Musick MA, Koenig HG, Hays JC, et al. Religious activity and depression among community-dwelling elderly persons with cancer: the moderating effect of race. *J Gerontol B Psychol Sci Soc Sci.* 1998;53(4):S218–S227.

29. Kurtz ME, Kurtz JC, Stommel M, et al. Predictors of depressive symptomatology of geriatric patients with lung cancer – a longitudinal analysis. *Psycho-Oncology.* 2002;11:12–22.

30. Kurtz ME, Kurtz JC, Stommel M, et al. Predictors of depressive symptomatology of geriatric patients with colorectal cancer: a longitudinal view. *Support Care Cancer.* 2002;10:494–501.

31. Perkins EA, Small BJ, Balducci L, et al. Individual differences in well-being in older breast cancer survivors. *Crit Rev Oncol Hematol.* 2007;62(1): 74–83.

32. Mols F, Coebergh JWW, van de Poll-Franse LV. Health-related quality of life and health care utilization among older long-term cancer survivors: a population-based study. *Eur J Cancer.* 2007;43:2211–2221.

33. Litwin MS, Lubeck DP, Spitalny GM, et al. Mental health in men treated for early stage prostate carcinoma posttreatment: longitudinal quality of life analysis from the Cancer of the Prostate Strategic Urologic Research Endeavor. *Cancer.* 2002;95:54–60.

34. Jayadevappa R, Chhatre S, Whittington R, et al. Health-related quality of life and satisfaction with care among older men treated for prostate cancer with either radical prostatectomy or external beam radiation therapy. *BJU Int.* 2006;97: 955–962.

35. Deimling GT, Bowman KF, Sterns S, et al. Cancer-related health worries and psychological distress among older adult, long-term cancer survivors. *Psycho-Oncology.* 2006;15:306–320.

36. Fehring RJ, Miller JF, Shaw C. Spiritual well-being, religiosity, hope, depression, and other mood states in elderly people coping with cancer. *Oncol Nurs Forum.* 1997;24:663–671.

37. Smith RL, Crane LA, Byers T, et al. An evaluation of the Man to Man self-help group in Colorado and Utah. *Cancer Pract.* 2002;10:234–239.

38. Coreil J, Behal R. Man to Man prostate cancer support groups. *Cancer Pract.* 1999;7(3):122–129.

39. Katz D, Koppie TM, Wu D, et al. Sociodemographic characteristics and health related quality of life in men attending prostate cancer support groups. *J Urol.* 2002;168: 2092–2096.

40. Templeton HRM, Coates VE. Development of an education package for men with prostate cancer on hormonal manipulation therapy. *Clin Effectiveness Nurs.* 2003;7:33–42.

41. Templeton H, Coates V. Evaluation of an evidence-based education package for men with prostate cancer on hormonal manipulation therapy. *Patient Educ Couns.* 2004;55:55–61.

42. Segal RJ, Reid RD, Courneya KS, et al. Resistance exercise in men receiving androgen deprivation therapy for prostate cancer. *J Clin Oncol.* 2003;21:1653–1659.

43. Bailey DE, Mishel MH, Belyea M, et al. Uncertainty intervention for watchful waiting in prostate cancer. *Cancer Nurs.* 2004;27: 339–346.

44. Lapid MI, Rummans TA, Brown PD, et al. Improving the quality of life of geriatric cancer patients with a structured multidisciplinary intervention: a randomized controlled trial. *Palliat Support Care.* 2007;5:107–114.

45. Mantovani G, Astara G, Lampis B, et al. Evaluation by multidimensional instruments of health-related quality of life of elderly cancer patients undergoing three different "psychosocial" treatment approaches: a randomized clinical trial. *Support Care Cancer.* 1996;4:129–140.

46. Duggleby WD, Degner L, Williams A, et al. Living with hope: initial evaluation of a psychosocial hope intervention for older palliative home care patients. *J Pain Symptom Manage.* 2007;33: 247–257.

47. Gottlieb BH, Wachala ED. Cancer support groups: a critical review of empirical studies. *Psycho-Oncology.* 2007;16:379–400.

48. Helgeson VS, Cohen S, Schulz R, et al. Education and peer discussion group interventions and adjustment to breast cancer. *Arch Gen Psychiatry.* 1999;56:340–347.

49. Helgeson VS, Cohen S, Schulz R, et al. Long-term effects of educational and peer discussion group interventions on adjustment to breast cancer. *Health Psychol.* 2001;20:387–392.

50. National Comprehensive Cancer Network. *NCCN Clinical Practice Guidelines in Oncology: Distress Management*: National Comprehensive Cancer Network; available at http://www.nccn.org/index. asp

51. Jacobsen PB, Donovan KA, Trask PC, et al. Screening for psychological distress in ambulatory cancer patients: a multicenter evaluation of the distress thermometer. *Cancer.* 2005;103: 1494–1502.

52. Zabora JR. Screening procedures for psychosocial distress. In: Holland JC, ed. *Psycho-oncology.* New York: Oxford University Press; 1998:653–661.

53. Courneya KS, Karvinen KH. Exercise, aging, and cancer. *Appl Physiol Nutr Metab.* 2007;32: 1001–1007.

54. Demark-Wahnefried W, Clipp EC, Morey MC, et al. Lifestyle intervention development study to improve physical function in older adults with cancer: outcomes from Project LEAD. *J Clin Oncol.* 2006;24:3465–3473.

55. Courneya KS, Segal RJ, Reid RD, et al. Three independent factors predicted adherence in a randomized controlled trial of resistance exercise

training among prostate cancer patients. *J Clin Epidemiol.* 2004;57:571–579.

56. Helgeson VS, Cohen S, Schulz R, et al. Group support interventions for women with breast cancer: who benefits from what? *Health Psychol.* 2000;19:107–114.

57. Sheard T, Maguire P. The effect of psychological interventions on anxiety and depression in cancer patients: results of two meta-analyses. *Br J Cancer.* 1999;80:1770–1880.

58. Linn MW, Linn BS, Harris R. Effects of counseling for late stage cancer patients. *Cancer.* 1982;49:1048–1055.

59. Worden JW, Weisman AD. Preventive psychosocial intervention with newly diagnosed cancer patients. *Gen Hosp Psychiatry.* 1984;6:243–249.

60. Telch CF, Telch MJ. Group coping skills instruction and supportive group therapy for cancer patients: a comparison of strategies. *J Consult Clin Psychol.* 1986;6:802–808.

61. Greer S, Moorey S, Baruch JDR, et al. Adjuvant psychological therapy for patients with cancer: a prospective randomised trial. *Br Med J.* 1992;304:675–680.

62. Roth AJ, Modi R. Psychiatric issues in older cancer patients. *Crit Rev in Oncol Hematol.* 2003;48:185–197.

63. U.S. Department of Commerce. A nation online: entering the broadband age. Available at: http://www.ntia.doc.gov/reports/anol/nationonlinebroadband04.pdf. September 2004.

64. Klemm P, Hurst M, Dearholt SL. Cyber solace: gender differences on Internet cancer support groups. *Comput Nurs.* 1999;17(2):65–72.

65. Gustafson DH, Hawkins R, Pingree S, et al. Effect of computer support on younger women with breast cancer. *J Gen Intern Med.* 2001;16:435–445.

66. Lieberman MA, Goldstein BA. Self-help on-line: an outcome evaluation of breast cancer bulletin boards. *J Health Psychol.* 2005;10:855–862.

67. Winzelberg AJ, Classes C, Alpers GW, et al. Evaluation of an Internet support group for women with primary breast cancer. *Cancer.* 2003;97:1164–1173.

68. Spiegel D, Classen C. *Group Therapy for Cancer Patients.* New York: Basic Books; 1997.

69. Classen C, Diamond S, Soleman H, et al. *Brief Supportive-Expressive Group Therapy for Women with Primary Breast Cancer: ATX Manual.* Stanford, CA: Stanford University School of Medicine; 1993.

70. Kreshka MA, Graddy K. *One in Eight: Women Speaking to Women, a Breast Cancer Workbook-Journal.* Grass Valley, CA: Sierra Nevada Cancer Center; 1997.

71. Bass SB, Ruzek SB, Gordon TF, et al. Relationship of Internet health information use with patient behavior and self-efficacy: experiences of newly diagnosed cancer patients who contact the National Cancer Institute's Cancer Information Service. *J Health Commun.* 2006;11:219–236.

72. Spiegel D, Bloom JR, Yalom I. Group support for patients with metastatic cancer: a randomized prospective outcome study. *Arch Gen Psychiatry.* 1981;38:527–533.

73. Goodwin PJ, Leszcz M, Ennis M, et al. The effect of group psychosocial support on survival in metastatic breast cancer. *N Engl J Med.* 2001;345:1719–1726.

74. Kissane DW, Grabsch B, Clarke DM, et al. Supportive-expressive group therapy for women with metastatic breast cancer: survival and psychosocial outcome from a randomized controlled trial. *Psycho-Oncology.* 2007;16:277–286.

75. Classen CC, Kramer HC, Blasey C, et al. Supportive-expressive group therapy for primary breast cancer patients: a randomized prospective multicenter trial. *Psycho-Oncology.* 2008;17:438–447.

76. Ferster CB. A functional analysis of depression. *Am Psychol.* 1973;28:857–870.

77. Jacobson NS, Dobson KS, Truax PA, et al. A component analysis of cognitive-behavioral treatment for depression. *J Consult Clin Psychol.* 1996;64:295–304.

78. Dimidjian S, Hollon SD, Dobson KS, et al. Randomized trial of behavioral activation, cognitive therapy, and antidepressant medication in the acute treatment of adults with major depression. *J Consult Clin Psychol.* 2006;74:658–670.

79. Lejuez CW, Hopko DR, Hopko SD. A brief behavioral activation treatment for depression: treatment manual. *Behav Modif.* 2001;25: 255–286.

80. Hopko DR, Bell JL, Armento ME, et al. Behavior therapy for depressed cancer patients. *Psychotherapy: Theory Res Pract Train.* 2005;42:236–243.

81. D'Zurilla T, Nezu A. *Problem Solving Therapy: A Social Competence Approach to Clinical Intervention.* New York: Springer; 1999.

82. Hegel MT, Imming J, Cyr-Provost M, et al. Role of behavioral health professionals in a collaborative stepped care treatment model for depression in primary care. *Fam Systems Health.* 2002;20(3):265–277.

83. Nezu CM, Nezu AM, Friedman SH, et al. Cancer and psychological distress: two investigations regarding the role of social problem-solving. *J Psychosocial Oncol.* 1999;16(3/4):27–40.

84. Arean PA, Hegel MT, Vannoy T, et al. The effectiveness of problem solving therapy for older, primary care patients with depression: results from the IMPACT Project. *Gerontologist.* 2008;48(3):311–323.

85. Rovner BW, Casten RJ, Hegel MT, et al. Preventing depression in age-related macular degeneration. *Arch Gen Psychiatry.* 2007;64(8):886–892.

86. Robinson RG, Ricardo RE, Moser D, et al. Escitalopram and problem solving therapy for prevention of poststroke depression: a randomized trial. *J Am Med Assoc.* 2008;299(20):2391–2400.

87. Nezu AM, Nezu CM, Felgoise SH, et al. Project Genesis: assessing the efficacy of problem-solving therapy for distressed adult cancer patients. *J Consult Clin Psychol.* 2003;71:1036–1048.

88. Serraino D, Fratino L, Zagonel V, et al. Prevalence of functional disability among elderly patients with cancer. *Crit Rev Oncol Hematol.* 2001;39:269–273.

89. Payne RA. *Relaxation Techniques: A Practical Handbook for the Health Care Professional.* 3rd ed. Edinburgh, Scotland: Elsevier Churchill Livingston; 2005.

90. Jacobsen PB, Donovan KA, Swaine ZN, et al. Management of anxiety and depression in adult cancer patients: toward an evidence-based approach. In: Chang AE, Ganz PA, Hayes DF, et al., eds. *Oncology: An Evidence-Based Approach.* Philadelphia: Springer; 2006:1552–1579.

91. Holland JC, Morrow GR, Schmale A, et al. A randomized clinical trial of alprazolam versus progressive muscle relaxation in cancer patients with anxiety and depressive symptoms. *J Clin Oncol.* 1991;9:1004–1011.

92. Yoo HJ, Ahn SH, Kim SB, et al. Efficacy of progressive muscle relaxation training and guided imagery in reducing chemotherapy side effects in patients with breast cancer and in improving their quality of life. *Support Care Cancer.* 2005;13:826–833.

93. Molassiotis A, Yung HP, Yam BMC, et al. The effectiveness of progressive muscle relaxation training in managing chemotherapy-induced nausea and vomiting in Chinese breast cancer patients: a randomized controlled trial. *Support Care Cancer.* 2002;10:237–246.

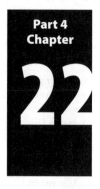

Symptom management and supportive care of older adults

22 Optimizing functional status in older adults with cancer

Gijsberta van Londen and Stephanie Studenski

A. Overview

Optimizing functional status should be a treatment goal during all phases of care of the older person with cancer. Functional status reflects the overall capacity of the individual to perform routine activities such as dressing or shopping. While function is important on its own, since it affects quality of life, it plays other useful roles in cancer care: (1) initial functional status is a powerful predictor of treatment tolerance and survival in general, (2) loss of function suggests a change in disease activity of the cancer or a comorbid condition and is an important indicator of the adverse effects of treatment, and (3) reduced functional status precipitates the need for help, whether by informal family caregivers or paid assistants.[1-3] Some forms of cancer in older persons, such as prostate cancer or some hematological malignancies, have become chronic conditions to be managed over years or decades, so the goals of cancer treatment have evolved from cure to chronic disease management. In the context of living with a chronic disease, the effects of treatment on function rather than on survival could be considered the most important outcome of care. The goal of this chapter is to provide a perspective on how knowledge about function can direct care planning at every phase of cancer care and to review the evidence about the effectiveness of potential interventions to promote function.

B. Rationale for care directed at functional status in older cancer patients

B.1. Linking disease and disability: Implications for cancer care

Functional status is the ability to perform daily activities important for independence. Elements of function include (1) basic or personal care such as eating, bathing, and dressing; (2) instrumental or household management, including shopping, meal preparation, financial management, and medication management; and (3) advanced activities such as travel, volunteering, or work. Knowledge about function plays a critical role in health care because it provides a way to link a medical perspective about disease to a patient management perspective about the consequences of illness. Models of disablement (Figure 22.1, far left column) posit that pathophysiological disease processes cause damage to organ systems (called *impairments*), which in turn produce symptoms and losses of abilities at the level of the organism (called *disability*), which can finally affect life roles (called *handicap*). In older persons with cancer, the disease that causes disability might be *the cancer itself* (e.g., lung cancer in second column, Figure 22.1) or an *adverse side effect of treatment* (e.g., taxane-induced peripheral neuropathy in the third column of Figure 22.1) and is often compounded by *chronic disease burden* in late life (far right column of Figure 22.1). Whatever the underlying disease process, the clinical manifestations are the organ system impairments (second row in Figure 22.1), which may be detected by physical examination, laboratory testing, imaging, or other modalities. These organ system impairments present as *symptoms* such as dyspnea, numbness, or fatigue. Such symptoms can be traced back up the chain of causation, using selected components of the diagnostic armamentarium, to the organ systems involved. The symptoms can also be traced downward toward the consequences for *function and disability* (third row in Figure 22.1) and handicap (fourth row in Figure 22.1). Thus the health care provider directs care using traditional medical skills integrated with the ability to link disease to function. A symptom or new physical finding can be traced back to its possible causes and forward to its impact on function. The provider uses this knowledge to assess disease severity and change over time, adverse effects, and comorbid status and plans medical and restorative services to prevent, treat, or adapt to the functional

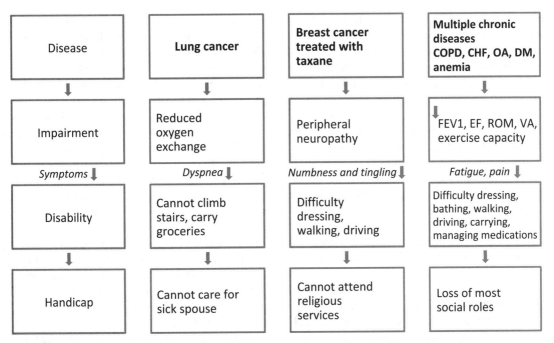

Figure 22.1 Linking disease to function. COPD = chronic obstructive lung disease; CHF = congestive heart failure; OA = osteoarthritis; DM = diabetes mellitus; FEV1 = forced expiratory volume in 1 second; EF = ejection fraction; ROM = range of motion; VA = visual acuity.

consequences of disease. This approach can be used at every phase of cancer care, from diagnosis to active cancer treatment to posttreatment recovery and long-term survivorship to terminal care.

B.2. Measuring function

Function can be assessed at widely varying levels of detail, from a global estimate based on indicators like the Karnofsky scale[4,5] or Eastern Cooperative Oncology Group (ECOG) status[6] to general health scales like the Short Form-36 (SF-36)[7] or cancer-specific scales like the Functional Assessment of Cancer Therapy FACT scales[8] to a full comprehensive geriatric assessment that assesses various physical, cognitive, emotional, social, and economic capacities as well as comorbid illnesses.[1-3] The level of detail should match the needs of the patient and the goals of care. It is possible that level of detail could change across the course of cancer care and be more comprehensive at initial assessment and perhaps immediately following intensive cancer interventions but more brief at other times. Please see Chapter 1 for additional details regarding geriatric assessment.

B.3. Prevalence of functional impairment in older cancer patients

The median age at cancer diagnosis for all sites is 67 years,[9] and about 60 percent of new can-

cer diagnoses are made in adults aged 65 years or older.[10] It is difficult to accurately estimate the extent of disability among older cancer patients for several reasons related to sampling, measurement, and timing of data collection. First, the data obviously depend on who, among the true population of older adults with cancer, are included in the sample to be studied. Since clinical trials notoriously select younger and healthier subjects for study,[11] the older cancer patient in a clinical trial is very likely to have better function than the overall population of older adults with cancer. Even referral to academic centers for cancer care (and inclusion in observational studies) is likely influenced by the health and function of the older adult. Second, the data available will depend on what data were collected. There may be global estimates of ECOG or Karnofsky status but much less known about activities of daily living, mobility, or cognitive status. Third, estimates will depend on the timing of data collection, whether prior, during, or after treatment. Changes over time during cancer treatment can be due to the cancer itself, treatment side effects, or exacerbation of comorbid conditions. In addition, participation in data collection over time is affected by changes in health and function. Participants whose health and function have worsened or who have died are no longer available to provide data about functional status. For all these reasons, longitudinal studies of functional status in the older cancer patient tend to start with better function than would be expected in the true population, tend to be global estimates of overall functional status, and tend to underestimate the onset or progression of disability since the sickest persons have withdrawn from study. For example, Given and colleagues followed SF-36 physical function in an observational study across diagnosis and treatment in older adults with several types of cancer.[12] They found that older cancer patients had better function than national norms at entry and that scores dropped across treatment cycles. In a cross-sectional study of metastatic breast cancer, in patients who had a mean age less than 60 years, the prevalence of functional impairment was 92 percent.[13] Among a cohort of prostate cancer patients aged 70 and older who were on long-term androgen deprivation therapy, about half had problems with physical function.[14] In a study of older women with cervical cancer who were entering a clinical trial, FACT scales indicated that function remained stable over time and pain decreased.[15] However, almost half of the participants dropped out over the course of the study, and the dropouts were developing worsening function prior to leaving the study. A summary of functional status among multiple studies that employed comprehensive geriatric assessment found that up to half of older cancer patients had limitations in instrumental activities of daily living.[16]

The older cancer survivor may be more medically and functionally stable compared to patients assessed during treatment and therefore somewhat more amenable to detailed studies of function. There have been several efforts to estimate disability in this population. Sixty percent of the current 10 million cancer survivors are aged 65 years or older.[17] The prevalence of functional impairment in cancer survivors is still difficult to estimate because functional problems in cancer survivors are diverse and multifactorial.[18] Survivors themselves are diverse; some patients have been cured or have an extended disease-free interval, some suffer from treatment-induced side effects, and some cannot be cured but are successfully controlled with chronic multidisciplinary interventions that may have adverse effects on function. In addition, coexisting unrelated conditions affect functional status as well. Nevertheless, functional impairment is common after cancer; in one study, up to 70 percent of cancer survivors aged 65 years and older at diagnosis were found to have at least one functional limitation.[17] In another study of women cancer survivors, about half had at least one functional limitation and, in analyses adjusted for age, health, and comorbid conditions, such limitations were more likely in survivors of hematopoietic, kidney, and lung cancer.[19] Since individuals who had cancer early in life are now surviving to old age, the issue of long-term disability after childhood cancer has become an important part of the knowledge base in cancer and aging survivorship. Childhood cancer survivors have physical performance limitations that may increase as they age. Performance deficits are more likely after a bone or brain tumor, Hodgkin's disease, radiation therapy, or a combination of alkylating agents and anthracyclines.[20]

B.4. Functional assessment across the phases of cancer care

Functional assessment serves different purposes across the phases of cancer care (Table 22.1).[18,21,22]

Prior to initiation of therapy

Knowledge about functional performance provides prognostic insight into the cancer patient's

Table 22.1 Functional assessment and treatment goals across the phases of care of the older cancer patient.

Care phase	Goals
Diagnosis	Assess causes of functional limitations, correct underlying problems as possible, predict treatment tolerance, tailor treatment plan
Active treatment	Assess consequences of treatment on function, adapt treatment, implement ancillary treatments to maximize function and treatment tolerance
Long-term survivorship	Assess long-term consequences of treatment, accelerate recovery of function, adapt to long-term disability
Palliative end-of-life care	Maximize function as tolerated, help caregivers

organ system impairment, potential to tolerate cancer therapy, and survival, allowing individualized treatment planning.[16,23,24] Baseline physical function in patients aged 65 years and over contributed significantly to level of physical function posttreatment.[25] Functional assessment is more related to physiological than biological age, guiding decision making about treatment tolerance and/or the need for chemotherapy dose adjustment.[26,27] Other clinical problems can be defined and stabilized so that cancer therapy is best tolerated and function is maximized during treatment.[28–30]

During cancer treatment

Tracking function across active treatments such as radiation or systemic chemo- or hormonal therapy can potentially increase treatment tolerance and minimize or shorten disability by proactively preventing side effects, attenuating already developed side effects, and providing adaptive mechanisms to cope with disability.[24,28,31] For example, monitoring function can help detect the consequences of muscle and strength loss because of long-term hormonal deprivation therapy.[32] It is possible that treatment decisions, especially for more chronic forms of cancer, could be made in part based on the consequences of various treatment strategies for function during treatment.

Survivorship

Functional status after the completion of active treatment can inform plans for rehabilitation and adaptation to any long-term disability.[33] Monitoring functional recovery after treatment could provide evidence to inform future patients about what to expect in terms of patterns of duration and extent of disability after various forms of treatment.

Palliative care

Even among cancer patients who are not likely to receive curative treatment and who are expected to die of their disease, functional assessment can guide palliative care for symptom control, plans for sites and types of personal care, caregiver training, and need for assistive equipment.

C. Interventions to promote function in the older cancer patient

Virtually all interventions targeted at the older cancer patient have implications for function as well as survival. For example, cancer chemother-

apy can be guided not only by the goal of cancer cure and survival but also, especially for potentially curable or chronic forms of cancer, by function during and after treatment. Similarly, there are long-term adverse functional consequences of chronic interventions such as hormone ablation[14] that might be anticipated and minimized with preventive medical interventions such as anabolic agents. The interventions examined in this chapter focus on strategies that are supplemental to the medical management of the cancer patient.

C.1. Comprehensive geriatric assessment

Comprehensive geriatric assessment (CGA) entails a thorough assessment of physical, cognitive, emotional, social, and economic function and a search for comorbid conditions and geriatric syndromes. Assessment is followed by a plan to implement corrective actions to improve function or reduce risk of future complications. CGA has high potential to serve as a function-promoting intervention in older cancer patients. A recent review of CGA in older cancer patients suggests that multiple problems that would otherwise be missed are detected and that several factors, especially capacity to perform instrumental activities and the presence of depression, are important prognostic indicators.[16] Some observational studies suggested that CGA might help predict adverse effects of treatment. The review emphasized that the effort of CGA should be targeted at high-risk elders based on the use of screening instruments to detect the older adult in need of full evaluation. Though CGA has been used to identify predictors, only a few trials of CGA have been performed to determine its effects on outcomes such as function. In a study of nurse-managed home care among older patients with cancer discharged from the hospital after surgery, survival was better for late-stage patients who received the intervention compared to those who did not, but effects on function are not reported.[34] In a substudy of CGA that targeted participants with cancer, the use of inpatient CGA resulted in better functional status at 6 months but no differences in survival.[35] A key issue in studies of CGA is whether the assessment is combined with control over delivery of recommended care.[36] Similarly, in cancer CGA, it will be important for trials of CGA to include the ability to implement the treatment recommendations. In addition, studies of CGA should include function at multiple time points as important outcomes.

Table 22.2 Select randomized controlled trials of exercise in cancer.

Trial reference	Type and number of cancer patients	Timing of exercise	Type of exercise	Main effects on function
Segal, 2009[43]	121 men, mean age 66 years, with prostate cancer with or without androgen deprivation	During radiation therapy	24-week supervised resistance or aerobic	Both prevented decline in fitness, improved perceived function, and reduced fatigue
Courneya, 2007[44,45]	242 women, mean age 49 years, with breast cancer	During chemotherapy	Supervised resistance or aerobic for the duration of chemotherapy	Reduced loss of fitness in aerobic group, better strength in resistance group, no differences in perceived fatigue or general health
Segal, 2003[42]	155 men, mean age 68 years, with prostate cancer	After starting androgen deprivation therapy	12-week supervised resistance training	Better self-reported function, increased strength
Courneya, 2003[82]	Postmenopausal women, mean age 59 years, with or without hormone therapy	After active therapy	Supervised aerobic	Fitness and perceived function were better with exercise
May, 2009[83]	147 cancer survivors, mean age 49 years	At least 3 months after active therapy	Home-based unsupervised aerobic plus strength with or without cognitive behavioral telephone support	Both arms had significant and sustained gains in self-reported functioning
Morey, 2009[41]	641 overweight long-term cancer survivors, mean age 73 years	At least 5 years since diagnosis with no evidence of disease	Telephone and printed material support for a self-managed diet and exercise program vs. wait list control	Less functional decline over 1 year

C.2. Exercise

Exercise has potential to promote improved function in older cancer patients. The evidence is difficult to interpret because studies do not systematically present data separately for older adults because the timing of exercise in relation to cancer treatment varies and because the type, intensity, duration, and degree of supervision of exercise differs among studies. Several recent reviews have summarized the evidence but often do not assess effects separately for older adults, report on different types of cancer, or distinguish the phase of treatment.[37–40] Studies of exercise with nonexercising controls are at risk to overestimate self-reported benefits because participants cannot be blinded and expectation bias influences perceived benefit. Nevertheless, in general, the studies suggest that exercise has benefits to strength, fitness, and self-perceived quality of life. Some studies report improved physical function. The following paragraphs will summarize evidence from select recent large, randomized clinical trials, first for interventions during cancer treatment and then for studies in cancer survivors. See Table 22.2 for details of the studies.

Studies during cancer treatment are challenging to implement, but several large trials have been completed. Randomized trials in men with prostate cancer[41–43] and women with breast cancer[44,45] suggest that both resistance and aerobic exercise are feasible during active treatment, even with chemotherapy. Compared to nonexercising controls, exercisers had better strength and endurance and reported better general functioning using FACT scales. Most of the exercise effects were prevention of decline among fairly high functioning adults.

Table 22.3 The roles of rehabilitation professionals in the care of older cancer patients.

Profession	Area of expertise	Sample services for older cancer patients
Physiatrist	Physical medicine	Evaluate impairments and prescribe an overall rehabilitation program, perform injections or other physical modalities, prescribe medications
Physical therapist	Mobility, therapeutic exercise, adaptive equipment	Assess and treat impairments, adapt therapeutic exercise to the individual, provide assistive devices for mobility, recommend splints or other supports
Occupational therapist	Self and household care adaptation, hand function	Provide energy-conserving strategies for personal and household management, adapt dressing, meal preparation, recommend and implement programs for hand and arm dysfunction
Speech therapist	Language, swallowing	Assess and treat swallowing disorders arising from radiation, chemotherapy, or local cancer
Nutritionist	Diet, food, and eating adaptations	Recommend dietary modifications for anorexia or dysphagia
Low-vision specialist	Strategies and equipment for blind or decreased vision	Adapt home for low vision, teach strategies for mobility and care with vision loss
Recreational therapist	Adapt personally meaningful activities	Develop adaptations for interests such as games, crafts, gardening
Rehabilitation nurse	Coordinate overall daily program and promote independence in self-care	Integrate therapeutic environment for self-care, recreation, family caregivers
Psychologist	Assess and treat cognition, mood, and other mental health issues	Evaluate cognition and mood, provide cognitive exercise, counseling
Social worker	Identify community resources, help caregiver planning	Discuss and implement home care plans with patient and family

Studies of cancer survivors similarly demonstrate expected benefits of exercise, with effects largely indicating prevention of decline. These trials are evolving toward self-regulated rather than supervised exercise.[41,46] A recent large multicenter study focused exclusively on older adult cancer survivors using a widely generalizable strategy of exercise and diet support using telephone counseling and printed materials.[41] This study demonstrated reduced decline in SF-36 physical function scores over 1 year.

Physical activity and exercise can play a helpful role during the phase of palliative cancer care as well. Though there are no reported clinical trials, there have been pilot studies of physical activity promotion during palliative care.[47] In general, these studies are small and preliminary but suggest that physical activity in multiple forms is feasible during this phase of cancer and has benefits in terms of physical function, quality of life, and fatigue.

C.3. Rehabilitation

Rehabilitation services encompass a wide range of therapeutic activities that can be helpful to the older cancer patient. Professionals with expertise in rehabilitation include physiatrists, physical therapists, occupational therapists, speech and language therapists, nutritionists, low-vision specialists, psychologists, recreation therapists, and rehabilitation nurses and social workers (Table 22.3). Each has a unique area of knowledge that can be used to promote function in older adults with cancer. For example, therapeutic exercise as a component of rehabilitation differs from the generic exercise described earlier. As opposed to the general strengthening and conditioning achieved with generic types of exercise, rehabilitative exercise tends to be more specifically prescribed, adapted, and delivered based on organ system impairments in the neurological, musculoskeletal, and cardiopulmonary systems. Exercises may be adapted to the special needs of the individual with paralysis, pain, or sensory disorders. Exercises may have specific purposes beyond fitness, such as decreasing spasticity, preventing contracture or increasing coordination. In addition to therapeutic exercise, physical and occupational therapists can develop programs to help older cancer patients adapt to impairments such as neuropathy, pulmonary insufficiency, or pathological bone fractures. Adaptations might include strategies for dressing, managing stairways, or preparing meals. Sometimes these adaptations include use of assistive devices for mobility or self-care. Speech therapists often lead programs to address swallowing problems during or after cancer treatment and are especially important in head and neck cancer. Low-vision specialists can help older adults develop strategies to maintain independent mobility, personal and household management, using techniques such as adapted lenses, environmental scanning, large print, and visual contrast. Nutritionists can evaluate and recommend dietary adaptations for anorexia or difficulty swallowing or for enteral feeding. Psychologists in rehabilitation can address issues related to cognition, mood, and anxiety. Recreation therapists can help adapt personally meaningful activities. For example, the older adult who has enjoyed gardening or sewing but who now has neuropathy or weight-bearing pain may be able to continue his or her preferred activity if the person uses adapted strategies or special equipment. Rehabilitation social workers can help identify community resources and assist caregivers in planning for needs in the home setting. Rehabilitation nurses can lead and integrate therapeutic environments to promote independence throughout the day and to advise caregivers on ways to assist the person with disability. Individual rehabilitation professional services can be provided in any setting or can be integrated into a therapeutic program, especially through inpatient programs. Traditional rehabilitation would be provided after completing a course of cancer treatments, but individual services might be appropriate at any time point from initial diagnosis through active treatment to recovery and long-term survival or palliative care at the end of life.

The evidence base is thin for the effect of rehabilitation services in cancer in general.[48] There are no publications that are specific to the older cancer patient. A survey of cancer patients who had received integrated hospital-based rehabilitation after cancer reported that patients found the services to be a helpful part of recovery.[49] They appreciated the coordinated services and found their interactions with other patients who were experiencing similar challenges to be helpful. A 6-week inpatient program for cancer patients that included individual exercise, sports, psychological education, and cancer information found improvements in endurance, strength, and health-related quality

of life.[50] The same research group carried out a 15-week controlled trial of their program and found gains in perceived quality of life to be greater with the integrated program compared to a less coordinated program.[33] Psychosocial support was found to be important to cancer patients after discharge from the hospital; patients reported needs for continuous support and information about rehabilitation, social support, advice about managing interactions with family and friends, counseling about fear of relapse, and family support.[51] An outpatient pulmonary rehabilitation program improved functional status and exercise tolerance in cancer patients with dyspnea and fatigue.[52] Rehabilitation can be provided in the palliative care setting to attempt to reduce the impact of increasing disability because of advanced, incurable cancer and its multitude of treatments.[56]

C.4. Pain management

Pain is ubiquitous in the older cancer patient. Independent of the status of the cancer, half of patients with cancer experience pain, and the rate increases to 74 percent in the terminal stage.[57] Pain has obvious effects on functioning as well as sleep, nutrition, and decreased socialization,[57] all of which can be magnified because of the presence of other age-related medical and psychosocial problems.[58] Pain control can improve function, but some forms of treatment such as opioid analgesics also have the potential for excess sedation, which can reduce function.[59,60] It is therefore important to have a comprehensive pain management plan throughout the cancer care continuum. This management plan should prioritize pain control while allowing the best possible function. Some individuals may choose to tolerate some pain to reduce treatment side effects and maximize function. A basic guideline is to use the World Health Organization ladder for pain management, which begins with nonopioid analgesics and progresses to weak opioids and eventually to strong opioids in conjunction with adjuvant analgesics and/or invasive analgesic procedures.[57,61,62]

C.5. Nutritional interventions

Patients with cancer have an increased risk of malnutrition and weight loss. Malnutrition occurs in up to 85 percent of patients with certain kinds of cancer such as pancreatic cancer. Malnutrition is often multifactorial, with contributions from interactions of the host and tumor. Factors include energy consumption from fast-growing tumors, secretion of catabolic cytokines by the host as a response to the tumor, and insufficient caloric intake because of anorexia or nausea and vomiting.[63–66] The most extreme form of malnutrition is cachexia, in which a patient experiences wasting of body tissues and develops immune, physical, and cognitive dysfunction.[67–69,71] Prevention and reversal of malnutrition is crucial to promote function and survival.[72] The large variety of causal factors requires an individual and often multimodal approach to nutritional support.[73] If the weight loss and malnutrition are suspected to be largely related to host-tumor interaction, anticancer therapy might be helpful but is limited because individuals with malnutrition respond less well to chemotherapy and may experience a higher complication rate.[67,74] Oral supplementation is the most natural, physiological, noninvasive method to increase intake of calories and essential nutrients. Appetite stimulants such as progestational agents, glucocorticoids, cannabinoids, cyproheptadine, olanzapine, and mirtazapine might be helpful as well.[75] If oral supplementation and appetite stimulants are unsuccessful or constrained by other factors, temporary enteral or even parenteral feeding may be appropriate. Some nutritional interventions have been shown to have beneficial effects on clinical outcomes and survival.[73] Evidence is lacking on functional outcomes or results specific to the older patient with cancer.

C.6. Psychological interventions

Fatigue, depression, and cognitive impairment can occur in anyone with cancer, but the underlying pathophysiology is poorly understood. A conceptual model has been proposed in which cytokines play a central causative role.[76] It is important to further unravel these relationships and identify potential methods of intervention because psychological impairment in cancer patients leads to worse outcomes than expected based on tumor characteristics.[77–79] In addition to standard interventions such as supportive counseling or the use of antidepressants, there is recent interest in cognitive rehabilitation for perceived cognitive effects of cancer and cancer treatment. Initial clinical trials of cognitive interventions have had disappointing results on objective tests of cognitive function.[80,81] These studies have not been targeted at the older cancer patient.

D. Priorities for future research

To develop a full armamentarium of interventions to promote function in the older patient with cancer, function must be measured as an outcome across all phases of cancer care to be able to determine contributors to loss of function and formally design individualized single and combined interventions in varying kinds of older adults with varying kinds of cancer. Function should become a high-priority outcome in all cancer studies, including clinical trials for pharmacological agents as well as more traditional rehabilitation interventions. Whether based on self-report of function, physical performance measures, or professional assessment, it would be helpful to know how function is affected at every time point from diagnosis through treatment, recovery, long-term survivorship, or the dying process. Novel forms of functional assessment that are well tolerated and easy to obtain are needed and might include activity monitors, reports of restricted activity or bed days, or wearable technology. Research could be done to better refine and operationalize the clinical assessment process that leads from symptoms and disabilities back through impairments and diseases. Such an evidence-based assessment process would allow more health professionals to be able to systematically link disease to function. Interventions such as CGA should be refined and modifications applied beyond the initiation of therapy through the phases of active treatment, recovery, and palliative care. Individual and combined interventions might be developed and tailored to the needs of specific classes of older adults. While there is great need to prevent functional decline in high-functioning older adults with cancer, there is also a great need to develop function-sparing interventions for vulnerable older adults with existing disabilities. Given the increasing chronicity or curability of many forms of cancer, it is more and more likely that an older adult will live with cancer rather than die from it. It is imperative that the care we offer the older patient surviving from or living with cancer be based on an informed treatment plan that optimizes both control of the cancer and independent function.

References

1. Balducci L, Beghe C. The application of the principles of geriatrics to the management of the older person with cancer. *Crit Rev Oncol Hematol.* 2000;35(3):147–154.

2. Hurria A. Incorporation of geriatric principles in oncology clinical trials. *J Clin Oncol.* 2007;25(34):5350–5351.

3. Schubert CC, Gross C, Hurria A. Functional assessment of the older patient with cancer. *Oncology.* 2008;22(8):916–922; discussion 925, 928.

4. Karnofsky D, Burchenal JH. *Evaluation of Chemotherapeutic Agents.* New York: Columbia University Press; 1949.

5. Mor V, Laliberte L, Morris JN, et al. The Karnofsky Performance Status Scale: an examination of its reliability and validity in a research setting. *Cancer.* 1984;53(9):2002–2007.

6. Oken MM, Creech RH, Tormey DC, et al. Toxicity and response criteria of the Eastern Cooperative Oncology Group. *Am J Clin Oncol.* 1982;5(6):649–655.

7. Hays RD, Sherbourne CD, Mazel RM. The RAND 36-item health survey 1.0. *Health Econ.* 1993;2(3):217–227.

8. Overcash J, Extermann M, Parr J, et al. Validity and reliability of the FACT-G scale for use in the older person with cancer. *Am J Clin Oncol.* 2001;24(6):591–596.

9. Jemal A, Center MM, Ward E, et al. Cancer occurrence. *Methods Mol Biol.* 2009;471:3–29.

10. Yancik R, Ries LA. Cancer in older persons: an international issue in an aging world. *Semin Oncol.* 2004;31(2):128–136.

11. Hurria A. Clinical trials in older adults with cancer: past and future. *Oncology.* 2007;21(3):351–358; discussion 363–364, 367.

12. Given B, Given C, Azzouz F, et al. Physical functioning of elderly cancer patients prior to diagnosis and following initial treatment. *Nurs Res.* 2001;50(4):222–232.

13. Cheville AL, Troxel AB, Basford JR, et al. Prevalence and treatment patterns of physical impairments in patients with metastatic breast cancer. *J Clin Oncol.* 2008;26(16):2621–2629.

14. Bylow K, Dale W, Mustian K, et al. Falls and physical performance deficits in older patients with prostate cancer undergoing androgen deprivation therapy. *Urology.* 2008;72(2):422–427.

15. McQuellon RP, Thaler HT, Cella D, et al. Quality of life (QOL) outcomes from a randomized trial of cisplatin versus cisplatin plus paclitaxel in advanced cervical cancer: a Gynecologic Oncology Group study. *Gynecol Oncol.* 2006;101(2):296–304.

16. Extermann M, Hurria A. Comprehensive geriatric assessment for older patients with cancer. *J Clin Oncol.* 2007;25(14):1824–1831.

17. Hewitt M, Rowland JH, Yancik R. Cancer survivors in the United States: age, health, and disability. *J Gerontol.* 2003;58(1):M82–M91.

18. Vikas Malhotra MCP. Functional problems in the patient with cancer. In: Rose BD, ed. UpToDate. Wellesley UpToDate, MA, 2008.

19. Sweeney C, Schmitz KH, Lazovich D, et al. Functional limitations in elderly female cancer survivors. *J Natl Cancer Inst.* 2006;98(8):521–529.

20. Ness KK, Hudson MM, Ginsberg JP, et al. Physical performance limitations in the Childhood Cancer Survivor Study cohort. *J Clin Oncol.* 2009;27(14):2382–2389.

21. Hurria A, Lichtman SM, Gardes J, et al. Identifying vulnerable older adults with cancer: integrating geriatric assessment into oncology practice. *J Am Geriatr Soc.* 2007;55(10):1604–1608.

22. Gosney MA. Clinical assessment of elderly people with cancer. *Lancet Oncol.* 2005;6(10):790–797.

23. Rodin MB, Mohile SG. A practical approach to geriatric assessment in oncology. *J Clin Oncol.* 2007;25(14):1936–1944.

24. Wildiers H. Mastering chemotherapy dose reduction in elderly cancer patients. *Eur J Cancer.* 2007;43(15):2235–2241.

25. Kurtz ME, Kurtz JC, Stommel M, et al. Loss of physical functioning among geriatric cancer patients: relationships to cancer site, treatment, comorbidity and age. *Eur J Cancer.* 1997;33(14):2352–2358.

26. Wedding U, Kodding D, Pientka L, et al. Physicians' judgement and comprehensive geriatric assessment (CGA) select different patients as fit for chemotherapy. *Crit Rev Oncol Hematol.* 2007;64(1):1–9.

27. Balducci L. Aging, frailty, and chemotherapy. *Cancer Control.* 2007;14(1):7–12.

28. Extermann M, Meyer J, McGinnis M, et al. A comprehensive geriatric intervention detects multiple problems in older breast cancer patients. *Crit Rev Oncol Hematol.* 2004;49(1):69–75.

29. Repetto L, Fratino L, Audisio RA. Comprehensive geriatric assessment adds information to Eastern Cooperative Oncology Group performance status in elderly cancer patients: an Italian Group for Geriatric Oncology study. *J Clin Oncol.* 2002;20(2):494–502.

30. Balducci L, Extermann M. Management of cancer in the older person: a practical approach. *Oncologist.* 2000;5(3):224–237.

31. Chen H, Cantor A, Meyer J. Can older cancer patients tolerate chemotherapy? A prospective

pilot study. *Cancer*. 2003;97(4): 1107–1114.

32. Galvao DA, Taaffe DR, Spry N, et al. Exercise can prevent and even reverse adverse effects of androgen suppression treatment in men with prostate cancer. *Prostate Cancer Prostatic Dis*. 2007;10(4):340–346.

33. van Weert E, Hoekstra-Weebers J, Grol B, et al. A multidimensional cancer rehabilitation program for cancer survivors: effectiveness on health-related quality of life. *J Psychosom Res*. 2005;58(6):485–496.

34. McCorkle R, Strumpf NE, Nuamah IF, et al. A specialized home care intervention improves survival among older post-surgical cancer patients. *J Am Geriatr Soc*. 2000;48(12): 1707–1713.

35. Rao AV, Hsieh F, Feussner JR, et al. Geriatric evaluation and management units in the care of the frail elderly cancer patient. *J Gerontol*. 2005;60(6):798–803.

36. Jahnigen DW, Applegate WB, Cohen HJ, et al. Working group recommendations: research on content and efficacy of geriatric evaluation and management interventions. *J Am Geriatr Soc*. 1991;39(9 Pt 2):42S–44S.

37. Cheema B, Gaul CA, Lane K, et al. Progressive resistance training in breast cancer: a systematic review of clinical trials. *Breast Cancer Res Treat*. 2008;109(1):9–26.

38. Liu RD, Chinapaw MJ, Huijgens PC, et al. Physical exercise interventions in haematological cancer patients, feasible to conduct but effectiveness to be established: a systematic literature review. *Cancer Treat Rev*. 2009;35(2):185–192.

39. Schmitz KH, Holtzman J, Courneya KS, et al. Controlled physical activity trials in cancer survivors: a systematic review and meta-analysis. *Cancer Epidemiol Biomarkers Prev*. 2005;14(7):1588–1595.

40. McNeely ML, Campbell KL, Rowe BH, et al. Effects of exercise on breast cancer patients and survivors: a systematic review and meta-analysis. *Can Med Assoc J*. 2006;175(1):34–41.

41. Morey MC, Snyder DC, Sloane R, et al. Effects of home-based diet and exercise on functional outcomes among older, overweight long-term cancer survivors: RENEW: a randomized controlled trial. *J Am Med Assoc*. 2009;301(18):1883–1891.

42. Segal RJ, Reid RD, Courneya KS, et al. Resistance exercise in men receiving androgen deprivation therapy for prostate cancer. *J Clin Oncol*. 2003;21(9):1653–1659.

43. Segal RJ, Reid RD, Courneya KS, et al. Randomized controlled trial of resistance or aerobic exercise in men receiving radiation therapy for prostate cancer. *J Clin Oncol*. 2009;27(3):344–351.

44. Courneya KS, Segal RJ, Mackey JR, et al. Effects of aerobic and resistance exercise in breast cancer patients receiving adjuvant chemotherapy: a multicenter randomized controlled trial. *J Clin Oncol*. 2007;25(28): 4396–4404.

45. Courneya KS, Segal RJ, Gelmon K, et al. Six-month follow-up of patient-rated outcomes in a randomized controlled trial of exercise training during breast cancer chemotherapy. *Cancer Epidemiol Biomarkers Prev*. 2007;16(12): 2572–2578.

46. May AM, Duivenvoorden HJ, Korstjens I, et al. The effect of group cohesion on rehabilitation outcome in cancer survivors. *Psychooncology*. 2008;17(9):917–925.

47. Lowe SS, Watanabe SM, Courneya KS. Physical activity as a supportive care intervention in palliative cancer patients: a systematic review. *J Support Oncol*. 2009;7(1):27–34.

48. Vargo MM. The oncology-rehabilitation interface: better systems needed. *J Clin Oncol*. 2008;26(16):2610–2611.

49. Korstjens I, Mesters I, Gijsen B, et al. Cancer patients' view on rehabilitation and quality of life: a programme audit. *Eur J Cancer Care (Engl)*. 2008;17(3):290–297.

50. van Weert E, Hoekstra-Weebers JE, Grol BM, et al. Physical functioning and quality of life after cancer rehabilitation. *Int J Rehabil Res*. 2004;27(1):27–35.

51. Mikkelsen TH, Sondergaard J, Jensen AB, et al. Cancer rehabilitation: psychosocial rehabilitation needs after discharge from hospital? *Scand J Prim Health Care*. 2008;26(4):216–221.

52. Morris GS, Gallagher GH, Baxter MF, et al. Pulmonary rehabilitation improves functional status in oncology patients. *Arch Phys Med Rehabil*. 2009;90(5):837–841.

53. Courneya KS, Vallance JKH, McNeely ML, et al. Exercise issues in older cancer survivors. *Crit Rev Oncol Hematol*. 2004;51(3):249–261.

54. Rao AV, Demark-Wahnfried W. The older cancer survivor. *Crit Rev Oncol Hematol*. 2006;60(2):131–143.

55. Ayanian JZ, Jacobsen PB. Enhancing research on cancer survivors. *J Clin Oncol*. 2006;24(32): 5149–5153.

56. Grunfeld E. Looking beyond survival: how are we looking at survivorship? *J Clin Oncol*. 2006; 24(32):5166–5169.

57. De Cicco M, Bortolussi R, Fantin D, et al. Supportive therapy of elderly cancer patients. *Crit Rev Oncol Hematol*. 2002;42(2):189–211.

58. Portenoy RK. Pain management in the older cancer patient. *Oncology*. 1992;6(2 suppl):86–98.

59. Delgado-Guay MO, Bruera E. Management of pain in the older person with cancer. *Oncology*. 2008;22(1):56–61.

60. Delgado-Guay MO, Bruera E. Management of pain in the older person with cancer. Part 2: treatment options. *Oncology*. 2008;22(2):148–152; discussion 152, 155, 160 passim.

61. Christo PJ, Mazloomdoost D. Interventional pain treatments for cancer pain. *Ann N Y Acad Sci*. 2008;1138:299–328.

62. Christo PJ, Mazloomdoost D. Cancer pain and analgesia. *Ann N Y Acad Sci*. 2008;1138:278–298.

63. Maarten von M. Cancer-associated malnutrition: an introduction. *Eur J Oncol Nurs*. 2005;9:S35–S38.

64. Skipworth RJ, Fearon KC. The scientific rationale for optimizing nutritional support in cancer. *Eur J Gastroenterol Hepatol*. 2007;19(5):371–377.

65. Skipworth RJ, Stewart GD, Dejong CH, et al. Pathophysiology of cancer cachexia: much more than host-tumour interaction? *Clin Nutr*. 2007;26(6):667–676.

66. Argiles JM, Busquets S, Moore-Carrasco R, et al. Targets in clinical oncology: the metabolic environment of the patient. *Front Biosci*. 2007;12:3024–3051.

67. Argiles JM. Cancer-associated malnutrition. *Eur J Oncol Nurs*. 2005;9(suppl 2):39–S50.

68. Toles M, Demark-Wahnefried W. Nutrition and the cancer survivor: evidence to guide oncology nursing practice. *Semin Oncol Nurs*. 2008;24(3):171–179.

69. Irwin ML, Mayne ST. Impact of nutrition and exercise on cancer survival. *Cancer J*. 2008;14(6):435–441.

70. Demark-Wahnefried W, Clipp EC, Morey MC, et al. Physical function and associations with diet and exercise: results of a cross-sectional survey among elders with breast or prostate cancer. *Int J Behav Nutr Phys Act*. 2004;1(1):16.

71. Ottery FD. Supportive nutrition to prevent cachexia and improve quality of life. *Semin Oncol*. 1995;22(2 suppl 3):98–111.

72. Michelle D. Nutritional screening and assessment in cancer-associated malnutrition. *Eur J Oncol Nurs*. 2005;9:S64–S73.

73. van Bokhorst-de van Der Schueren MA. Nutritional support strategies for malnourished cancer patients. *Eur J Oncol Nurs*. 2005;9 (suppl):74–83.

74. Bosaeus I. Nutritional support in multimodal therapy for cancer cachexia. *Support Care Cancer*. 2008;16(5):447–451.

75. Mattox TW. Treatment of unintentional weight loss in patients with cancer. *Nutr Clin Pract*. 2005;20(4):400–410.

76. Seruga B, Zhang H, Bernstein LJ, et al. Cytokines and their relationship to the symptoms and outcome of cancer. *Nat Rev Cancer*. 2008;8(11):887–899.

77. Stommel M, Given BA, Given CW. Depression and functional status as predictors of death among cancer patients. *Cancer*. 2002;94(10):2719–2727.

78. Raji MA, Kuo YF, Freeman JL, et al. Effect of a dementia diagnosis on survival of older patients after a diagnosis of breast, colon, or prostate cancer: implications for cancer care. *Arch Intern Med*. 2008;168(18):2033–2040.

79. Kurtz ME, Kurtz JC, Stommel M, et al. The influence of symptoms, age, comorbidity and cancer site on physical functioning and mental health of geriatric women patients. *Women Health*. 1999;29(3):1–12.

80. Poppelreuter M, Weis J, Bartsch HH. Effects of specific neuropsychological training programs for breast cancer patients after adjuvant chemotherapy. *J Psychosoc Oncol*. 2009;27(2):274–296.

81. Poppelreuter M, Weis J, Mumm A, et al. Rehabilitation of therapy-related cognitive deficits in patients after hematopoietic stem cell transplantation. *Bone Marrow Transplant*. 2008;41(1):79–90.

82. Courneya KS, Mackey JR, Bell GJ, et al. Randomized controlled trial of exercise training in postmenopausal breast cancer survivors: cardiopulmonary and quality of life outcomes. *J Clin Oncol*. 2003;21(9):1660–1668.

83. May AM, Korstjens I, van Weert E, et al. Long-term effects on cancer survivors' quality of life of physical training versus physical training combined with cognitive-behavioral therapy: results from a randomized trial. *Support Care Cancer*. 2009;17(6):653–663.

The myeloid growth factors in older adults with cancer

Gary H. Lyman and Nicole M. Kuderer

A. Introduction

Myelosuppression represents the major dose-limiting toxicity of cancer chemotherapy regimens, particularly in older cancer patients. In addition, aging is associated with a progressive decline in the functional reserve of the bone marrow as well as other organ systems. Such age-related reductions of hematopoietic stem cells, including a progressive restriction in hematopoietic tissue, may result in an increased risk of death from infection, particularly among older patients under stress such as treatment with myelosuppressive chemotherapy. Neutropenic complications, most notably febrile neutropenia, are accompanied by considerable morbidity, mortality, and cost. The myeloid growth factors have been shown to significantly reduce the risk of neutropenic complications, including febrile neutropenia and its consequences. These agents have been integrated in modern oncology practice with recommendations based on clinical practice guidelines from several professional organizations. This chapter summarizes the rationale and potential value of these agents in the management of elderly patients receiving cancer chemotherapy.

B. Chemotherapy-induced neutropenic complications

B.1. Risk of neutropenic complications

Despite improved supportive care, including a broad array of active antibiotics, febrile neutropenia and its consequences continue to be associated with frequent and prolonged hospitalization, sometimes resulting in infection-related mortality.[1] The risk of hematologic toxicity associated with systemic chemotherapy is greatest during the initial cycles of treatment.[2-5] The likelihood that patients developing neutropenic complications will experience those events during the first treatment cycle ranges from 50 to 80 percent across cancer types (Figure 23.1). The real

or perceived risk of neutropenic complications also frequently results in subsequent reductions in chemotherapy dose intensity, potentially compromising survival in patients treated with curative intent.[6-10] Therefore the apparent decrease in febrile neutropenia risk beyond the initial cycle of chemotherapy appears to be largely the result of interventions to reduce the risk, including dose reductions or delays or secondary prophylaxis with myeloid growth factors.[2,11]

B.2. Age and the risk of neutropenic complications

The majority of malignancies occur in older patients who appear to derive similar benefit from systemic chemotherapy as younger cancer patients, provided comparable treatment is administered and similar doses are used.[12,13] However, increasing age is accompanied by a reduction in bone marrow reserves as well as an increase in the prevalence of comorbid medical conditions. Older individuals may also have a reduced ability to increase hematopoiesis in response to infection or cytotoxic chemotherapy due in part to a decrease in cytokine production. Increased circulating levels of proinflammatory cytokines may also limit hematopoietic progenitor response as well as interfere with hematopoietic growth factor precursors in older persons.[14] Nevertheless, evidence suggests that older cancer patients remain responsive to the hematopoietic growth factors.[15] Increasing age has been consistently identified as a predictor of neutropenic complications including febrile neutropenia, infection-related mortality, and subsequent dose reductions and delays. The impact of age or the comorbid conditions that often accompany aging on risk of neutropenic complications is perhaps most evident in the first cycle of chemotherapy, when most patients are receiving relative full treatment dose intensity. As shown in Figure 23.2, the risk of febrile neutropenia is greater in patients aged 65 years and older, with most

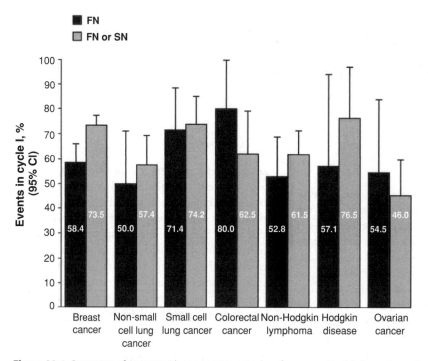

Figure 23.1 Proportion of patients with one or more episodes of severe and/or febrile neutropenia who experienced their initial event in cycle 1 by cancer type from a prospective population study of patients initiating chemotherapy at 117 U.S. oncology practices.[2] FN = febrile neutropenia; SN = severe neutropenia.

of the excess risk evident early in the course of treatment. Elderly patients with diffuse large-cell lymphoma receiving cyclophosphamide, doxorubicin, vincristine, and prednisone (CHOP) or CHOP-like chemotherapy experience nearly twice the risk of febrile neutropenia in the first cycle compared to younger patients.[3,4] The lower risk of neutropenic events in subsequent cycles appears to relate to reductions in chemotherapy dose intensity or the addition of secondary prophylaxis with a myeloid growth factor or occasionally the

use of prophylactic antibiotics. Though rarely employed in practice, continued administration of full-dose-intensity chemotherapy without growth factor support in the face of neutropenic events results in a persistent high risk of febrile neutropenia over subsequent cycles.

Increasing age is also associated with a decline in glomerular filtration rate, which may result in increased toxicity from renally excreted chemotherapeutic agents. Reduction in hepatic metabolism may exist in older patients along with

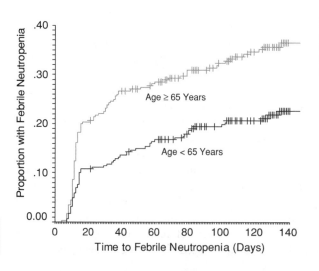

Figure 23.2 Kaplan-Meier plot of the cumulative risk of febrile neutropenia in 577 patients with aggressive non-Hodgkin's lymphoma receiving CHOP-like chemotherapy by age group. Tick marks indicate censored patients.[4]

reduced volume of distribution because of loss of body protein and low serum albumin and red cell mass resulting in higher serum levels of water-soluble drugs and greater toxicity.[16] While the risks of severe and febrile neutropenia, including infection-related mortality, appear to be greater in older cancer patients, the response to comparable modern cancer chemotherapy seems to be similar to that in younger patients.[17,18]

B.3. Risk of serious complications of febrile neutropenia

The consequence of severe and febrile neutropenia in older individuals may lead to early death or to serious illness associated with loss of functional independence. The risk of serious medical complications also appears to be greater among older cancer patients. In a study by the Multinational Association of Supportive Care in Cancer of over 1,100 patients diagnosed with febrile neutropenia from some 15 countries, 339 experienced serious medical complications, including death.[19] Patients over 60 years of age experienced a greater risk of adverse outcomes even after adjustment for severe burden of illness, complexity of infection, uncontrolled cancer, and neutrophil count on admission (odds ratio [OR] 4.36, $p < .004$). In another study of nearly 42,000 unselected hospitalized cancer patients with febrile neutropenia, those aged 65 years and older experienced a mortality rate

of 12.7 percent (95% confidence interval [CI] 12.1–13.3) compared to 8.2 percent (95% CI 7.9–8.5) among younger patients.[1] The excess mortality among elderly cancer patients hospitalized with febrile neutropenia remained significant after adjustment for major comorbidities and infection-related complications. In addition to the impact of reduced organ reserves and increased frailty associated with aging, the risk of mortality increases progressively with the numbers of major comorbidities (Figure 23.3).[1]

B.4. Reduced chemotherapy dose intensity

An additional and potentially serious consequence of severe or febrile neutropenia relates to the risk of chemotherapy dose reductions and treatment delays causing reduced delivered dose intensity, potentially compromising treatment effectiveness.[20] Nevertheless, modification of chemotherapy dose and schedule is a common strategy for reducing the anticipated toxicity of chemotherapy among older patients. In a population study of women receiving adjuvant breast cancer chemotherapy at some 1,200 U.S. oncology practices, overall, 53 percent received less than 85 percent of standard chemotherapy dose intensity compared to 67 percent among women aged 65 years and over ($p < .001$).[9] More recent follow-up of women with early-stage breast cancer from

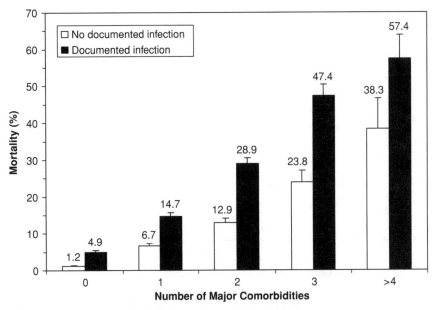

Figure 23.3 Impact of major comorbidities on mortality in 41,779 patients hospitalized at 115 academic health sciences centers over a 6-year period either with documented infection (solid bars) or without documented infection (open bars).[1]

the same practices along with results from a separate prospective cohort study confirm the persistent impact of older age on reductions in delivered chemotherapy dose intensity.[21,22] Likewise, in a retrospective study of patients with aggressive non-Hodgkin's lymphoma receiving CHOP or CHOP-like chemotherapy treated at 567 U.S. practices, 60 percent of patients over 60 years of age received less than 85 percent of standard dose intensity chemotherapy compared to 44 percent in those aged 60 years or younger.[10] Following adjustment for gender, stage, performance status, pretreatment blood counts, and myeloid growth factor use, older age remained a highly significant determinant of reduced relative dose intensity (OR 1.57, 95% CI 1.34–1.84, $p < .001$).

C. The myeloid growth factors

Recombinant human myeloid growth factors have been shown to reduce the incidence and severity of neutropenic complications across a range of malignancies and regimens, often facilitating the delivery of full chemotherapy dose intensity.[23–25] Multiple randomized controlled trials (RCTs) have confirmed the efficacy and safety of these agents in both adult and pediatric cancer patients receiving myelosuppressive chemotherapy.[26,27] In the systematic review of granulocyte colony-stimulating factor (G-CSF) by Kuderer and

colleagues, conducted in support of the American Society of Clinical Oncology (ASCO) White Blood Cell Growth Factor Guidelines, a significant reduction in risk of febrile neutropenia was observed across a broad range of baseline risk ranging from 17 percent to 80 percent in different study populations (Figure 23.4).[26] The long-acting myeloid growth factor pegfilgrastim appears to have several advantages related to patient convenience, improved compliance, and potentially greater potency.[26,28–30]

C.1. Myeloid growth factor use in older cancer patients

Although the sensitivity of myeloid progenitors to endogenous cytokines may be compromised in older individuals, responsiveness to exogenously administered recombinant myeloid growth factors appears well maintained. The effectiveness of G-CSF in older patients has been well established in a number of studies.[18,31–33] In the recent G-CSF meta-analysis, significant reductions in the risk of febrile neutropenia were found in studies that included all adult age groups (relative risk [RR] = 0.47; 95% CI 0.34–0.66, $p < .001$) as well as among the four RCTs in patients with non-Hodgkin's lymphoma restricted to elderly patients (RR 0.68, 95% CI 0.53–0.87, $p = .003$) (Figure 23.5).[26] These results were recently confirmed in an updated

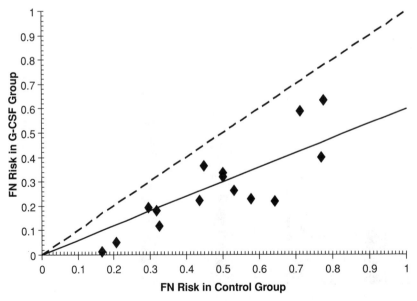

Figure 23.4 Scatter plot of the risk of febrile neutropenia in randomized controlled trials of cancer patients receiving chemotherapy with or without primary G-CSF prophylaxis comparing control patients (horizontal axis) and G-CSF patients (vertical axis). The dashed line represents equal risk in both study arms, whereas the solid line represents a weighted linear regression line through the observed data points (solid diamonds).[26] FN = febrile neutropenia; G-CSF = granulocyte colony-stimulating factor.

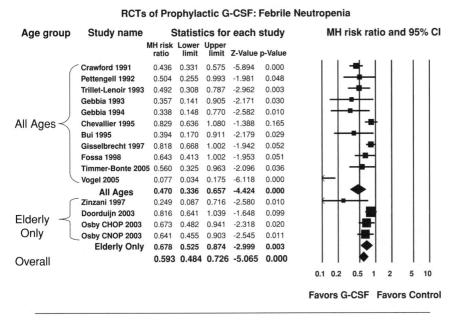

RCTs of Prophylactic G-CSF: Febrile Neutropenia

Age group	Study name	MH risk ratio	Lower limit	Upper limit	Z-Value	p-Value
	Crawford 1991	0.436	0.331	0.575	-5.894	0.000
	Pettengell 1992	0.504	0.255	0.993	-1.981	0.048
	Trillet-Lenoir 1993	0.492	0.308	0.787	-2.962	0.003
	Gebbia 1993	0.357	0.141	0.905	-2.171	0.030
	Gebbia 1994	0.338	0.148	0.770	-2.582	0.010
All Ages	Chevallier 1995	0.829	0.636	1.080	-1.388	0.165
	Bui 1995	0.394	0.170	0.911	-2.179	0.029
	Gisselbrecht 1997	0.818	0.668	1.002	-1.942	0.052
	Fossa 1998	0.643	0.413	1.002	-1.953	0.051
	Timmer-Bonte 2005	0.560	0.325	0.963	-2.096	0.036
	Vogel 2005	0.077	0.034	0.175	-6.118	0.000
	All Ages	**0.470**	**0.336**	**0.657**	**-4.424**	**0.000**
	Zinzani 1997	0.249	0.087	0.716	-2.580	0.010
Elderly	Doorduijn 2003	0.816	0.641	1.039	-1.648	0.099
Only	Osby CHOP 2003	0.673	0.482	0.941	-2.318	0.020
	Osby CNOP 2003	0.641	0.455	0.903	-2.545	0.011
	Elderly Only	**0.678**	**0.525**	**0.874**	**-2.999**	**0.003**
Overall		**0.593**	**0.484**	**0.726**	**-5.065**	**0.000**

Figure 23.5 Forest plot of the relative risk for febrile neutropenia in randomized controlled trials comparing adult patients receiving G-CSF versus no G-CSF patients grouped by age group eligibility criteria (all ages vs. elderly only). Relative risk estimates are shown as solid boxes with size inversely proportional to study variance, with 95% confidence limits on estimates.[26] RCT = randomized controlled trial; G-CSF = granulocyte colony-stimulating factor.

Cochrane systematic review of the CSFs in non-Hodgkin's lymphoma.[34] Absolute risk reductions for febrile neutropenia in the meta-analysis were 21.8 percent (95% CI 14.7–28.8, $p < .001$) in studies allowing all adult age groups and 13.7 percent (95% CI 7.9–19.4, $p < .001$) among studies of elderly patients. Although a significant reduction in all-cause early mortality was observed in patients receiving G-CSF support, this treatment effect reached statistical significance in studies allowing all age groups (RR 0.63; 95% CI 0.43–0.91) but did not among the three reporting lymphoma studies limited to elderly patients (RR 0.52, 95% CI 0.27–1.02). While no significant impact on overall survival was observed in the systematic review, a study from the Nordic Lymphoma Group in elderly patients receiving CHOP chemotherapy reported a significant increase in delivered relative dose intensity as well as overall survival in those randomized to receive prophylactic G-CSF with a median follow-up of approximately 5 years ($p = .045$).[32] This was not seen in the study by Doorduijn and colleagues utilizing a fixed G-CSF dose instead of weight-based dosing in elderly lymphoma patients.[31] No increase in the risk of second malignancies or long-term mortality has been seen in the RCTs, although most studies were not adequately powered to address these outcomes definitively.

In a recent study, 852 patients aged 65 years and older with solid tumors or non-Hodgkin's lymphoma were randomized to primary prophylaxis with pegfilgrastim or physician discretion after cycle 1 such as dose reductions, treatment delays, or the administration of secondary pegfilgrastim prophylaxis.[35] Patients randomized to receive primary prophylaxis experienced significantly fewer episodes of febrile neutropenia, hospitalization for febrile neutropenia, and dose reductions and delays (Figure 23.6).[35]

Despite these observations, only a minority of elderly cancer patients initiating systemic chemotherapy are offered myeloid growth factor support. Instead, reduced dose intensity is more commonly employed in older patients to reduce the risk of neutropenia.[9,10,21,22]

D. Clinical practice guidelines for the myeloid growth factors

D.1. Overview of clinical practice guidelines

Clinical practice guidelines have been developed by several professional organizations based on evidence from the RCTs and meta-analyses of RCTs that these agents reduce the incidence of febrile

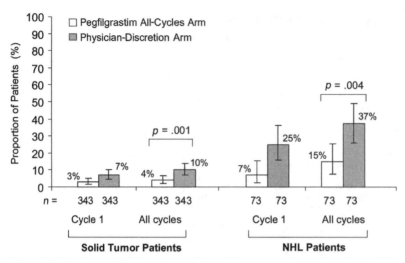

Figure 23.6 Incidence of febrile neutropenia in cycle 1 and across all cycles in patients with solid tumors and in patients with non-Hodgkin's lymphoma.[35]

neutropenia and its complications. These guidelines include those from the ASCO, the National Comprehensive Cancer Network (NCCN), and the European Organisation for Research and Treatment of Cancer (EORTC).[23–25] ASCO published the first CSF guidelines in 1994, which it updated in 1996, 1997, and 2000.[36,37] In 2006, ASCO completed the most comprehensive update of the guidelines presented to date.[25] In 2005, the NCCN published myeloid growth factor guidelines that have been updated annually through 2009.[38,39] In 2006, the EORTC published G-CSF guidelines for adults with solid tumors and malignant lymphoma.[23] These general G-CSF guidelines complement previous EORTC guidelines on the use of these agents specifically in elderly cancer patients.[40]

D.2. Comparison of recent myeloid growth factor guidelines

The 2006 ASCO White Blood Cell Growth Factor Guidelines altered the recommended threshold for consideration of primary CSF prophylaxis from the previous 40 percent febrile neutropenia risk to 20 percent.[25] The updated guidelines also address the use of these agents with less intensive regimens under special circumstances, including older age and major comorbid illnesses that place a patient at increased risk of febrile neutropenia.[25] This major update in the ASCO guidelines was based on a review of recent RCTs and the meta-analysis of 17 RCTs of prophylactic G-CSF described earlier.[26,41] The summary analysis of these trials demonstrated that patients randomized to primary G-CSF prophylaxis experienced not only a reduction in the risk of febrile neutropenia but also significant reductions in infection-related and early all-cause mortality during chemotherapy, while significantly increasing the chemotherapy dose intensity delivered. A wide range of additional topics are summarized in the ASCO guideline update, including their specific use in older patients (Table 23.1).

The EORTC guidelines published in 2006 also recommend routine prophylactic use of G-CSF in those receiving a regimen with a 20 percent or greater risk of febrile neutropenia.[23] As earlier, the guidelines recommend an individual risk assessment in those receiving a regimen associated with a risk of 10–20 percent and no use of prophylactic G-CSF in patients with a risk <10 percent (Figure 23.7). As with the other guidelines, prophylactic G-CSF is recommended with dose-dense or dose-intense chemotherapy. Likewise, where a reduction in chemotherapy dose intensity may be associated with a poor outcome, consideration of G-CSF prophylaxis to maintain dose intensity is recommended. Previous EORTC guidelines were published that specifically addressed the role of the myeloid growth factors in older patients.[40] Those guidelines highlight that while the risk of febrile neutropenia is increased in the elderly, particularly early in the course of treatment, older age is not a contraindication to modern cancer chemotherapy. The guidelines conclude that there is sufficient evidence of therapeutic efficacy to recommend prophylactic G-CSF support to reduce the incidence of chemotherapy-associated neutropenic complications including

Table 23.1 American Society of Clinical Oncology 2006 White Blood Cell Growth Factor Guidelines update summary.

Setting/indication	Recommended	Not recommended
General circumstances	FN risk in the range of 20% or higher	
Special circumstances	Clinical factors dictate use	
Secondary prophylaxis	Based on chemotherapy reaction among other factors	
Therapy of afebrile neutropenia		Not to be used routinely
Therapy of febrile neutropenia	If high-risk for complications or poor clinical outcomes	Not to be used routinely as adjunctive treatment with antibiotic therapy
Acute myeloid leukemia	Following induction therapy, patients >55 years old most likely to benefit	Not to be used for priming effects
	After the completion of consolidation chemotherapy	
Myelodysplastic syndrome		Intermittent administration for a subset of patients with severe neutropenia and recurrent infection
Acute lymphocytic leukemia	After the completion of initial chemotherapy or first postremission course	
Radiotherapy	Consider if receiving radiation therapy alone and prolonged delays are expected	Avoid patients receiving concomitant chemotherapy and radiation therapy
Older patients	If ≥65 years old with diffuse aggressive lymphoma and treated with curative chemotherapy	
Pediatric population	For the primary prophylaxis of pediatric patients with a likelihood of FN and the secondary prophylaxis or therapy for high-risk patients	G-CSF use in children with ALL should be considered carefully
Radiation injury	Prompt administration of CSF or pegylated G-CSF if exposed to lethal doses of total-body radiotherapy	

Note. Please note that proper use of CSF happens in conjunction with consideration of varied factors and circumstances. This summary table is provided to assist in summarizing the guideline slide set. There are additional recommendations not presented in this table. Modified from Smith et al.[25] FN = febrile neutropenia; G-CSF = granulocyte colony-stimulating factor.

febrile neutropenia in older patients receiving systemic chemotherapy for non-Hodgkin's lymphoma, small-cell lung cancer, and genitourinary tumors. Though available data in other cancer settings are limited, the guidelines suggest that similar levels of efficacy with prophylactic growth factors are likely. Though there is also insufficient evidence to conclude that the CSFs improve overall survival, the authors argue that maintaining dose intensity with primary CSF prophylaxis is reasonable in elderly patients receiving curative myelosuppressive chemotherapy. A systematic review conducted in support of the 2006 EORTC CSF guidelines concluded that older age, particu-

larly age 65 years or older, was consistently associated with an increased risk of neutropenic complications across a range of tumor types and treatment regimens.[23] The guidelines recommend that age 65 years or older be considered a high-risk factor for consideration of G-CSF support even when the regimen-reported risk is less than 20 percent.

The myeloid growth factor guidelines from the NCCN, since their inception in 2005, have encouraged a process starting with an initial evaluation based on the type of cancer, chemotherapy regimen, patient-specific risk factors, and treatment intention.[38,39] After assessing a patient's risk, the guidelines recommend the use of primary G-CSF prophylaxis in patients with an individual risk of 20 percent or greater. Patients at intermediate risk in the range of 10–20 percent may be considered for prophylactic G-CSF if there are clinical factors such as age that place the patient at greater risk for febrile neutropenia or serious consequences such as prolonged hospitalization or death. Though the NCCN guidelines differ from those of both ASCO and EORTC in that they are largely based on a consensus process of experts in the field rather than an extensive evidence-based review, they are updated on an annual basis.

A comprehensive overview of the major myeloid growth factor guidelines has recently been conducted, including a comparison of the actual recommendations and the comparative strengths and weaknesses.[42] The ASCO and EORTC guidelines are accompanied by a more rigorous evaluation of the evidence, whereas the NCCN guidelines are more concise and algorithm oriented. Recommendations, however, appear to be remarkably consistent across the guidelines for primary prophylaxis, secondary prophylaxis, and their value in the care of elderly cancer patients.[42] All guidelines make note of the importance of patient risk factors, including older age, the presence of major comorbidities as well as prior febrile neutropenia, advanced stage, poor performance or nutritional status, and low baseline blood counts. All guidelines recognize as well the increased risk for neutropenic complications among older cancer patients. The NCCN has a specific guideline for managing chemotherapy in older patients and recommends prophylactic G-CSF in patients aged 65 years and older receiving chemotherapy with a dose intensity equivalent to CHOP.[43] Similarly, EORTC specifies age over 65 as a high-risk criterion for the occurrence of febrile neutropenia and has specific myeloid growth factor guidelines for the elderly cancer patients (Figure 23.7).[40]

D.3. Recommendations for the myeloid growth factors in the elderly cancer patient

The updated ASCO guidelines indicate that older age is a factor often warranting the use of prophylactic CSFs even when the risk of febrile neutropenia–associated chemotherapy is less than 20 percent.[25] Multiple studies among older patients with lymphoma that have found an increased risk of neutropenia and its complications are cited. While the alternative methods for reducing the risk of FN, including dose reduction and delays, are discussed, the guidelines

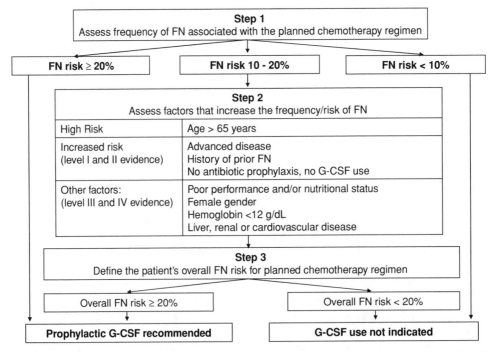

Figure 23.7 Patient assessment algorithm to decide prophylactic G-CSF use from the clinical practice guidelines developed by the European Organisation for Research and Treatment of Cancer (EORTC).[23] FN = febrile neutropenia; G-CSF = granulocyte colony-stimulating factor.

note that these strategies have been associated with reduced response and survival in RCTs of lymphoma patients undergoing curative therapy. Therefore the ASCO guidelines specifically recommend the use of prophylactic CSF for reducing the occurrence of febrile neutropenia or infection in patients aged 65 years and older with diffuse aggressive lymphoma treated with curative chemotherapy. Further clinical trials to address the value of prophylactic CSFs in other settings based solely on age are encouraged. The NCCN Myeloid Growth Factor Guidelines also identify increasing age as a predictor of severe and febrile neutropenia and subsequent serious medical consequences.[11,39] The guidelines point out that older patients are often treated with lower chemotherapy doses to minimize the occurrence of neutropenic complications. Since older patients with cancer can obtain the same benefit from aggressive chemotherapy as younger patients, effective management of the risk of neutropenic complications is crucial to enabling full-dose chemotherapy in this population. The updated ASCO guidelines note that reduced renal function accompanying the aging process may account in part for the impact of older age on the risk of neutropenic complications from myelosuppressive chemotherapy.[25]

E. Clinical decision support for myeloid growth factors

The decision to initiate prophylactic myeloid growth factor support is commonly based on the intensity of the chemotherapy regimen, a prior episode of febrile neutropenia, or a subjective clinical assessment of patient risk. In malignancies treated with curative intent requiring full-dose-intensity chemotherapy, older age is often associated with sufficient risk of early febrile neutropenia to warrant primary prophylaxis with a CSF. In addition to older age, variables that contribute to an increased risk of neutropenic complications include the cancer type and treatment regimen, various comorbidities, and measures of renal and hepatic function (Figure 23.8). A number of studies have attempted to assess risk based on retrospective observations to enhance clinical assessment.[44] These efforts have uniformly concluded that increasing age is an important risk factor for the occurrence of neutropenic complications.

Multivariate risk models are undergoing validation and may soon be available to assist clinical decision making in clinical oncology in the selection of high-risk patients for targeted use of G-CSF prophylaxis. Utilizing a prospective study of U.S. community oncology practices,

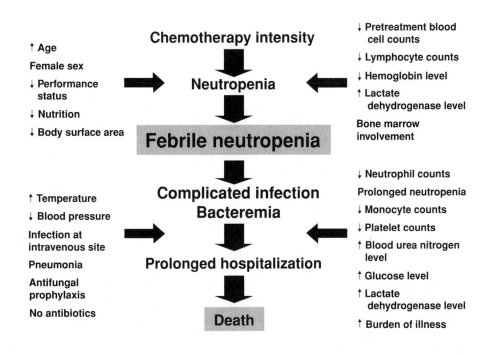

Figure 23.8 Risk factors for chemotherapy-induced neutropenia, including (top) febrile neutropenia or (bottom) severe and potentially fatal complications identified in a review of the medical literature.[44]

Table 23.2 Multivariate logistic regression model for severe or febrile neutropenia over cycles 1–4 in cancer patients ≥70 years of age (n = 928).

Variable	Odds ratio (95% CI)	p value
Cancer type		<.0001
Colon	1.35 (0.52–3.52)	.5373
Lung small-cell	7.26 (2.82–18.74)	<.0001
Lung non-small-cell	0.92 (0.38–2.20)	.8468
Ovary	1.01 (0.39–2.63)	.9783
Breast	2.76 (1.10–6.92)	.0299
Lymphoma	3.36 (1.41–8.02)	.0063
Other tumors	1.00–	–
Age		.1414
70–74	1.63 (0.99–2.67)	.0546
75–79	1.55 (0.93–2.59)	.0815
80 and above	1.00–	–
Planned RDI		.0794
<85%	1.00–	–
≥85%	1.69 (1.06–2.67)	.0263
Unknown	1.64 (0.77–3.52)	.2009
Anthracycline-based regimen	6.30 (3.76–10.57)	<.0001
Platinum-based regimen	3.84 (2.34–6.31)	<.0001
BSA ≤ 2 m²	1.91 (1.13–3.26)	.0167
Previous chemotherapy	1.87 (1.27–2.77)	.0016
Elevated BUN	1.52 (1.05–2.21)	.0272
Elevated alkaline phosphatase	1.60 (1.07–2.41)	.0264
Prophylactic CSF	0.36 (0.21–0.62)	.0002

Note. Results are adjusted for ECOG PS ≥ 2 and number of comorbidities ≥ 2, neither of which was statistically significant. RDI = relative dose intensity; BSA = body surface area; BUN = blood urea nitrogen; CSF = colony-stimulating factor. Model's R^2 = 0.26; c = 0.782. Modified from Shayne et al.[22]

a multivariate risk model has been developed that identifies significant independent risk factors for neutropenic events among patients aged 70 years and older (Table 23.2).[22] As in younger patients, the period of greatest risk of neutropenic events in elderly patients receiving chemotherapy is in the initial cycle of treatment. Significant predictors of severe or febrile neutropenia in elderly patients with solid tumors and malignant lymphoma adjusted for body surface area included cancer type, especially small-cell lung cancer, breast cancer, and malignant lymphoma;

prior chemotherapy; planned chemotherapy dose intensity 85 percent or more of standard dosing; anthracycline- or platinum-based chemotherapy; and elevated blood urea nitrogen or alkaline phosphatase. Following adjustment for these factors, prophylactic myeloid growth factor was associated with a significant reduction in risk of neutropenic complications (OR 0.36, 95% CI 0.21–0.62, p = .0002). While no increase in risk of neutropenic events was observed with age in this study, a significant trend toward increasing reductions in delivered chemotherapy dose intensity was reported with increasing age in both early-stage and advanced-stage patients. There remains a need for additional well-designed studies to better identify elderly patients receiving cancer chemotherapy who are at greatest risk for febrile neutropenia and most likely to benefit from prophylactic CSF. As accurate risk models for neutropenic complications are developed and independently validated in older patients receiving systemic chemotherapy, they should provide a valuable tool for practicing oncologists in providing optimal care to older patients receiving cancer chemotherapy.

F. Economic considerations for the myeloid growth factors

Management of older individuals with cancer is often considered to be more costly and less effective than that of managing younger patients because of the increased risk of therapeutic complications and the reduced potential for benefit associated with limited life expectancy and less responsive malignancies.[45] The decision to utilize a colony-stimulating factor in patients receiving cancer chemotherapy should be based primarily on clinical indications including patient risk and the potential benefit of treatment, including a reduction in the risk of febrile neutropenia and early infection-related mortality as well as any impact on chemotherapy dose intensity and long-term survival.[46,47] Nevertheless, the cost of myeloid growth factors often raises economic concerns at the institutional, payor, and societal level.[48] The direct costs of the myeloid growth factors should be balanced against any reduction in costs associated with the treatment of febrile neutropenia and its sequelae.[49] The cost of hospitalization for febrile neutropenia has been reported to vary between $10,000 and $20,000 in the United States.[1,50] A small proportion of hospitalized patients with febrile neutropenia account for the majority of the total cost because of long lengths of stay associated with comorbidities and treatment-related complications.[1]

Economic models have been developed on the basis of the level of risk of febrile neutropenia and the clinical efficacy associated with prophylactic CSFs demonstrated in RCTs.[46,49] The trade-off between costs of growth factor use and the reduction in costs associated with the prevention of febrile neutropenia have provided estimates of overall expected costs or savings.[49,51,52] Such models have demonstrated that primary prophylaxis with G-CSF may actually reduce overall health care costs in many clinical settings. Though clinical practice guidelines often discuss these economic models, none of the current myeloid growth factor guideline recommendations are based on cost considerations. Febrile neutropenia risk threshold estimates associated with a net cost savings in the range of 20 percent or less are conservative projections based on average U.S. direct medical costs for hospitalization for febrile neutropenia, thus indirectly supporting the recommendations of the myeloid growth factor guidelines.[51–53] These projections do not consider emergency room care, physician fees, follow-up care, medications, or indirect and out-of-pocket costs.[54] Consideration of indirect and out-of-pocket costs results in even lower risk threshold estimates favoring the use of the CSFs.[55,56] Though outpatient management of febrile neutropenia may reduce individual costs, the overall cost savings appears small because of the shifting of low-risk patients with small influence on the total costs to the outpatient setting, leaving the more costly febrile neutropenia episodes to be dealt with in the inpatient setting.[57] Risk models for patient selection for the targeted application of the myeloid growth factors in the high-risk setting may improve the cost efficiency or cost effectiveness of their use further.[19,44] Though further investigation is needed, myeloid growth factors used along with antibiotics at the time of hospitalization for treatment of febrile neutropenia may also reduce the length of hospitalization and associated costs.[58,59]

There have been few studies of the economic impact of febrile neutropenia or the myeloid growth factors specifically in older patients with cancer.[18] As discussed earlier, the risk of febrile neutropenia in older cancer patients may be greater, whereas frequent dose reductions and delays may modulate short-term risk while increasing the potential for subsequent disease recurrence or progression.[20,22]

G. Safety of the myeloid growth factors

Despite demonstrating efficacy in multiple RCTs and nearly 20 years of clinical experience with the myeloid growth factors in support of patients receiving cancer chemotherapy, safety concerns have occasionally surfaced based largely on anecdotal case reports and retrospective population studies. The most commonly reported toxicity associated with these agents is that of bone pain, which is generally mild to moderate in intensity and self-limited. However, the presence of G-CSF receptors on the surface of leukemic cells in some patients with acute myeloid leukemia has led some authors to express concern about a possible increased risk of acute myelogenous leukemia (AML) and other preleukemic myeloid disorders such as the myelodysplastic syndrome in patients receiving G-CSF. Using Surveillance, Epidemiology, and End Results (SEER)-Medicare-linked data, Hershman and colleagues recently reported on 5,510 elderly women with early-stage breast cancer who received adjuvant chemotherapy.[60] Of the 906 women (16%) receiving G-CSF or GM-CSF, 16 (1.77%) developed AML or myelodysplastic syndrome (MDS) compared to 48 of the 4,604 not receiving G-CSF (1.04%), for a hazard rate ratio of 2.14 (95% CI 1.12–4.08). Among other factors, the use of G-CSF and GM-CSF was associated with receipt of radiation therapy and cyclophosphamide treatment.

The interpretation of such retrospective studies is complicated by their post hoc analysis and limited ability to identify many or most relevant confounding factors. In addition to age, selection bias may have occurred in patients selected nonrandomly to receive G-CSF because of undiagnosed but preexisting hematologic disorders, prior chemotherapy and radiation therapy, low baseline blood parameters, and other recognized inherited and acquired risk factors for neutropenia. Complicating the assessment of any risk associated with these agents is the recognized carcinogenicity and leukemogenicity of ionizing radiation and many of the commonly employed cancer chemotherapeutic agents given in conjunction with G-CSF. Many of the RCTs of G-CSF in patients receiving cancer chemotherapy demonstrated an ability to sustain or increase the dose intensity and delivered a total dose of cancer chemotherapy, further confounding any separate influence of G-CSF on the risk of AML, MDS, or other second malignancies. In a systematic review of RCTs of

G-CSF-supported chemotherapy with at least 2 years of follow-up, 24 trials were identified.[61] Though no difference in all second malignancies was observed in patients receiving G-CSF, an increase in AML or MDS was seen with an absolute increase in risk of 4 cases per 1,000 treated. However, patients in the G-CSF treatment arms consistently received greater chemotherapy dose or dose intensity, making interpretation difficult. At the same time, G-CSF-treated patients in these trials experienced a lower mortality rate, presumably because of better tumor control, with a median duration of follow-up of 5 years. It will be difficult with the data available to distinguish any risk for AML or MDS associated with G-CSF from that related to greater chemotherapy dose and intensity.

H. Conclusions

Myelosuppression, including neutropenic complications, continues to represent the major dose-limiting toxicity associated with cancer chemotherapy, which most often occurs early in the course of treatment. Nowhere is this more evident than in the treatment of older cancer patients with responsive and potentially curable malignancies. Though reductions in chemotherapy dose intensity by decreasing chemotherapy dose or delaying treatment may reduce the immediate risk of neutropenic events including febrile neutropenia, the impact of such actions on long-term disease control and survival remains of concern. While prophylactic antibiotics appear to reduce the risk of fever, such strategies have no impact on the underlying neutropenia and may contribute to the major problem associated with emerging antimicrobial resistance in both gram-positive and gram-negative bacteria. Primary prophylaxis with the myeloid growth factors represents an effective and cost-effective approach for reducing the risk of febrile neutropenia in older cancer patients receiving chemotherapy, while enabling delivery of full dose intensity in most patients. The use of prophylactic G-CSF is currently recommended by clinical practice guidelines developed by the ASCO, the NCCN, and the EORTC when the risk of febrile neutropenia is 20 percent or greater as well as in certain special circumstances, including the treatment of older cancer patients. Further investigation of risk factors and the development and validation of risk models for febrile neutropenia are needed. Such models should enable a more individualized assessment of risk as well as more appropriate and cost-effective use of these agents in patients at greatest risk and most likely to benefit. While the indications for the use of these agents have expanded considerably, continued safety monitoring and identification of better strategies for selecting patients at increased risk for febrile neutropenia and most likely to benefit from such support are needed.

References

1. Kuderer NM, Dale DC, Crawford J, et al. Mortality, morbidity, and cost associated with febrile neutropenia in adult cancer patients. *Cancer*. 2006;106(10):2258–2266.

2. Crawford J, Dale DC, Kuderer NM, et al. Risk and timing of neutropenic events in adult cancer patients receiving chemotherapy: the results of a prospective nationwide study of oncology practice. *J Natl Compr Canc Netw*. 2008;6(2):109–118.

3. Lyman GH, Delgado DJ. Risk and timing of hospitalization for febrile neutropenia in patients receiving CHOP, CHOP-R, or CNOP chemotherapy for intermediate-grade non-Hodgkin lymphoma. *Cancer*. 2003;98(11):2402–2409.

4. Lyman GH, Morrison VA, Dale DC, et al. Risk of febrile neutropenia among patients with intermediate-grade non-Hodgkin's lymphoma receiving CHOP chemotherapy. *Leuk Lymphoma*. 2003;44(12):2069–2076.

5. Timmer-Bonte JN, de Boo TM, Smit HJ, et al. Prevention of chemotherapy-induced febrile neutropenia by prophylactic antibiotics plus or minus granulocyte colony-stimulating factor in small-cell lung cancer: a Dutch randomized phase III study. *J Clin Oncol*. 2005;23(31):7974–7984.

6. Bonneterre J, Roche H, Kerbrat P, et al. Epirubicin increases long-term survival in adjuvant chemotherapy of patients with poor-prognosis, node-positive, early breast cancer: 10-year follow-up results of the French Adjuvant Study Group 05 randomized trial. *J Clin Oncol*. 2005;23(12):2686–2693.

7. Budman DR, Berry DA, Cirrincione CT, et al. Dose and dose intensity as determinants of outcome in the adjuvant treatment of breast cancer. The Cancer and Leukemia Group B. *J Natl Cancer Inst*. 1998;90(16):1205–1211.

8. Chu E, DeVita V. *Principles of Medical Oncology*. 7th ed. Philadelphia: Lippincott; 2006.

9. Lyman GH, Dale DC, Crawford J. Incidence and predictors of low dose-intensity in adjuvant breast cancer chemotherapy: a nationwide study of community practices. *J Clin Oncol*. 2003;21(24):4524–4531.

10. Lyman GH, Dale DC, Friedberg J, et al. Incidence and predictors of low chemotherapy dose-intensity in aggressive non-Hodgkin's lymphoma: a nationwide study. *J Clin Oncol*. 2004;22(21):4302–4311.

11. Lyman GH. Guidelines of the National Comprehensive Cancer Network on the use of myeloid growth factors with cancer chemotherapy: a review of the evidence. *J Natl Compr Canc Netw*. 2005;3(4):557–571.

12. Balducci L, Lyman GH. Patients aged > or = 70 are at high risk for neutropenic infection and should receive hemopoietic growth factors when treated with moderately toxic chemotherapy. *J Clin Oncol*. 2001;19(5):1583–1585.

13. Balducci L, Yates J. General guidelines for the management of older patients with cancer. *Oncology*. 2000;14(11A):221–227.

14. Balducci L, Hardy CL, Lyman GH. Hemopoiesis and aging. *Cancer Treat Res*. 2005;124:109–134.

15. Shank Jr WA, Balducci L. Recombinant hemopoietic growth factors: comparative hemopoietic response in younger and older subjects. *J Am Geriatr Soc*. 1992;40(2):151–154.

16. Baker SD, Grochow LB. Pharmacology of cancer chemotherapy in the older person. *Clin Geriatr Med*. 1997;13(1):169–183.

17. Coiffier B, Lepage E, Briere J, et al. CHOP chemotherapy plus rituximab compared with CHOP alone in elderly patients with diffuse large-B-cell lymphoma. *N Engl J Med*. 2002;346(4):235–242.

18. Lyman GH, Kuderer N, Agboola O, et al. Evidence-based use of colony-stimulating factors in elderly cancer patients. *Cancer Control*. 2003;10(6):487–499.

19. Klastersky J, Paesmans M, Rubenstein EB, et al. The Multinational Association for Supportive Care in Cancer risk index: a multinational scoring system for identifying low-risk febrile neutropenic cancer patients. *J Clin Oncol*. 2000;18(16):3038–3051.

20. Lyman GH. Impact of chemotherapy dose intensity on cancer patient outcomes. *J Natl Compr Canc Netw*. 2009;7:99–108.

21. Shayne M, Crawford J, Dale DC, et al. Predictors of reduced dose intensity in patients with early-stage breast cancer receiving adjuvant chemotherapy. *Breast Cancer Res Treat*. 2006;100(3):255–262.

22. Shayne M, Culakova E, Poniewierski MS, et al. Dose intensity and hematologic toxicity in older cancer patients receiving systemic chemotherapy. *Cancer*. 2007;110(7):1611–1620.

23. Aapro MS, Cameron DA, Pettengell R, et al. EORTC guidelines for the use of granulocyte-colony stimulating factor to reduce the incidence of chemotherapy-induced febrile neutropenia in adult patients with lymphomas and solid tumours. *Eur J Cancer*. 2006;42(15):2433–2453.

24. Crawford J, Althaus B, Armitage J, et al. Myeloid growth factors: clinical practice guidelines in oncology. *J Natl Compr Canc Netw*. 2007;5(2):188–202.

25. Smith TJ, Khatcheressian J, Lyman GH, et al. 2006 update of recommendations for the use of white

blood cell growth factors: an evidence-based clinical practice guideline. *J Clin Oncol.* 2006;24(19):3187–3205.

26. Kuderer NM, Dale DC, Crawford J, et al. Impact of primary prophylaxis with granulocyte colony-stimulating factor on febrile neutropenia and mortality in adult cancer patients receiving chemotherapy: a systematic review. *J Clin Oncol.* 2007;25(21):3158–3167.

27. Wittman B, Horan J, Lyman GH. Prophylactic colony-stimulating factors in children receiving myelosuppressive chemotherapy: a meta-analysis of randomized controlled trials. *Cancer Treat Rev.* 2006;32(4):289–303.

28. Green MD, Koelbl H, Baselga J, et al. A randomized double-blind multicenter phase III study of fixed-dose single-administration pegfilgrastim versus daily filgrastim in patients receiving myelosuppressive chemotherapy. *Ann Oncol.* 2003;14(1):29–35.

29. Holmes FA, O'Shaughnessy JA, Vukelja S, et al. Blinded, randomized, multicenter study to evaluate single administration pegfilgrastim once per cycle versus daily filgrastim as an adjunct to chemotherapy in patients with high-risk stage II or stage III/IV breast cancer. *J Clin Oncol.* 2002;20(3):727–731.

30. Pinto L, Liu Z, Doan Q, et al. Comparison of pegfilgrastim with filgrastim on febrile neutropenia, grade IV neutropenia and bone pain: a meta-analysis of randomized controlled trials. *Curr Med Res Opin.* 2007;23(9):2283–2295.

31. Doorduijn JK, Van Der Holt B, van Imhoff GW, et al. CHOP compared with CHOP plus granulocyte colony-stimulating factor in elderly patients with aggressive non-Hodgkin's lymphoma. *J Clin Oncol.* 2003;21(16):3041–3050.

32. Osby E, Hagberg H, Kvaloy S, et al. CHOP is superior to CNOP in elderly patients with aggressive lymphoma while outcome is unaffected by filgrastim treatment: results of a Nordic Lymphoma Group randomized trial. *Blood.* 2003;101(10):3840–3848.

33. Zinzani PL, Storti S, Zaccaria A, et al. Elderly aggressive-histology non-Hodgkin's lymphoma: first-line VNCOP-B regimen experience on 350 patients. *Blood.* 1999;94(1):33–38.

34. Bohlius J, Herbst C, Reiser M, et al. Granulopoiesis-stimulating factors to prevent adverse effects in the treatment of malignant lymphoma. *Cochrane Database Syst Rev.* 2008;4:CD003189.

35. Balducci L, Al-Halawani H, Charu V, et al. Elderly cancer patients receiving chemotherapy benefit from first-cycle pegfilgrastim. *Oncologist.* 2007;12(12):1416–1424.

36. American Society of Clinical Oncology. Recommendations for the use of hematopoietic colony-stimulating factors: evidence-based, clinical practice guidelines. *J Clin Oncol.* 1994;12(11):2471–2508.

37. Ozer H, Armitage JO, Bennett CL, et al. 2000 update of recommendations for the use of hematopoietic colony-stimulating factors: evidence-based, clinical practice guidelines. American Society of Clinical Oncology Growth Factors Expert Panel. *J Clin Oncol.* 2000;18(20):3558–3585.

38. Crawford J, Althaus B, Armitage J, et al. Myeloid growth factors clinical practice guidelines in oncology. *J Natl Compr Canc Netw.* 2005;3(4):540–555.

39. Crawford J, Armitage J, Balducci L, et al. Myeloid growth factors. *J Natl Compr Canc Netw.* 2009;7(1):64–83.

40. Repetto L, Biganzoli L, Koehne CH, et al. EORTC Cancer in the Elderly Task Force guidelines for the use of colony-stimulating factors in elderly patients with cancer. *Eur J Cancer.* 2003;39(16):2264–2272.

41. Vogel CL, Wojtukiewicz MZ, Carroll RR, et al. First and subsequent cycle use of pegfilgrastim prevents febrile neutropenia in patients with breast cancer: a multicenter, double-blind, placebo-controlled phase III study. *J Clin Oncol.* 2005;23(6):1178–1184.

42. Lyman GH, Kleiner JM. Summary and comparison of myeloid growth factor guidelines in patients receiving cancer chemotherapy. *J Natl Compr Canc Netw.* 2007;5(2):217–228.

43. Balducci L, Cohen HJ, Engstrom PF, et al. Senior adult oncology clinical practice guidelines in oncology. *J Natl Compr Canc Netw.* 2005;3(4):572–590.

44. Lyman GH, Lyman CH, Agboola O. Risk models for predicting chemotherapy-induced neutropenia. *Oncologist.* 2005;10(6):427–437.

45. Lyman GH, Kuderer NM. The diagnosis and treatment of cancer in the elderly: cost effectiveness considerations. In: Lodovico Balducci, Gary H Lyman, William B Ershler, Martine Extermann, eds. *Comprehensive Geriatric Oncology.* 2nd ed. London: Taylor and Francis; 2004:pp 510–524.

46. Lyman GH, Kuderer N, Greene J, et al. The economics of febrile neutropenia: implications for the use of colony-stimulating factors. *Eur J Cancer.* 1998;34(12):1857–1864.

47. Lyman GH, Kuderer NM. Epidemiology of febrile neutropenia. *Support Cancer Ther.* 2003;1:1–12.

48. Lyman GH, Kuderer NM. The economics of the colony-stimulating factors in the prevention and treatment of febrile neutropenia. *Crit Rev Oncol Hematol.* 2004;50(2):129–146.

49. Lyman GH, Lyman CG, Sanderson RA, et al. Decision analysis of hematopoietic growth factor use in patients receiving cancer chemotherapy. *J Natl Cancer Inst.* 1993;85(6):488–493.

50. Caggiano V, Weiss RV, Rickert TS, et al. Incidence, cost, and mortality of neutropenia hospitalization associated with chemotherapy. *Cancer.* 2005;103(9):1916–1924.

51. Eldar-Lissai A, Cosler LE, Culakova E, et al. Economic analysis of prophylactic pegfilgrastim in adult cancer patients receiving chemotherapy. *Value Health.* 2008;11(2):172–179.

52. Ramsey SD, Liu Z, Boer R, et al. Cost-effectiveness of primary versus secondary prophylaxis with pegfilgrastim in women with early-stage breast cancer receiving chemotherapy. *Value Health.* 2009;12:217–225.

53. Lyman G, Lalla A, Barron R, et al. Cost-effectiveness of pegfilgrastim versus 6-day filgrastim primary prophylaxis in patients with non-Hodgkin's lymphoma receiving CHOP-21 in United States. *Curr Med Res Opin.* 2009;25(2):401–411.

54. Hassett MJ, O'Malley AJ, Pakes JR, et al. Frequency and cost of chemotherapy-related serious adverse effects in a population sample of women with breast cancer. *J Natl Cancer Inst.* 2006;98(16):1108–1117.

55. Cosler LE, Calhoun EA, Agboola O, et al. Effects of indirect and additional direct costs on the risk threshold for prophylaxis with colony-stimulating factors in patients at risk for severe neutropenia from cancer chemotherapy. *Pharmacotherapy.* 2004;24(4):488–494.

56. Lyman GH. Time is money for both the healthy and the sick. *Med Care.* 2005;43(7):637–639.

57. Cosler LE, Sivasubramaniam V, Agboola O, et al. Effect of outpatient treatment of febrile neutropenia on the risk threshold for the use of CSF in patients with cancer treated with chemotherapy. *Value Health.* 2005;8(1): 47–52.

58. Clark OA, Lyman GH, Castro AA, et al. Colony-stimulating factors for chemotherapy-induced febrile neutropenia: a meta-analysis of randomized controlled trials. *J Clin Oncol.* 2005;23(18):4198–4214.

59. Cosler LE, Eldar-Lissai A, Culakova E, et al. Therapeutic use of granulocyte colony-stimulating factors for established febrile neutropenia: effect on costs from a hospital perspective. *Pharmacoeconomics.* 2007;25(4):343–351.

60. Hershman D, Neugut AI, Jacobson JS, et al. Acute myeloid leukemia or myelodysplastic syndrome following use of granulocyte colony-stimulating factors during breast cancer adjuvant chemotherapy. *J Natl Cancer Inst.* 2007;99(3):196–205.

61. Lyman GH, Dale DC, Culakova E, et al. Acute Myeloid Leukemia or Myelodysplastic Syndrome in Randomized Controlled Clinical Trials of Cancer Chemotherapy With Granulocyte Colony-Stimulating Factor: A Systematic Review. *J Clin Oncol.* 2010 (in press).

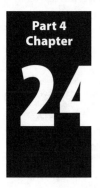

Symptom management and supportive care of older adults

Erythropoiesis-stimulating agents in older adults with cancer

Matthew S. McKinney and Jeffrey Crawford

A. Introduction

The prevalence of anemia in older persons is higher than in the general population and is associated with significant clinical symptoms and poorer prognosis in this group. An increased incidence of cancer and the use of cytotoxic agents in this population also places patients at increased risk of development of anemia and consequently may also increase their morbidity/mortality risk. Since the introduction of erythropoiesis-stimulating agents (ESAs), clinicians have sought potential uses of these agents to treat cancer-related anemia. Though studies demonstrated an improvement in anemia, reduction in blood transfusion, and improved quality of life, there was hope that mortality would also be improved. However, some recent reports have shown possible adverse effects of ESAs on tumor progression and survival in patients being treated for cancer. In this chapter, we review the effects of anemia on the prognosis of geriatric cancer patients, consider the rationale for use of ESAs versus other therapies for cancer-related anemia, and discuss some of the recent reports regarding potential adverse effects of ESAs, resulting in current guidelines of usage of ESAs.

B. Prevalence and morbidity/mortality associated with anemia in the aged

Anemia is significantly more prevalent in the aged population, and there are ample data to suggest that this is associated with poor outcomes. The prevalence of anemia by World Health Organization criteria (hgb less than 13 gm/dL in men and hgb less than 12 gm/dL in women) in the geriatric population has been reported to be approximately 11–28 percent in persons over 65 years of age.[1,2] The incidence rises with advancing age, and there appears to be an increased incidence/prevalence in men.[3] Anemia in the elderly

is often related to a higher prevalence of chronic diseases such as chronic kidney disease, arthritis, and malignancy; however, a significant portion (20–30%) of cases of anemia in this population remain unexplained.[4–7] Since the increased mortality rates occur at similar hemoglobin values in young and older persons, it is assumed that anemia represents a disease state and not a normal physiologic consequence of aging.

The prevalence of anemia among patients with cancer is also high and further complicates the treatment of older cancer patients. Reports have documented rates of anemia as high as 40 percent in patients with solid tumors,[8,9] and 60–70 percent of patients with hematologic malignancies such as multiple myeloma and chronic lymphocytic leukemia may be anemic at time of diagnosis.

Treatment with cytotoxic agents further predisposes patients with cancer to anemia. The usual mechanism underlying anemia in this setting is myelosuppression,[10,11] although hemolytic processes may also play a role.[12,13] While not as rapid in onset or recovery as granulocytopenia or thrombocytopenia, anemia affects a significant proportion of patients undergoing cancer treatment and is generally cumulative over treatment cycles. Particular cytotoxic agents appear more likely to cause anemia, but dose and dose intensity are major risk factors. Several reviews and meta-analyses document significantly higher rates of chemotherapy-related anemia in patients being treated for lung, ovarian, and genitourinary malignancies.[14,15] Up to 60 percent of patients treated with cisplatin-paclitaxel for non-small-cell lung cancer (NSCLC) may experience grade 1–2 anemia (hgb less than 10.0 gm/dL),[16] and a U.K. study involving 2,821 solid tumor patients undergoing chemotherapy treatment for various malignancies found that 33 percent of patients required blood transfusion.[17]

Cisplatin and carboplatin tend to cause anemia, requiring transfusion more frequently than other agents.[18–20] The degree of anemia caused by these agents does not correlate well to the development of thrombocytopenia or granulocy-topenia[20–22] or to the severity of cisplatin-induced renal dysfunction.[23] The mechanism seems to be related to the suppression of erythropoietin in the peritubular cells of the nephron as opposed to suppression of bone marrow erythroid precursors.[22] Anthracyclines and taxanes also appear to cause disproportionately higher rates of anemia than regimens containing other agents, but anemia has been reported with a variety of other agents, including vinorelbine, 5-fluorouracil (5-FU), methotrexate, and gemcitabine.[24]

It is unclear to what degree older age may influence the development of anemia in untreated or treated cancer patients as several studies have shown no link between age and development of cancer-associated anemia,[25] while others have incorporated age into risk-assessment models for chemotherapy-associated anemia.[26,27] Because pretreatment hemoglobin levels tend to predict the development of chemotherapy-associated anemia,[15] one could anticipate a higher prevalence of this problem in the geriatric cancer patient population. More prospective clinical studies are needed to clarify the link between age and chemotherapy-associated anemia as this may have important consequences for treatment in this population.

C. Mechanisms of aging-related anemia

A variety of underlying mechanisms may account for the increased prevalence of anemia in aged persons. Several studies have examined the erythropoietin response to anemia and subsequent hematopoiesis. Whereas erythropoietin levels are consistently similar among young healthy adults and across (in response to) various levels of anemia, erythropoietin levels in older persons are highly variable and tend to be higher than in younger patients with similar degrees of anemia.[28] Alternatively, some groups have shown decreased erythropoietin levels in elderly patients with unexplained anemia,[29] and an inappropriately low rise of erythropoietin in response to anemia has been documented.[30] Ershler and colleagues followed a group of 143 healthy subjects over a period of 8–31 years and found significant declines in hemoglobin and increased erythropoietin levels, even in patients who did not develop anemia by the standard definition.[31] This suggests that older patients may require higher systemic erythropoietin levels to compensate for underly-

ing processes predisposing them to anemia; they may also paradoxically produce less erythropoietin in response to anemia.

Hematopoietic changes secondary to the aging process may correlate with this rise in erythropoietin in the aged and help account for the increased prevalence of anemia in this population. This also likely limits the ability of the older patient to compensate for insults caused by cytotoxic chemotherapy and is an important consideration for clinicians caring for this patient population. With aging, the number of hematopoietic progenitors remains intact[32]; however, the ability of animals and humans to replenish blood cells under times of stress appears diminished.[33–35] Baraldi-Junkins and colleagues showed impaired erythocytosis in response to anemia in a group of 40 anemic geriatric patients. Overall, they cited an age-related decline in hematopoietic reserve as the reason for this finding.[36] Aged animals and humans also appear to secrete less colony-stimulating agents such as erythropoietin and granulocyte colony-stimulating factor (G-CSF) and other growth cytokines in response to anemia and other stressors than do younger subjects, which complicates this scenario.[37]

The incidence of myelodysplastic syndrome (MDS) rises in the elderly as a consequence of cumulative DNA and cellular damage.[38,39] More subtle age-related changes may hamper the marrow response to anemia. IL-6, a cytokine that plays a role in mediating bone marrow resistance to erythropoietin, also becomes elevated as persons age and may contribute to aging-related anemia.[31] These findings solidify the argument that a latent defect of hematopoiesis may exist in the geriatric population and accounts for a portion of the increased prevalence of anemia in older populations. This also demonstrates that the etiology for poor hematopoietic reserve is multifactorial in origin. Regardless of the mechanism of anemia in older persons, it is paramount that oncologists be aware of the increased prevalence of anemia in the geriatric population and its impact on morbidity and mortality.

D. Morbidity and mortality of anemia among the geriatric population

Anemia has a significant physiologic impact on a number of organ systems and consequently correlates with a poorer quality of life and worse prognosis in the geriatric cancer patient. Overall quality of life (QOL), while often difficult to measure, is a major focus of oncologic care, particularly in elderly patients and those not treated with curative regimens.[40] Several authors have documented relatively lower QOL score in elderly patients with cancer as opposed to the general population.[41] Global QOL may correlate to overall functional status, whereas anemia has been shown to particularly worsen symptoms such as fatigue,[42] while other QOL parameters may be relatively maintained. Mancuso and colleagues found a significant correlation between development of anemia and lower functional and cognitive measures using the geriatric comprehensive assessment (GCA) tool in a group of patients aged over 70 years being treated for NSCLC.[43] Interestingly, these declines tended to reverse with improvement in anemia in individual patients. In elderly patients without cancer, anemia has been linked to increased falls,[44] physical decline,[45] objective muscle weakness,[46] increased resting heart rate,[47] and a predisposition to Alzheimer's disease,[48] among other effects. Patients consistently rate maintenance of QOL as one of the main goals of cancer treatment,[49] so it seems logical to focus on treatment of cancer and chemotherapy-related anemia to optimize the care of the older patient population.

The presence of anemia at the time of cancer diagnosis as well as development of anemia during chemotherapy or as a consequence of the disease has significant prognostic implications as well. The Rai,[50] Binet,[51] and Durie-Salmon[52] classifications directly link anemia with poor prognosis in well-known staging systems for chronic lymphocytic leukemia (CLL) and multiple myeloma, respectively. Additionally, anemia has been incorporated into prognostic models for Hodgkin's[53] and non-Hodgkin's lymphoma (NHL), and in one study, anemia was associated with a shorter duration of progression-free survival (PFS) across all NHL subtypes except marginal zone lymphoma.[54] Numerous studies also show a link between anemia and poor prognosis in solid tumors including NSCLC,[55] head and neck malignancies,[56] prostate adenocarcinoma,[57] transitional cell carcinoma,[58] renal cell carcinoma,[59] ovarian cancer,[60] and cancer of the cervix.[61] Data from these and other cohorts suggest that development of anemia has prognostic value independent of stage of disease in patients with malignancies. One comprehensive review that included over 60 such studies confirmed that

anemia (defined arbitrarily among studies with hemoglobin values from 8.5–14.0 gm/dL) was associated with significantly decreased survival times in the previously listed malignancies and further quantitated a 65 percent increased hazard of death across the 14 malignancies represented in the study.[62]

There are also concerns that anemia may abrogate the response of tumors to chemotherapy, radiation, or chemoradiotherapy. Oxygenation and the tumor response to hypoxia are very important aspects underlying the effectiveness of radiation on a pathophysiologic level, and so it makes sense that anemia may reduce the benefit of radiotherapy.[63] There is further evidence that development of anemia in patients undergoing treatment with radiation is a marker of poor outcome as there are data showing a worse treatment response in patients with cervical carcinoma[61] and head and neck cancer[56] among patients who developed anemia during their treatment course, as opposed to those who did not. Whether this poorer response is due to the anemia per se or whether anemia is serving as a marker of more aggressive disease or comorbidity has not been fully resolved.

Overall it is clear that the presence and development of anemia has important prognostic significance in patients with cancer and particularly in the geriatric population. Anemia also adversely affects QOL in this patient population and is an important consideration in the treatment of older cancer patients. Given these factors, clinicians have focused much attention on the use of recombinant human erythropoietin for correction of cancer-related anemia; recent research has defined the pleomorphic role of erythropoietin in maintaining homeostasis in diverse organ systems and has better defined the clinical applications for its usage.

E. Erythropoietin structure, function, and pharmacology

Erythropoietin is a 34 kDa glycoprotein hormone that controls red blood cell production in the bone marrow by acting on late erythroid progenitors (CFU-E). Interstitial peritubular cells in the kidney produce erythropoietin in response to hypoxemia.[64] Erythropoietin therefore serves as the principal regulator of erythropoiesis.[65] The cloning of erythropoietin in 1985 led to the development of recombinant pharmaceutical preparations that could then be used to increase reticulocytosis and reduce anemia.[66,67] Recombinant human erythropoietin (rhEPO) exists in several isoforms (most commonly erythropoietin alpha and beta as well as darbepoetin alpha). Collectively, these agents are known as ESAs.[68,69] Darbepoetin alpha is an isoform that is more heavily glycosylated than EPO-alpha and -beta; epoetins contain 3N- and 1 O-linked carbohydrate groups, whereas darbepoetin contains two additional N-glycosylated chains. No clinically significant difference has been observed among the three ESAs with regard to erythropoietic response when pharmacologically equivalent doses have been studied side by side. Epoetin-alpha and darbepoetin-alpha are approved for use in the United States, Canada, and Europe, whereas epoetin-beta is approved in Europe and Canada but not in the United States.

Epoetin-alpha (and -beta) has a half-life ($t_{1/2}$) of approximately 10 hours when injected intravenously (IV) and is not removed by hemodialysis; $t_{1/2}$ in end-stage renal disease (ESRD) patients is approximately 20 percent longer than in persons with intact renal function. High plasma levels are reached immediately with IV infusion; however, subcutaneous administration results in longer sustained response (with subcutaneous injection, peak levels are obtained after 5–24 hours). The extensive glycosylation of darbepoetin-alpha results in much slower subcutaneous absorption and a long $t_{1/2}$; peak levels occur 71–123 hours after subcutaneous administration in cancer patients, and the $t_{1/2}$ after IV administration is 21 hours. Erythropoietin and darbepoetin distribute strictly in the vascular compartment, and relatively small amounts (10–20%) are excreted through the urine. The underlying mechanism of the remainder of erythropoietin metabolism is unknown.

A clear dose-response relationship is seen with administration of EPO-alpha and EPO-beta with doses 50–300 U/kg three times weekly, and a greater response to EPO is generally not seen with doses over 300 U/kg three times weekly. These agents are both dosed at an initial dose of 150 U/kg or 40,000 U weekly for anemia associated with solid malignancies, and the dose may be increased to 300 U/kg three times weekly or 60,000 U weekly if the hemoglobin does not rise by more than 1 gm/dL after 4 weeks and if the hemoglobin concentration is not sufficient to avoid red blood cell transfusion. Similar dosage schemes have been used for anemia associated with myelodysplastic syndromes.[70]

Darbepoetin-alpha has similar indications to other rhEPO agents and is dosed based on pharmacologically equivalent dosage schemes similar to the regimens described earlier. The clinical activity of darbepoetin-alpha is similar to EPO-alpha and EPO-beta when dosed at a 260:1 ratio (1 mg darbepoetin per 260 U EPO by Medicare payment guidelines). Three resultant darbepoetin-alpha dosage schemes utilizing different intervals have been evaluated as treatment for cancer-associated and chemotherapy-associated anemia: 2.25 mcg/kg subcutaneously once weekly,[71] 200 mcg subcutaneously once every 2 weeks weeks,[72] and 6.75 mcg/kg subcutaneously once every 3 weeks.[73] Similar dosage adjustments are advised to bring hemoglobin to a range (usually 10–12 gm/dL) that will avoid transfusion, with a decrease in the dose once the target hemoglobin is achieved.

Side effects, including hypertension, headaches, seizures, and pure red cell aplasia, associated with ESA administration have been documented, largely in the ESRD population. Pure red cell aplasia associated with ESAs appears to be due to a formulation issue leading to the development of antierythropoietin antibodies that has been resolved.[74] ESAs may be associated with a flulike illness on initiation and may also cause an injection site reaction as well as other side effects such as dizziness, cough, peripheral edema, and fatigue. Overall, these agents are generally well tolerated, and the percentage of patients who discontinue these medications because of adverse events is low.

Given that pharmacologically equivalent dosages of ESAs are clinically equivalent, the decision to use a particular agent may depend on clinician preference, patient characteristics, and considerations regarding cost-effectiveness.[75]

F. Use of erythropoiesis-stimulating agents (ESAs) in cancer- and chemotherapy-associated anemia

Since ESAs were approved for use to decrease transfusion requirements in patients receiving chemotherapy for cancer in 1993 by the U.S. Food and Drug Administration (FDA), a number of clinical trials have attempted to determine the effect these agents have on lowering transfusion requirements, improving QOL, and lengthening survival. Early optimism regarding ESAs for cancer-associated anemia has been tempered by more recent data suggesting possible harm associated with their use, particularly when treating to high hemoglobin targets. These data prompted a change to the drugs' labeling to include the FDA's 2007 black-box warning concerning ESAs and increased risk of venous thromboembolic events (VTE) and mortality risks. Given these concerns, it is important that the geriatric oncologist understand the evidence regarding the rationale for ESA use in cancer-related anemia and gain an appreciation for possible future directions regarding these drugs.

Most early studies of rhEPO used reduction in number of red blood cell transfusions as the primary end point. It became clear from these trials that ESAs reduce transfusion requirements in cancer patients significantly. A 2001 meta-analysis by Seidenfeld and colleagues showed an odds ratio (OR) of requiring transfusion of 0.38 across 22 clinical trials involving rhEPO utilized in cancer-related anemia when therapy is initiated at hemoglobin values below 10 gm/dL.[76] These studies were not designed to detect mortality differences between strategies involving rhEPO versus transfusion, nor did they fully address possible QOL differences. Though more than a dozen further trials have addressed QOL with ESA administration, there is still controversy regarding the impact of ESAs in QOL. There are a number of reasons for this, including employment of heterogeneous QOL measures, incomplete reporting of QOL metrics, and the inherent difficulties in quantifying QOL outcomes. When assessed with standard QOL measurement tools such as the FACT scale,[77] there was no significant difference in QOL between rhEPO and transfusion-based strategies for management of cancer-associated anemia, although this trended toward improved QOL for ESAs in two different meta-analyses.[76,78] Individual trials have documented QOL benefits with ESA use in chemotherapy-associated anemia in older persons[79–81] as well as anemia associated with aging.[79,82–84] As we learn more about the effects of ESAs on cancer patients with anemia, future clinical trials focusing on QOL measures in specific situations (e.g., for anemia associated with individual malignancies or particular chemotherapeutic regimens) may become important in defining the role of these agents in patients more prone to morbid outcomes from anemia such as the aged.

G. ESAs and impact on survival in patients with cancer

Recent trials designed to analyze the effect of ESAs on cancer progression and mortality have shown possible deleterious effects on survival and possibly increased risks for adverse events such as VTE, cardiovascular events, and increased tumor progression in cancer patients treated with ESA. Studies showing adverse events in noncancer patients point toward increased risk of cardiovascular disease and thrombotic disorders separate from risk associated with tumor effects. As early as 1998, data from the nephrology literature suggested a possible hypercoagulable state associated with ESA use. A trial involving 1,233 hemodialysis-dependent ESRD patients was halted early when increased mortality in the normal hematocrit (hematocrit levels of 42 ± 3% vs. 30 ± 3%) arm was noted.[85] Increased thrombosis of dialysis vascular access was also noted in this study among the higher hematocrit group, and other studies have suggested a similar correlation to EPO use and thrombotic events in this population.[85] Two further studies, the Correction of Hemoglobin and Outcomes in Renal Insufficiency (CHOIR) trial[86] and the Cardiovascular Risk Reduction by Early Anemia Treatment with Epoetin-beta (CREATE) trial,[87] showed increases in mortality or cardiovascular events and VTE, respectively, among hemodialysis patients treated to normal hemoglobin levels. In the CHOIR study, there was a hazard ratio (HR) of 1.48 for all-cause mortality among patients randomized to higher hemoglobin values (13.5 gm/dL vs. 11.3 gm/dL); however, this difference was not significantly different from the lower-hemoglobin group ($p = .07$).[86]

Recent clinical data involving patients with cancer- and chemotherapy-related anemia have shown similar adverse effects associated with ESA use in cancer patients and point toward specific effects of ESAs on tumor progression. Since 2003, eight randomized controlled trials (RCTs) have noted similar increases in VTE and/or mortality in patients treated with ESAs for cancer-related anemia. The ENHANCE trial enrolled 351 anemic patients with head and neck cancer and randomized them to treatment with epoetin-beta 300 U/kg or placebo while undergoing curative radiotherapy regimens.[88] Locoregional progression was worse with epoetin-beta than placebo (relative risk [RR] 1.62), and overall survival (OS) was worse (RR 1.39). Increased vascular events (including VTE) were also increased in the epoetin-beta group, and more patients in the treatment group died because of cardiovascular disease.[88] In the Breast Cancer Erythropoietin Trial (BEST) reported by Leyland-Jones in 2005, 939 women with metastatic breast cancer were randomized to treatment with epoetin-alpha versus placebo if the hemoglobin fell to below 13 gm/dL. The study was stopped early because of higher mortality in the epoetin-alpha group (12-month OS 70% vs. 76% in ESA vs. placebo arm, respectively). Time to disease progression was similar in both groups, although there was an increased early risk of death from cancer in the ESA group, suggesting progression of disease associated with epoetin-alpha.[89] Other studies involving patients undergoing treatment for head and neck cancer,[90] cervix cancer,[91] and NSCLC[92] have either been halted early because of increased interim mortality or adverse events or have shown unfavorable results in the ESA arms at completion. A study involving 989 patients with diverse malignancies not undergoing chemotherapy or radiation treatment that randomized patients to darbepoetin 6.75 mcg/kg every fourth week or placebo found no statistically significant difference in transfusion requirements but did document poorer survival in the darbepoetin arm.[93] Furthermore, a large meta-analysis from Bennett and colleagues including 4,610 patients with cancer treated in RCTs with ESAs versus placebo revealed a RR of 1.57 for VTE development and found a significant increase in the risk of mortality (HR 1.10) for patients treated with ESAs.[94] Other systematic reviews from 2006 and 2007 confirmed a significantly increased risk of VTE in cancer patients treated with ESAs and trends toward increased mortality that were not statistically significant.[95,96]

This emerging data led the FDA to declare a black-box warning regarding ESAs and the risk of VTE and death in cancer patients. Clinicians have been warned by the FDA to maintain hemoglobin levels as low as possible with these agents and not to exceed hemoglobin values of more than 12 gm/dL when using ESAs. The FDA has stated that ESAs should be avoided when cancer is being treated with curative regimens given the preceding data. Overall, these trials and the resultant FDA warning have led to significant changes in the clinical usage of ESAs in the past few years. There is clearly a great deal still to learn regarding the pathophysiology of these agents as the mechanisms underlying the increased mortality associated with ESA use are unknown; whether ESA usage in specific malignancies or in specific situations is appropriate is also an unanswered question. Many of the preceding trials have been criticized for unbalanced randomization and for targeting excessively high hemoglobin targets or treating patients with ESAs empirically while dis-

regarding hemoglobin values. Most of the aforementioned RCTs targeted hemoglobin values in the range of 13–14 gm/dL, which is well above the usual target value, which may account for the increase in mortality seen in these studies. It is unclear if ESAs affect mortality when used to target lower hemoglobin values of approximately 10–11 gm/dL, similar to the lower thresholds used in the CHOIR trial as opposed to higher values. Other data analysis suggests that there is no negative survival impact associated with attaining high hemoglobin values; rather, the adverse events tend to occur in patients unable to attain higher hemoglobin values while receiving high doses of ESAs.[97] This suggests either a toxic effect from excessive doses of ESAs or that the patients unable to achieve higher hemoglobin levels simply have a poorer outcome. More prospective studies are needed to fully delineate this relationship of morbidity/mortality with ESA dosing and hemoglobin levels.

H. Biology of erythropoietin receptors

These studies do emphasize the need to consider the pleomorphic effects of ESAs on cancer patients. Erythropoietin has effects on diverse organ systems throughout the body, including the immune system, the vascular compartment, and the central nervous system. Erythropoietin receptors (EpoR) are present on erythroid cells,[98] megakaryocytes,[99] endothelial cells,[100] and some neuronal cells.[101] EpoR belongs to the cytokine family of receptors and signals intracellularly through Jak2 tyrosine kinases activated after erythropoietin binding and EpoR dimerization.[102] Signaling then occurs through the PI-3/Akt,[103] Ras/MAP,[104] and STAT pathways,[105,106] which have considerable overlap with cellular machinery necessary for proliferation and antiapoptosis. It is then intuitive that EpoR signaling could be linked to cancer cell proliferation and invasion given these properties. EpoR mRNA transcripts have been found within cancer cells in cell cultures[107,108]; however, in vitro ligand studies using monoclonal antibodies have shown variable expression within these cell lines and have not documented the quantities of EpoR thought to be sufficient for triggering proliferation in these models.[109] Immunohistochemical assays on patient tumor samples have shown binding to EpoR antibodies[110]; however, there are concerns that cross-reactivity to heat shock proteins exists and that these reagents exist.[111] It is also unclear if EpoR mRNA quantification directly correlates to proliferation signaling on the cellular level as EpoRs may serve diverse purposes within tumor cells. Preclinical studies involving animal models have found varying effects on cellular proliferation,[112] tumor invasion,[113] and chemoradiotherapy sensitivity,[114] although these models are limited by significant physiological side effects associated with ESA administration as well as other difficulties with animal models. Other studies involving ESAs in cell culture models have documented enhanced proliferation[115] and antiapoptotic signaling[116] in models of various solid tumor types. Alternatively, some groups have postulated that increased oxygenation related to rhEPO may decrease production of tumor cytokines and angiogenesis through downregulation of hypoxia-inducible factor-1 (HIF-1) and other mechanisms.[117]

Erythropoietin contributes to thrombosis, likely through multiple effects. Reports link rhEPO to increased platelet aggregation[118] and decreased protein C concentrations.[119] Increased blood viscosity associated with higher hemoglobin values may also contribute to this effect; however, clinical studies have disputed the link between hemoglobin level and thrombosis in hemodialysis patients. Endothelial proliferative effects may also play a role in cardiovascular effects of ESAs, but the exact mechanism of this effect is unclear.[120]

Cellular signaling mechanisms at the receptor level may explain the adverse events associated with ESAs in patients with cancer seen in recent clinical trials. However, more data at the clinical and basic science level are needed to better define the role of EpoR signaling with regard to the increase in mortality and cancer progression.

I. Positive ESA clinical studies

Though concerns have been raised, it is important also to consider specific indications for ESA use with a positive risk-benefit for cancer-associated anemia that may be applicable in the geriatric population. ESAs have been used to treat the anemia associated with myelodysplastic syndromes, a disease predominantly of the elderly. Since the early 1990s, more than 50 clinical trials involving epoetin and darbepoetin have been published, and a 2008 meta-analysis showed approximately 60 percent erythroid response rates with these agents and no significant difference with regard to epoetin versus darbepoetin.[121] A clin-ical trial involving 358 MDS patients treated with either G-CSF and erythropoietin or placebo revealed improved survival (HR 0.6 after approximately 14-year follow-up) among G-CSF/ESA-treated patients, particularly in patients needing relatively few red blood cell transfusions (less than two per month).[122] MDS patients with lower erythropoietin levels tend to have a more robust response to treatment with rhEPO, and current NCCN guidelines[123] call for ESA treatment in MDS patients with symptomatic anemia who have EPO levels of under 500 mU/mL.

A trial involving anemic patients with small-cell lung cancer, with an average of greater than 60, beginning chemotherapy also showed a possible role for ESAs in this patient group. Grote and colleagues randomized 224 patients with hemoglobin less than 14.5 gm/dL to epoetin-alpha 150 U/kg or placebo three times weekly prior to initiating chemotherapy for small-cell lung cancer and found similar OS and rates of tumor response. There were significantly fewer transfusions in the ESA arm for this trial, and patients randomized to epoetin had significantly higher hemoglobin levels.[124] This suggests that there may be specific tumor types or chemotherapy regimens for which ESAs are particularly well suited and may not have deleterious effects on survival or tumor progression while helping to avoid cancer-related and chemotherapy-related anemia.

These studies also show that it is very important to critically appraise the recent studies showing worsened mortality with ESA use. Critics have pointed out a number of problems with using these data to assume increased mortality with ESA use in current practice. First, these trials either used ESAs empirically or targeted hemoglobin values much higher than advised in the drug packaging or than has been FDA approved. Heterogeneous and unbalanced patient groups may also cloud the picture. It is also unknown if rhEPO dose plays a role as there has been a suggestion in other trials that adverse effects may be increased at higher ESA doses; patients with poor responses to ESAs initially may thus be exposed to higher doses of these medications and potentially higher VTE or cancer progression risk. Overall, we do not know if these agents are cost-effective or decrease morbidity/mortality when used in more conservative schemes that focus on achieving lower hemoglobin goals and avoidance of transfusions. Since red blood cell transfusion carries its own accompanying risk, including increased risk of VTE, it is unknown what transfusion strategy is best in this situation. Future studies in specific patient populations will be needed to define the role of ESAs in supportive oncologic care in the future, and clinicians should be cautious concerning their use currently, given the possibility of adverse effects, until more studies of this nature are completed.

There are a paucity of data regarding the specific use of ESAs in older populations. Some authors report decreased responsiveness to rhEPO in the aged, while there are small clinical trials that show excellent hemoglobin increases and anecdotal clinical responses to ESAs in this population, particularly in frail patients with underlying comorbidities. Most of the trials involving ESAs in cancer patients have included a large proportion of elderly patients given the high prevalence of cancer and anemia in this group, and so it is assumed that similar risk-benefit ratios are likely to exist in the geriatric cancer population. More clinical trials are needed, however, to better guide clinicians with regard to the use of these agents as the frailty and relative increase in comorbid conditions in the aged cancer patient population may represent a situation where ESAs have a significant impact on morbidity/mortality.

J. Conclusions

The geriatric cancer population has a higher prevalence of anemia related to multiple factors, including possible erythropoietin resistance and reduced bone marrow reserve associated with aging. Anemia has been associated with increased morbidity/mortality risks. In the treatment of chemotherapy-induced anemia, ESAs reduce the adverse effects of anemia in this population by reducing transfusion and potentially improving QOL. However, clinical data recently suggested adverse effects on cancer progression and VTE risk, particularly at high hemoglobin targets. Currently clinicians should use these agents according to practice guidelines, with more conservative targets of a hemoglobin of 10 gm/dL. Treatment is not recommended in the setting of ongoing treatment with a curative cure with chemotherapy, or in the palliative setting in the treatment of cancer-related anemia in the absence of chemotherapy. Further studies are needed to more clearly define the use of ESAs in the aged population as well as in specific clinical situations where anemia predisposes patients to especially high morbidity/mortality risks.

References

1. Guralnik JM, Eisenstaedt RS, Ferrucci L, et al. Prevalence of anemia in persons 65 years and older in the United States: evidence for a high rate of unexplained anemia. *Blood*. 2004;104(8):2263–2268.

2. Salive ME, Cornoni-Huntley J, Guralnik JM, et al. Anemia and hemoglobin levels in older persons: relationship with age, gender, and health status. *J Am Geriatr Soc*. 1992;40(5):489–496.

3. Ania BJ, Suman VJ, Fairbanks VF, et al. Prevalence of anemia in medical practice: community versus referral patients. *Mayo Clin Proc*. 1994;69(8):730–735.

4. Joosten E, Pelemans W, Hiele M, et al. Prevalence and causes of anaemia in a geriatric hospitalized population. *Gerontology*. 1992;38(1–2):111–117.

5. Ania BJ, Suman VJ, Fairbanks VF, et al. Incidence of anemia in older people: an epidemiologic study in a well defined population. *J Am Geriatr Soc*. 1997;45(7):825–831.

6. Nilsson-Ehle H, Jagenburg R, Landahl S, et al. Haematological abnormalities and reference intervals in the elderly: a cross-sectional comparative study of three urban Swedish population samples aged 70, 75 and 81 years. *Acta Med Scand*. 1988;224(6):595–604.

7. Artz AS, Fergusson D, Drinka PJ, et al. Mechanisms of unexplained anemia in the nursing home. *J Am Geriatr Soc*. 2004;52(3):423–427.

8. Coiffier B, Guastalla JP, Pujade-Lauraine E, et al. Anemia Study Group. Predicting cancer-associated anaemia in patients receiving non-platinum chemotherapy: results of a retrospective survey. *Eur J Cancer*. 2001;37(13):1617–1623.

9. Kyle RA. Multiple myeloma: review of 869 cases. *Mayo Clin Proc*. 1975;50(1):29–40.

10. Bokemeyer C, Oechsle K, Hartmann JT. Anaemia in cancer patients: pathophysiology, incidence and treatment. *Eur J Clin Invest*. 2005;35(suppl 3):26–31.

11. Dainiak N, Kulkarni V, Howard D, et al. Mechanisms of abnormal erythropoiesis in malignancy. *Cancer*. 1983;51(6):1101–1106.

12. Hamblin TJ, Orchard JA, Myint H, et al. Fludarabine and hemolytic anemia in chronic lymphocytic leukemia. *J Clin Oncol*. 1998;16(9):3209–3210.

13. Rytting M, Worth L, Jaffe N. Hemolytic disorders associated with cancer. *Hematol Oncol Clin North Am*. 1996;10(2):365–376.

14. Ludwig H, Fritz E. Anemia in cancer patients. *Semin Oncol*. 1998;25(3 suppl 7):2–6.

15. Skillings JR, Sridhar FG, Wong C, et al. The frequency of red cell transfusion for anemia in patients receiving chemotherapy: a retrospective cohort study. *Am J Clin Oncol*. 1993;16(1):22–25.

16. Pirker R, Krajnik G, Zochbauer S, et al. Paclitaxel/cisplatin in advanced non-small-cell lung cancer (NSCLC). *Ann Oncol*. 1995;6(8):833–835.

17. Dalton JD, Bailey NP, Barrett-Lee PJ, et al. Multicenter UK audit of anemia in patients receiving cytotoxic. *Proc Am Soc Clin Oncol*. 1998;17:418a.

18. Hensley ML, Lebeau D, Leon LF, et al. Identification of risk factors for requiring transfusion during front-line chemotherapy for ovarian cancer. *Gynecol Oncol*. 2001;81(3):485–489.

19. Pivot X, Guardiola E, Etienne M, et al. An analysis of potential factors allowing an individual prediction of cisplatin-induced anaemia. *Eur J Cancer*. 2000;36(7):852–857.

20. Wiltshaw E, Kroner T. Phase II study of cis-dichlorodiammineplatinum(II) (NSC-119875) in advanced adenocarcinoma of the ovary. *Cancer Treat Rep*. 1976;60(1):55–60.

21. Rossof AH, Slayton RE, Perlia CP. Preliminary clinical experience with cis-diamminedichloro-platinum (II) (NSC 119875, CACP). *Cancer*. 1972;30(6):1451–1456.

22. Wood PA, Hrushesky WJ. Cisplatin-associated anemia: an erythropoietin deficiency syndrome. *J Clin Invest*. 1995;95(4):1650–1659.

23. Ahn SH, Garewal HS. Low erythropoietin level can cause anemia in patients without advanced renal failure. *Am J Med*. 2004;116(4):280–281.

24. Coskun HS, Yilmaz O, Alanoglu G, et al. Chemotherapy-associated anemia in solid tumors patients from Anatolia. *Proc Am Soc Clin Oncol*. 2005;23(16S):8257.

25. Barrett-Lee PJ, Ludwig H, Birgegard G, et al. Independent risk factors for anemia in cancer patients receiving chemotherapy: results from the European Cancer Anaemia Survey. *Oncology*. 2006;70(1):34–48.

26. Vincent M, Dranitsaris G, Clemons M, et al. The development of a prediction tool for chemotherapy-induced anemia in patients with advanced non-small cell lung cancer (NSCLC) palliative receiving chemotherapy [abstract]. *J Clin Oncol Meet Abstr*. 2006;24(18 suppl): 8600.

27. Du XL, Osborne C, Goodwin JS. Population-based assessment of hospitalizations for toxicity from chemotherapy in older women with breast cancer. *J Clin Oncol*. 2002;20(24):4636–4642.

28. Kario K, Matsuo T, Nakao K. Serum erythropoietin levels in the elderly. *Gerontology*. 1991;37(6):345–348.

29. Joosten E, Van Hove L, Lesaffre E, et al. Serum erythropoietin levels in elderly inpatients with anemia of chronic disorders and iron deficiency anemia. *J Am Geriatr Soc.* 1993;41(12):1301–1304.

30. Matsuo T, Kario K, Kodoma K, et al. An inappropriate erythropoietic response to iron deficiency anaemia in the elderly. *Clin Lab Haematol.* 1995;17(4):317–321.

31. Ershler WB, Sheng S, McKelvey J, et al. Serum erythropoietin and aging: a longitudinal analysis. *J Am Geriatr Soc.* 2005;53(8):1360–1365.

32. Lipschitz DA, Udupa KB, Milton KY, et al. Effect of age on hematopoiesis in man. *Blood.* 1984;63(3):502–509.

33. Rothstein G. Disordered hematopoiesis and myelodysplasia in the elderly. *J Am Geriatr Soc.* 2003;51(3 suppl):S22–S26.

34. Boggs DR, Patrene KD. Hematopoiesis and aging III: anemia and a blunted erythropoietic response to hemorrhage in aged mice. *Am J Hematol.* 1985;19(4):327–338.

35. Rothstein G, Christensen RD, Nielsen BR. Kinetic evaluation of the pool sizes and proliferative response of neutrophils in bacterially challenged aging mice. *Blood.* 1987;70(6):1836–1841.

36. Baraldi-Junkins CA, Beck AC, Rothstein G. Hematopoiesis and cytokines: relevance to cancer and aging. *Hematol Oncol Clin North Am.* 2000;14(1):45–61.

37. Buchanan JP, Peters CA, Rasmussen CJ, et al. Impaired expression of hematopoietic growth factors: a candidate mechanism for the hematopoietic defect of aging. *Exp Gerontol.* 1996;31(1–2):135–144.

38. Aul C, Gattermann N, Schneider W. Age-related incidence and other epidemiological aspects of myelodysplastic syndromes. *Br J Haematol.* 1992;82(2):358–367.

39. Quesnel B, Guillerm G, Vereecque R, et al. Methylation of the p15(INK4b) gene in myelodysplastic syndromes is frequent and acquired during disease progression. *Blood.* 1998;91(8):2985–2990.

40. Bottomley A, Vanvoorden V, Flechtner H, et al. EORTC Quality of Life Group EORTC Data Center. The challenges and achievements involved in implementing quality of life research in cancer clinical trials. *Eur J Cancer.* 2003;39(3):275–285.

41. Boogaerts M, Coiffier B, Kainz C. Epoetin beta QOL Working Group. Impact of epoetin beta on quality of life in patients with malignant disease. *Br J Cancer.* 2003;88(7):988–995.

42. Wedding U, Rohrig B, Pientka L, et al. Anaemia-related impairment in quality of life in elderly cancer patients prior to chemotherapy. *J Cancer Res Clin Oncol.* 2007;133(5):279–286.

43. Mancuso A, Migliorino M, De Santis S, et al. Correlation between anemia and functional/cognitive capacity in elderly lung cancer patients treated with chemotherapy. *Ann Oncol.* 2006;17(1):146–150.

44. Penninx BW, Pluijm SM, Lips P, et al. Late-life anemia is associated with increased risk of recurrent falls. *J Am Geriatr Soc.* 2005;53(12):2106–2111.

45. Penninx BW, Guralnik JM, Onder G, et al. Anemia and decline in physical performance among older persons. *Am J Med.* 2003;115(2):104–110.

46. Chaves PH, Ashar B, Guralnik JM, et al. Looking at the relationship between hemoglobin concentration and prevalent mobility difficulty in older women: should the criteria currently used to define anemia in older people be reevaluated? *J Am Geriatr Soc.* 2002;50(7):1257–1264.

47. Wu WC, Rathore SS, Wang Y, et al. Blood transfusion in elderly patients with acute myocardial infarction. *N Engl J Med.* 2001;345(17):1230–1236.

48. Beard CM, Kokmen E, O'Brien PC, et al. Risk of Alzheimer's disease among elderly patients with anemia: population-based investigations in Olmsted County, Minnesota. *Ann Epidemiol.* 1997;7(3):219–224.

49. Pinquart M, Duberstein PR. Information needs and decision-making processes in older cancer patients. *Crit Rev Oncol Hematol.* 2004;51(1):69–80.

50. Rai KR, Sawitsky A, Cronkite EP, et al. Clinical staging of chronic lymphocytic leukemia. *Blood.* 1975;46(2):219–234.

51. Binet JL, Auquier A, Dighiero G, et al. A new prognostic classification of chronic lymphocytic leukemia derived from a multivariate survival analysis. *Cancer.* 1981;48(1):198–206.

52. Durie BG, Salmon SE. A clinical staging system for multiple myeloma: correlation of measured myeloma cell mass with presenting clinical features, response to treatment, and survival. *Cancer.* 1975;36(3):842–854.

53. Gobbi PG, Zinzani PL, Broglia C, et al. Comparison of prognostic models in patients with advanced Hodgkin disease: promising results from integration of the best three systems. *Cancer.* 2001;91(8):1467–1478.

54. Moullet I, Salles G, Ketterer N, et al. Frequency and significance of anemia in non-Hodgkin's lymphoma patients. *Ann Oncol.* 1998;9(10):1109–1115.

55. Wigren T, Oksanen H, Kellokumpu-Lehtinen P. A practical prognostic index for inoperable non-small-cell lung cancer. *J Cancer Res Clin Oncol.* 1997;123(5):259–266.

56. Lee WR, Berkey B, Marcial V, et al. Anemia is associated with decreased survival and increased locoregional failure in patients with locally advanced head and neck carcinoma: a secondary analysis of RTOG 85–27. *Int J Radiat Oncol Biol Phys.* 1998;42(5):1069–1075.

57. Berry WR, Laszlo J, Cox E, et al. Prognostic factors in metastatic and hormonally unresponsive carcinoma of the prostate. *Cancer.* 1979;44(2):763–775.

58. Gospodarowicz MK, Hawkins NV, Rawlings GA, et al. Radical radiotherapy for muscle invasive transitional cell carcinoma of the bladder: failure analysis. *J Urol.* 1989;142(6):1448–1453; discussion 1453–1454.

59. Citterio G, Bertuzzi A, Tresoldi M, et al. Prognostic factors for survival in metastatic renal cell carcinoma: retrospective analysis from 109 consecutive patients. *Eur Urol.* 1997;31(3):286–291.

60. Obermair A, Handisurya A, Kaider A, et al. The relationship of pretreatment serum hemoglobin level to the survival of epithelial ovarian carcinoma patients: a prospective review. *Cancer.* 1998;83(4):726–731.

61. Pedersen D, Sogaard H, Overgaard J, et al. Prognostic value of pretreatment factors in patients with locally advanced carcinoma of the uterine cervix treated by radiotherapy alone. *Acta Oncol.* 1995;34(6):787–795.

62. Caro JJ, Salas M, Ward A, et al. Anemia as an independent prognostic factor for survival in patients with cancer: a systemic, quantitative review. *Cancer.* 2001;91(12):2214–2221.

63. Harrison LB, Shasha D, Homel P. Prevalence of anemia in cancer patients undergoing radiotherapy: prognostic significance and treatment. *Oncology.* 2002;63(suppl 2):11–18.

64. Lacombe C, Da Silva JL, Bruneval P, et al. Peritubular cells are the site of erythropoietin synthesis in the murine hypoxic kidney. *J Clin Invest.* 1988;81(2):620–623.

65. Krantz SB. Erythropoietin. *Blood.* 1991;77(3):419–434.

66. Jacobs K, Shoemaker C, Rudersdorf R, et al. Isolation and characterization of genomic and cDNA clones of human erythropoietin. *Nature.* 1985;313(6005):806–810.

67. Lin FK, Suggs S, Lin CH, et al. Cloning and expression of the human erythropoietin gene. *Proc Natl Acad Sci U S A.* 1985;82(22):7580–7584.

68. Storring PL, Tiplady RJ, Gaines Das RE, et al. Epoetin alfa and beta differ in their erythropoietin isoform compositions and biological properties. *Br J Haematol.* 1998;100(1):79–89.

69. Macdougall IC, Gray SJ, Elston O, et al. Pharmacokinetics of novel erythropoiesis stimulating protein compared with epoetin alfa in dialysis patients. *J Am Soc Nephrol.* 1999;10(11):2392–2395.

70. Rizzo JD, Somerfield MR, Hagerty KL, et al. Use of epoetin and darbepoetin in patients with cancer: 2007 American Society of Hematology/American Society of Clinical Oncology clinical practice guideline update. *Blood.* 2008;111(1):25–41.

71. Vansteenkiste J, Pirker R, Massuti B, et al. Double-blind, placebo-controlled, randomized phase III trial of darbepoetin alfa in lung cancer patients receiving chemotherapy. *J Natl Cancer Inst.* 2002;94(16):1211–1220.

72. Schwartzberg LS, Yee LK, Senecal FM, et al. A randomized comparison of every-2-week darbepoetin alfa and weekly epoetin alfa for the treatment of chemotherapy-induced anemia in patients with breast, lung, or gynecologic cancer. *Oncologist.* 2004;9(6):696–707.

73. Kotasek D, Steger G, Faught W, et al. Darbepoetin alfa administered every 3 weeks alleviates anaemia in patients with solid tumours receiving chemotherapy; results of a double-blind, placebo-controlled, randomised study. *Eur J Cancer.* 2003;39(14):2026–2034.

74. Bennett CL, Luminari S, Nissenson AR, et al. Pure red-cell aplasia and epoetin therapy. *N Engl J Med.* 2004;351(14):1403–1408.

75. Ben-Hamadi R, Duh MS, Aggarwal J, et al. The cost-effectiveness of weekly epoetin alfa relative to weekly darbepoetin alfa in patients with chemotherapy-induced anemia. *Curr Med Res Opin.* 2005;21(10):1677–1682.

76. Seidenfeld J, Piper M, Flamm C, et al. Epoetin treatment of anemia associated with cancer therapy: a systematic review and meta-analysis of controlled clinical trials. *J Natl Cancer Inst.* 2001;93(16):1204–1214.

77. Yellen SB, Cella DF, Webster K, et al. Measuring fatigue and other anemia-related symptoms with the Functional Assessment of Cancer Therapy (FACT) measurement system. *J Pain Symptom Manage.* 1997;13(2):63–74.

78. Bohlius J, Wilson J, Seidenfeld J, et al. Recombinant human erythropoietins and cancer patients: updated meta-analysis of 57 studies including 9353 patients. *J Natl Cancer Inst.* 2006;98(10):708–714.

79. Aapro MS, Dale DC, Blasi M, et al. Epoetin alfa increases hemoglobin levels and improves quality of life in anemic geriatric cancer patients receiving chemotherapy. *Support Care Cancer.* 2006;14(12):1184–1194.

80. Boccia R, Lillie T, Tomita D, et al. The effectiveness of darbepoetin alfa administered every 3 weeks on hematologic outcomes and quality of life in older patients with

chemotherapy-induced anemia. *Oncologist.* 2007;12(5):584–593.

81. Cascinu S, Del Ferro E, Fedeli A, et al. Recombinant human erythropoietin treatment in elderly cancer patients with cisplatin-associated anemia. *Oncology.* 1995;52(5):422–426.

82. Agnihotri P, Telfer M, Butt Z, et al. Chronic anemia and fatigue in elderly patients: results of a randomized, double-blind, placebo-controlled, crossover exploratory study with epoetin alfa. *J Am Geriatr Soc.* 2007;55(10):1557–1565.

83. Ershler WB, Artz AS, Kandahari MM. Recombinant erythropoietin treatment of anemia in older adults. *J Am Geriatr Soc.* 2001;49(10):1396–1397.

84. Moreno F, Aracil FJ, Perez R, et al. Controlled study on the improvement of quality of life in elderly hemodialysis patients after correcting end-stage renal disease-related anemia with erythropoietin. *Am J Kidney Dis.* 1996;27(4):548–556.

85. Besarab A, Bolton WK, Browne JK, et al. The effects of normal as compared with low hematocrit values in patients with cardiac disease who are receiving hemodialysis and epoetin. *N Engl J Med.* 1998;339(9):584–590.

86. Singh AK, Szczech L, Tang KL, et al. Correction of anemia with epoetin alfa in chronic kidney disease. *N Engl J Med.* 2006;355(20):2085–2098.

87. Drueke TB, Locatelli F, Clyne N, et al. Normalization of hemoglobin level in patients with chronic kidney disease and anemia. *N Engl J Med.* 2006;355(20):2071–2084.

88. Henke M, Laszig R, Rube C, et al. Erythropoietin to treat head and neck cancer patients with anaemia undergoing radiotherapy: randomised, double-blind, placebo-controlled trial. *Lancet.* 2003;362(9392):1255–1260.

89. Leyland-Jones B, Semiglazov V, Pawlicki M, et al. Maintaining normal hemoglobin levels with epoetin alfa in mainly nonanemic patients with metastatic breast cancer receiving first-line chemotherapy: a survival study. *J Clin Oncol.* 2005;23(25):5960–5972.

90. Overgaard J, Hoff C, Sand HH, et al. Randomized study of the importance of novel erythropoiesis stimulating protein (Aranesp) for the effect of radiotherapy in patients with primary squamous cell carcinoma of the head and neck (HNSCC) – the Danish Head and Neck Cancer Group DAHANCA 10 randomized trial. *Eur J Cancer.* 2007;5(suppl):7.

91. Thomas G, Ali S, Hoebers FJ, et al. Phase III trial to evaluate the efficacy of maintaining hemoglobin levels above 12.0 g/dL with erythropoietin vs above 10.0 g/dL without erythropoietin in anemic patients receiving concurrent radiation and cisplatin for cervical cancer. *Gynecol Oncol.* 2008;108(2):317–325.

92. Wright JR, Ung YC, Julian JA, et al. Randomized, double-blind, placebo-controlled trial of erythropoietin in non-small-cell lung cancer with disease-related anemia. *J Clin Oncol.* 2007;25(9):1027–1032.

93. Smith Jr RE, Aapro MS, Ludwig H, et al. Darbepoetin alpha for the treatment of anemia in patients with active cancer not receiving chemotherapy or radiotherapy: results of a phase III, multicenter, randomized, double-blind, placebo-controlled study. *J Clin Oncol.* 2008;26(7):1040–1050.

94. Bennett CL, Silver SM, Djulbegovic B, et al. Venous thromboembolism and mortality associated with recombinant erythropoietin and darbepoetin administration for the treatment of cancer-associated anemia. *J Am Med Assoc.* 2008;299(8):914–924.

95. Wilson J, Yao GL, Raftery J, et al. A systematic review and economic evaluation of epoetin alpha, epoetin beta and darbepoetin alpha in anaemia associated with cancer, especially that attributable to cancer treatment. *Health Technol Assess.* 2007;11(13):1–202.

96. Rizzo JD, Somerfield MR, Hagerty KL, et al. Use of epoetin and darbepoetin in patients with cancer: 2007 American Society of Clinical Oncology/American Society of Hematology clinical practice guideline update. *J Clin Oncol.* 2008;26(1):132–149.

97. Szczech LA, Barnhart HX, Inrig JK, et al. Secondary analysis of the CHOIR trial epoetin-alpha dose and achieved hemoglobin outcomes. *Kidney Int.* 2008;74(6):791–798.

98. Broudy VC, Lin N, Brice M, et al. Erythropoietin receptor characteristics on primary human erythroid cells. *Blood.* 1991;77(12):2583–2590.

99. Fraser JK, Tan AS, Lin FK, et al. Expression of specific high-affinity binding sites for erythropoietin on rat and mouse megakaryocytes. *Exp Hematol.* 1989;17(1):10–16.

100. Anagnostou A, Liu Z, Steiner M, et al. Erythropoietin receptor mRNA expression in human endothelial cells. *Proc Natl Acad Sci U S A.* 1994;91(9):3974–3978.

101. Masuda S, Nagao M, Takahata K, et al. Functional erythropoietin receptor of the cells with neural characteristics: comparison with receptor properties of erythroid cells. *J Biol Chem.* 1993;268(15):11208–11216.

102. Witthuhn BA, Quelle FW, Silvennoinen O, et al. JAK2 associates with the erythropoietin receptor and is tyrosine phosphorylated and activated following stimulation with erythropoietin. *Cell.* 1993;74(2):227–236.

103. Mayeux P, Dusanter-Fourt I, Muller O, et al. Erythropoietin induces the association of phosphatidylinositol 3′-kinase with a tyrosine-phosphorylated protein complex containing the erythropoietin receptor. *Eur J Biochem*. 1993;216(3):821–828.

104. Gobert S, Duprez V, Lacombe C, et al. The signal transduction pathway of erythropoietin involves three forms of mitogen-activated protein (MAP) kinase in UT7 erythroleukemia cells. *Eur J Biochem*. 1995;234(1):75–83.

105. Gouilleux F, Pallard C, Dusanter-Fourt I, et al. Prolactin, growth hormone, erythropoietin and granulocyte-macrophage colony stimulating factor induce MGF-Stat5 DNA binding activity. *EMBO J*. 1995;14(9):2005–2013.

106. Pallard C, Gouilleux F, Charon M, et al. Interleukin-3, erythropoietin, and prolactin activate a STAT5-like factor in lymphoid cells. *J Biol Chem*. 1995;270(27):15942–15945.

107. Acs G, Acs P, Beckwith SM, et al. Erythropoietin and erythropoietin receptor expression in human cancer. *Cancer Res*. 2001;61(9):3561–3565.

108. Arcasoy MO, Amin K, Karayal AF, et al. Functional significance of erythropoietin receptor expression in breast cancer. *Lab Invest*. 2002;82(7):911–918.

109. Elliott S, Busse L, Bass MB, et al. Anti-Epo receptor antibodies do not predict Epo receptor expression. *Blood*. 2006;107(5):1892–1895.

110. Acs G, Zhang PJ, Rebbeck TR, et al. Immunohistochemical expression of erythropoietin and erythropoietin receptor in breast carcinoma. *Cancer*. 2002;95(5):969–981.

111. Brown WM, Maxwell P, Graham AN, et al. Erythropoietin receptor expression in non-small cell lung carcinoma: a question of antibody specificity. *Stem Cells*. 2007;25(3):718–722.

112. LaMontagne KR, Butler J, Marshall DJ, et al. Recombinant epoetins do not stimulate tumor growth in erythropoietin receptor-positive breast carcinoma models. *Mol Cancer Ther*. 2006;5(2):347–355.

113. Mohyeldin A, Dalgard CL, Lu H, et al. Survival and invasiveness of astrocytomas promoted by erythropoietin. *J Neurosurg*. 2007;106(2):338–350.

114. Gewirtz DA, Di X, Walker TD, et al. Erythropoietin fails to interfere with the antiproliferative and cytotoxic effects of antitumor drugs. *Clin Cancer Res*. 2006;12(7 Pt 1):2232–2238.

115. Westenfelder C, Baranowski RL. Erythropoietin stimulates proliferation of human renal carcinoma cells. *Kidney Int*. 2000;58(2):647–657.

116. Liu WM, Powles T, Shamash J, et al. Effect of haemopoietic growth factors on cancer cell lines and their role in chemosensitivity. *Oncogene*. 2004;23(4):981–990.

117. Hale SA, Wong C, Lounsbury KM. Erythropoietin disrupts hypoxia-inducible factor signaling in ovarian cancer cells. *Gynecol Oncol*. 2006;100(1):14–19.

118. Taylor JE, Henderson IS, Stewart WK, et al. Erythropoietin and spontaneous platelet aggregation in haemodialysis patients. *Lancet*. 1991;338(8779):1361–1362.

119. Macdougall IC, Davies ME, Hallett I, et al. Coagulation studies and fistula blood flow during erythropoietin therapy in haemodialysis patients. *Nephrol Dial Transplant*. 1991;6(11):862–867.

120. Diskin CJ, Stokes Jr TJ, Pennell AT. Pharmacologic intervention to prevent hemodialysis vascular access thrombosis. *Nephron*. 1993;64(1):1–26.

121. Moyo V, Lefebvre P, Duh MS, et al. Erythropoiesis-stimulating agents in the treatment of anemia in myelodysplastic syndromes: a meta-analysis. *Ann Hematol*. 2008;87(7):527–536.

122. Jadersten M, Malcovati L, Dybedal I, et al. Erythropoietin and granulocyte-colony stimulating factor treatment associated with improved survival in myelodysplastic syndrome. *J Clin Oncol*. 2008;26(21):3607–3613.

123. Greenberg PL, Attar E, Battiwalla M, et. al. NCCN Guidelines in Clinical Oncology: myelodysplastic syndromes. National Comprehensive Cancer Network Web site. Available at: http://www.nccn.org/professionals/physician_gls/PDF/mds.pdf.

124. Grote T, Yeilding AL, Castillo R, et al. Efficacy and safety analysis of epoetin alfa in patients with small-cell lung cancer: a randomized, double-blind, placebo-controlled trial. *J Clin Oncol*. 2005;23(36):9377–9386.

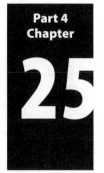

25 Management of depression and anxiety in older adults with cancer

Mark I. Weinberger, Christian J. Nelson, and Andrew J. Roth

A. Introduction

Depression and anxiety are common among patients with cancer. Given the severity of a cancer diagnosis, it is understandable for patients to experience symptoms of distress. Yet distress is often experienced on a continuum from situational anxiety and depressive symptoms to more severe disorders that require more extensive treatment. At various times during a cancer experience, patients may experience brief periods of denial or despair followed by distress with a mixture of depressed mood and anxiety, insomnia, and irritability. These symptoms may last for days to several weeks, after which usual patterns of adaptation return. This response is highly variable; however, it is important to remember that consistent symptoms of depression or anxiety are not part of a normal adjustment process for older patients with cancer. In this chapter, we will present information on the unique issues regarding prevalence, phenomenology, and treatment recommendations for depression and anxiety in older patients with cancer.

B. Depression

When considering psychiatric symptoms in cancer, depression receives the most attention because of its high prevalence, cost, and enormous impact on the individual and family.[1] Despite the high prevalence rates and deleterious effects of depression, elderly patients are far less likely to be diagnosed with major depression or dysthymia than any other age group,[2] and depression is thus frequently undertreated in older patients with cancer.[3-5] In fact, oncologists and oncology nurses often underestimate the morbidity caused by depression.[6]

One potential reason for the underdiagnosis of depression in older cancer patients is that depressive symptoms manifest themselves differently in both later adulthood and in patients with cancer. For example, the symptoms of cancer and the side effects of treatment often overlap with many symptoms of depression. Therefore depressive symptoms may be difficult to separate from other problems associated with cancer such as pain, anxiety, or adjustment to the cancer diagnosis.[1] For older patients, symptom profiles of depression may differ from younger adults as older adults often present with more somatic complaints (such as body aches and malaise) as opposed to affective complaints (i.e., sadness, guilt, and self-criticism). Taken together, diagnosing depression in older patients with cancer is specifically challenging.[7]

B.1. Depression in patients with cancer

Like all psychiatric disorders, a diagnosis of major depressive disorder (MDD) has specific criteria. The two most important symptoms are depressed mood and loss of interest or pleasure (i.e., anhedonia). These are generally referred to as the gateway symptoms of depression (for a list of all criteria for MDD, see Table 25.1). At least five of the symptoms of depression in Table 25.1, including one gateway symptom, need to be endorsed by the patient to qualify for a diagnosis of major depression. The prevalence of depression in patients with cancer has ranged from 6 to 25 percent.[8] The diversity in these rates is due to the use of dissimilar methodologies, the depression criteria measured, and nonuniformity in the cancer sites studied. It is likely, though, that many patients with cancer demonstrate distressing subsyndromal depressive symptoms that also go undiagnosed and would also benefit from proper treatment.[9]

Depression is associated with decreased quality of life, significant deterioration in recreational and physical activities, relationship difficulties, sleep problems, more rapidly progressing cancer symptoms, and more advanced disease and pain compared with nondepressed cancer patients.[10] Depression may not cause these issues, but the presence of depression typically worsens the distress experienced from these physical and psychosocial symptoms and can interfere with effective coping and cancer treatment. In a recent

Table 25.1 *DSM-IV* criteria for major depressive disorder.

Five of the following symptoms must be present:
Gateway symptoms
• Depressed mood
• Diminished interest/loss of pleasure in all or almost all activities (i.e., anhedonia)
Other symptoms of depression
• Weight loss or gain (more than 5% of body weight)
• Insomnia or hypersomnia
• Psychomotor agitation or retardation
• Fatigue
• Feelings of worthlessness or inappropriate guilt
• Reduced ability to concentrate
• Recurrent thoughts of death or suicide

Note. Shading represents symptoms that may overlap with symptoms of cancer or cancer treatment. Adapted from Weinberger et al.[37]

Table 25.2 Diagnosing depression in patients with cancer.

Step 1: Gateway symptoms of depression
First assess the two gateway symptoms of depression:
• Depressed mood
• Diminished interest and/or pleasure
Step 2: Additional symptoms of depression
Attempt to differentiate these symptoms from common symptoms of cancer:
• Weight loss or gain
• Insomnia or hypersomnia
• Psychomotor agitation or retardation
• Fatigue
• Feelings of worthlessness or inappropriate guilt
• Reduced ability to concentrate
• Recurrent thoughts of death or suicide
Step 3: Differentiating depression
Focus on the following symptoms to help differentiate depressive symptoms from cancer symptoms:
• Late insomnia: Waking up in the middle of the night with difficulty getting back to sleep because of worry or concern
• Mood variation: The patient may not report being depressed all the time but may report consistent depressed mood in the morning or evening
• Anxiety
• Agitation
• Loss of sexual interest

Note. Adapted from Weinberger et al.[37]

study, depression was found to be an independent predictor of poor survival in patients with advanced cancer,[11] and suicide risk in patients with cancer is higher compared to patients with other medical illnesses.[12] This emphasizes the point that proper assessment of depressive symptoms in patients with cancer is critical so that appropriate interventions can be offered in a timely fashion.[11]

Unfortunately, depression is one of the most challenging psychiatric problems to diagnose in patients with cancer.[13] As mentioned earlier, the primary complexity is that many symptoms of cancer and side effects of treatment overlap with the symptoms of depression. For example, significant weight loss, sleep problems, fatigue, and difficulty concentrating may be symptoms of depression *or* symptoms of cancer and/or its accompanying treatment side effects. The shaded symptoms in Table 25.1 are all symptoms that overlap with depression and cancer or side effects of treatment, leaving only the gateway symptoms of depressed mood and loss of interest or pleasure as the two pure symptoms of depression in patients with cancer.

For the oncologist, busy clinics and lack of specific training in identifying depression make it unrealistic to conduct a complete diagnostic interview for depression with recognition of different diagnostic schemas. To screen cancer patients for depression (see Table 25.2), we suggest asking the two gateway questions of depressed mood and loss of interest or pleasure because these are the two pure symptoms of depression in patients with cancer. Screening patients for depression using these

two symptoms – depressed mood and anhedonia – may indicate to a busy clinician the patients who require more in-depth psychiatric assessment and possible intervention. To help distinguish between the somatic symptoms of depression versus side effects of disease, it may also be helpful to discuss symptoms suggested by Guo and colleagues such as late insomnia, mood variation, anxiety, and loss of sexual interest, which may offer succinct and specific evidence for a diagnosis of depression in patients with cancer.[14]

Validated questionnaires may also be useful to help oncologists screen for depression. There are five well-validated self-report measures that are commonly used to assess depression: the Hospital Anxiety and Depression Scale (HADS), the Center for Epidemiologic Studies on Depression (CESD-20), the Beck Depression Inventory (BDI) and the Geriatric Depression Scale (GDS), and the Patient Health Questionnaire. All these measures are easy and quick to administer and will likely provide a clinician with a baseline measure of depressive symptoms. If a patient endorses either sad mood or loss of interest, administering one of these self-report measures can establish the diagnosis of depression and a baseline from which to measure symptomatic improvement.

Another option for oncologists is to screen for general psychological distress. This can be assessed using the Distress Thermometer, a brief, self-administered scale that has been used extensively and is well validated in patients with cancer.[5] The measure requires patients to rate their level of distress from 0 (no distress) to 10 (extreme distress) on a thermometer and then identify domains that are causing the distress. This tool may be a good gateway for more elaborate screening for anxiety and depression.

B.2. Depression in geriatric patients with cancer

Identifying depression in older patients with cancer presents a unique challenge to clinicians and researchers as it combines the difficulty of diagnosing depression in patients with cancer with the complexities of detecting depression in older adults. Symptoms of depression can be caused by several medical conditions. The most common physical cause of depression in older patients is uncontrolled pain. It is accompanied by anxiety and a sense of anguish that life is intolerable unless the pain is relieved. Patients also interpret new or increasingly severe pain as a sign that the cancer has progressed, causing greater depression and hopelessness. Other physical causes of depressed mood include hypercalcemia from bone metastasis, other electrolyte imbalances, deficient vitamin B_{12} or folate, hypothyroidism or adrenal insufficiency, and paraneoplastic syndromes.

Despite these intricacies, the research in this area provides a guide for specific suggestions for identifying depression in older cancer patients (see Table 25.3). A screen of the two gateway symptoms of depression should be administered first (i.e., depressed mood and loss of interest). Even though it is less common for older adults to endorse these two symptoms, a proper and thorough assessment of depression should still begin with asking about these two symptoms. Even if the patient denies these gateway questions, it is important to elicit information about other potential symptoms of depression in this sample, including general malaise as opposed to being depressed or loss of interest, or general aches and pains or stom-

Table 25.3 Diagnosing depression in geriatric patients with cancer.

Step 1: Gateway symptoms of depression
First assess the two gateway symptoms of depression:
- Depressed mood
- Diminished interest and/or pleasure

Step 2: Additional symptoms of depression
Assess other symptoms of depression that may help differentiate depressive from cancer symptoms:
- Weight loss or gain
- Insomnia or hypersomnia
- Psychomotor agitation or retardation
- Fatigue
- Feelings of worthlessness or inappropriate guilt
- Reduced ability to concentrate
- Recurrent thoughts of death or suicide

Step 3: Differentiating depression
Assess symptoms to focus on differentiating cancer and depressive symptoms in older patients with cancer:
- General malaise: Older patients may be less likely to report loss of interest and sad mood and more likely to report a general malaise or dissatisfaction
- General aches and pains/stomachaches, as opposed to cancer or tumor-specific pain
- Diffuse somatic complaints, as opposed to specific complaints associated with treatment side effects
- Hopelessness: Most patients with cancer are somewhat hopeful about the upcoming treatment and potential outcome; however, older depressed adults may see little purpose or hope to treatments
- Late insomnia: Waking up in the middle of the night with difficulty getting back to sleep because of worry or concern
- Mood variation: The reported mood changes throughout the day
- Change/loss of sexual interest

Note. Adapted from Weinberger et al.[37]

achaches as opposed to specific tumor-site pain or specific side effects of cancer treatment. Hopelessness is also an important aspect to discuss; many patients with cancer express some hope for a meaningful future or a cure of their cancer; thus reporting little or no hope for either may be a sign of depression. Sleep may be problematic for both patients with cancer and older patients; however, it is important to ask if the patient wakes up in the middle of the night (middle insomnia) and has difficulty getting back to sleep because he or she worries or feels anxious or wakes up too early in the morning. An older depressed patient may also report mood variation during the day. For example, the patient may report that during part of the day, his or her mood is fine (i.e., euthymic), however, the patient may spend most of the day with a general malaise. Establishing a good rapport in a more open-ended manner with older patients is essential as this helps the patient feel comfortable reporting depressive symptoms.

B.3. Treatment for depressed patients with cancer

Though there is evidence about the efficacy of treatments for geriatric depression, there is minimal evidence specifically demonstrating the effectiveness of psychological and pharmacologic treatments in depressed patients with cancer.[15] The level of distress, the inability to carry out daily activities, and the response to psychotherapeutic interventions are the signs used to determine when a psychotropic medication is needed. It is important to educate patients about the therapeutic response time of these medications. It can take up to 2 weeks for most antidepressants to work and possibly up to 5–6 weeks for a good trial at any dose. If there is no response or insufficient response by this time, the dose may be increased as indicated and tolerated. If patients are not aware of this time frame, they may become prematurely noncompliant with the drug.

Medications that are typically used to treat depression in patients with cancer are those that are used in treating depression in general. Most commonly, serotonin specific reuptake inhibitors (SSRIs) and serotonin-norepinephrine reuptake inhibitors (SNRIs) are prescribed for older patients with cancer. The SSRIs do not have the same risks of cardiac arrhythmias, hypotension, and troublesome anticholinergic effects such as urinary retention, memory impairment, sedation, and reduced awareness as do the tricyclic antidepressants (TCAs). The most common side effects of the SSRIs, usually dose related, include mild gastric distress and nausea, increased intestinal motility, and brief periods of increased headache and insomnia (and sometimes hypersomnia). Some patients may experience anxiety, tremor, restlessness, and akathisia (which, though rare, can be problematic for the patient with comorbid Parkinson's disease). SSRIs can cause sexual dysfunction in men and women, a side effect that often leads to cessation of the medication. Though some patients can have some transient appetite suppression and subsequent weight loss, the anorectic properties of these drugs have not been a limiting factor in this population. The SSRIs have a wider margin of safety than the TCAs in the event of an overdose. The shorter half-life of some SSRIs, such as sertraline, citalopram, and escitalopram, allows for faster clearance should this be necessary in the medically ill. Paroxetine has no active metabolites and therefore is also removed from a patient's system relatively quickly on discontinuation. Because most of these drugs are strongly protein-bound, consideration must be given to their interactions with other medications such as coumadin, digoxin, and cisplatin. If there is no response to an SSRI after 4–6 weeks, the dose may be increased by 25–50 percent, if tolerated, to obtain a better outcome. Paroxetine and citalopram are now available in new formulations that are reported to improve their side effect profiles.

All the SSRIs have the ability to inhibit the hepatic isoenzyme P450 2D6. This is important with respect to dose/plasma-level ratios and drug interactions because the SSRIs are dependent on hepatic metabolism. It is important to consider drug-drug interactions, especially in the elderly, who may be on multiple medication regimens and have various physicians. This has become especially important recently as the interactions of these medications, which decrease effective levels of tamoxifen, a hormonal agent used in breast cancer, have been elucidated. It appears that venlafaxine and mirtazapine are least interactive with tamoxifen, though further research is needed. SSRIs should be avoided with the chemotherapeutic agent procarbazine, which has monamine oxidase inhibitor (MAOI)-like properties.

Venlafaxine and duloxetine are potent inhibitors of neuronal serotonin and norepinephrine reuptake.[16] They are similar to TCAs in terms of efficacy, without the same uncomfortable side effects. Like other antidepressants, venlafaxine should not be used in patients receiving MAOIs. Its side effect profile tends to be generally well tolerated. At higher doses, there is the potential side effect of hypertension, which must be looked for. Mirtazapine is a sedating antidepressant useful in depressed patients with associated anxiety and insomnia. It has few gastrointestinal and sexual side effects and may induce weight gain. It is usually dosed at bedtime because it can be sedating.

Bupropion has an activating profile that makes it useful in lethargic medically ill patients yet should be avoided in patients with a history of seizure disorders and brain tumors and in those who are malnourished; it may cause anxiety or restlessness in some patients. Bupropion is less cardiotoxic than the TCAs. It is also commonly used for smoking cessation.

TCAs may be used when patients have severe treatment-resistant depression or have concomitant neuropathic pain syndromes; however, they are difficult for the elderly to tolerate at therapeutic doses. Patients receiving TCAs should have a baseline electrocardiogram (EKG) for cardiac clearance with caution in patients with bundle branch blocks and QTc prolongation. These medications have a quinidine-like effect at therapeutic plasma levels. There are no strict guidelines for EKG monitoring over time. At high plasma doses, the drugs can become arrhythmogenic. The anticholinergic actions of TCAs can cause confusion as well as serious tachycardia, and the quinidine-like effects of TCAs can lead to arrhythmias. Postural hypotension and dizziness may also occur; these are of particular concern for the frail, volume-depleted patient who is at risk for falls and possible osteoporosis-related fractures. For patients already exposed to a variety of sedating agents (e.g., narcotic analgesics, antiemetics, anxiolytics, and neuroleptics), TCAs can accentuate the overall cumulative sedating effects of these medications. Urinary retention and constipation are also problematic side effects. It is for these reasons that studies using the Beers criteria[17] for inappropriate medication prescribing in older adults have noted the dangers of using highly anticholinergic antidepressants (i.e., amitriptyline and doxepin). These issues become even more problematic in those among the elderly who are on multiple medications.[18]

If indicated, TCAs should also be started at low doses and increased slowly every 5–7 days, until a therapeutic dose is attained or side effects become a dose-limiting factor. Dosages may be monitored by blood levels.

Psychostimulants may be used when there is coexisting fatigue or malaise. There is growing experience for supporting the use of Ritalin (methylphenidate), dextroamphetamine, or Provigil (modafinil) to treat depressive symptoms in patients with cancer based on their quick response time and alleviation of concomitant symptoms including fatigue, sedation, and poor concentration. They may be useful early in the treatment of depression until an antidepressant has a chance to become therapeutic. They are most helpful in the treatment of depression in patients with advanced cancer and in those in whom dysphoric mood is associated with severe psychomotor slowing, decreased motivation, apathy, and even mild cognitive impairment. Psychostimulants have been shown to improve attention, concentration, and overall performance on neuropsychological testing in the medically ill.[19] In relatively low doses, psychostimulants stimulate appetite, promote a sense of well-being, and decrease feelings of weakness and fatigue in patients with cancer. Psychostimulants are usually dosed in the morning, and at noon if needed, to avoid sleep problems. The dosage is slowly increased over several days until a desired effect is achieved or until side effects, such as overstimulation, anxiety, tremor, insomnia, mild increase in blood pressure and pulse rate, or confusion decrease. Tolerance will develop, and adjustment of dose may be necessary. An additional benefit of such stimulants as methylphenidate and dextroamphetamine is that they have been shown to reduce sedation secondary to opioid analgesics and provide adjuvant analgesics in patients with cancer.[20] However, the safety of psychostimulants in older patients with cancer has not been studied extensively. Patients receiving Ritalin should have no history of seizures or arrhythmias. Pulse and blood pressure should be monitored regularly in the elderly.

Choosing an antidepressant in the elderly cancer population may be based on whether a patient or family member has responded well to an antidepressant in the past. Other factors that should be considered include the patient's overall health and cognitive abilities; social and financial resources, which are often limited in this patient population; and any other existing psychiatric conditions (i.e., substance abuse, psychosis, or anxiety disorders). The elderly might require longer treatment trials than other patient populations, so patience is important for both the patient and practitioner. Antidepressant selection in the elderly cancer population may also be based on a number of physical variables. It is useful to note if there is a need for physical symptom control (i.e., neuropathic pain, fatigue, and insomnia) in addition to treatment for the psychiatric symptoms. These symptoms may be treated, at least in part, by the antidepressant. In addition, it is helpful to consider the side effect profiles of different antidepressants, including those side effects that may be useful as well as those that should be avoided. For example, if a patient presents with fatigue or sedation, the most appropriate agent may be an energizing SSRI (i.e., fluoxetine and paroxetine), bupropion, or a psychostimulant. Consider mirtazapine or a calming SSRI like citalopram in a patient who is experiencing anxiety. If the patient presents with gastric problems, an appropriate agent may be mirtazapine or a TCA. Either mirtazapine, a TCA, or a psychostimulant can be used in patients complaining of loss of appetite.

Patients who are unable to swallow pills may be able to take an antidepressant in an elixir (fluoxetine, paroxetine, sertraline, nortriptyline, and amitriptyline) or mirtazapine, which comes in a soluble tablet preparation. Patients with stomatitis secondary to chemotherapy or radiotherapy or those who have slow intestinal motility or urinary retention should receive an antidepressant with the least anticholinergic side effects.

Psychotherapy, including supportive therapy; psychoeducational interventions; cognitive-behavioral therapy (CBT); interpersonal therapy; and problem-solving therapy also appear to help depressed patients with cancer. Supportive techniques, such as active listening with supportive comments, can be readily applied by oncologists and oncology nurses. Cognitive therapy, which focuses on how an individual's inaccurate thoughts or assessments of his or her situation lead to anxious and depressed feelings, can be used to help a patient develop an adaptive perspective on his or her circumstances. Faulty thought processes such as "my PSA just increased – I'm going to die" or "my doctor didn't set up a firm follow-up appointment; he must think I'm going to die soon" will likely lead to depressed emotions, but they may be challenged with attempts to reframe them in a healthier manner: "if my doctor can identify a progression of disease by a PSA before there are clear metastases, perhaps she can do something to prevent worsening of the illness" or "my doctor needs to wait until certain tests are completed and results returned before making a firm, meaningful follow-up appointment"; similarly, "what's the point in living any longer if I am going to die soon" may be reframed to "there is still more that can be meaningful and fulfilling in my life no matter how much longer I may have to live." CBT has been found to help depressed patients with cancer, in particular, combining behavioral activation with cognitive techniques. Group therapy for patients with cancer, caregivers, and families may be advantageous, allowing individuals to receive support from others facing similar problems. Further research is warranted to better document more ideal psychotherapeutic treatments for elderly cancer patients with depression. A combined treatment including both pharmacologic and psychotherapeutic techniques is likely the best option for older patients with cancer.

C. Anxiety

Anxiety disorders in older cancer patients are common. As with depression, there needs to be greater attention on understanding and recognizing anxiety disorders in older adults with cancer.

C.1. Anxiety in patients with cancer

Stark and House discuss dimensions of anxiety in patients with cancer.[21] The authors believe that pathological anxiety can be recognized when it is either out of proportion compared to the level of threat, when it persists or leads to deterioration without intervention, or when there is a disruption of usual or desirable functioning. Anxiety that endures and causes impairment should be treated.[22] The anxiety disorders most common in patients with cancer are panic disorder, adjustment disorder with anxiety, phobias, and generalized anxiety disorder (GAD). Similar to depression, these disorders are difficult to assess in patients with cancer.[22]

The evaluation of anxiety symptoms is a frequent reason for requesting a psychiatric consultation. Anxiety may increase as cancer progresses and with a decline in physical status. The most common symptoms are feelings of hyperarousal, irritability, and uncontrollable negative thoughts. In severe form, anxiety symptoms may include tachycardia, shortness of breath, diaphoresis, gastrointestinal distress, and nausea. Prevalence rates of anxiety vary widely in studies of patients with cancer. Studies have shown rates anywhere between 1 and 23% across anxiety disorders and cancer types.[23–26] In patients with advanced cancer, rates of anxiety have been found to be close to 30 percent.[27]

C.2. Anxiety in geriatric patients with cancer

Older adults with cancer often have multiple medical conditions and complex polypharmacy issues that may blur the clinical presentation of anxiety.[22] Several factors that can complicate the diagnosis of anxiety in older patients with cancer include pain, respiratory distress, sepsis, endocrine abnormalities, hypoglycemia, hyper- and hypocalcemia, hormone-secreting tumors, and pancreatic cancer.[22] A change in metabolic state or an impending medical catastrophe may be heralded by symptoms of anxiety. Suddenly occurring symptoms of anxiety with chest pain, respiratory distress, restlessness, and a feeling of "jumping out of one's skin" may indicate a pulmonary embolus. Patients who are hypoxic often appear anxious and fear that they are suffocating or dying.

Medications, such as bronchodilators and (β)-adrenergic receptor stimulants, that are commonly used for chronic respiratory conditions may cause anxiety, irritability, and tremulousness. The use of steroids, antiemetics, and withdrawal from narcotics, benzodiazepines, and alcohol can all cause anxiety. The psychiatric symptoms associated with the use of steroids such as dexamethasone are dose related and often persist even after the medications have been tapered. Akathisia, a common side effect of neuroleptic drugs (e.g., metoclopramide and prochlorperazine) used to control nausea and to treat the symptoms of a delirium, may often manifest as anxiety and restlessness.[28] These symptoms can be controlled by the addition of a benzodiazepine, a beta-blocker, or an antiparkinsonian agent. Given the common use of these medications in later adulthood, diagnosing anxiety in these patients is complicated but very important. Patients who have a delirium often manifest symptoms of anxiety, restlessness, and agitation. These confusional states generally have multiple causes, including hypoglycemia, organ failure, electrolyte imbalance, nutritional failure, and infection.[29]

Withdrawal states from alcohol, opioids, and benzodiazepines are often overlooked as causes of anxiety and agitation, even in older patients. Patients with head and neck cancers often have unreported or underreported histories of alcohol abuse[1] and may have increased anxiety and agitation as signs of a withdrawal state.[30] Patients in the palliative-care setting may have been prescribed shorter-acting benzodiazepines (e.g., lorazepam, alprazolam, and oxazepam) to control both anxiety and nausea. With inadequate dosing regimens, these patients often have rebound anxiety between doses. These patients may benefit from an increase in the dosing frequency of the short-acting benzodiazepine or from a switch to a longer-acting benzodiazepine (e.g., clonazepam). Bronchodilators and (β)-adrenergic stimulants, psychostimulants, and caffeine can all cause anxiety, irritability, and tremulousness.[31]

The diagnosis of anxiety in older patients with cancer is usually determined by questions asked in a clinical interview. In patients who are less debilitated and who are cognitively intact, the use of assessment instruments improves screening for symptoms and facilitates the monitoring of treatment progress. Several instruments have been used to measure anxiety. The Hospital Anxiety and Depression Scale (HADS) is a self-report measure that assesses the cognitive items associated with depression and anxiety and thus avoids the confound of physical symptoms in medically ill patients.[32] State-Trait Anxiety Inventory[33] and the General Health Questionnaire[34] have also been used. As stated earlier, the Distress Thermometer,[35] a one-item visual analog scale in the form of a thermometer, may be a more feasible screening tool for older patients.

Panic disorder often presents as a sudden, unpredictable episode of intense discomfort and fear with thoughts of impending doom. Those patients who already have compromised respiratory function may have cyclical exacerbations of their anxiety and breathing problems. Symptoms of a preexisting panic disorder may intensify during the palliative-care phase, when patients are confronting increasing physical symptoms and disability and their own mortality. Generalized anxiety disorder is characterized by ongoing excessive worry, difficulty controlling the worry or apprehension, and the presence of symptoms of autonomic hyperactivity and hypervigilance.

C.3. Treatment for anxious older patients with cancer

Psychotherapeutic and pharmacologic approaches have been shown to successfully treat anxiety disorders in older adults. A number of psychotherapeutic modalities help achieve this goal. Cognitive-behavioral interventions and supportive therapy, interpersonal therapy, problem-solving therapy, and insight-oriented therapy have been used successfully with older patients to relieve anxiety.

For patients with mild to moderate anxiety, the use of psychological techniques alone may be sufficient to assist them in managing anxiety. Psychoeducational interventions are particularly useful for anxious patients who have difficulty understanding medical information about their prognoses and symptoms. Explaining the predictable emotional phases through which patients pass as they face new and frightening information may also alleviate anxiety. Providing information to patients' families enables them to cope more effectively, which in turn enhances patients' sense of support. Patients with anxiety may benefit from specific cognitive-behavioral interventions, including reframing negative, irrational thought processes, progressive relaxation, distraction, guided imagery, meditation, biofeedback, and hypnosis. Other psychotherapeutic techniques, such as supportive and insight-oriented therapy, may be helpful to reduce anxiety symptoms and allow for better coping with the cancer.

Several medications have been used in older patients with cancer, including benzodiazepines, buspirone, neuroleptics, and hypnotics. A variety of anxiolytic drugs are prescribed for older patients with cancer; one-quarter to one-third of patients with advanced cancer receive antianxiety medication during their hospitalizations.[36] In deciding whether a pharmacological approach to the management of anxiety may be useful, the severity of the patient's symptoms and the degree to which they interfere with overall well-being are the most reliable guides. Given the possibility of compromised hepatic and renal functioning as well as increased sensitivity to pharmacological interventions, if drugs are to be used in older patients, the rubric of starting with lower doses than would be used with younger, physically healthy patients and increasing these doses more cautiously will lead to more manageable side effects.

The first-line antianxiety drugs are the benzodiazepines. In older patients, however, these medications may result in mental status changes such as confusion or impaired concentration or memory. These changes are more often seen in those with advanced disease and those with impaired hepatic or brain function. Dose-dependent side effects, such as drowsiness, confusion, and decreased motor coordination, must be monitored carefully in the elderly patient. Benzodiazepine use represents an important iatrogenic risk factor for falls for older adults. Falls are an important cause of mortality for those aged over 75 years. One must keep in mind the synergistic effects of the benzodiazepines with other medications that have central nervous system–depressant properties such as narcotics and some antidepressants. Elderly patients with dementia or brain injury who are administered benzodiazepines may experience paradoxical behavioral disturbances such as aggressiveness, irritability, and agitation. For patients with compromised hepatic function, the use of shorter-acting benzodiazepines, such as lorazepam and oxazepam, for anxiety and temazepam for sleep is preferred

because these drugs are metabolized by conjugation with glucuronic acid and have no active metabolites. Lorazepam and alprazolam are useful not only for anxiety but also as antiemetic (lorazepam) and antipanic (alprazolam) drugs. A longer-acting benzodiazepine, such as clonazepam, may provide more consistent relief of anxiety symptoms and may have mood-stabilizing effects as well.

For insomnia, the benzodiazepine temazepam as well as the nonbenzodiazepine hypnotics zolpidem, zaleplon, eszopiclone, and rozerem may be effective. In addition, sedating antidepressants, such as trazodone or mirtazapine, may also help patients with persistent anxiety and insomnia. Duloxetine may be helpful for patients with anxiety and neuropathic pain syndromes. A relatively nonsedating neuroleptic such as haloperidol or a sedating atypical neuroleptic such as olanzapine or quetiapine may be more effective for the patient who is anxious or has trouble sleeping and is confused. Neuroleptics may also be useful for the patient whose anxiety is substance induced (e.g., steroids). Drowsiness and somnolence are the most common adverse effects of benzodiazepines; reductions in dose and the passage of time eliminate these effects. In anxious patients with severely compromised pulmonary function, the use of benzodiazepines that suppress central respiratory mechanisms may be unsafe. Low doses of atypical neuroleptics such as olanzapine or quetiapine or a low dose of an antihistamine can be useful for these individuals. The anticholinergic effects of these medications must be monitored carefully in the debilitated patient who is prone to developing delirium. Structurally unlike other anxiolytics, buspirone is useful for patients with generalized anxiety disorder and for those at risk for abuse. Buspirone is not effective on an as-needed basis, and its effects are not apparent for 1–2 weeks, which may be problematic in patients who have significant anxiety and who do not have long to live.

For the treatment of panic disorder, the benzodiazepines alprazolam and clonazepam and antidepressant medications (i.e., SSRIs, TCAs, and MAOIs) have demonstrated effectiveness. Alprazolam rapidly blocks panic attacks. The TCA imipramine is effective in the management of panic disorder; its anticholinergic side effects, however, are not well tolerated by debilitated or older cancer patients. In the oncology setting, the SSRIs sertraline, paroxetine, citalopram, and escitalopram, which have fewer side effects than the TCAs, are effective in the management of depression, generalized anxiety, and panic disorder. Newer antidepressants such as mirtazapine and venlafaxine are also useful for anxious patients. Antidepressants, however, require from 1 to 4 weeks or more to reach therapeutic levels and therefore may be less useful in the palliative-care setting. Although monoamine oxidase inhibitors are effective in the management of panic disorder and depression, the risk of hypertensive crisis from concomitant ingestion of sympathomimetics (e.g., amphetamines and meperidine) commonly used in the oncology setting, coupled with the need for a low-tyramine diet, make these medications less desirable for patients with advanced cancer.

D. Summary and conclusion

Anxiety and depression are highly prevalent in older patients with cancer. This chapter has provided a summary of the issues that need to be considered when diagnosing and treating older cancer patients with anxiety and depression. Yet diagnosing depression and anxiety in older patients with cancer is difficult because cancer and these syndromes have distinct but overlapping symptom profiles. Therefore clinicians need to be able to recognize symptoms of depression and anxiety in older patients with cancer to improve recognition, diagnosis, and treatment.

Psychotherapeutic and psychopharmacological interventions are optimal in treating anxiety and depression in older patients with cancer, though they may be more resistant to accepting these treatments. Antidepressants and neuroleptic medications in particular have an important role in treating depression and delirium. Oncologists should be aware of the indications for psychotropic medications, of the possible side effects or drug interactions of psychiatric medications, and how to obtain psychiatric consultation if needed. Last, more psycho-oncological intervention research is needed to better assess the efficacy and safety of these therapies in older adults with cancer.

References

1. Massie MJ. Prevalence of depression in patients with cancer. *J Natl Cancer Inst Monogr.* 2004;32:57–71.

2. Extermann M, Hurria A. Comprehensive geriatric assessment for older patients with cancer. *J Clin Oncol.* 2007;25(14):1824–1831.

3. Henderson S. Epidemiology of psychiatric disorders. In: Sadock BJ and Saddock VA, eds. *Comprehensive Textbook of Psychiatry.* 7th ed. Philadelphia: Lippincott Williams & Wilkins; 2000.

4. Yesavage JA, Brink TL, Rose TL, et al. Development and validation of a geriatric depression screening scale: a preliminary report. *J Psychiatr Res.* 1983;17(1):37–49.

5. Morley JE. The top 10 hot topics in aging. *J Gerontol.* 2004;59(1):24–33.

6. Passik S, Donaghy KB, Theobald DE, et al. Oncology staff recognition of depressive symptoms on videotaped interviews of depressed cancer patients: implication for designing a training program. *J Pain Symptom Manage.* 2000;19:329–338.

7. Spoletini I, Gianni W, Repetto L, et al. Depression and cancer: an unexplored and unresolved emergent issue in elderly patients. *Crit Rev Oncol Hematol.* 2008;65:143–155.

8. Bottomley A. A depression in cancer patients: a literature review. *Eur J Cancer Care.* 1998;7:181–191.

9. Reich M. Depression and cancer: recent data on clinical issues, research challenges and treatment approaches. *Curr Opin Oncol.* 2008;20:353–359.

10. Hopko D, Bell JL, Armento ME, et al. The phenomenology and screening of clinical depression in cancer patients. *J Psychosoc Oncol.* 2008;26:31–51.

11. Lloyd-Williams M, Shiels C, Taylor F, et al. Depression: an independent predictor of early death in patients with advanced cancer. *J Affect Disord.* 2009;113(1-2):127–132

12. Walker J, Waters RA, Murray G, et al. Better off dead: suicidal thoughts in cancer patients. *J Clin Oncol.* 2008;26:4725–4730.

13. Trask PC. Assessment of depression in cancer patients. *J Natl Cancer Inst Monogr.* 2004;32:80–92.

14. Guo Y, Musselman DL, Manatunga AK, et al. The diagnosis of major depression in patients with cancer: a comparative approach. *Psychosomatics.* 2006;47:376–384.

15. Rodin G, Katz M, Lloyd N, et al. Treatment of depression in cancer patients. *Curr Oncol.* 2007;14:180–188.

16. Schatzberg A. Pharmacological priniciples of antidepressant efficacy. *Hum Psychopharmacol.* 2002;17(suppl 1):17–22.

17. Beers MH. Explicit criteria for determining potentially inappropriate medication use by the elderly: an update. *Arch Intern Med.* 1997;157(14):1531–1536.

18. Golden A, Preston RA, Barnett SD, et al. Inappropriate medication prescribing in homebound older adults. *J Am Geriatr Soc.* 1999;47:948–953.

19. Fernandez F, Adams F, Levy J, et al. Cognitive impairment due to AIDS related complex and its response to psychostimulants. *Psychosomatics.* 1988;29:38–46.

20. Bruera E, Chadwick S, Brennels C, et al. Methylphenidate associated with narcotics for the management of depressive disorders in cancer patients. *Psychosomatics.* 1992;33:352–356.

21. Stark D, House A. Anxiety in cancer patients. *Br J Cancer.* 2000;83:1261–1267.

22. Roth A, Modi R. Psychiatric issues in older cancer patients. *Crit Rev Oncol Hematol.* 2003;48:185–197.

23. Harrison J, Maguire P. Predictors of psychiatric morbidity in cancer patients. *Br J Psychiatry.* 1994;165:593–598.

24. Kissane D, Clarke DM, Ikin J, et al. Psychological morbidity and quality of life in Australian women with early-staged breast cancer: a cross-sectional survey. *Med J Aust.* 1998;169:192–196.

25. Lee M, Love SB, Mitchell JB, et al. Mastectomy or conservation for early breast cancer: psychological morbidity. *Eur J Cancer.* 1992;28A:1340–1344.

26. Fallowfield LJ, Hall A, Maguire P, et al. Psychological effects of being offered choice of surgery for breast cancer. *Br Med J.* 1994;309(6952):448.

27. Brandenberg Y, Bolund C, Sigurdardottir V. Anxiety and depressive symptoms at different stages of malignant melanoma. *Psychooncology.* 1992;1:71–78.

28. Fleishman S, Lavin M, Sattler M, et al. Antiemetic-induded akathisia in cancer patients. *Am J Psychiatry.* 1994;151:763–765.

29. Massie M, Holland JC, Glass E. Delirium in terminally ill cancer patients. *Am J Psychiatry.* 1983;140:1048–1050.

30. Holland J, Breitbart WS, Jacobsen PJ, et al., eds. *Alcoholism and Cancer.* New York: Oxford University Press; 1998.

31. Levy M, Catalino RB. Control of common physical symptoms other than pain in patients with terminal disease. *Semin Oncol.* 1985;12:411–430.

32. Zigmond A, Snaith R. The Hospital Anxiety and Depression Scale. *Acta Psych Scand.* 1983;67:361–370.

33. Spielberger C. *The Manual for the State Trait Anxiety Inventory.* Palo Alto, CA: Consulting Psychological Press; 1983.

34. Goldberg D, Gater R, Sartorius N, et al. The validity of two versions of the GHQ in the WHO study of mental illness in general health care. *Psychol Med.* 1997;27:191–197.

35. Jacobsen P, Donovan KA, Trask PC, et al. Screening for psychological distress in ambulatory cancer patients. *Cancer.* 2005;103:1494–1502.

36. Stiefel F, Kornblith A, Holland J. Changes in the prescription patterns of psychotropic drugs for cancer patients during a 10 year period. *Cancer.* 1990;65:1048–1053.

37. Weinberger MI, Roth AJ, Nelson CJ. Untangling the complexities of depression diagnosis in older cancer patients. *Oncologist.* 2009;14(1):60–66.

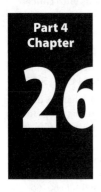

Management of pain in older adults with cancer

Anthony Nicholas Galanos, Katja Elbert-Avila, and Leslie J. Bryan

Although the world is full of suffering, it is also full of the overcoming of it.
– *Helen Keller, Optimism (1903)*

A. Why focus on the elderly?

Geriatric patients are complex, do not fit in the traditional biomedical model, and are underrepresented in cancer research trials; thus guidance for the practicing oncologist is not abundant, and myths and misunderstandings about older people are even more abundant. Why should the practicing oncologist give special attention to this population and their issues?

First is the so-called demographic imperative.[1] The fastest-growing segment of the U.S. population is the cohort who are greater than or equal to 65 years of age. Indeed, by the year 2030, this segment will comprise 20 percent of the U.S. population.[2] Furthermore, the incidence of cancer in the United States dramatically increases with age, with a median age at diagnosis of 67 years and a median age at death of 73 years.[3] Mortality rates show a dramatic difference by age if one is over 65 years of age, and the absolute number of deaths and the age at death have continued to increase from 1970 to 2002. At present, about 25 percent of new cancer diagnoses are in patients aged 65–74 years, about 22 percent in patients aged 75–84 years, and about 7.5 percent in those aged 85 years and older. This burden of cancer will lead to even more pressure on an already stressed medical care system and is especially distressing as when compared with younger patients, older patients have consistently received less screening, less aggressive surgery, less systemic therapy, and less participation in clinical trials.[3]

The prevalence of cancer pain is compelling. In a systematic review of the literature that included statistical pooling of the study results, a compendium of 52 studies pointed to the following.

Pain prevalence in cancer patients was high: 64 percent in patients with metastatic, advanced, or terminal disease; 59 percent in patients on anti-cancer treatment; and 33 percent in patients who had been cured of cancer.[4] The provider is further misled by the notion that older cancer patients either have less pain than younger cancer patients or, because of age, feel it less or suffer less from it. However, there are no data to support these misconceptions.

Experimental studies of pain sensitivity and pain tolerance across all ages have had mixed results. Overall, the data suggest that age-related changes in pain perception are probably not clinically significant.[5] One criticism of the studies cited is that the painful stimulus used to cause pain in the laboratory is so low that lack of its perception, a myth of aging, may be irrelevant to the recognition of clinically meaningful pain. Indeed, a wide range of individual variation was observed, indicating that age was, at most, just one of the variables affecting perception of pain.[6]

To confuse the oncologist further, elderly patients are also characterized by atypical disease presentation, and pain symptoms may not belie the severity of pathology in the elderly. In fact, what can cause clear and ongoing expressions of pain in young adults may manifest as confusion, restlessness, aggression, or fatigue in an older person.[5]

Another difference between older and younger cancer patients is comorbidities. Over half of patients with cancer who are aged between 70 and 90 years are functionally dependent or require assistance with activities of daily living.[7] Most are taking multiple medications, and the mean number of associated comorbid conditions is 3.5.[7]

The atypical presentation of disease, the polypharmacy, and the comorbidities lead us to another concept in geriatric medicine: *decreased physiologic reserve.*[8] That is to say, age alone does not predict physiologic decline, but as we age, the ability to compensate for and bounce back from physiologic insults such as cancer declines. The more the physiologic reserves of an elderly person are depleted, the more likely the person is to become functionally dependent. Age-related

Table 26.1 Partial list of guidelines for the management of cancer pain.

Organization	Focus on elderly	Year	Web site
World Health Organization (WHO)	Yes	2007	http://www.who.org/
National Comprehensive Cancer Network (NCCN)	Yes	2008	http://www.nccn.org/
American Pain Society	No	2005	http://www.ampainsoc.org/
Joint Commission on Accreditation of Health Organizations (JCAHO)	No	2001	http://www.jcaho.org/
National Pharmaceutical Council (NPC)	No	2005	http://www.npcnow.org/
American Geriatrics Society (AGS)	Yes	2002	http://www.americangeriatrics.org/
American College of Physicians (ACP)	No	2008	http://www.acponline.org/
European Society for Medical Oncology (ESMO)	No	2008	http://www.esmo.org/
International Association for the Study of Pain (IASP)	Yes	2008	http://www.iasp-pain.org/
Agency for Healthcare Research and Quality (AHRQ)	Yes	2006	http://www.ahrq.gov/

changes occur at different rates in different persons, and the extent of their presence is poorly reflected in chronologic age. This is the concept of *heterogeneity of aging*.[6,9] The ability to compensate for these insults manifests itself in the functional status of the patient. So it is better to approach the geriatric patient from a functional viewpoint than from the traditional approach of disease and cure. This functional approach to the patient has been in the geriatric medicine literature since the early 1980s[8,10] and has profound implications for how to assess and treat the elderly patient with cancer pain.

So there is great heterogeneity in the physiology of older patients, and there are also several different populations of elders to consider when it comes to pain management. An overview of cancer patients in the long-term care setting, for example, is beyond the scope of this chapter. The authors acknowledge these different populations and remind the practicing oncologist that there are data in all three of these settings highlighting the *undertreatment* of pain. Despite national guidelines, consensus panels, and standards (see Table 26.1), we present data to show that cancer pain remains undertreated.

B. Undertreatment of pain

In one recent Medline search, the authors sought to identify and describe all studies conducted between 1987 and 2007 that assessed undertreatment of pain and tried to identify factors that predicted such undertreatment. Twenty-six studies met their criteria and revealed that 43 percent of cancer patients were undertreated.[11] Patients who were rated less ill (better performance status) and

at an early stage of disease were more likely to receive inadequate analgesia.[11]

A classic paper in the *Journal of the American Medical Association* in 1998 evaluated the adequacy of pain management in elderly and minority cancer patients admitted to nursing homes. Data were from the multilinked Systematic Assessment of Geriatric Drug Use via Epidemiology (SAGE) database. More than one-fourth of patients in daily pain did not receive any analgesic agent. Patients older than 85 years in daily pain were more likely to receive no analgesics. Other independent predictors of failing to receive any analgesic agent were minority race, low cognitive performance, and how many other medications the patient received. The authors concluded that daily pain was prevalent among nursing home residents with cancer and was often untreated, particularly among the older and minority patients.[12]

In outpatients with metastatic cancer, the picture was not much brighter. Cleeland and colleagues looked at over 1,300 outpatients with metastatic cancer affiliated with the Eastern Cooperative Oncology Group (ECOG). Sixty-seven percent of the patients reported that they had pain or had taken analgesic drugs daily during the week preceding the study, and 36 percent had pain severe enough to impair their ability to function. However, 42 percent were not given adequate analgesic therapy. Of note, patients seen at centers that treated predominantly minorities were 3 times more likely than those treated elsewhere to have inadequate pain management.[13]

More recently, a review was conducted to see if pain management in cancer patients with bone metastases improved over a 7-year time period. Per the study, patients who experienced moderate or severe pain and were prescribed no pain medication, nonopioids, or weak opioids were considered to be undermedicated. The median age was 68 years, with a range of up to 95 years of age, and no appreciable decline was noted in the proportion of patients with moderate to severe pain who received no pain medication, nonopioids, or weak opioids during the study period. The authors concluded that despite published guidelines and the dissemination of data about bone metastases and the need for analgesia, a significant proportion of patients continue to be undermedicated.[14]

Even the hospital setting is disheartening in this regard. Dating back to the 1990s, Desbiens and colleagues looked at pain in 1,266 patients at least 80 years of age in the Hospitalized Elderly Longitudinal Project (HELP). HELP enrolled patients at four teaching hospitals and excluded trauma patients. In this study of the oldest old, 45.8 percent complained of pain and 19 percent reported extremely severe pain of any frequency or moderately severe pain occurring at least half the time.[15] Interventions to improve pain scores in a large university hospital failed,[16] and a recent systematic review looked at institutional interventions to improve the assessment and treatment of pain in hospitalized cancer patients.[17] Sadly, though the review identified effective interventions to improve both nursing knowledge and assessment of pain, it was unable to identify any study that demonstrated improvements in the patients' pain experience.[17] The authors recommended that future research specifically target physicians.

C. Barriers

Barriers to good pain management in cancer patients have been studied.[18] The barriers to optimum pain relief have been classified into three categories: patient, professional, and system barriers.[19] Simply put, physicians, nurses, and other medical personnel both lack knowledge in pain management and hold many misconceptions about the effects of available therapies. In addition, patients themselves hamper their own treatment because of similar misconceptions about opioids and other drugs and lack of reporting to medical personnel that pain is an issue. Older patients may expect to have pain and will not report symptoms. Also, older patients value being a "good patient" and do not wish to use clinic time with problems that they themselves can handle or endure.[20] In order to improve patient comfort with disclosing

this information, one of the authors routinely asks patients, "If you were having pain, would you tell me?"[21]

It seems like not much has changed since the early 1990s. The ECOG conducted a group-wide survey to determine the amount of knowledge about cancer pain and its treatment among physicians practicing in ECOG-affiliated institutions and to determine the methods of pain control being used by these physicians.[22] Roughly one-half of the 1,800 surveys were returned. Eighty-six percent felt that the majority of patients were undermedicated for their pain, and 31 percent would wait until the patient's prognosis was 6 months or less before they would start maximal analgesia. *Poor pain assessment* was rated by 76 percent of the physicians as the single most important barrier to adequate pain management. Given the multiple complexities of the elderly cancer patient, what is the best way to do an adequate assessment?

D. Assessment

Acknowledging that pain assessment in older adults is a multidimensional and often multidisciplinary event,[23] reliance on self-report remains the most reliable measure of the pain complaint.[24] The sheer range and choice of pain assessment instruments can be daunting for the clinician (the consensus statement mentioned earlier had over 400 references), but the data clearly support self-report as the method of choice.[2,25] This behooves the clinician to believe the patient, even in the setting of mild to moderate cognitive impairment.

Furthermore, the expression of cancer pain is not simple biology (a direct representation of somatosensory cortex impact by afferent stimuli) but rather a multidimensional construct.[26] For example, cultural beliefs, psychological states including depression and delirium, and other cancer symptoms (e.g., fatigue, nausea, dyspnea) all affect the expression of pain.[26] More important, the "meaning of the pain" to the patient is absolutely crucial.[27] What are the patient's previous experiences with pain? Was it controlled or not? Does the pain serve as a metaphor for impending death? The nature of cancer pain can change during the course of disease, further complicating the clinician's task. In summary, all pain is real, and all pain means something to the patient.

E. It is more than just pain

It has been proposed that the approach favored in geriatric medicine, the comprehensive geriatric assessment, would allow for better management of elderly patients with cancer.[28] This is an extension of the work of Karnofsky, with its emphasis on functional status, to a more extensive assessment of the domains contributing not only to pain but to quality of life: physical and mental health, behavioral symptoms, social and economic resources, and so on. This more global approach has met with success in both the outpatient[29] and inpatient settings.[30] One caveat is that though comprehensive geriatric assessment has aided in understanding and managing the quality-of-life issues and functional needs of older patients, it can be time consuming and difficult to reimburse. However, data support this approach with outpatient older cancer patients using a self-administered questionnaire in a self-report format, thus bypassing the preceding concerns.[31] These data suggest that the assessment of pain does not need to be too time or labor intensive.

F. Heterogeneity in aging

This returns us to the gerontological principle of heterogeneity in aging. In no domain is this concept more relevant than in the physiological changes with aging that influence pain management. Thus the oncologist must be mindful of changes in drug metabolism, other comorbidities, and polypharmacy when prescribing medications for older patients. In a review in the *Journal of the American Geriatrics Society*, on average, a 70-year-old takes seven different medications.[32] Chronologic age is not the same as physiological age, and this accounts for the wide interindividual variation and unpredictable nature of adverse effects as a result of divergent individual patient therapeutic indexes.[7]

G. Aging physiology: Pain management

Physiological changes with age include a decreased cardiac index of 1 percent per year and reduced renal function of 1 percent per year after the age of 50 years, decreased hepatic blood flow, decreased hepatic mass, reduced hepatic cytochrome enzymes, and decreased plasma protein binding. Hepatic metabolism is reduced by 30–40 percent, so some opioids have increased oral bioavailability because of reduced hepatic extraction. Also of importance is that aging is associated with increased body fat, which increases the volume of distribution of lipophilic medications and delays both elimination and the onset of drug action without changing serum concentrations. Age-related reduced volume of distribution increases plasma concentrations of hydrophilic drugs, which secondarily increases drug diffusion to receptor sites. Polypharmacy because of multiple comorbidities increases the potential for pharmacokinetic and pharmacodynamic drug-drug interactions.[7]

Clinically, what this means is that if body fat increases as a proportion of total body weight, then a lipophilic drug such as fentanyl would have greater distribution, and conversely, a less extensive distribution would result for a hydrophilic drug like morphine.[33] The age-related decrements in glomerular filtration are of equal clinical importance. Drug and metabolite accumulation can occur in folks who are taking drugs that are renally excreted. So in considering the pharmacotherapy of pain, the nonsteroidal anti-inflammatory drugs (NSAIDs), morphine (with its metabolites morphine-6-glucuronide and morphine-3-glucuronide), meperidine (with its metabolite normeperidine), and propoxyphene (with its metabolite norpropoxyphene) are clinically important.[33] Keeping potential side effects and age-related changes in mind, two opioids that should be avoided in all elderly patients are meperidine and propoxyphene. Meperidine has a low potency relative to morphine and a toxic metabolite, normeperidine. Normeperidine is neurotoxic and can cause generalized seizures. Since normeperidine is eliminated renally, it is to be avoided in elderly patients.[33] Similarly for propoxyphene, it has a toxic metabolite, norpropoxyphene. Whereas the half-life of propoxyphene is 6–12 hours, the half-life of norpropoxyphene is 30–36 hours, and this can be prolonged further in those with decreased renal function or those exposed to repeated doses. Thus propoxyphene should not be prescribed in the elderly.[33]

The decrement in renal function with aging cannot be overemphasized. Specifically, with respect to opioids, some metabolites have greater potency than the parent compound or produce greater adverse effects on accumulation, as noted earlier.[33] There should be an increased awareness that in elderly patients, normal serum creatinine concentrations do not exclude renal impairment and that several commonly prescribed drugs require dose adjustments or should be avoided in the presence of renal insufficiency. Please note that the reduction in muscle mass in the elderly limits the value of serum creatinine in predicting glomerular filtration. Furthermore, as glomerular filtration rate (GFR) decreases, serum creatinine becomes less predictable as a means of determining drug excretion.[34]

H. Management

Though the elderly represent a unique population with a heterogeneity in their responses to therapy because of age-related change in pharmacokinetics and pharmacodynamics, there are principles and guidelines dating back to the 1980s and the World Health Organization (WHO) that provide evidence-based guidance. Cancer pain can be controlled with simple treatments in more than 80 percent of cases,[26] and research continues to show that the WHO ladder is more effective than standard community oncology practice for managing cancer pain.[35] In 1986 WHO published a set of guidelines for cancer pain management based on the three-step analgesic ladder.[36] Validation studies show that this approach works.[37,38] More recent studies are more critical because of strict evidence-based standards yet are generally supportive of the guidelines. In a rigorous review of the literature utilizing systematic databases to study cancer pain, Ferreira and colleagues concluded that the studies demonstrate that anywhere from 45–100 percent of the patients with pain who were using the WHO ladder had adequate analgesia. The authors conclude that though more evidence-based studies are needed, the WHO guidelines can be clinically useful.[39] Even the most rigorous and critical of authors conclude that the WHO guidelines are valid and are likely to remain the cornerstone of cancer pain management in the future.[40,41]

With this background on the principles and framework for pain management in the elderly, it is instructive to review the efforts of the American Geriatrics Society in addressing pain and cancer pain, in particular. A panel of experts, convened in 2001, revised earlier recommendations and exhaustively reviewed the literature. In its publication, "The Management of Persistent Pain in Older Persons," this panel reviewed both the quality of evidence (levels 1–3) and strength of evidence (A–E).[25] The panel recommended to combine pharmacologic and nonpharmacologic treatments, and this chapter will emphasize the pharmacologic. Furthermore, the admonition to "start low and go slow" was articulated: "Start with the lowest anticipated effective dose, monitor

frequently on the basis of expected absorption and known pharmacokinetics of the agent(s), and then titrate the dose on the basis of likely steady-state blood levels and clinically demonstrated effects."[25] What follows is the presentation of individual analgesics by drug class.

I. Nonopioid analgesics

I.1. Acetaminophen

Acetaminophen (also referred to as paracetamol) is preferred to NSAIDs in the elderly because of its low gastrointestinal and renal toxicity.[7] Acetaminophen is not a peripheral anti-inflammatory agent but is centrally acting and, in this sense, is a weaker analgesic than the cyclo-oxygenase inhibitors. Metabolized by glucuronidation, there are no age-related reductions in the clearance of acetaminophen; however, dosages above 2.6 g/d are unlikely to produce further analgesic benefit. Hepatic toxicity can occur at lower dosages than 4 g/d if there is coexisting liver disease, fasting, or regular alcohol consumption.[7]

I.2. Nonsteroidal anti-inflammatory drugs

The NSAIDs are a large group of agents widely used for their anti-inflammatory properties to reduce fever and pain. There is speculation that NSAIDs provide synergistic analgesia when used in combination with opioids (described later). This class of drug has a ceiling effect so that increases in the dose will not result in further improvement of the pain and numerous adverse effects in the elderly: gastrointestinal toxicity (bleeding and perforation), renal toxicity, and platelet aggregation inhibition. Of note, renal toxicity may appear at lower doses in the elderly with subclinical renal insufficiency, more frequently than in younger patients. Even the newer COX-2 inhibitors may have similar renal effects and certainly can affect cardiovascular status, a common comorbidity in the elderly.[33]

The evidence for efficacy and safety of NSAIDs in the treatment of cancer-related pain via meta-analysis from published randomized controlled trials appeared in 1994.[42] The article concluded that NSAIDs reduce cancer-related pain significantly more than placebo and supported the WHO recommendation to avoid the use of placebo in treating cancer pain. The studies were not sufficient to recommend NSAIDs for malignant bone pain in particular.

Subsequently, a much more rigorous review of 42 trials assessed the safety and efficacy of NSAIDs alone or combined with opioids in the treatment of cancer pain. Heterogeneity of study methods and outcomes precluded meta-analyses. Clear evidence to support superior safety or efficacy of one NSAID over another was lacking, and trials of combinations of an NSAID with an opioid showed no significant advantage, or at most a slight but statistically significant advantage, compared with either single entity.[43] The authors of this article state, "By combining an NSAID with an opioid, one should hope to achieve a reduction in the dose of opioid required to control pain, a reduction in side effects, or both. The 10 studies comparing NSAID versus opioid had conflicting results."[43] However, the article concludes by raising the question that the cyclo-oxygenase-2 inhibitors had potentially antiangiogenic properties and needed further study. Two articles in the *British Journal of Cancer* specifically look at the COX-2 inhibitor celecoxib and its effect on angiogenesis, tumor growth, metastasis, and mortality.[44,45] This clearly is an area ripe for future research.

The American Geriatrics Society has once again updated its Clinical Practice Guideline: Pharmacological Management of Persistent Pain in Older Persons. This guideline, and the data that support it, were presented in May 2009 at a plenary session of the society's national meeting.[46] Specifically, the guideline recommends that acetaminophen be considered as initial and ongoing pharmacotherapy of patients with mild to moderate musculoskeletal pain but – in a significant departure from the 2002 guideline – recommends that nonselective NSAIDs and COX-2 selective inhibitors be considered rarely and with caution. The new guideline recommends that all patients with moderate to severe pain, pain-related functional impairment, or diminished quality of life due to pain be considered for opioid therapy.[47] The guideline did not comment on opioids and NSAIDs together or the efficacy of NSAIDs in the setting of metastatic bone pain. Therefore a brief mention of bisphosphonates is appropriate.

I.3. Bisphosphonates

Metastatic bone disease occurs in more than 500,000 patients, including almost all patients with myeloma, two-thirds of patients with breast and prostate cancers, and one-third of patients with lung cancer.[48] Bisphosphonates bind to hydroxyapatite crystals, preventing resorption directly and inhibiting osteoclastic activity. For patients with metastasis to the bone, intravenous bisphosphonates reduce skeletal morbidity and may also possess significant antitumor effects. Both pamidronic acid (pamidronate) and zoledronic acid (zoledronate) are indicated for cancer-related hypercalcemia. Of note, pamidronic acid relieves pain associated with bone metastases and reduces opioid requirements by 30–50 percent of baseline. This drug is approved for long-term monthly administration in myeloma and in breast cancer with bone metastasis.

By far the most potent agent is zoledronic acid, whose relative potency is 1,000 times greater than pamidronate and 100,000 times greater than etidronate, an early bisphosphonate that contains no nitrogen. The potency of bisphosphonates varies greatly depending on their R1 and R2 side chains and the inclusion of nitrogen.[48] One significant but rare complication of bisphosphonates is osteonecrosis of the jaw.[49] Usually, jaw necrosis is characterized clinically by chronically exposed jawbone, up to and including suppuration and sequestration. The lesions are markedly refractory to treatment, including intensive antibiotic therapy and repeated jaw surgery. These features are reminiscent of osteoradionecrosis.[49] Clinicians are encouraged to be vigilant for conditions that might render patients more susceptible to this complication such as preexisting dental or periodontal disease, older age, potency and duration of the bisphosphonate administered, cancer chemotherapy, smoking, and a history of corticosteroid therapy.[50]

J. Opioids

For a comprehensive and thorough review of opioids and pain in the elderly, the reader is referred to a lengthy manuscript generated by the multidisciplinary group that attended the International Forum on Pain Medicine in 2005. Acknowledging that WHO step III opioids are the mainstay of pain treatment for cancer patients, with morphine as the paradigm, they reviewed the strength of evidence for opioids for cancer-related pain in the elderly, non-cancer-related pain, and neuropathic pain, citing over 250 references.[51] This chapter will review opioids in relation to cancer pain and will address common side effects from these agents in a proactive manner.

Table 26.2 Opioid routes of administration.

Route of administration	Opioid
PO, PR	Codeine
PO, IV	Oxycodone
PO	Hydrocodone
IV, PO, PR	Methadone
SC, IV, PR, PO, SL Epidural/intrathecal	Hydromorphone
PO, PR	Tramadol
IV, SC Epidural/intrathecal	Fentanyl
PO, SL, SC, IV Epidural/intrathecal	Morphine

Note. Oral = PO; PR = per rectum; SL = sublingual; SC = subcutaneous; IV = intravenous. Modified from Davis and Srivastava.[7]

Opioids are the cornerstone of the analgesic regimen for moderate to severe pain, though not all persons will respond similarly. Thus close follow-up and regular assessment are necessary. Opioids and related drugs can be described in several ways, including their activity at opioid receptors. The three main types of opioid receptors are mu, delta, and kappa receptors.[33] Mu-receptor agonists generally produce analgesia, affect numerous body systems, and influence mood. Mu-receptor agonists have no therapeutic ceiling effect and can be adjusted upward until pain is controlled or adverse effects ensue. And the inability of one opioid to attain analgesia does not preclude the use of another. There are a number of mu-receptor agonists with a variety of routes of administration (see Table 26.2)

The weak opioids codeine and tramadol have ceiling effects, resulting in limited analgesia and dose-related adverse effects. Both tramadol and codeine are converted to mu agonists by CYP2D6, so patients receiving medications that block CYP2D6 fail to experience analgesia with either of these opioids.[7] Codeine is metabolized by the liver to codeine-6-glucuronide, and most of the analgesic effect offered by codeine is due to the relatively small amount of morphine produced.[34]

Tramadol is a centrally acting analgesic with two mechanisms of action: weak opioid agonist activity and inhibition of monoamine uptake. Because the elimination half-life of tramadol is increased approximately twofold in patients with impaired hepatic or renal function, multiple administration of tramadol in such patients requires increased dosage intervals.[34]

If an older patient is having severe pain, there is no reason for delaying strong opioid therapy. Strong opioids include morphine, oxycodone, hydromorphone, fentanyl, and methadone. When strong opioids are given to elderly patients, the admonition of "start low and go slow" is imperative.[34]

The gold standard, morphine, is available in oral, rectal, sublingual, and parenteral forms. Morphine is highly extracted by the liver and is metabolized into two major metabolites, morphine-3-glucuronide (M3G) and morphine-6-glucuronide (M6G), which account for approximately 40 percent and 10 percent of the morphine dose recovered in the urine, respectively.[34] Hepatic impairment has been reported to be nonsignificant with respect to the pharmacokinetics of morphine as there is a relatively large hepatic reserve for glucuronidation. However, in patients with renal failure, the ratios of M3G and M6G to morphine accumulate substantially, making opioid toxicity more likely.[34]

Hydromorphone is more potent and soluble than morphine. An analog of morphine, hydromorphone is transformed in the liver to hydromorphone-3-glucuronide and hydromorphone-6-glucuronide, which are eliminated by the kidney. Thus these metabolites also accumulate in renal failure, and the same concerns for morphine apply here as well. Indeed, the metabolites of hydromorphone are active and can contribute to the production of toxic effects.[34]

A different kind of opioid with less concern for renal function is oxycodone. A semisynthetic opioid receptor agonist, oxycodone can be used as an alternative to morphine, and the pharmacokinetics of oxycodone are mostly independent of age, renal function, and serum albumin, so it is an attractive drug in the elderly.[34]

Yet another alternative to morphine is methadone, and it has gained popularity with regard to cancer pain. Methadone is a mu opioid receptor agonist with NMDA (N-methyl-D-aspartic acid) receptor antagonist affinity and has demonstrated positive results in controlling pain no longer responsive to morphine, hydromorphone, and fentanyl.[52] Its pharmacokinetics vary extremely among individuals, probably because of its metabolism through the cytochrome P450 enzyme family. At least four P450 proteins are involved in the methylation of methadone, so caution should be used in elderly cancer patients taking other medications because the P450 system can be inhibited or stimulated by these drug-drug interactions.[53] Advantages of methadone are that it can be given orally, intravenously, or rectally and its oral and rectal bioavailability is greater than 85 percent. It may have a role in the treatment of neuropathic pain because of its action as an antagonist of the NMDA receptor. Patients with renal impairment on maintenance methadone do not have higher plasma concentrations than those with normal renal function. However, because of its long half-life and propensity to accumulate, elderly patients receiving methadone should be monitored carefully.[53] Indeed, let the reader be aware that the use of methadone is limited by its remarkably long and unpredictable half-life, large interindividual variations in pharmacokinetics, the potential for delayed toxicity, and above all the limited knowledge of the correct administration intervals and the equianalgesic ratio with other opioids when administered long term.[52] Finally, not a small issue but one specific to methadone is the issue of the QTc interval.[54] Methadone may prolong the rate-corrected QT (QTc) and result in *torsade de pointes*. Patients should have an electrocardiogram (ECG) prior to initiating methadone, again at 30 days, and yearly thereafter to measure the QTc interval (QT interval corrected for heart rate).[54] If the QTc interval exceeds 500 ms, consider discontinuing or reducing the methadone dose and discontinuing drugs that promote hypokalemia. The expert panel concludes that "nonetheless, with regard to cardiac arrhythmia risk, standardized methadone can be safely administered as long as the potential for QTc interval prolongation is recognized through ECG screening and appropriate clinical actions are taken in the presence of QTc interval prolongation."[54]

Fentanyl may be an alternative to morphine in older patients with reduced renal clearance because of lack of accumulation of important metabolites but should not be used in opioid-naive patients.[34] Fentanyl is a synthetic opioid, a potent mu-receptor agonist. It can be delivered as an intravenous, transdermal, or oral transmucosal preparation. Fentanyl is metabolized by the liver via CYP3A4 to compounds that are inactive and nontoxic. Patches should be used cautiously in older cancer patients because these patients have a relatively low ratio of lean body mass to fat, which alters absorption and increases chances of drug accumulation once fat and muscle stores have been saturated. So beware of its use in cachectic patients and in opioid-naive patients.[34] Indeed, in the presence of hypoalbuminemia, both the effec-

tiveness and toxicity of fentanyl via any route may be increased as the drug is highly protein bound. However, compared with morphine, fentanyl is less likely to cause side effects, including pruritus, nausea, and constipation.[7]

K. Opioid adverse effects

The most common adverse effects are constipation, sedation, nausea, and vomiting. Adverse effects are to be anticipated and treated proactively.[27]

To prevent opioid constipation, prophylactic laxatives and stool softeners are started at the initiation of opioid administration. Softeners such as docusate sodium, 100 mg two to three times daily, are combined with a stimulant laxative or osmotic laxative. As with the opioid, dosage and schedule must be individualized, particularly in the elderly.[7] When nausea and vomiting are related to constipation, a prokinetic agent such as metoclopramide is a good consideration. Another approach to refractory constipation is rotation to another opioid, specifically methadone, which appears to cause less constipation than other opioids but does have its own issues, as outlined ealier.[53]

One author states that "mild sedation and transient cognitive impairment are common with initiation of opioids in the elderly."[7] The reader is asked to note that poor pain control leads to delirium and other cognitive effects independent of opioid use in older persons, and impaired cognition is not a contraindication to starting opioids.[7] For example, this chapter alluded to delirium in those elders with decreased physiologic reserve and renal function, but it should be noted that in a prospective cohort study at four New York hospitals that enrolled over 500 patients with hip fracture and without delirium, patients who received less than 10 mg of parenteral morphine sulfate equivalents per day were more likely to develop delirium than patients who received more analgesia. In short, avoiding opioids or using very low doses of opioids increased the risk of delirium. For cognitively intact patients with undertreated pain, their risk of delirium was 9 times higher than for those whose pain was adequately treated.[55] This study is yet another example of preventable suffering in our older population. If confusion does develop, one can reduce the dose, rotate to another opioid, alter the route of administration, and look to discontinue other drugs that could be contributing to the confusion such as anticholinergics, benzodiazepines, or tricyclic antidepressants. Note that opioid antagonists such as naloxone do not reverse confusion, delirium, or myoclonus and are not used solely for that indication.[7] If death is imminent, opioids are generally not rotated, and haloperidol is used for agitation/hallucinations, and benzodiazepines have a role for myoclonus and/or seizure activity.[7]

Nausea has three potential mechanisms vis-à-vis opioids: stimulation from the chemoreceptor trigger zone located in the postrema of the fourth ventricle, vertigo from cochlear stimulation, and gastroparesis.[7] Treatment with antiemetics can be tried; however, most reviews suggest that if nausea is persistent, reduce the dosage, try an alternative route, or rotate opioids.[7]

Myoclonus is a common, usually mild reaction to opioids. Generally, myoclonus is not a harbinger of seizure.[7] The drug list should be reviewed and any offending antipsychotic medication should be deleted. If not successful, then an opioid switch may be necessary. The addition of a benzodiazepine may reduce myoclonus, although increased sedation may be a side effect.

Respiratory depression, though feared, is rare in opioid-naive persons if low starting dosages are used and titrated judiciously. When respiratory depression does occur, it is often in opioid-naive patients who have received a brief course of an opioid and have other signs such as sedation and mental clouding.[33] Respiratory depression generally occurs more rapidly with lipid-soluble agents and with large, rapid dose escalation.[33]

Under some circumstances naloxone may be used to reverse opioid toxicity; however, the literature is replete with warnings about its use. If naloxone is used, its dosage should be adjusted *slowly* to reverse respiratory depression and decrease the chance of antagonizing analgesic effects. One way to achieve this is to dilute 0.4 mg of naloxone hydrochloride to a volume of 10 mL and then give the patient 1 mL of this solution at a time. The reader is cautioned that if a large bolus of naloxone is given, severe worsening of pain may occur that will be difficult to treat.[33] As one author put it, "if naloxone is to be used in a person who has been taking opioids for pain for a long time, administration can result in agony."[32] Furthermore, opioid withdrawal may occur in patients who have opioid physical dependence. Hypertension, tachycardia, and pulmonary edema may result as well as seizures if naloxone is administered after receiving meperidine.[33]

Two other side effects of note are urinary retention and pruritus (itching). Opioids may increase smooth muscle tone (leading to bladder spasms) and sphincter tone, a more frequent event in the elderly. Catheterization may be required.

The mechanism for the pruritus is not fully known, though mast cell release of histamine is part of the equation.[33] Switching to a different opioid may be necessary, and sedating antihistamines should be avoided or used with caution in older adults.

The literature is also in agreement that psychostimulants have a role to play for the mild sedation expected of opioids. Amphetamine, methylphenidate, and caffeine all have supporting literature to counteract opioid-induced sedative effects.[27] Psychostimulants also have a positive effect on cognition in the elderly and help keep the sleep-wake cycle intact by keeping the patient awake during the day with dosing of Ritalin, for example, at 8 A.M. and 12 noon. Personal experience with our palliative-care database shows that dosages as little as 2.5 mg of Ritalin at 8 A.M. and 12 noon are highly effective and show results within 48 hours.[56]

The switching and rotation of opioids is an excellent strategy in the management of opioid side effects. Converting from one opioid to another is a separate skill set, and the reader is directed to a recent publication in the Journal of Opioid Management, "Opioid Rotation in Patients with Cancer: A Review of the Current Literature," for detailed steps and guidelines in this regard.[57] Suffice it to say that opioid conversion should not be a mere mathematical calculation but part of a larger and more comprehensive assessment of the patient's current opioid therapy, pain, and adverse effect profile; comorbidities; and use of concomitant drugs. Furthermore, given the wide variability in conversion ratios reported in the literature, the optimal dose must be highly individualized. Though no long-term data are available, it is reported that opioid switching may improve the balance between pain relief and adverse effects in approximately 70–80 percent of patients.[34]

Finally, a discussion regarding the word *opiophobia*: "Opioids, Pain and Fear" was a recent editorial in the Annals of Oncology,[20] and a recent update in the Annals of Internal Medicine highlighted pain management and referred to this term as well.[58] In that review, a study by Portenoy and colleagues utilizing a hospice population was highlighted.[59] The study question asked whether opioid use hastens death in patients with advanced disease. The concern was that undertreatment of pain was secondary to fears that opioids would hasten death. The patients were older, with a mean age of 77 years, and came from 13 hospices across the United States. There was no association between percentage change in opioid dose and time until death. This study's findings help strengthen the existing claims that opioids are safe to use in patients with advanced illness.[59]

K.1. Nonpharmacological treatment

Although medications are the foundation of cancer pain management, recognition of the limitations of pharmacologic therapy and psychosocial factors involved in pain has led to the development of psychosocial interventions.[60,61] Although further testing in clinical trials is needed to establish evidence-based recommendations for the use of psychosocial interventions in treating older cancer patients, such interventions may be useful adjuvants in a comprehensive pain treatment plan. A systematic review and meta-analysis of behavioral therapies for cancer pain management found that these interventions as a group generally led to improved pain control (effect size 0.232, 95% confidence interval 0.072–0.392).[62] In addition, quality and strength of evidence ratings for a variety of nonpharmacological approaches are provided by the 2002 American Geriatrics Society's panel on persistent pain.[25]

The same report alerts the provider that unrelieved persistent pain commonly causes patients to seek relief with alternative medicine, including homeopathy, naturopathy, and chiropractic and spiritual healing.[25] Indeed, patients are seeking help, with or without the knowledge of their oncologists. The 2002 National Health Survey of over 31,000 U.S. adults found that 40 percent of patients with a current or former cancer diagnosis affirmed complementary and alternative medicine (CAM) use within the last year. Of note, cancer and pain were two of the most commonly cited reasons for CAM use.[63] From this, it is clear that the nonpharmacological approaches have evidenced-based merit and that our patients are not as concerned about the evidence as they are about seeking treatments for their pain that we have either undertreated or not treated at all.

L. The future

A recent review in *Drugs* gave an overview of the latest developments in routes of administration and associated drugs used to treat pain: intravenous, transdermal with iontophoresis, transdermal, pulmonary, microspheres, topical, subcutaneous, intranasal spray, sublingual spray, and oral transmucosal.[64] Under its "Evidence-Based Practice Program," the Agency for Healthcare Research and Quality is developing scientific information on which to base clinical guidelines, performance measures, and other quality-improvement tools.[65] Cohen, in a thoughtful review, laid out a research agenda in the *Journal of Clinical Oncology* that recommended research agendas in the areas of basic biology, societal aspects, and clinical aspects of cancer and aging.[66]

What is clear is that the demographic imperative will only exacerbate and highlight the situation we have now and any deficiencies that we have vis-à-vis pain management in the elderly cancer patient. This population has not been enrolled in clinical studies, and clinical trials are needed that are specific to elderly patients and that include assessments that go beyond performance status and incorporate features of comprehensive geriatric assessment. Studies in the areas of the selective COX-2 inhibitors and their impact on tumor biology as well as the new field of pharmacogenetics will have direct applicability to the aged patient with cancer pain. Perhaps what is needed most are studies targeted at how to improve education and implementation of guidelines regarding evaluation and treatment of pain by physicians and other health care providers.

The older patient with cancer represents a complexity not found in the rest of medicine, and as such, the traditional biomedical model fails to assist the clinician. However, there is evidence for a more comprehensive approach that emphasizes function and quality of life. To that end, the presence of pain and other symptoms behoove the practitioner to be aggressive in management, while always being aware of the physiological changes that accompany aging and the context and meaning in which the pain occurs. And though more research is needed in this underrepresented population, we do know that older patients with cancer suffer when we do not treat their pain and that this suffering can be overcome.

References

1. Galanos AN, Gardner WA, Riddick L. Forensic autopsy in the elderly. *South Med J.* 1989;82:462–466.

2. Rao A, Cohen HJ. Symptom management in the elderly cancer patient: Fatigue, pain, and depression. *J Natl Cancer Inst Monogr.* 2004;32:150–157.

3. Muss HB. Cancer in the elderly: a societal perspective from the United States. *Clin Oncol.* 2009;21:92–98.

4. Van Den Beuken E, de Rijke JM, Kessels AG, et al. Prevalence of pain in patients with cancer: a systematic review of the past 40 years. *Ann Oncol.* 2007;18:1437–1449.

5. Gibson SJ, Helme RD. Age-related differences in pain perception and report. *Clin Geriatr Med.* 2001;17:433–456.

6. Balducci L. Management of cancer pain in geriatric patients. *J Support Oncol.* 2003;1:175–191.

7. Davis MP, Srivastava M. Demographics, assessment and management of pain in the elderly. *Drugs Aging.* 2003;20(1):24–57.

8. Becker PM, Cohen HJ. The functional approach to the care of the elderly: a conceptual framework. *J Am Geriatr Soc.* 1984;32:923–929.

9. Nelson EA, Dannefer D. Aged heterogeneity: fact or fiction? The fate of diversity in gerontological research. *Gerontologist.* 1992;32:17–23.

10. Kennie DC. Good health care of the aged. *J Am Med Assoc.* 1983;249:770–773.

11. Deandrea S, Montanari M, Moja L, Apolone G. Prevalence of undertreatment in cancer pain: a review of published literature. *Ann Oncol.* 2008;19(12):1985–1991.

12. Bernabei R, Gambassi G, Lapane K, et al. Management of pain in elderly patients with cancer. SAGE Study Group. Systematic Assessment of Geriatric Drug Use via Epidemiology. *J Am Med Assoc.* 1998;279:1877–1882.

13. Cleeland CS, Gonin R, Hatfield AK, et al. Pain and its treatment in outpatients with metastatic cancer. *N Engl J Med.* 1994;330:592–596.

14. Kirou-Mauro AM, Hird A, Wong J, et al. Has pain management in cancer patients with bone metastases improved? A seven year review at an outpatient palliative radiotherapy clinic. *J Pain Symptom Manage.* 2009;37:77–84.

15. Desbiens NA, Meuller-Rizner N, Connors AF, et al. Pain in the oldest-old during hospitalization and up to one year later. HELP Investigators. Hospitalized Elderly Longitudinal Project. *J Am Geriatr Soc.* 1997;45:1167–1172.

16. Morrison RS, Meier DE, Fischberg D, et al. Improving the management of pain in hospitalized adults. *Arch Intern Med.* 2006;166:1033–1039.

17. Goldberg G, Morrison SR. Pain management in hospitalized cancer patients: a systematic review. *J Clin Oncol.* 2007;25:1792–1802.

18. Pargeon KL, Hailey BJ. Barriers to effective cancer pain management: a review of the literature. *J Pain Symptom Manage.* 1999;18:358–368.

19. Sun VC, Borneman T, Berrell B, et al. Overcoming barriers to cancer pain management: an institutional change model. *J Pain Symptom Manage.* 2007;34:359–369.

20. Maltoni M. Opioids, pain and fear. *Ann Oncol.* 2008;19:5–7.

21. Galanos, AN; Personal communication. April 2009

22. Von Roenn JH, Cleeland CS, Gonin R, et al. Physician attitudes and practice in cancer pain management: a survey from the Eastern Cooperative Oncology Group. *Ann Intern Med.* 1993;119:121–126.

23. An interdisciplinary expert consensus statement on assessment of pain in older persons. *Clin J Pain.* 2007;23(suppl 1):S1–S43.

24. Bruckenthal P. Assessment of pain in the elderly adult. *Clin Geriatr Med.* 2008;24:213–236.

25. The management of persistent pain in older persons: AGS panel on persistent pain in older persons. *J Am Geriatr Soc.* 2002;50:S205–S224.

26. Bruera E, Kim HK. Cancer pain. *J Am Med Assoc.* 2003;290:2476–2479.

27. Abernethy A. Older Patients with Cancer: A Framework for Managing Pain. In: *American Society of Clinical Oncology Educational Book: 43rd Annual Meeting.* Chicago: American Society of Clinical Oncology; 2007:301–306.

28. Bernabei R, Venturiero V, Tarsitani P, et al. The comprehensive geriatric assessment: when, where, how. *Crit Rev Oncol Hematol.* 2000;33:45–56.

29. Prevalence and pattern of symptoms in patients with cancer pain: a prospective evaluation of 1635 cancer patients referred to a pain clinic. *J Pain Symptom Manage.* 1994;9:372–382.

30. Rao AV, Hsieh F, Feussner JR, et al. Geriatric evaluation and management units in the care of the frail elderly cancer patient. *J Gerontol.* 2005;60A:798–803.

31. Ingram SS, Seo PH, Martell RE, et al. Comprehensive assessment of the elderly cancer patient: the feasibility of self-report methodology. *J Clin Oncol.* 2002;20:770–775.

32. Gloth FM. Pain management in older adults: prevention and treatment. *J Am Geriatr Soc.* 2001;49:188–199.

33. Strassels SA, McNicol E, Suleman R. Pharmacotherapy of pain in older adults. *Clin Geriatr Med*. 2008;24:275–298.

34. Mercadante S, Arcuri E. Pharmacological management of cancer pain in the elderly. *Drugs Aging*. 2007;24:761–776.

35. Du Pen SL, Du Pen AR, Polissar N, et al. Implementing guidelines for cancer pain management: results of a randomized controlled clinical trial. *J Clin Oncol*. 1999;17:361–370.

36. World Health Organization. *Cancer Pain Relief and Palliative Care*. Geneva, Switzerland: World Health Organization; 1990.

37. Zech DF, Grond S, Lynch UJ, et al. Validation of World Health Organization guidelines for cancer pain relief: a 10-year prospective study. *Pain*. 1995;63:65–76.

38. Ventafridda V, Tamburini M, Caraceni A, et al. A validation study of the WHO method for cancer pain relief. *Cancer*. 1987;59:850–856.

39. Ferreira K, Kimura M, Teixeira MJ. The WHO analgesic ladder for cancer pain control, twenty years of use. How much pain relief does one get from using it? *Support Care Cancer*. 2006;14:1086–1093.

40. Reid C, Davies A. The World Health Organization three-step analgesic ladder comes of age. *Palliative Med*. 2004;18:175–176.

41. Mercadante S, Fulfaro F. World Health Organization guidelines for cancer pain: a reappraisal. *Ann Oncol*. 2005;16(suppl 4):132–135.

42. Eisenberg E, Berkey CS, Carr DB, et al. Efficacy and safety of nonsteroidal anti-inflammatory drugs for cancer pain: a meta-analysis. *J Clin Oncol*. 1994;12:2756–2765.

43. McNicol E, Strassels S, Goudas L, et al. Nonsteroidal anti-inflammatory drugs, alone or combined with opioids, for cancer pain: a systematic review. *J Clin Oncol*. 2004;22:1975–1992.

44. Farooqui M, Li Y, Rogers T, et al. COX-2 inhibitor celecoxib prevents chronic morphine – induced promotion of angiogenesis, tumour growth, metastasis, and mortality without compromising analgesia. *Br J Cancer*. 2007;97:1523–1531.

45. AH Schontal. Direct non-cyclooxygenase-2 targets of celecoxib and their potential relevance for cancer therapy. *Br J Cancer*. 2007;97:1465–1468.

46. Release of the AGS guideline: pharmacological management of persistent pain in older persons. Paper presented at: American Geriatrics Society 2009 Annual Scientific Meeting; May 1, 2009; Chicago, IL.

47. American Geriatrics Society Panel on the Pharmacological Management of Persistent Pain in Older Persons. Pharmacological Management of Persistent Pain in Older Persons. *Journal of the American Geriatrics Society*. 2009;57(8):1331–1346.

48. Berenson JR. Metastatic bone disease: zoledronic acid and beyond. *J Support Oncol*. 2009;7(suppl 1):6–7.

49. Diel IJ, Bergner P, Grotz KA. Adverse effects of bisphosphonates: current issues. *J Support Oncol*. 2007;5:475–482.

50. Eisenberg E. Osteonecrosis of the jaw: significant but rare complication of bisphosphonates. *J Support Oncol*. 2009;7(suppl 1):8–9.

51. Pergolizzi J, Boger RH, Budd K, et al. Opioids and the management of chronic severe pain in the elderly: consensus statement of an international expert panel with focus on the six clinically most often used World Health Organization step III opioids. *Pain Practice*. 2008;4:287–313.

52. Ripamonti C, Duke DE. Strategies for the treatment of cancer pain in the new millennium. *Drugs*. 2001;61:955–977.

53. Delgado-Guay MO, Bruera E. Management of pain in the older person with cancer: Part 2: treatment options. *Oncology*. 2008;22:148-152.

54. Krantz MJ, Martin J, Stimmel B, et al. QTc interval screening in methadone treatment. *Ann Intern Med*. 2009;150:387–395.

55. Morrison RS, Magaziner J, Gilbert M, et al. Relationship between pain and opioid analgesics on the development of delirium following hip fracture. *J Gerontol*. 2003;58A:76–81.

56. Galanos, AN; Personal communication. April 2009

57. Vadalouca A, Moka E, Argyra E, et al. Opioid rotation in patients with cancer: a review of the current literature. *J Opioid Manage*. 2008;4:213–249.

58. Goldstein NE, Fischberg D. Update in palliative medicine. *Ann Intern Med*. 2008;148:135-140.

59. Portenoy RK, Sibirceva U, Smout R, et al. Opioid use and survival at the end of life: a survey of a hospice population. *J Pain Symptom Manage*. 2006;32:532–540.

60. Keefe FJ, Abernethy AP, Campbell LC. Psychological approaches to understanding and treating disease-related pain. *Annu Rev Psychol*. 2005;56:601–630.

61. Zaza C, Baine N. Cancer pain and psychological factors: a critical review of the literature. *J Pain Symptom Manage*. 2002;24:526–542.

62. Abernethy AP, Keefe FJ, McCrory DC, et al. *Technology Assessment on the Use of Behavioral Therapies for Treatment of Medical Disorders: Part 2 - Impact on Management of Patients with Cancer Pain*. Durham, North Carolina: Duke Center for Clinical Health Policy Research. As cited in Abernethy AP, Keefe FJ, McCrory DC,

et al. Behavioral therapies for the management of cancer pain: a systematic review. In: Flor H, Kalso E, Dostrovsky JO, eds. *Proceedings of the 11th World Congress on Pain.* Seattle, WA: IASP Press; 2006:789–798.

63. Corbin LW, Mellis BK, Kutner JS. Letter to the editor: the use of complementary and alternative medicine therapies by patients with advanced cancer and pain in a hospice setting: a multicentered, descriptive study. *J Palliative Med.* 2009;12:7–8.

64. Guindon J, Walczak J, Beaulieu P. Recent advances in the pharmacological management of pain. *Drugs.* 2007;67(15):2121–2133.

65. *Management of Cancer Pain: Summary, Evidence Report/Technology Assessment.* Report 35, Publication 01-E033. Washington, DC: Agency for Healthcare Research and Quality; 2001.

66. Cohen HJ. The cancer aging interface: a research agenda. *J Clin Oncol.* 2007;25:1945–1948.

27 Management of fatigue in older adults with cancer

Tami Borneman, Virginia Sun, and Betty Ferrell

A. Introduction

The global and U.S. population is aging at an unprecedented rate.[1,1a] Cancer is a disease affecting predominantly older persons with incidence and prevalence increasing with age.[2-6] Fifty-seven percent of newly diagnosed cancers and 71 percent of cancer deaths occur in those aged 65 years or older.[7] In addition to cancer, many older persons have comorbid medical conditions (e.g., cardiomyopathies, diabetes, depression), rendering them more susceptible to illness and treatment as well as limiting their functional capacities.[8,9] Fatigue from cancer and/or its treatment is the most commonly reported symptom by older cancer patients and affects 70–100 percent of those receiving treatment for cancer.[5-7] This chapter discusses the current evidence regarding cancer-related fatigue in the elderly and provides recommendations for the assessment and management of this distressing symptom in the elderly cancer population as well as future areas of research that are needed to further the science.

B. Review of the current evidence

As society ages, the number of older adults with cancer will continue to increase, and 70–100 percent of those receiving treatment for cancer will experience fatigue.[5-10] Cancer-related fatigue (CRF) is defined by the National Comprehensive Cancer Network (NCCN) as "a distressing persistent, subjective sense of physical, emotional and/or cognitive tiredness or exhaustion related to cancer or cancer treatment that is not proportional to recent activity and interferes with usual functioning."[11] Because CRF is an individual experience perceived by the patient and is more severe, more distressing, and less likely to be relieved by rest than fatigue in healthy patients, it is best described by self-report. All other sources of data are important additional information.[11] CRF affects all aspects of the patient's quality of life and can persist 5–10 years following completion of treatment.[12,13] The impact on the patient's physi-

cal functioning is exceptionally distressing and has been reported as being more distressing than pain or nausea.[13-15] CRF may be caused by treatments such as chemotherapy, radiation therapy, bone marrow transplantation, biological response modifiers, or contributing factors such as pain, emotional distress, anemia, altered nutritional status, sleep disturbance, decreased activity, and comorbidities.[11]

CRF affects physical functioning and can be very debilitating.[16] For the general geriatric population, the need for assistance with activities of daily living (ADLs) and instrumental ADLs (IADLs) is an independent predictor of morbidity and mortality. The older cancer patient is more likely to have functional limitations in ADLs than the noncancer patient.[17] For many patients, physical activity levels decrease during and after treatment, with some patients not returning to prior treatment levels. This can lead to a cycle of declining physical activity leading to increased fatigue, which leads to further decreased conditioning and increased weakness and fatigue during any physical activity.[5]

Luciani and colleagues[4] conducted a retrospective cross-sectional study of 214 patients aged 70 years or older seen over 3 months in the authors' Senior Adult Oncology Program. Patients were screened with a questionnaire assessing ADLs, IADLs, performance status (PS), cognitive impairment, depression, and malnutrition. Additionally, each patient was assessed for fatigue using the Fatigue Symptom Inventory, which measures four aspects of fatigue – severity, frequency, daily patterns of fatigue, and interference with daily activities – as well as complete blood counts and chemical panels. Eighty-one percent of the patients reported fatigue, and the interference score of fatigue was a probable mediator for dependencies in ADLs ($p < .001$) and IADLs ($p < .001$) and poorer PS ($p < .001$). Data revealed a correlation between severity, interference, and frequency of fatigue and depression, but only hemoglobin partially correlated with fatigue.

Anemia expression was correlated to functional status. All fatigue dimensions were significantly associated with ADL and IADL dependencies and with the Geriatric Depression Scale. The authors concluded that fatigue in the elderly could represent a long-term complication of cancer and cancer treatment that may accelerate functional decline.[4]

Comorbid conditions in the older cancer patient are also causes of morbidity and mortality, impacting life expectancy and tolerance to treatment and quality of life.[2,6] Those over the age of 65 have an average of three comorbidities, with the most common being cardiovascular disease, hypertension, chronic obstructive pulmonary disease (COPD), arthritis, and depression.[18] Comorbidities were found to be a prevailing issue among 867 elderly patients with newly diagnosed breast, prostate, lung, or colorectal cancer. Kozachik and Bandeen-Roche[3] conducted a secondary analysis on this population and followed the patients at four points in time (6–8 weeks, 12–16 weeks, 24 weeks, and 52 weeks) during the year after their diagnosis. The patients also completed a demographic questionnaire, the Comorbidity Index, and the Patient Symptom Experience. The researchers sought to determine if a patient's sex, age, comorbidity status, cancer site, stage of disease, or treatment regimen predicted patterns of pain, fatigue, and insomnia over time. The mean patient age was slightly over 72, most patients were men, and most reported a mean of more than two comorbidities. Twenty-seven percent reported four or more comorbidities. The top four comorbid conditions reported were heart problems (31%), arthritis (20%), high blood pressure (50%), and chronic lung disease (16%). Results revealed that advanced age was not significantly associated with increased patterns of pain, fatigue, and insomnia. Comorbidities were correlated with pain, fatigue, and insomnia only at wave 1 and 4 observation times. Sex was associated with significant risks of reporting fatigue/insomnia or fatigue/pain, with women reporting the most fatigue and sleep disturbance. Treatment modality was associated with significantly increased risks of pain/fatigue/insomnia. Having late-stage lung cancer and reporting pain/fatigue/insomnia at wave 2, 3, and 4 observation times were significantly associated with death.[3]

The psychological impact of CRF in older cancer patients can greatly diminish their quality of life. CRF affects the patient's social activities, leisure time, and responsibilities.[19] There is debate as to whether a correlation exists between fatigue and depression. However, depression occurs in approximately 20–50 percent of patients with cancer.[20-27] It is the most common psychiatric disorder among cancer patients and yet is frequently undiagnosed because of the oftentimes coexistent symptoms from cancer and/or cancer treatment such as fatigue, pain, and appetite loss.[22,23,28-30]

Hwang and colleagues[31] assessed multidimensional independent predictors of CRF and found that dyspnea, pain, lack of appetite, feeling drowsy, feeling sad, and feeling irritable predicted fatigue independently. Physical and psychological symptoms predict fatigue independently in the multidimensional model and supersede laboratory data.[31] Liao and Ferrell[32] assessed fatigue in the elderly and found a significant relationship between fatigue and depression, pain, number of medications, and physical function.[32] Respini and colleagues[6] found that fatigue correlated with depression in older cancer patients to a degree comparable to that in younger patients.[6] This study assessed the prevalence and correlates of fatigue in 77 cancer patients aged 60 or older during outpatient treatment with chemotherapy or pamidronate. An older study conducted by Hickie and colleagues[33] examined the prevalence and sociodemographic and psychiatric correlates of prolonged fatigue syndromes of 1,593 patients attending four general primary care practice settings. Twenty-five percent reported prolonged fatigue, and 37 percent had a psychological disorder. Of the 25 percent with fatigue, 70 percent had both fatigue and psychological disorder, whereas 30 percent had fatigue only. Data revealed that patients with fatigue were more likely to also have a depressive disorder.[33] The literature clearly shows the interrelationship between fatigue and psychological disorders.

C. Practical recommendations for managing fatigue in the elderly

An essential component of managing CRF in the elderly is a thorough assessment. Table 27.1 provides the fatigue assessment form used in our current National Institutes of Health–funded study to improve pain and fatigue management in the oncology setting.[34,35] The form was created based on recommendations from the NCCN CRF guidelines[11] and is used and completed by treating clinicians during clinic visits to document in a systematic manner the comprehensive assessment of fatigue. First, comorbidities need to be assessed

Table 27.1 Doctor/Nurse fatigue assessment.

Comorbidities
__ COPD   __ CAD   __ HTN   __ Diabetes   __ Other

Fatigue
- Level 0–10   __/10
- Are you having pain?   __ Yes (see other side)

Anemia
- Labs __ Hb level __ Iron panel (__Serum ferritin __TIBC __Transferrin saturation)
- Iron supplementation   __Yes   __No (__Oral __IV)
- Erythropoietic therapy   __Yes   __No

Nutrition
- Weight loss > 5%   __Yes   __No
- Appetite stimulants   __Megace   __Dronabinol   __Other

Sleep problems
- Sleep strategies
- Sleep medications _____

Depression/anxiety
- Do you feel depressed?   __Yes   __No   __Sometimes
- Medications _____

Referrals
- __Nutrition   __PT/OT   __SW   __Psychology   __Psychiatry
  __Support group

and addressed to determine other factors that may be contributing to fatigue related to cancer treatments. Elderly patients with a history of COPD or diabetes may be at higher risk for experiencing debilitating fatigue if treatment is planned. After assessing for comorbidities, patients should be asked to rate their fatigue level on a numerical analog scale (0–10). The NCCN guidelines recommend the following cutoffs for fatigue severity: 0–3 for "none to mild," 4–6 for "moderate," and 7–10 for "severe."[11] The guidelines recommend that all patients with a reported fatigue severity of moderate to severe intensity should be assessed using a focused history and examination to pinpoint treatable causes.[11] Treatable causes include anemia, pain, insomnia, malnutrition, and emotional distress. Finally, any referrals made to a supportive care expert, such as a dietitian, rehabilitation worker, social worker, psychologist or psychiatrist, or a support group, should be documented. The NCCN guidelines recommend using an interdisciplinary model for managing CRF.[11]

Another cornerstone of a successful fatigue management plan is to empower patients and families through education that provides them with knowledge on managing fatigue. Patients should be instructed on the definition of CRF, its causes, and how long patients are expected to experience fatigue. Second, a list of common causes of CRF should be provided to include anemia, pain, emotional distress, sleep problems, poor nutrition, inactivity, and other illnesses or comorbidities. Patients should be instructed on when to contact their clinicians about fatigue and the common questions that clinicians might ask to assess and manage the symptom. A list of energy-conservation tips should be provided to help patients with self-management of fatigue. The NCCN suggests the following as tips on energy conservation: setting priorities, delegating tasks, establishing a structured daily routine, balancing rest and activities, and limiting naps to 45 minutes to maintain nighttime sleep quality.[11] For patients with moderate to severe fatigue, the NCCN guidelines recommend interventions such as exercise, stress management, relaxation, support groups, sleep hygiene techniques, and treatment of anemia. Finally, the principles of exercise and tips on staying active should be included.

A number of systematic reviews and one Cochrane review have been undertaken to examine the efficacy of exercise in fatigue management.[36–38] A detailed assessment by a rehabilitation expert such as a physical therapist should be accessed if available to prescribe a comprehensive and safe exercise regimen. The prescribed exercise regimen should be initiated gradually and at a pace based on the individual's capabilities. Table 27.2 provides an outline of key concepts to be included in patient education for CRF. The outline includes education points on what fatigue is, common causes of fatigue, common words

Table 27.2 Managing fatigue.

What is fatigue?
- An overwhelming sense of exhaustion physically, mentally, emotionally
- Can occur with cancer or cancer treatment
- Can persist over time and interfere with usual activities
- Differs from the tiredness of everyday life, which is usually temporary and relieved by rest
- More distressing and not always relieved by rest
- Can vary in its unpleasantness and severity
- Can make being with friends/family difficult
- Can make it difficult to follow your treatment plan

Common causes of cancer-related fatigue
- Anemia (low red blood cell count)
- Pain
- Emotional distress
- Sleep problems
- Poor nutrition
- Lack of exercise
- Other illnesses such as infection, hypertension, diabetes

Common words used to describe cancer-related fatigue
- Feeling tired, weak, exhausted, weary, worn out
- Having no energy, not being able to concentrate
- Feelings of heaviness in arms and legs, feeling little to no motivation, sadness and/or irritability, and unable to sleep or sleeping too much

What to tell your doctor
- When did the fatigue start?
- Has it progressed over the course of your treatment?
- What makes your fatigue better?
- What makes your fatigue worse?
- How has the fatigue affected your daily activities?

Energy conservation principles
- Prioritize your activities in order of importance
- Ask for help and delegate tasks when you can
- Place items you use often within easy reach
- Establish a structured routine
- Balance rest and activities, performing activities during times of higher energy
- Establish a regular bedtime
- Whenever possible, sit instead of standing when performing tasks

Principles of exercise
- Your heart, lungs, and muscles require a daily workout. When you are less active, especially while in bed, your heart, lungs, and muscles have very little work to do. Over time, your heart pumps less forcefully, your lungs expand less fully, and your muscles will become weak and tight. This causes a drop in your energy level, which affects your ability to carry out your daily routine.
- The following tips should be considered:
  - Check with your doctor before exercising
  - Do exercises slowly and completely
  - If too tired to finish exercises, do what you can
  - Always work at your own pace; do not rush
  - Work within your own target heart rate (see your doctor for details)
  - Remember to breathe while you exercise
  - Walk!

no problem   0   1   2   3   4   5   6   7   8   9   10   **severe problem**

Table 27.3 Nutrition to manage fatigue.

Managing and optimizing your nutrition can help to
- Prevent or reverse nutrient deficiencies (e.g., too little calcium or vitamins)
- Preserve lean body mass
- Better tolerate treatments
- Minimize nutrition-related side effects and complications (nausea, vomiting, and dehydration)
- Maintain strength and energy
- Protect immune function, decreasing risk of infection
- Aid in recovery and healing
- Maximize quality of life

Poor Nutrition: Its Effects
In people with cancer, certain changes in nutrition can affect fatigue levels. These changes include the ability to process nutrients, increase energy requirements, and decrease intake of food, fluids, and some minerals.

These changes can be caused by the following:
- Changes in the body's ability to break down food products (metabolism)
- Competition between your cancer and your body for nutrients
- Poor appetite
- Nausea/vomiting
- Diarrhea or bowel obstruction

Fatigue can affect your interest in food, ability to shop, and ability to prepare healthy meals. Some suggestions include the following:
- Be familiar with your treatment and possible side effects
- Make sure you get enough rest
- Save favorite foods for nontreatment days so they won't be linked to an unfavorable event
- Poor nutrition and not eating can increase your fatigue
- If unable to eat regular-sized meals, eat small meals more often
- Include protein in your diet (fish, beans, milk, cheese)
- Drink plenty of fluids (8–10 cups per day)
- If unable to eat, drink high-calorie, high-protein drinks (milk, juices, smoothies, milkshakes, nutrition supplements)
- Stock your pantry to avoid extra shopping trips
- Keep foods handy that need little to no preparation (pudding, peanut butter, tuna fish, cheese, eggs)
- Do some cooking in advance and freeze meal-sized portions
- Eat larger meals when feeling better
- Talk to family/friends about help with shopping/cooking

Please ask your physician to refer you to a dietitian if you
- Have had minimal food intake for 5 days or more
- Have difficulties with chewing or swallowing
- Are receiving tube feedings or IV nutrition (total parenteral nutrition)
- Have a pressure ulcer or skin breakdown
- Are not able to maintain weight
- Wish to see a dietitian about your nutrition concerns

used to describe fatigue, what patients should tell their clinicians about fatigue, energy-conservation principles, and the principles of exercise.

As previously discussed, there are several treatable causes that impact CRF. Nutrition is a cause that is of particular importance for the elderly cancer patient. Geriatric patients may also be at higher risk for malnutrition. Potential reasons include more difficulty accessing healthy food items, poorly fitted dentures, or inability to prepare healthy meals secondary to functional limits. Geriatric oncology patients may be at par-

ticular risk because of gastrointestinal side effects (nausea, diarrhea) as well as poor appetite secondary to cancer treatment.[39] Table 27.3 provides a detailed guide on nutrition in the management of CRF that can be used as educational material for patients. It is important to stress the importance of optimizing nutrition in oncology, particularly in relation to fatigue management. Patients should be provided with adequate information on potential side effects so that they are aware of what to expect during treatment. If unable to eat regularly, patients can be advised to switch their eating habits from three large meals per day to six smaller meals spread throughout the day. The importance of maintaining adequate fluid intake should be emphasized, unless contraindicated. Finally, if available, referrals to nutrition experts such as dietitians should be initiated to aid elderly patients in optimizing their nutrition as a strategy for fatigue management.

Another treatable cause that may aggravate CRF is sleep deprivation. Owing to natural courses of aging, the length and quality of REM sleep decreases as the aging process continues.[8] Elderly cancer patients may be at higher risk for greater sleep disturbance. Table 27.4 provides a patient education guide for strategies to promote sleep. Patients can be instructed on the principles of sleep hygiene. These principles include the avoidance of caffeinated drinks or intense exercise before going to bed. Maintaining a dark, cool, and quiet sleep environment may help with inducing and enhancing sleep.[40] If possible, patients should be strongly encouraged to limit their daily nap times to no more than two 60-minute naps per day. This strategy will help in maintaining the quality of nighttime sleep. Relaxation or sleep-inducing strategies, such as taking warm baths, drinking a glass of warm milk, or listening to soothing music, can be used.

Stress management strategies, such as meditation, massage, or muscle relaxation, may also manage cancer-related fatigue.[41–43] Any contributing factors, such as anxiety, should be addressed by supportive care experts and assessed as a possible contributor to sleep disturbance. Patients should be assessed for any other symptoms, such as uncontrolled pain, that may be interfering with the quality of sleep. Maintaining physical activity during the day may help with promoting sleep at night, and patients, if possible, should be encouraged to remain as active as possible. Finally, if pharmacologic intervention is warranted, clinicians can discuss the various options available either over the counter or prescribed, and a pharmacologic agent should be chosen together with the patient that will provide the greatest benefit without debilitating side effects.

A number of pharmacologic agents have been evaluated for the treatment of cancer-related fatigue. The class of pharmacologic agents that shows the most promise in managing CRF are psychostimulants, which are known to increase alertness and motivation. Methylphenidate has been evaluated in HIV patients[44] and advanced cancer patients.[45] In a pilot study by Bruera and col-

Table 27.4 Strategies to help with promoting sleep.

Sleep hygiene strategies
- Avoid coffee, tea, chocolate, and soft drinks before going to bed.
- Avoid exercising 2–4 hours before bedtime.
- Sleep in a dark, cool, quiet, and relaxing room.
- Develop a bedtime ritual (i.e., warm milk before bedtime).
- Use your bed only for sleeping and intimacy.
- If possible, go to bed at the same time each night.

Sleep restriction strategies
- Add 1 additional of hour of sleep if you feel ill or unable to get up at the scheduled time in the morning.
- Limit naps to no more than two everyday, each lasting less than an hour.

Relaxation strategies
- Take a warm shower or bath before going to bed.
- Listen to soothing music.
- Use meditation, massage, progressive relaxation, or other strategies to decrease stress.

Other strategies
- Keeping yourself as active as possible during the day will help with promoting sleep at night (discuss with your health provider what forms of exercise are safest for you).
- Having other symptoms, such as pain or fatigue, can affect your sleep. If you are currently experiencing other symptoms, please talk to your provider about how to best manage these symptoms.
- If you are worried, depressed, or anxious, talk to your provider about resources to help you cope with these concerns.
- A variety of sleep medications (over the counter or prescribed) are available to help you sleep. Please ask your provider about which sleep medications would be best for you to take.

leagues,[46] an improvement was shown in general well-being, depression, and fatigue scores as measured by the Functional Assessment of Chronic Illness Therapy - Fatigue (FACIT-F) scale.[46] Because of the rapid onset of action and short half-life of methylphenidate,[47] a subsequent double-blind, randomized, placebo-controlled trial by Bruera and colleagues[48] tested a patient-controlled methylphenidate protocol for patients with a self-reported fatigue intensity of 4 or greater as measured by the FACIT-F scale. Dosage tested in this study was methylphenidate 5 mg or placebo every 2 hours as needed, up to four tablets per day, with fatigue assessment at day 8, 15, and 36.[48] Fatigue intensity decreased significantly at day 8 in both groups, but there was no significant difference in fatigue improvement.[48] However, in the open-label phase, a significant difference in fatigue improvement was found between groups and was sustained through days 15 and 36.[48] It was unclear whether the extended improvement during the open-label phase was an independent result or due to placebo effect. Although there is evidence on a preliminary level to support the effectiveness of psychostimulants for the treatment of CRF, some caution needs to be taken, particularly for geriatric oncology patients. Owing to their rapid onset, behavioral effects, and tolerance issues, there is an increased risk for experiencing side effects. The most common side effects of psychostimulants include agitation and insomnia, which may cause more harm than benefit for elderly cancer patients. Cardiovascular issues, such as hypertension, palpitations, and arrhythmias, as well as confusion, psychosis, and tremors are rare side effects but again may be potentially dangerous for elderly cancer patients. These common and potential side effects limit the use of this class of agents for elderly cancer patients because of contraindications for cardiovascular as well as other comorbid conditions.[47]

Modafinil has been tested as a fatigue treatment option. In a study with breast cancer survivors, Morrow and colleagues[49] reported an 86 percent reduction of fatigue intensity with a modafinil dosage of 200 mg/d. Donepezil, an agent used in the treatment of Alzheimer's dementia, was evaluated by Bruera and colleagues[50] in a double-blind placebo-controlled trial of donepezil 5 mg/d compared to placebo. The study results were negative, with no statistically significant difference shown between groups. Toxicities are also a problem for this drug and include nausea, vomiting, diarrhea, muscle and abdominal cramps, and anorexia, which may limit its use in the geriatric oncology setting.[47] Studies exploring the use of antidepressants as a possible mechanism for managing fatigue demonstrated no differences in fatigue scores.[51]

The following case examples are used to illustrate practical recommendations on fatigue management for the elderly in a realistic clinical setting.

C.1. Case 1: Mr. L

Mr. L is an 80-year-old male who is diagnosed with stage II colon cancer. He has a history of chronic arthritis and is a diabetic. His blood sugar is not optimally controlled, and Mr. L has had two recent visits to the emergency room for uncontrolled blood glucose. Over the years, because of his uncontrolled diabetes, Mr. L gradually developed diabetic peripheral neuropathy, and he uses a walker to help with ambulation. The neuropathy has interfered significantly with Mr. L's functional status, and he relies on a niece who lives close by to shop for food and everyday essentials. Mr. L's wife passed away 1 year ago, and Mr. L admits that he is still "mourning" his loss. Mr. L has agreed to receive chemotherapy to treat his colon cancer. He comes to the clinic today for his third course of chemotherapy and reports that he has been "very tired" for the past week. When asked to rate his fatigue intensity over the past 7 days, Mr. L reports that it is a 6 out of 10.

Discussion

According to the NCCN guidelines, Mr. L is currently suffering from moderate fatigue. This rating alone should trigger a red flag, and a more focused fatigue history and examination should be conducted, in addition to a comprehensive geriatric assessment. An in-depth fatigue history should be collected. This history should include the onset, pattern, and duration of fatigue over the past 7 days; changes over time; associated or alleviating factors; and the amount of interference that fatigue has on functional status. Next, a thorough assessment of treatable contributing factors should occur. Given Mr. L's history, a number of areas should warrant further evaluation: the status of his known comorbidities, possible pain from his chronic arthritis and neuropathy, activity level, nutrition status, possible depression secondary to complicated bereavement, and possible anemia secondary to three courses of chemotherapy. Referrals to supportive care experts such as a dietitian, physical therapist, psychologist, social worker, or pain specialist should be considered to manage the treatable causes. An endocrinologist may be needed if Mr. L's diabetes continues to be poorly controlled. Patient education materials should be accessed, and education on strategies of fatigue management, such as energy conservation and physical activity, should be provided. Finally, reassessment should occur at each clinic visit for Mr. L, given the many treatable causes that may be contributing to his fatigue. The clinician should maintain constant communication with any supportive care experts managing Mr. L's fatigue to better reassess and update the treatment plan, if needed.

C.2. Case 2: Mrs. J

Mrs. J is a 75-year-old female recently diagnosed with stage III pancreatic cancer. She has a history of COPD, having had a 20-year history of smoking. She is scheduled to begin chemotherapy treatment after being told that her tumor is unresectable. Mrs. J reports abdominal pain that is rated at 5 out of 10. She has also lost a substantial amount of weight since her diagnosis. Mrs. J reports feeling stressed and anxious because she is worried that she will not be able to care for her husband with Alzheimer's. Mrs. J's only son passed away from a car accident 3 years ago, and she is her husband's primary caregiver.

Discussion

Given the history of the patient, it can be predicted that Mrs. J is at higher risk for developing CRF. In this situation, the treatable causes (comorbidities, pain, weight loss, emotional distress) should all be assessed through a focused history and examination. If possible, referrals to a pain specialist, dietitian, and psychologist should be considered to manage the potential treatable causes of fatigue. Mrs. J's COPD should be evaluated to assess whether optimal control is achieved. The most important issue to address in Mrs. J's case would be her role as primary caregiver for her husband with Alzheimer's. In this case, a consultation with social work would aid in addressing some of these issues. It is essential to secure some care assistance for Mrs. J while she is receiving treatment. Psychosocial interventions such as stress management techniques, relaxation, or support groups might be beneficial for Mrs. J as well.

D. The future of fatigue-related research in the elderly

There are several important areas of research that are needed to further understand fatigue in elderly cancer patients and to further enhance assessment and management. First, CRF research should be designed specifically to target the elderly population. By doing so, the specific needs of elderly cancer patients can be better elucidated. Armed with more descriptive studies to explore the needs, attitudes, knowledge, and experience of CRF in the elderly, tailored patient education in assessment and management of fatigue can be developed.

Patient education for the elderly cancer patient must acknowledge the fact that fatigue is common in cancer and that elderly patients should be encouraged to discuss the symptom with their clinicians. Functional status should be assessed in detail for the elderly cancer patient because a limit in function may lead to inactivity or malnutrition, which can aggravate fatigue. Loss of functional independence has been associated with reduced survival, diminished quality of life, depression, and financial burden for patients, and fatigue is a primary cause of functional dependence for elderly cancer patients.[4] It has been reported that fatigue may accelerate the functional decline of elderly cancer patients.[4] Although evidence-based clinical guidelines are available for managing CRF, it is unclear whether these guidelines are generalizable to elderly cancer patients because the majority of the evidence has not been tested specifically in an elderly sample population. While the majority of recommendations can be applied to the elderly population, there may be issues that are specific to the elderly that are not thoroughly addressed in the guidelines.

Over the last decade, exercise and physical activity has emerged as a potentially effective strategy for managing CRF. The abundance of evidence can be recognized by the publication of numerous systematic reviews and a Cochrane review to determine the scientific evidence behind the efficacy of exercise. However, many limitations still exist in the current evidence on exercise. The quality of studies published thus far is widely variable.[36] There are issues with statistical power because many studies were limited by a small sample size.[36,52] In RCTs conducted on activity-based interventions, a variety of regimens were used. This variation makes it difficult to determine the most effective type of exercise for fatigue management. Future research is necessary to determine which parameters of exercise are most effective in managing fatigue. These parameters include type of exercise (aerobic or resistance), mode of exercise, length and frequency of sessions, and the amount of intensity that needs to be carried out.[36,53,54] These parameters should also apply for developing activity-based interventions for the elderly cancer patient. Because comorbidities and functional dependence are common in the elderly population, it is crucial to develop modes of activity that are realistically feasible for this understudied population. Although experts are calling for research that produces more long-term follow-up outcomes of activity-based interventions, it may be equally important to focus on short-term outcomes in the elderly population. Finally, outcome measures used to assess fatigue in research should be psychometrically tested in elderly populations to establish reliability and validity as perceptions of fatigue may be different.

E. Conclusion

Cancer is primarily a disease of the older population. As the geriatric population of the United States increases, it is expected that more elderly individuals will be treated with cancer. Fatigue continues to be recognized as the most common and distressing chronic complication of cancer and its treatments. Fatigue affects all aspects of quality of life and can lead to reduced social interactions and functional independence for the elderly. Clinicians should be aware of evidence-based strategies to assess and manage CRF. An interdisciplinary, comprehensive model of fatigue management incorporating focused assessment and patient education can be helpful in supporting elderly patients and families who are experiencing fatigue. Future research in fatigue should focus on describing the unique aspect of fatigue in the elderly cancer population and developing tailored interventions that are specific and realistic for this understudied population.

References

1. United Nations. World population aging: 1950–2050. United Nations Web site. Available at: http://www.un.org/esa/population/publications/worldageing19502050/.

1a. United Nations. World population prospects: the 2006 revision. United Nations Web site. Available at: http://www.un.org/esa/population/publications/wpp2006/WPP2006_Highlights_rev.pdf.

2. Hurria A. We need a geriatric assessment for oncologists. *Nat Clin Pract Oncol*. 2006;3:642–643.

3. Kozachik SL, Bandeen-Roche K. Predictors of patterns of pain, fatigue, and insomnia during the first year after a cancer diagnosis in the elderly. *Cancer Nurs*. 2008;31:334–344.

4. Luciani A, Jacobsen PB, Extermann M, et al. Fatigue and functional dependence in older cancer patients. *Am J Clin Oncol*. 2008;31:424–430.

5. Luctkar-Flude MF, Groll DL, Tranmer JE, et al. Fatigue and physical activity in older adults with cancer: a systematic review of the literature. *Cancer Nurs*. 2007;30:E35–E45.

6. Respini D, Jacobsen PB, Thors C, et al. The prevalence and correlates of fatigue in older cancer patients. *Crit Rev Oncol Hematol*. 2003;47:273–279.

7. Rao A, Cohen HJ. Symptom management in the elderly cancer patient: fatigue, pain, and depression. *J Natl Cancer Inst Monogr*. 2004;32:150–157.

8. Balducci L. *NCCN Clinical Practice Guidelines in Oncology: Senior Adult Oncology*. National Comprehensive Cancer Network Website. 2010. Accessed 3/23/10. Available at http://www.nccn.org/professionals/physician_gls/PDF/senior.pdf.

9. Penedo FJ, Schneiderman N, Dahn JR, et al. Physical activity interventions in the elderly: cancer and comorbidity. *Cancer Invest*. 2004;22:51–67.

10. Berger AM, Abernathy AP, Atkinson A, et al. NCCN clinical practice guidelines in oncology: cancer-related fatigue. National Comprehensive Cancer Network Web site. Available at: http://www.nccn.org/professionals/physician_gls/PDF/fatigue.pdf.

11. National Comprehensive Cancer Network. NCCN clinical practice guidelines in oncology: Cancer-related fatigue. National Comprehensive Cancer Network Web site. 2010. Accessed 3/23/10. Available at: http://www.nccn.org/professionals/physician_gls/PDF/fatigue.pdf.

12. Berger AM, Mitchell SA. Modifying cancer-related fatigue by optimizing sleep quality. *J Natl Compr Canc Netw*. 2008;6:3–13.

13. Mustian KM, Palesh O, Heckler CE, et al. Cancer-related fatigue interferes with activities of daily living among 753 patients receiving chemotherapy: A URCC CCOP study [abstract]. *J Clin Oncol*. 2008;26:15S.

14. Mallinson T, Cella D, Cashy J, et al. Giving meaning to measure: linking self-reported fatigue and function to performance of everyday activities. *J Pain Symptom Manage*. 2006;31:229–241.

15. Stone P, Richardson A, Ream E, et al. Cancer-related fatigue: inevitable, unimportant and untreatable? Results of a multi-centre patient survey. Cancer Fatigue Forum. *Ann Oncol*. 2000;11:971–975.

16. Hofman M, Ryan JL, Figueroa-Moseley CD, et al. Cancer-related fatigue: the scale of the problem. *Oncologist*. 2007;12(suppl 1):4–10.

17. Keating NL, Norredam M, Landrum MB, et al. Physical and mental health status of older long-term cancer survivors. *J Am Geriatr Soc*. 2005;53:2145–2152.

18. Repetto L. Greater risks of chemotherapy toxicity in elderly patients with cancer. *J Support Oncol*. 2003;1(4 suppl 2):18–24.

19. Romito F, Montanaro R, Corvasce C, et al. Is cancer-related fatigue more strongly correlated to haematological or to psychological factors in cancer patients? *Support Care Cancer*. 2008;16:943–946.

20. Akechi T, Okuyama T, Onishi J, et al. Psychotherapy for depression among incurable cancer patients. *Cochrane Database Syst Rev*. 2008;2:CD005537.

21. Bowers L, Boyle DA. Depression in patients with advanced cancer. *Clin J Oncol Nurs*. 2003;7:281–288.

22. Chochinov HM. Depression in cancer patients. *Lancet Oncol*. 2001;2:499–505.

23. Fulcher CD. Depression management during cancer treatment. *Oncol Nurs Forum*. 2006;33:33–35.

24. Lloyd-Williams M. Screening for depression in palliative care. *Am J Hosp Palliat Care*. 2001;18:79–80.

25. Miller K, Massie MJ. Depression and anxiety. In: Berger AM, Shuster JL, Von Roen JH, eds. *Principles and Practice of Palliative Care and Supportive Oncology*. 3rd ed. Philadelphia: Lippincott, Williams & Wilkins; 2007:445–456.

26. Schneider KL, Shenassa E. Correlates of suicide ideation in a population-based sample of cancer patients. *J Psychosoc Oncol*. 2008;26:49–62.

27. Deimling GT. The effects of cancer-related pain and fatigue on functioning of older adult, long-term care survivors. *Cancer Nursing* 2007;30:421-433.

28. Lawrie I, Lloyd-Williams M, Taylor F. How do palliative medicine physicians assess and manage depression. *Palliat Med.* 2004;18:234–238.

29. Massie MJ. Prevalence of depression in patients with cancer. *J Natl Cancer Inst Monogr.* 2004;32:57–71.

30. Pirl WF. Evidence report on the occurrence, assessment, and treatment of depression in cancer patients. *J Natl Cancer Inst Monogr.* 2004;32:32–39.

31. Hwang SS, Chang VT, Rue M, et al. Multidimensional independent predictors of cancer-related fatigue. *J Pain Symptom Manage.* 2003;26:604–614.

32. Liao S, Ferrell BA. Fatigue in an older population. *J Am Geriatr Soc.* 2000;48:426–430.

33. Hickie IB, Hooker AW, Hadzi-Pavlovic D, et al. Fatigue in selected primary care settings: sociodemographic and psychiatric correlates. *Med J Aust.* 2006;164:585–588.

34. Borneman T, Piper BF, Sun VC, et al. Implementing the Fatigue Guidelines at one NCCN member institution: process and outcomes. *J Natl Compr Canc Netw.* 2007;5:1092–1101.

35. Piper BF, Borneman T, Sun VC, et al. Cancer-related fatigue: role of oncology nurses in translating national comprehensive cancer network assessment guidelines into practice. *Clin J Oncol Nurs.* 2008;12(5 suppl):37–47.

36. Cramp F, Daniel J. Exercise for the management of cancer-related fatigue in adults. *Cochrane Database Syst Rev.* 2008;2:CD006145.

37. Knols R, Aaronson NK, Uebelhart D, et al. Physical exercise in cancer patients during and after medical treatment: a systematic review of randomized and controlled clinical trials. *J Clin Oncol.* 2005;23:3830–3842.

38. Stricker CT, Drake D, Hoyer KA, Mock V. Evidence-based practice for fatigue management in adults with cancer: exercise as an intervention. *Oncol Nurs Forum.* 2004;31:963-976.

39. Brown JK. A systematic review of the evidence on symptom management of cancer-related anorexia and cachexia. *Oncol Nurs Forum.* 2002;29:517–532.

40. Berger AM, VonEssen S, Khun BR, et al. Feasibilty of a sleep intervention during adjuvant breast cancer chemotherapy. *Oncol Nurs Forum.* 2002;29:1431–1441.

41. Spiegel D, Bloom JR, Yalom I. Group support for patients with metastatic cancer: a randomized outcome study. *Arch Gen Psychiatry.* 1981;38:527–533.

42. Yates P, Aranda S, Hargraves M, et al. Randomized controlled trial of an educational intervention for managing fatigue in women receiving adjuvant chemotherapy for early-stage breast cancer. *J Clin Oncol.* 2005;23:6027–6036.

43. Ream E, Richardson A, Alexander-Dann C. Supportive intervention for fatigue in patients undergoing chemotherapy: a randomized controlled trial. *J Pain Symptom Manage.* 2006;31:148–161.

44. Breitbart W, Rosenfeld B, Kaim M, et al. A randomized, double-blind, placebo-controlled trial of psychostimulants for the treatment of fatigue in ambulatory patients with human immunodeficiency virus disease. *Arch Intern Med.* 2001;161:411–420.

45. Sarhill N, Walsh D, Nelson KA, et al. Methylphenidate for fatigue in advanced cancer: a prospective open-label pilot study. *Am J Hosp Palliat Care.* 2001;18:187–192.

46. Bruera E, Driver L, Barnes EA, et al. Patient-controlled methylphenidate for the management of fatigue in patients with advanced cancer: a preliminary report. *J Clin Oncol.* 2003;21:4439–4443.

47. Breitbart W, Alici Y. Pharmacologic treatment options for cancer-related fatigue: current state of clinical research. *Clin J Oncol Nurs.* 2008;12(5 suppl):27–36.

48. Bruera E, Valero V, Driver L, et al. Patient-controlled methylphenidate for cancer fatigue: a double-blind, randomized, placebo-controlled trial. *J Clin Oncol.* 2006;24:2073–2078.

49. Morrow GR, Gillies LJ, Hickok JT, et al. The positive effect of the psychostimulant modafinil on fatigue from cancer that persists after treatment is completed. *ASCO Annu Meet Proc, Part I.* 2005;23:729s.

50. Bruera E, El Osta B, Valero V, et al. Donepezil for cancer fatigue: a double-blind, randomized, placebo-controlled trial. *J Clin Oncol.* 2007;25:3475–3481.

51. Rao AV, Cohen HJ. Fatigue in older cancer patients: etiology, assessment, and treatment. *Semin Oncol.* 2008;35:633–642.

52. Jacobsen PB, Donovan KA, Vadaparampil ST, et al. Systematic review and meta-analysis of psychological and activity-based interventions for cancer-related fatigue. *Health Psychol.* 2007;26:660–667.

53. Kangas M, Bovbjerg DH, Montgomery GH. Cancer-related fatigue: a systematic and meta-analytic review of non-pharmacological therapies for cancer patients. *Psychol Bull.* 2008;134:700–741.

54. Stone PC, Minton O. Cancer-related fatigue. *Eur J Cancer.* 2008;44:1097–1104.

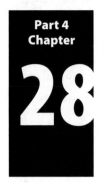

Management of dyspnea in older adults with cancer

Amy P. Abernethy, Jane L. Wheeler, and David C. Currow

Dyspnea, a complex psychophysiologic phenomenon characterized by the sensation of breathlessness, afflicts a substantial proportion of advanced cancer patients. Reported prevalences range from 15 to 79 percent, depending on the primary tumor site and other factors.[1-7] A prospective study of 1,860 adult patients with advanced cancer found an overall prevalence of 19 percent, with highest prevalence (46%) among lung cancer patients and lowest (6%) among head and neck cancer patients.[1] Another prospective study in a general cancer population ($n = 923$) reported an overall dyspnea prevalence of 46 percent.[8] Among a general population in the community ($n = 8,396$), the prevalence of substantial breathlessness that limits exertion is 9 percent.[9] Among terminally ill cancer patients, a retrospective analysis of National Hospice Study data found that prevalence rates generally exceeded 50 percent.[7]

For elderly cancer patients, dyspnea can be especially troubling. In a Finnish study of consecutive cancer patients with heterogeneous diagnoses ($n = 203$, mean age 65 years), dyspnea ranked among the four most disturbing symptoms as reported by patients on the Edmonton Symptom Assessment System, ranking symptoms on a scale of 0–10. Forty-nine percent of total respondents reported experiencing dyspnea; 18 percent reported a dyspnea score of 4 or greater.[10] A Taiwanese study of symptom patterns of advanced cancer patients in a palliative care unit ($n = 77$, mean age 62 years) found that dyspnea was experienced by 49 percent of patients on admission, 42 percent 1 week after admission, and 67 percent 2 days before death; of 19 symptoms monitored, only dyspnea and anorexia exhibited a pattern of decrease then increase.[11] An earlier Taiwanese study ($n = 125$, mean age 62 years) performed at the same institution reported similar results: 59 percent frequency of dyspnea on admission, with 39 percent of symptoms rated moderate or severe, and a decreasing then increasing pattern from admission to death.[12] Similarly, in a longitu-

dinal study of advanced cancer patients followed at home ($n = 373$, mean age 66 years), dyspnea was among a handful of symptoms that tended to increase over time and to peak at lower levels of performance status.[13] In multiple studies enrolling advanced and/or elderly cancer patients, dyspnea has been found to be significantly correlated with psychological distress and anxiety[8,12,14-17] as well as with spiritual distress.[18]

Although widely recognized, dyspnea has proven difficult to define for several reasons. The physical mechanisms and parameters of dyspnea may or may not be attributable to measurable physiologic factors. Dyspnea contains a significant subjective component; moreover, the patient's experience of breathlessness varies widely, depending on factors such as the individual's underlying disease, ethnic/racial background, previous health experiences, and emotional state. Reflecting this complexity, an American Thoracic Society consensus panel defined dyspnea as "a subjective experience of breathing discomfort that consists of qualitatively distinct sensations that vary in intensity. The experience derives from interactions among multiple physiological, psychological, social, and environmental factors, and may induce secondary physiological and behavioral responses."[19]

A. Etiology of dyspnea

Rather than developing along a straightforward pathophysiologic pathway, the etiology of dyspnea appears to entail multiple, potentially interrelated mechanisms that remain as yet poorly understood.[20] The sensation can originate in the central and peripheral chemoreceptors in response to increases in P_aCO_2 and decreases in P_aO_2 and pH[19]; it may be aggravated by activation of mechanical receptors in the chest wall and respiratory muscles and of vagal receptors in the airways and lungs.[21-23] Dyspnea may result when respiratory motor activity fails to meet incoming afferent activity such as information from chemo-, vagal, mechano-, pulmonary stretch, and muscle receptors.[19] This response failure may occur when ventilatory impedance increases, as during bronchoconstriction; when ventilatory demand increases, as during exercise; when respiratory muscle function is abnormal, as during lung hyperinflation; and when central perception of dyspnea increases, as during an anxiety attack. Potentially modifiable causes of dyspnea include hypoxia, anemia, and bronchospasm.[16] The various pathways of dyspnea development appear to interact in ways that are only starting to be understood, and it is reasonable to assume that additional factors will be identified that further explain the etiology of dyspnea.

B. Goals of care for the elderly patient with dyspnea

Discussion of dyspnea management for the elderly cancer patient must take into account the unique characteristics of this population and its correspondingly distinct goals of care. Typically, cancer patients over age 65 years present with multiple comorbidities; their care regimens often include several medications; they often rely on a caregiver who is also elderly. High frequencies of cognitive impairment and increased sensitivity to drug side effects also complicate symptom management in the elderly.[24] These patients rarely possess a robust and resilient physiologic constitution with which to combat a symptom such as breathlessness.[25] Their understanding of prognosis and their expectations for achievable physical function may differ from those of younger patients.[15]

In treating an older population, particularly patients transitioning to palliative care, the clinician should reconsider goals of care. In many cases, reduction of symptom burden and improvement in quality of life will outweigh cure or extension of survival as primary treatment goals. In the case of the older adult with dyspnea, treatment may thus focus on interventions seeking to relieve the patient's sensation of breathlessness, to improve his or her functional status and thereby, presumably, to enhance quality of life.

It is not unusual for patients to complain of dyspnea out of proportion to their objective physical disability or functional impairment. Because symptom relief, functional status, and quality of life are defined as primary goals of care in the palliative phase, a discrepancy between the patient's experience of breathlessness and physical measures of the phenomenon is irrelevant. The clinician accepts the patient's report of his or her symptom as the target of treatment and evaluates which palliative intervention(s) will be most likely to improve those symptoms.

C. Assessment of dyspnea

Good clinical management of dyspnea begins with a full assessment, with a first intention of identifying potentially reversible causes that might be corrected. Because the patient's dyspnea is likely to be multifactorial in origin, full assessment should address a comprehensive array of potential etiologies, as suggested in Table 28.1.

To quantify the functional impact of dyspnea, clinicians can use physical measures such as a 6-minute walk test or an endurance shuttle walking test (an externally paced field walking test) if the patient is physically capable. For the profoundly breathless, reading or simple isometric

Table 28.1 Checklist for dyspnea assessment: Identify and resolve potentially modifiable causes of dyspnea.

Pulmonary
- ☐ Lung tumor
- ☐ Pneumonia
- ☐ Pleural effusion: if recurrent, consider pleurodesis
- ☐ Lymphangitis carcinomatosa
- ☐ Obstruction of large airways, with or without distal collapse
- ☐ Chronic obstructive pulmonary disease (COPD)

Cardiovascular
- ☐ Pericardial effusion
- ☐ Congestive cardiac failure
- ☐ Pulmonary emboli
- ☐ Superior vena cava obstruction
- ☐ Anemia
- ☐ Arrythmias

Neuromuscular
- ☐ Muscle weakness/fatigue (may be due to or aggravated by anorexia/cachexia syndrome)
- ☐ Carcinoma en cuirasse, i.e., restrictive malignant infiltration of the chest wall
- ☐ Reduced respiratory drive (e.g., due to opiates)
- ☐ Peripheral nerve palsies (e.g., phrenic nerve)
- ☐ Malignant infiltration of cranial nerve: hoarse voice ± "bovine" cough; ENT referral; palliative injection of bulk material into vocal cord may help

Psychological
- ☐ Anxiety
- ☐ Fear

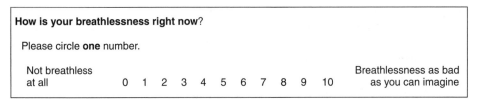

How is your breathlessness right now?

Please circle **one** number.

Not breathless at all		0 1 2 3 4 5 6 7 8 9 10	Breathlessness as bad as you can imagine

Figure 28.1 Numerical rating scale.

exercises present more appropriate measures of functional impact. Categorical functional scales such as the Medical Research Council Chronic Dyspnea Scale have long been used to score the effect of breathlessness on daily activities. These sorts of scales are easy to administer and provide a simple assessment of the functional impact of dyspnea.[26]

Because symptom relief is a principal goal of dyspnea management, a valid measure of patient-reported symptom intensity is integral to assessment. A variety of instruments are available for this purpose. Single-item scales such as a visual analog scale or numerical rating scale (Figure 28.1), or the Borg scale (Table 28.2) or Modified Medical Research Council Dyspnea Scale (Table 28.3), are useful in the clinical setting for longitudinal monitoring of the symptom and response to therapy. The Cancer Dyspnea Scale (CDS) developed by Tanaka and colleagues defines dyspnea from the patient's perspective and encompasses effort, anxiety, and discomfort; it is suitable for assessment of patients' experiences in real-world clinical settings.[17] The CDS was originally developed and validated in Japanese; an English-language validation study has been completed, led by Uronis. Preliminary results indicate that the CDS can be incorporated into a busy oncology clinic and that this scale with high face validity also has construct validity.[27]

Careful assessment of dyspnea is especially important in older adults because of its prognostic significance. A study of 107 palliative care patients with median age of 63 years found that dyspnea increased relative risk of death more than twofold (hazard ratio 2.04; 95% confidence interval [CI] 1.26–3.31, $p < .01$).[28] Dyspnea may be related to survival through its impact on quality of life, which has been shown to predict survival: colon, breast, ovarian, and prostate cancer patients (122 inpatients, 96 outpatients) participated in a cross-sectional validation study of the Memorial Symptom Assessment Scale (MSAS), a multidimensional quality-of-life instrument that measures the frequency of, severity of, and distress caused by physical symptoms. In multivariate analysis, decreased survival was independently predicted by higher physical symptom subscale score ($p = .004$) and lower performance status score (Karnofsky Performance Status, $p = .009$).[29]

Table 28.2 Borg Scale.[91]

Score	Severity
0	No breathlessness at all
0.5	Very very slight (just noticeable)
1	Very slight
2	Slight breathlessness
3	Moderate
4	Somewhat severe
5	Severe breathlessness
6	
7	Very severe breathlessness
8	
9	Very very severe (almost maximum)
10	Maximum

Table 28.3 Modified Medical Research Council Dyspnea Scale.[92]

Grade	Description of symptom
0	"I only get breathless with strenuous exercise"
1	"I get short of breath when hurrying on the level or walking up a slight hill"
2	"I walk slower than people of the same age on the level because of breathlessness or have to stop for breath when walking at my own pace on the level"
3	"I stop for breath after walking about 100 yards or after a few minutes on the level"
4	"I am too breathless to leave the house" or "I am breathless when dressing"

Note. This modified Medical Research Council scale uses the same descriptors as the original Medical Research Council scale in which the descriptors are numbered 1–5.

D. Evidence-based pharmacologic strategies for management of dyspnea

The first principle of treatment for dyspnea is management of the underlying disease; however, in palliative care, underlying etiologies are rarely modifiable. When the underlying etiology of the dyspnea has been maximally treated but the patient is still breathless, the dyspnea is generally called *intractable* or *refractory*.[30] Pharmacologic interventions for the symptom of breathlessness are typically divided into those directed at the underlying disease, such as steroids, diuretics, and bronchodilators, and more general interventions indicated by the symptom without respect for underlying disease, such as opioids and oxygen. This review focuses on the general treatments for refractory dyspnea that can be employed regardless of etiology.

E. Oral and parenteral opioids

Opioids are a common approach to management of refractory dyspnea; although they have been well studied for this purpose, their use nonetheless remains controversial. Opponents raise safety as the primary concern and suggest respiratory depression as the predominant risk.[31,32]

The mechanisms of action through which opioids relieve dyspnea are potentially complex; they may act centrally, peripherally, or by reducing anxiety.[33] Existing evidence confirms that opioids reduce ventilatory response to carbon dioxide,[34] hypoxia,[35,36] inspiratory flow-resistive loading,[37] and exercise.[38] Morphine decreases oxygen consumption both at rest and with exercise in healthy individuals.[38]

The efficacy of opioids for relief of dyspnea has been evaluated in a systematic review and meta-analysis conducted by Jennings and colleagues. The authors found a highly statistically significant effect of regular oral and parenteral opioids on the sensation of breathlessness (overall pooled effect size -0.31, 95% CI $-0.50-[-0.13]$, $p = .0008$). However, the clinical effect was relatively small (approximately 8 mm on a 100-mm visual analog scale, with baseline levels of dyspnea of 50 mm).[39] Reasons proposed by the authors for this small effect included small doses, doses that were not titrated, long dosing intervals, and inability to achieve steady state with single-dose studies. The authors' evaluation of the data did not suggest an association between opioid use and changes in arterial blood gas measurements or oxygen saturation.

In a parallel study, Abernethy and colleagues conducted a trial using oral morphine in opioid-naive adults with refractory dyspnea, defined as dyspnea at rest despite maximal treatment for reversible factors.[30] Eligible patients had serum concentration of creatinine within twice the normal range, stable needs for oxygen and medication, and ability to fill out diary cards. This 8-day, randomized, double-blind crossover study of 20 mg once-daily sustained-release oral morphine sulfate or placebo enrolled 48 outpatients with refractory dyspnea. The primary outcome was the sensation of breathlessness measured on a 100-mm visual analog scale. Participants were elderly (mean age 76, standard deviation [SD] 5); 71 percent were receiving oxygen therapy. The mean baseline morning dyspnea score was 43 (SD 26). Patients receiving morphine had a significant decrease in dyspnea, with mean improvements in dyspnea intensity of 6.6 mm in the morning ($p = .011$) and 9.5 mm in the evening ($p = .006$), when plasma levels were close to their peak. Relative improvement over baseline dyspnea was 15–22 percent, and patients were more likely to prefer morphine than placebo. These results were similar to the estimate of efficacy for oral and parenteral opioids generated by Jennings and colleagues. Morphine did not depress the respiratory rate (mean respiratory rate for morphine vs. placebo was 20 [SD 5] vs. 21 [SD 4], $p = .143$); no episodes of sedation or obtundation were recorded. The main side effect was constipation ($p = .021$); neither treatment caused more vomiting, confusion, sedation, or appetite suppression. Participants who received morphine also described better sleep at night ($p = .039$).

When considering the prescription of oral morphine in the opioid-naive older person with breathlessness, we suggest that the prescriber check the patient's renal and hepatic function and also consider that elderly individuals may be more sensitive to opiates. The prescriber may want to start off at a lower morphine dose, for example, 15 mg of sustained release product, and then titrate upward to effect. Presumptive treatment for constipation is critical.

A systematic review of the literature through July 2006 evaluated the effectiveness of four drug classes – opioids, phenothiazines, benzodiazepines, and systemic corticosteroids – for relieving dyspnea in advanced cancer patients.

This systematic review and meta-analysis confirmed the findings of Jennings and Abernethy that systemic opioids conferred significant benefit for relief of dyspnea. Evidence that systemic morphine reduced dyspnea came from two small placebo-controlled trials in cancer patients[40,41]; dihydrocodeine also significantly reduced dyspnea in four placebo-controlled trials.[42–45] The authors concluded that oral or parenteral systemic opioids can be used to manage dyspnea in cancer patients and that oral promethazine may be used as a second-line agent if systemic opioids cannot be used or in addition to systemic opioids.[46]

F. Palliative oxygen

Palliative oxygen is prescribed when the primary treatment goal is relief of breathlessness. A systematic review through 2003 examined the use of palliative oxygen for the management of breathlessness in cancer, chronic obstructive pulmonary disease (COPD), and heart failure. Results were inconsistent and remarkably patient-dependent; most studies were small (range 5–50 patients) and poorly controlled.[47] The authors concluded that oxygen at rest may have a role in palliative treatment for COPD patients but that palliative oxygen should be used only after conducting an n-of-1 assessment to evaluate the impact of oxygen on both breathlessness and quality of life.[14] In 2008, Uronis and colleagues updated this work with a systematic review and meta-analysis of palliative oxygen to manage cancer-related dyspnea.[48] Five studies were included, and the authors analyzed primary data obtained from three of the original study investigators. A total of 134 patients were included in the meta-analysis. Oxygen failed to improve dyspnea in mildly or nonhypoxemic cancer patients (standardized mean difference –0.09, 95% CI –0.22–0.04, $p = .16$).

Despite an historical lack of evidence to demonstrate its benefit, palliative oxygen has been commonly prescribed for dyspnea management – even in patients not meeting criteria for domiciliary oxygen therapy. In a Canadian study, over 40 percent of patients receiving long-term oxygen therapy ($n = 237$) did not meet current guidelines stipulated in the Ontario Ministry of Health Home Oxygen Program.[49] In a survey of palliative care specialists and respiratory physicians in Australia and New Zealand ($n = 214$), 58 percent of respondents (69% of palliative medicine clinicians and 48% of respiratory physicians) reported a belief that palliative oxygen is beneficial; 65 percent of respondents cited intractable dyspnea as the most common reason for prescription.[50] Canadian clinicians reported similar convictions.[51]

To resolve the uncertainty regarding efficacy of palliative oxygen for refractory dyspnea, Abernethy and colleagues conducted a large, international, randomized, controlled, double-blind study of palliative oxygen versus medical air (i.e., room air with ambient partial pressure of oxygen delivered via nasal cannulae at the same flow rate as oxygen) for patients with PaO_2 greater than 55 mmHg.[52] Neither gas proved superior in relieving the sensation of dyspnea ($p = .456$) or for improving quality of life ($p = .281$). Dyspnea and quality of life improved over the 7-day study period in both arms ($p < .0001$ for each outcome); the positive effect of medical air delivered by nasal cannulae suggests that the benefit of palliative gases may be due to the mechanics of gas delivery rather than to the gas itself. Results of the Abernethy trial indicated that patients with more severe breathlessness, defined as a high baseline breathlessness score of 7 or more on a 0–10 numerical rating scale, may derive greater benefit from palliative oxygen. Furthermore, an interim assessment found that patients could differentiate whether they symptomatically improved after a trial of medical gas and that patients not deriving benefit were unlikely to continue therapy, perhaps because of its significant logistical and personal burden.[53] Given these results, it is recommended that the clinician consider an n-of-1 trial of palliative oxygen for patients with high baseline, and modify the treatment plan based on the patient's response and desire to continue this therapy.

G. Psychotropic drugs

Psychotropic agents have been used to treat refractory dyspnea based on the assumptions that (1) dyspnea contains a large psychological, and (2) anxiety significantly contributes to the functional impairment associated with breathlessness.[54] Psychotropic drugs used in dyspnea management have included anxiolytics, phenothiazines, and selective serotonin reuptake inhibitors (SSRIs). In practice, and until further data from high-quality randomized controlled trials become available, the clinician should consider an n- of-1 trial for the patient who may be a candidate for these treatment approaches. In such a scenario, the clinician carefully monitors the patient for relief of dyspnea, improvement in performance status/function, and adverse effects. When placebos are not available, clinicians should consider a single-sided *n*-of-1 trial in which they carefully document outcomes in concert with the patient and caregiver(s).

G.1. Benzodiazepines

Diazepam, commonly used for treating anxiety, has been studied for effect on dyspnea. A small study by Mitchell-Heggs and colleagues reported "striking reduction in dyspnea" from treating four patients severely disabled from chronic airflow obstruction with diazepam.[55] Subsequent studies failed to replicate these results.[56,57] The systematic review by Viola and colleagues identified only one benzodiazepine trial specific to cancer patients.[58] The investigators randomized patients ($n = 101$) in the terminal stages of cancer to morphine 2.5 mg 4 hourly, midazolam 5.0 mg 4 hourly, or the combination. They found an improvement in dyspnea intensity from baseline with morphine, midazolam, and the two-agent combination but no between-treatment differences. Man and colleagues investigated the use of alprazolam, a shorter-acting and potentially less sedating benzodiazepine medication than diazepam, for relief of dyspnea. This placebo-controlled, double-blind study randomized patients ($n = 24$) with chronic obstructive lung disease to alprazolam (0.5 mg once daily) or placebo administered for 1 week, followed by placebo for 1 week, then either placebo or alprazolam for 1 week. The maximum exercise level attained, distance covered in the 12-minute walk test, and subjective perception of dyspnea remained unchanged before and after alprazolam.[59] A study by Eimer and colleagues of clorazepate was closed because of intolerable side effects.[60]

Practically, benzodiazepines can be prescribed for individuals where anxiety obviously and substantially aggravates dyspnea. Because midazolam can be dangerous when used in uncontrolled settings and may not be allowed in some clinical areas, alprazolam as a short-acting product or clonazepam for longer-acting control may be substituted.

G.2. Other anxiolytics

Buspirone, a serotonergic anxiolytic agent, is a respiratory stimulant in animals.[61,62] Two small studies enrolling patients with severe COPD[63,64] evaluated the effects of buspirone on breathlessness, exercise tolerance, and anxiety. The study populations differed: Singh and colleagues required that participants exhibit baseline anxiety as measured by the Spielberger State-Trait Anxiety Inventory Scale; Argyropoulou and colleagues did not require baseline anxiety assessment. The studies yielded conflicting results: Argyropoulou and colleagues documented improvement in all three domains, whereas Singh and colleagues found no difference. These data, though inconsistent, suggest that there may be a role for anxiolytic agents in *selected* patients with refractory dyspnea.

G.3. Selective serotonin reuptake inhibitors

The 1990s saw a surge in interest surrounding the use of SSRIs to treat dyspnea, and indeed, a small body of weak evidence may suggest efficacy. SSRIs may improve dyspnea by relieving anxiety symptoms or by directly impacting respiration. Many patients who have dyspnea that seems disproportionate to their pulmonary compromise experience depression and/or anxiety; data suggest that treatment of these symptoms may help to relieve dyspnea.[65] Studies in animal models suggest that serotonin acts at the level of the brain stem respiratory center; this action may affect the sensation of breathlessness.[66] A small pilot study conducted by Papp and colleagues[67] ($n = 6$) and a case series reported by Smoller and colleagues[68] ($n = 7$) found that patients taking sertraline experienced a "decrease" in breathlessness and "improvements" in exercise tolerance, though these studies lacked control arms or formal measures of dyspnea. Currently, in the absence of an underlying psychiatric indication, there is insufficient evidence to recommend the use of SSRIs to relieve dyspnea.

G.4. Inhaled furosemide

Furosemide has been suggested as a potential intervention for dyspnea because of the inhibitory effect it exerts on the cough response, induced by its low chloride content,[69] and its preventive effect on bronchoconstriction in asthma.[70–72] Inhaled furosemide may also act indirectly on the vagally mediated sensory nerve ending in airway epithelium.[73] In healthy subjects, inhaled furosemide can prolong breath-holding time and the period of no respiratory sensation and has slowed the development of discomfort during loaded breathing.[23] In patients with moderate to severe COPD (FEV_1 less than 70%) and moderate-to-severe chronic breathlessness ($n = 19$), a randomized study evaluated the effects of inhaled furosemide versus placebo on exercise-induced dyspnea.[74] Mean dyspnea scores on a visual analog scale after exercise were lower in the furosemide group (34 mm [SD 25] vs. 42 [SD 24], $p = .014$). Exercise-related FEV_1 and FVC also improved after furosemide inhalation ($p = .038$ and $.005$, respectively) but not after placebo. Inhaled furosemide appears promising for treatment of dyspnea but further evidence is required to demonstrate its benefit.

G.5. Heliox28

Heliox28, a mixture of 72 percent helium and 28 percent oxygen, also shows promise of efficacy for relief of dyspnea; the suggested mechanism of action is that the low density of helium, when replacing nitrogen in air, may reduce the effort of breathing and improve alveolar ventilation.[75] A phase II crossover study in lung cancer patients with refractory dyspnea ($n = 12$) assessed the palliative role of Heliox28.[75] Breathlessness during a 6-minute walk test was evaluated while patients breathed Heliox28, 28 percent oxygen, or medical air. Dyspnea scores on a visual analog scale were significantly lower when patients breathed Heliox28 than medical air (40.2% [SD 4.8] vs. 59.3% [SD 5.3], $p < .05$), but there was no significant difference between Heliox28 and oxygen (47.0% [SD 5.6]) or between oxygen and medical air. Borg scores also did not differ significantly, though participants did walk farther breathing Heliox28 than oxygen (214.2 m [SD 9.6] vs. 174.6 m [SD 11.2], $p < .05$) or medical air (128.8 m [SD 10.3], $p < .0001$). This study suggests that Heliox28 may offer a treatment option for patients with refractory dyspnea, but further evidence is needed, and issues of cost and feasibility may diminish the usefulness of this treatment in the geriatric population.

H. Pharmacologic strategies not supported by current evidence

For the oncologist managing a complex clinical scenario such as dyspnea, the injunction "do no harm" holds special meaning. Recent evidence has helped clarify those interventions that do not benefit the patient with dyspnea as well as those that do. Viola and colleagues, in a systematic review of the literature through July 2006, found that neb-

ulized morphine was not effective in controlling dyspnea in any individual study or at the level of meta-analysis. No controlled trials examined systemic corticosteroids in the treatment of cancer patients. Of the other nonopioid drugs examined, only oral promethazine, a phenothiazine, showed benefit for relieving breathlessness. Presumably the mechanism of action here is indirect; promethazine blocks dopamine, producing sedation, and thus may alleviate the anxiety that underlies or exacerbates dyspnea in some patients. The authors concluded that nebulized morphine, prochlorperazine, and benzodiazepines are not recommended for management of dyspnea and that promethazine must not be used parenterally.[46]

I. Nonpharmacologic approaches to dyspnea management

Though some patients experience relief with opioids or palliative oxygen, adequate management of dyspnea remains a challenge to the clinician, in large part because of the complex nature of this phenomenon. Parallel to pharmacologic strategies, several nonpharmacologic approaches warrant consideration for their potential benefits in relieving dyspnea experienced by specific patients. These approaches include breathlessness clinics, pulmonary rehabilitation, pleurodesis for malignant pleural effusions, and breathing techniques. For geriatric patients, who may have limited ability to travel to specialized pulmonary rehabilitation or breathlessness clinics, current nonpharmacologic interventions that offer greatest promise include psychosocial support and breathing techniques.

J. Breathlessness clinics

In the United Kingdom, breathlessness clinics have become standard treatment for lung cancer patients. Weekly sessions focus on counseling, breathing retraining, relaxation, and coping/adaptation strategies for dealing with breathlessness. Data from randomized trials support this model,[76] but thus far the model is limited by its focus on lung cancer and its regional development.

K. Breathing techniques

Several controlled breathing techniques, including positioning and pursed-lip breathing, are useful in managing dyspnea. In the most commonly used breathing position to alleviate breathlessness, the patient leans forward and supports his or her weight with the arms and upper body. This position increases abdominal pressure and may improve respiratory muscle function.[19] Use of the forward-leaning position has also been reported to improve inspiratory muscle strength[77] and diaphragmatic function,[78] reduce the use of accessory muscles, and decrease abdominal breathing.[78–80]

Pursed-lip breathing involves inhalation through the nose followed by a slow exhalation, usually of 4–6 seconds, through pursed lips. It has been shown to decrease air trapping by stenting the airways and preventing dynamic airway collapse.[81] This procedure often helps to avert panic attacks brought on by severe breathlessness.[82] Clinicians should be advised, however, that despite studies demonstrating the benefit of breathing techniques for relieving dyspnea, results in actual clinical practice vary.[19]

L. Psychosocial support

Fundamental to the treatment of any cancer patient, psychosocial support becomes more important as patients' physical statuses begin to decline and as they experience more functional limitations. Patients often need psychological help in coping with their illness, the changes occurring in their lives, and the emotions associated with particular symptoms such as dyspnea. Fear and anxiety are logical responses to restrictions on one's breathing and may in turn fuel an increase in symptoms. Anxiety, one particularly common psychological correlate of dyspnea, can lead to a progressive spiral of worsening breathlessness and greater psychological distress. The literature bears out this relationship between dyspnea and anxiety. A prospective study of terminally ill cancer patients ($n = 100$; 49 with lung cancer) reported a significant association between dyspnea and anxiety ($p < .001$)[16]; a prospective study of lung cancer patients of all stages ($n = 120$) demonstrated a relationship between increasing dyspnea and anxiety ($p = .03$) and panic ($p = .01$). Not surprisingly, patients with worse dyspnea have lower reported quality of life ($p = .04$).[83]

No existing guidelines describe the provision of psychosocial support for either dyspnea patients or their informal caregivers. Clinicians caring for these patients must be conscious of the potential need for increased support, respond to patient and family concerns when they arise, and be prepared to refer patients and caregivers to appropriate professionals as warranted.

M. Caregiver support

Spouses and other family members, informal caregivers, clinical care providers, and community members close to the patient may all bear various logistical, financial, and/or emotional burdens because of their relationship with the dyspnea sufferer. When relationships and family roles change as a result of disease progression and increasing symptom burden, relatives and family members may require support.[33] Several qualitative studies have highlighted the support needs of caregivers of patients with dyspnea. Booth and colleagues investigated the experience of living with breathlessness, both for patients with cancer or COPD and for their informal caregivers.[84] The investigators interviewed 10 COPD patients and their caregivers and reported that many caregivers found taking care of a breathless person to be "pre-occupying, restricting, and a major cause of anxiety." They concluded that clinicians must not forget about the needs of their patients' families and that patients with disabling symptoms are often best cared for through a multidisciplinary approach. A similar study, also describing the experiences of 10 patients with COPD and their caregivers, revealed that caregivers experienced losses similar to those of the patients, felt burdened by multiple roles, and had a sense of unfairness that introduced tension into the patient-caregiver relationship.[85]

N. Global intervention strategies

In recent years, a wide range of interventions have been studied as possible management strategies for dyspnea. This breadth of inquiry points to the emergence of a new, more expansive way of thinking about the complex phenomenon of dyspnea. Indeed, the term *total dyspnea* has been used to describe a new perspective on the phenomenon, one patterned after the *total pain* concept articulated in the early 1960s by Dame Cecily Saunders.[86] In the *total dyspnea* framework, dyspnea encompasses suffering in four realms: physical, psychological, interpersonal, and existential. Correspondingly, treatment of dyspnea must address the individual patient's needs in each area (Figure 28.2). The resulting approach is comprehensive, multidimensional, multidisciplinary, and patient centered (Table 28.4).[87]

Physical care has been discussed earlier. Psychological care in the total dyspnea approach begins with assessment using a validated instrument such as the Hospital Anxiety and Depression

Table 28.4   Checklist for comprehensive, patient-centered management of dyspnea in older adults.

General management principles

☐ Begin with a comprehensive assessment, including patient-reported (subjective) and psychological measures.
☐ Identify and treat reversible causes.
☐ Adopt a multidisciplinary approach that incorporates nonpharmacological strategies.
☐ Communicate realistically with patients to help them modify expectations.
☐ Respond according to the patient's place in the disease continuum and to his or her preferred goals of care.

Pharmacologic management

☐ Opioids are the mainstay of treatment. Low-dose morphine has been demonstrated to be safe and effective even in elderly patients with COPD.
☐ In opioid-naive patients, start with a dose of 15-mg sustained-release morphine once daily (if no contraindications). Increase dose frequency to twice per day after 5–7 days if the patient tolerates the medication but has residual breathlessness.
☐ For severe, acute dyspnea, administer 2–5 mg IV morphine every 5–10 minutes.
☐ In patients with contraindication to morphine, use long-acting oxycodone, starting at 10 mg once per day and increasing to twice per day after 5–7 days, as tolerated and needed.
☐ If an opioid-tolerant patient is already on a regular dose of morphine or another opioid, sequentially increase the opioid by 20% of total daily dose every 3–5 days until breathlessness is relieved or side effects occur.[93]
☐ Consider benzodiazepines only for individuals in whom anxiety causes obvious and substantial aggravation of dyspnea; use alprazolam for short-acting, and clonazepam for longer-acting, control.
☐ Use other drugs as appropriate to address additional dyspnea-related symptoms such as antitussives (coughing), anticholinergics (secretions), diuretics, bronchodilators, and corticosteroids.

Oxygen and nonpharmacologic management

☐ Palliative oxygen or medical air may relieve symptoms in certain patients with refractory dyspnea. Treatment should be based on symptom relief rather than on pulse oximetry.
☐ Patients generally prefer to use a nasal cannula than a mask; claustrophobic patients may best be served by a face tent. For the dying patient, there is no need to administer more than 4–6 L/min of oxygen via nasal cannula.
☐ Symptom management discussions should include caregivers and family members to alleviate any concerns they may have about treatment, especially opioids, and to inform them of nonpharmacologic approaches they can support.
☐ Positioning the patient in a forward-leaning posture, with weight supported by the arms and upper body, often helps relieve dyspnea.
☐ Pursed-lip breathing, in which the patient inhales through the nose and exhales slowly (4–6 seconds) through pursed lips, can help relieve dyspnea.
☐ Relaxation techniques (e.g., massage, guided imagery) can reduce distress and thereby dyspnea.
☐ Psychosocial support can alleviate distress, which may in turn reduce the sensation of breathlessness where anxiety exacerbates the patient's experience of it.
☐ Spiritual and existential aspects of dyspnea and its management should be addressed, engaging professional, community, and family resources where possible and appropriate.
☐ Caregiver needs should be discussed, along with ways to minimize caregiver burden and distress associated with managing dyspnea in a loved one.

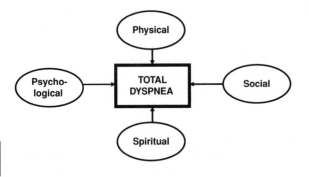

Figure 28.2 Total dyspnea model.

The case of James, Jerri Mae, and Dr. Inspired

James is an 82-year-old African American man with recurrent non-small-cell lung cancer. His wife, Jerri Mae, brings him to the Emergency Department one evening when he experiences extreme difficulty catching his breath. The on-call resident notes that both patient and caregiver appear severely distressed, that James walks very laboriously with a cane, that he is overweight, and that he takes asthma medications but no medications specifically for dyspnea. The attending, Dr. Inspired, arrives and performs a full assessment to evaluate possible causes of James's breathlessness, identify remediable factors, and develop an integrated plan that helps relieve James's symptoms while also attending to the physical, logistical, existential, and psychosocial impact of his situation. Dr. Inspired rules out modifiable cardiovascular and pulmonary factors. He prescribes low-dose morphine at 15 mg twice daily for the breathlessness. Having addressed the potential physiologic causes of the immediate dyspnea episode, Dr. Inspired proceeds to explore the patient's experience of dyspnea. He asks James to rate his current dyspnea using the Cancer Dyspnea Scale, and evaluates the more stable picture of his symptoms by having him grade his functional impairment over the past week using the Modified Medical Research Council's Chronic Dyspnea Scale. This assessment gives him a better understanding of James's experience, thus guiding the choice of further inquiry and intervention. James rates his dyspnea as 7 on a 0–10 numerical rating scale, and describes the anxiety associated with the sensation of smothering. Given this symptom severity, Dr. Inspired refers James and Jerri Mae to a physical therapist who can teach them breathing techniques to use when James's dyspnea intensifies, and to regain a sense of calm around baseline symptoms. He talks with James and his wife together about the psychological component of dyspnea, without negating the very real physical nature of the phenomenon, and asks if he would like to speak with a counselor. James indicates that he would prefer not to talk to a psychologist, but might be open to medications that alleviate distress. This option is left open for discussion at a follow-up visit in one week. Dr. Inspired asks James if he believes in a higher power or has another source of spiritual strength to call upon; James and Jerri Mae describe their involvement in the local Southern Baptist church, and the threesome discuss how James's beliefs and his pastor might help him manage fear and anxiety surrounding his physical circumstances. Dr. Inspired, James, and Jerri Mae discuss the very real concern that James is going to die, advance directives (James has a living will), finding meaning in life, and support for Jerri Mae. Finally, Dr. Inspired connects Jerri Mae to the cancer center's patient and family support program, where volunteers are available to provide caregivers with support such as phone check-ins, transportation, and help with grocery shopping. James and Jerri Mae leave the hospital much relieved, and feeling empowered to manage James's symptoms day by day with multidisciplinary help, a sense that there are options available if needs intensify, and a confidence that they will receive the support they need.

Figure 28.3 Total dyspnea: Example of the global approach to dyspnea management in action.

Scale[88] or the National Comprehensive Cancer Network Distress Scale,[89] featuring the well-recognized distress "thermometer." Targeted to needs thus identified, psychological care should be individualized, provided by appropriate trained professionals, and coordinated with medical care. Interpersonal needs are often readily identified through communication with family members and caregivers in the clinical visit. Sometimes the act of inquiring itself can be a powerful intervention; at other times, referral to available community resources, local agencies, or support groups can help alleviate interpersonal stress. Finally, existential or spiritual concerns can be identified through evaluation instruments such as the Functional Assessment of Chronic Illness Therapy Spirituality subscale.[90] Identified concerns should be handled in a manner compatible with the patient's and/or family's belief structure and spiritual orientation, with patients referred to appropriate professionals for follow-up. The story of James, Jerri Mae, and Dr. Inspired highlights this patient-centered approach (Figure 28.3).

References

1. Vainio A, Auvinen A. Prevalence of symptoms among patients with advanced cancer: an international collaborative study. Symptom Prevalence Group. *J Pain Symptom Manage*. 1996;12(1):3–10.

2. Krech RL, Walsh D. Symptoms of pancreatic cancer. *J Pain Symptom Manage*. 1991;6(6):360–367.

3. Brescia FJ, Adler D, Gray G, et al. Hospitalized advanced cancer patients: a profile. *J Pain Symptom Manage*. 1990;5(4):221–227.

4. Coyle N, Adelhardt J, Foley KM, et al. Character of terminal illness in the advanced cancer patient: pain and other symptoms during the last four weeks of life. *J Pain Symptom Manage*. 1990;5(2):83–93.

5. Higginson I, McCarthy M. Measuring symptoms in terminal cancer: are pain and dyspnoea controlled? *J R Soc Med*. 1989;82(5):264–267.

6. Reuben DB, Mor V, Hiris J. Clinical symptoms and length of survival in patients with terminal cancer. *Arch Intern Med*. 1988;148(7):1586–1591.

7. Reuben DB, Mor V. Dyspnea in terminally ill cancer patients. *Chest*. 1986;89(2):234–236.

8. Dudgeon DJ, Kristjanson L, Sloan JA, et al. Dyspnea in cancer patients: prevalence and associated factors. *J Pain Symptom Manage*. 2001;21(2):95–102.

9. Currow DC, Plummer JL, Crockett A, et al. A community population survey of prevalence and severity of dyspnea in adults. *J Pain Symptom Manage*. 2009;38(4):533–545.

10. Salminen E, Clemens KE, Syrjanen K, et al. Needs of developing the skills of palliative care at the oncology ward: an audit of symptoms among 203 consecutive cancer patients in Finland. *Supportive Care Cancer*. 2008;16(1):3–8.

11. Tsai J-S, Wu C-H, Chiu T-Y, et al. Symptom patterns of advanced cancer patients in a palliative care unit. *Palliative Med*. 2006;20(6):617–622.

12. Chiu T-Y, Hu W-Y, Lue B-H, et al. Dyspnea and its correlates in Taiwanese patients with terminal cancer. *J Pain Symptom Manage*. 2004;28(2):123–132.

13. Mercadante S, Casuccio A, Fulfaro F. The course of symptom frequency and intensity in advanced cancer patients followed at home. *J Pain Symptom Manage*. 2000;20(2):104–112.

14. Bruera E, Schoeller T, MacEachern T. Symptomatic benefit of supplemental oxygen in hypoxemic patients with terminal cancer: the use of the N of 1 randomized controlled trial. *J Pain Symptom Manage*. 1992;7(6):365–368.

15. Dudgeon DJ. Managing dyspnea and cough. *Hematol Oncol Clin N Am*. 2002;16(3):557–577.

16. Dudgeon DJ, Lertzman M, Dudgeon DJ, et al. Dyspnea in the advanced cancer patient. *J Pain Symptom Manage*. 1998;16(4):212–219.

17. Tanaka K, Akechi T, Okuyama T, et al. Development and validation of the Cancer Dyspnoea Scale: a multidimensional, brief, self-rating scale. *Br J Cancer*. 2000;82(4):800–805.

18. Edmonds P, Higginson I, Altmann D, et al. Is the presence of dyspnea a risk factor for morbidity in cancer patients? *J Pain Symptom Manage*. 2000;19(1):15–22.

19. Dyspnea: mechanisms, assessment, and management: a consensus statement. American Thoracic Society. *Am J Respir Crit Care Med*. 1999;159(1):321–340.

20. Luce JM, Luce JA, Luce JM, et al. Perspectives on care at the close of life: management of dyspnea in patients with far-advanced lung disease: "once I lose it, it's kind of hard to catch it. . . ." *J Am Med Assoc*. 2001;285(10):1331–1337.

21. Cristiano LM, Schwartzstein RM, Cristiano LM, et al. Effect of chest wall vibration on dyspnea during hypercapnia and exercise in chronic obstructive pulmonary disease. *Am J Respir Crit Care Med*. 1997;155(5):1552–1559.

22. O'Donnell DE, Webb KA, O'Donnell DE, et al. Exertional breathlessness in patients with chronic airflow limitation: the role of lung hyperinflation. *Am Rev Respir Dis*. 1993;148(5):1351–1357.

23. Nishino T, Ide T, Sudo T, et al. Inhaled furosemide greatly alleviates the sensation of experimentally induced dyspnea. *Am J Respir Crit Care Med*. 2000;161(6):1963–1967.

24. Ferrell BA. Pain evaluation and management in the nursing home. *Ann Intern Med*. 1995;123(9):681–687.

25. Rao AV, Hsieh F, Feussner JR, et al. Geriatric evaluation and management units in the care of the frail elderly cancer patient. *J Gerontol*. 2005;60(6):798–803.

26. Papiris SA, Daniil ZD, Malagari K, et al. The Medical Research Council dyspnea scale in the estimation of disease severity in idiopathic pulmonary fibrosis. *Respir Med*. 2005;99(6):755–761.

27. Uronis HE, Blackwell S, Bosworth H, et al. An examination of the psychometric properties of an English version of the Cancer Dyspnea Scale (CDS) for evaluating dyspnea in patients with advanced lung cancer. *Support Care Cancer*. 2007;15:728.

28. Hardy JR, Turner R, Saunders M, et al. Prediction of survival in a hospital-based continuing care unit. *Eur J Cancer*. 1994;30A(3):284–288.

29. Chang VT, Thaler HT, Polyak TA, et al. Quality of life and survival: the role of multidimensional symptom assessment. *Cancer.* 1998;83(1): 173–179.

30. Abernethy AP, Currow DC, Frith P, et al. Randomised, double blind, placebo controlled crossover trial of sustained release morphine for the management of refractory dyspnoea [see comment]. *Br Med J.* 2003;327(7414):523–528.

31. Currow DC, Abernethy AP, Frith P. Morphine for management of refractory dyspnoea. *Br Med J.* 2003;327:1288–1289.

32. Pauwels RA, Buist AS, Calverley PM, et al. Global strategy for the diagnosis, management, and prevention of chronic obstructive pulmonary disease. NHLBI/WHO Global Initiative for Chronic Obstructive Lung Disease (GOLD) Workshop summary. *Am J Respir Crit Care Med.* 2001;163(5):1256–1276.

33. Leach RM. Palliative medicine and non-malignant, end-stage respiratory disease. In: Doyle D, Hanks G, Cherny N, eds. *Oxford Textbook of Palliative Medicine.* 3rd ed. New York: Oxford University Press; 2005:895–916.

34. Eckenhoff JE, Oech SR. The effects of narcotics and antagonists upon respiration and circulation in man: a review. *Clin Pharmacol Ther.* 1960;1:483–524.

35. Santiago TV, Pugliese AC, Edelman NH. Control of breathing during methadone addiction. *Am J Med.* 1977;62(3):347–354.

36. Weil JV, McCullough RE, Kline JS, et al. Diminished ventilatory response to hypoxia and hypercapnia after morphine in normal man. *N Engl J Med.* 1975;292(21):1103–1106.

37. Kryger MH, Yacoub O, Dosman J, et al. Effect of meperidine on occlusion pressure responses to hypercapnia and hypoxia with and without external inspiratory resistance. *Am Rev Respir Dis.* 1976;114(2):333–340.

38. Santiago TV, Johnson J, Riley DJ, et al. Effects of morphine on ventilatory response to exercise. *J Appl Physiol.* 1979;47(1):112–118.

39. Jennings AL, Davies AN, Higgins JP, et al. A systematic review of the use of opioids in the management of dyspnoea. *Thorax.* 2002;57(11): 939–944.

40. Bruera E, MacEachern T, Ripamonti C, et al. Subcutaneous morphine for dyspnea in cancer patients. *Ann Intern Med.* 1993;119(9):906–907.

41. Mazzocato C, Buclin T, Rapin CH. The effects of morphine on dyspnea and ventilatory function in elderly patients with advanced cancer: a randomized double-blind controlled trial. *Ann Oncol.* 1999;10(12):1511–1514.

42. Buck C, Laier-Groeneveld G, Criee CP. The effect of dihydrocodeine and terbutaline on breathlessness and inspiratory muscle function in normal subjects and patients with COPD [abstract]. *Eur Respir J.* 1996;9:344S.

43. Chua TP, Harrington D, Ponikowski P, et al. Effects of dihydrocodeine on chemosensitivity and exercise tolerance in patients with chronic heart failure. *J Am Coll Cardiol.* 1997;29(1):147–152.

44. Johnson MA, Woodcock AA, Geddes DM. Dihydrocodeine for breathlessness in "pink puffers." *Br Med J Clin Res Ed.* 1983;286(6366):675–677.

45. Woodcock AA, Gross ER, Gellert A, et al. Effects of dihydrocodeine, alcohol, and caffeine on breathlessness and exercise tolerance in patients with chronic obstructive lung disease and normal blood gases. *N Engl J Med.* 1981;305(27):1611–1616.

46. Viola R, Kiteley C, Lloyd NS, et al. The management of dyspnea in cancer patients: a systematic review. *Support Care Cancer.* 2008;16(4):329–337.

47. Booth S, Anderson H, Swannick M, et al. The use of oxygen in the palliation of breathlessness: a report of the expert working group of the Scientific Committee of the Association of Palliative Medicine. *Respir Med.* 2004;98(1): 66–77.

48. Uronis HE, Currow DC, McCrory DC, et al. Oxygen for relief of dyspnoea in mildly- or non-hypoxaemic patients with cancer: a systematic review and meta-analysis. *Br J Cancer.* 2008;98(2):294–299.

49. Guyatt GH, McKim DA, Austin P, et al. Appropriateness of domiciliary oxygen delivery. *Chest.* 2000;118(5):1303–1308.

50. Abernethy AP, Currow DC, Frith PA, et al. Prescribing palliative oxygen: a clinician survey of expected benefit and patterns of use. *Palliative Med.* 2005;19:165–172.

51. Stringer E, McParland C, Hernandez P. Physician practices for prescribing supplemental oxygen in the palliative care setting. *J Palliative Care.* 2004;20(4):303–307.

52. Abernethy AP, McDonald C, Frith P, et al. Palliative oxygen versus medical air for relief of dyspnea: results of an international, multi-site, randomized controlled trial. Paper presented at: Annual Assembly of the American Academy of Hospice and Palliative Medicine and Hospice and Palliative Nurses Association; March 27, 2009; Austin, TX.

53. Currow DC, Fazekas B, Abernethy AP. Oxygen use – patients define symptomatic benefit discerningly. *J Pain Symptom Manage.* 2007;34(2):113–114.

54. Kim HF, Kunik ME, Molinari VA, et al. Functional impairment in COPD patients: the impact of anxiety and depression. *Psychosomatics.* 2000;41(6):465–471.

55. Mitchell-Heggs P, Murphy K, Minty K, et al. Diazepam in the treatment of dyspnoea in the "Pink Puffer" syndrome. *Q J Med.* 1980;49(193):9–20.

56. Sen D, Jones G, Leggat PO. The response of the breathless patient treated with diazepam. *Br J Clin Pract.* 1983;37(6):232–233.

57. Woodcock AA, Gross ER, Geddes DM. Drug treatment of breathlessness: contrasting effects of diazepam and promethazine in pink puffers. *Br Med J Clin Res Ed.* 1981;283(6287): 343–346.

58. Navigante AH, Cerchietti LC, Castro MA, et al. Midazolam as adjunct therapy to morphine in the alleviation of severe dyspnea perception in patients with advanced cancer. *J Pain Symptom Manage.* 2006;31(1):38–47.

59. Man GC, Hsu K, Sproule BJ. Effect of alprazolam on exercise and dyspnea in patients with chronic obstructive pulmonary disease. *Chest.* 1986;90(6):832–836.

60. Eimer M, Cable T, Gal P, et al. Effects of clorazepate on breathlessness and exercise tolerance in patients with chronic airflow obstruction. *J Fam Pract.* 1985;21(5): 359–362.

61. Garner SJ, Eldridge FL, Wagner PG, et al. Buspirone, an anxiolytic drug that stimulates respiration. *Am Rev Respir Dis.* 1989;139(4):946–950.

62. Mendelson WB, Martin JV, Rapoport DM. Effects of buspirone on sleep and respiration. *Am Rev Respir Dis.* 1990;141(6):1527–1530.

63. Argyropoulou P, Patakas D, Koukou A, et al. Buspirone effect on breathlessness and exercise performance in patients with chronic obstructive pulmonary disease. *Respiration.* 1993;60(4):216–220.

64. Singh NP, Despars JA, Stansbury DW, et al. Effects of buspirone on anxiety levels and exercise tolerance in patients with chronic airflow obstruction and mild anxiety. *Chest.* 1993;103(3):800–804.

65. Burns BH, Howell JB. Disproportionately severe breathlessness in chronic bronchitis. *Q J Med.* 1969;38(151):277–294.

66. Mueller RA, Lundberg DB, Breese GR, et al. The neuropharmacology of respiratory control. *Pharmacol Rev.* 1982;34(3):255–285.

67. Papp LA, Weiss JR, Greenberg HE, et al. Sertraline for chronic obstructive pulmonary disease and comorbid anxiety and mood disorders. *Am J Psychiatry.* 1995;152(10):1531.

68. Smoller JW, Pollack MH, Systrom D, et al. Sertraline effects on dyspnea in patients with obstructive airway disease. *Psychosomatics.* 1998;39(1):24–29.

69. Ventresca PG, Nichol GM, Barnes PJ, et al. Inhaled furosemide inhibits cough induced by low chloride content solutions but not by capsaicin. *Am Rev Respir Dis.* 1990;142(1):143–146.

70. Bianco S, Pieroni MG, Refini RM, et al. Protective effect of inhaled furosemide on allergen-induced early and late asthmatic reactions. *N Engl J Med.* 1989;321(16):1069–1073.

71. Bianco S, Vaghi A, Robuschi M, et al. Prevention of exercise-induced bronchoconstriction by inhaled frusemide. *Lancet.* 1988;2(8605): 252–255.

72. Robuschi M, Gambaro G, Spagnotto S, et al. Inhaled frusemide is highly effective in preventing ultrasonically nebulised water bronchoconstriction. *Pulm Pharmacol.* 1989;1(4): 187–191.

73. Chung KF, Barnes PJ. Loop diuretics and asthma. *Pulm Pharmacol.* 1992;5(1):1–7.

74. Ong K-C, Kor A-C, Chong W-F, et al. Effects of inhaled furosemide on exertional dyspnea in chronic obstructive pulmonary disease. *Am J Respir Crit Care Med.* 2004;169(9):1028–1033.

75. Ahmedzai SH, Laude E, Robertson A, et al. A double-blind, randomised, controlled phase II trial of Heliox28 gas mixture in lung cancer patients with dyspnoea on exertion. *Br J Cancer.* 2004;90(2):366–371.

76. Corner J, O'Driscoll M. Development of a breathlessness assessment guide for use in palliative care. *Palliative Med.* 1999;13(5):375–384.

77. O'Neill S, McCarthy DS. Postural relief of dyspnoea in severe chronic airflow limitation: relationship to respiratory muscle strength. *Thorax.* 1983;38(8):595–600.

78. Sharp JT, Drutz WS, Moisan T, et al. Postural relief of dyspnea in severe chronic obstructive pulmonary disease. *Am Rev Respir Dis.* 1980;122(2):201–211.

79. Barach AL. Chronic obstructive lung disease: postural relief of dyspnea. *Arch Phys Med Rehab.* 1974;55(11):494–504.

80. Barach AL, Beck GJ. The ventilatory effects of the head-down position in pulmonary emphysema. *Am J Med.* 1954;16(1):55–60.

81. Tiep BL, Burns M, Kao D, et al. Pursed lips breathing training using ear oximetry. *Chest.* 1986;90(2):218–221.

82. Madge S, Edmond G. End-stage management of respiratory disease. In: Esmond G, ed. *Respiratory Nursing.* London: Bailliere Tindall; 2001: 229–240.

83. Smith EL, Hann DM, Ahles TA, et al. Dyspnea, anxiety, body consciousness, and quality of life in patients with lung cancer. *J Pain Symptom Manage.* 2001;21(4):323–329.

84. Booth S, Silvester S, Todd C. Breathlessness in cancer and chronic obstructive pulmonary disease: using a qualitative approach to describe the experience of patients and carers. *Palliative Support Care.* 2003;1(4):337–344.

85. Seamark DA, Blake SD, Seamark CJ, et al. Living with severe chronic obstructive pulmonary disease (COPD): perceptions of patients and their carers. An interpretative phenomenological analysis. *Palliative Med.* 2004;18(7):619–625.

86. Saunders C. Care of patients suffering from terminal illness at St. Joseph's Hospice, Hackney, London. *Nursing Mirror.* 1964;14:vii–x.

87. Abernethy AP, Wheeler JL. Total dyspnoea. *Curr Opin Support Palliative Care.* 2008;2(2):110–113.

88. Zigmond AS, Snaith RP, Zigmond AS, et al. The Hospital Anxiety and Depression Scale. *Acta Psych Scand.* 1983;67(6):361–370.

89. *NCCN Clinical Practice Guidelines in Oncology: Distress Management.* Fort Washington, PA: National Comprehensive Cancer Network; 2007.

90. Peterman AH, Fitchett G, Brady MJ, et al. Measuring spiritual well-being in people with cancer: the functional assessment of chronic illness therapy – Spiritual Well-being Scale (FACIT-Sp). *Ann Behav Med.* 2002;24(1):49–58.

91. VNAA Chronic Care Clearinghouse home page. Available at: http://www.chronicconditions.org/.

92. Pulmonary Rehabilitation Toolkit home page. Available at: http://www.pulmonaryrehab.com.au/.

93. Bruera E, MacEachern T, Ripamonti C, et al. Subcutaneous morphine for dyspnea in cancer patients. *Ann Intern Med.* 1993;119(9):906–907.

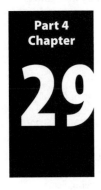

29

Management of the gastrointestinal side effects of therapy in older adults with cancer

Laura Raftery, Stephen A. Bernard, and Richard M. Goldberg

The treatment of cancer often leads to gastrointestinal (GI) side effects. There are few dedicated studies to guide therapy and management of toxicity in elderly patients who are receiving cancer therapy. Consequently, conclusions regarding symptomatic management of GI-related adverse events are largely derived from subset or pooled analyses. The need for supportive cancer care in this population equals or exceeds that of the younger patient.

The burden of a cancer diagnosis, treatment, and potential toxicities of therapy can deplete the limited physical, emotional, and financial reserves of an older patient, especially a frail one. Even a seemingly robust older patient may show a more rapid decline compared to a younger individual receiving similar therapy. The volume of information from clinical trials concerning the toxicity of cancer therapy in older adults is limited. Many trials have had limited enrollment of elderly patients or an age cutoff between 60 and 70 years; extrapolation of these data to an older age group may not be appropriate. Use of post hoc subset analysis from larger studies may produce selection bias, and individuals enrolled in clinical trials are often more medically fit than the general population of older adults and as such are not representative. Despite these limitations, a number of conclusions about managing GI side effects of cancer therapy can be derived from available data.

Aging is associated with a decrement in glomerular filtration rate (GFR), total body water, plasma protein concentration, and muscle mass, which can affect the pharmacokinetics of antineoplastic agents and increase susceptibility of normal tissues to injury. Managing older cancer patients demands a composite assessment of a patient's comorbid illnesses, medications, cognitive ability, functional limitations, nutritional state, and psychological and socioeconomic status to individualize management strategies in a way that permits optimal therapy to be delivered with acceptable side effects.

Ideally, oncologists managing older patients are well aware of the diversity of the older population; they weigh the costs and benefits of therapy for each individual and devise thoughtful treatment plans as complications and toxicities arise. Withholding therapy or reducing drug doses out of a desire to avoid toxic side effects certainly can minimize toxicity but also limits the possibility for remission or cure. Assuming that older patients will be intolerant of intensive therapy often does them a disservice as a number of studies indicate that tolerance is not a function of age alone. Physicians may choose to recommend attenuated therapies, and older patients may choose to forego relatively intensive therapy because of assumptions about toxicity based on other patients' experiences of debilitating side effects. In many cases, these regimens can be effectively delivered to older patients without excessive side effects; that is, when comorbid conditions are thoughtfully considered and controlled, many elderly can be treated just as younger patients are treated. Thus conscientious attention to supportive care is arguably one of the most important interventions an oncologist can make to preserve quality of life, influence a favorable outcome, and ultimately, conserve health care resources spent on toxicity management.

In this chapter, we describe some of the common gastrointestinal side effects seen with treatment of cancer and management of these side effects. We focus on studies with information on adults aged 65 years and older and use the term *elderly* to describe this group collectively. Specific data on individuals of older age groups are more limited but will also be discussed.

A. Diarrhea

Diarrhea is a common problem in cancer patients who have received chemotherapy, biologic therapy (Tables 29.1 and 29.2), or radiation therapy to the abdomen and pelvis. Severe diarrhea can be life threatening or lethal, particularly in the elderly

Table 29.1 Chemotherapeutic agents that can cause diarrhea (does not include biologic agents).

Capecitabine
Cisplatin
Cytarabine
Cyclophosphamide
Daunorubicin
Docetaxel
Doxorubicin
5-Fluorouracil
Interferon
Irinotecan
Leucovorin
Methotrexate
Oxaliplatin
Paclitaxel
Topotecan

Note. From Mercadante.[106]

Table 29.2 Biologic agents that cause diarrhea.

Biologic agent	Diarrhea (%)
Sorafenib[106]	35–40 (grade 3–4 = 10%)
Imatinib[107]	30
Lapatinib[108]	40
Bortezomib[109]	57 (grade 3–4 = 7%)
Erlotinib[110]	56 (grade 3–4 = 6%)
Cetuximab[111]	23 (grade 3–4 = 2%)
Panitumumab[112]	21 (grade 3–4 = 1%)

Table 29.3 NCI Common Toxicity Criteria Grading of Diarrhea Version 3.

Grade 1 = increase of 2–3 stools per day
Grade 2 = increase of 4–6 stools per day or nocturnal stools or moderate cramping, not interfering with normal activity
Grade 3 = increase of 7–9 stools per day or severe cramping and incontinence and interfering with normal activity
Grade 4 = increase of 10 stools per day or grossly bloody stools and need for parenteral support

Note. From http://www.cancer.gov/cancertopics/pdq/supportivecare/gastrointestinalcomplications.

and sepsis. 5-FU and the oral 5-FU pro-drug capecitabine impair DNA synthesis by inhibiting thymidylate synthase and RNA synthesis.[3]

Leucovorin (LV) enhances the efficacy of 5-FU by interacting with thymidylate synthase to form a stable ternary complex that potentiates the effects of 5-FU. The 5-FU-LV combination alone or in multidrug regimens is used widely and may produce additional mucosal injury compared to 5-FU alone.[4] Diarrhea occurs more often with coadministration of LV and especially with bolus rather than infusional administration of 5-FU. In one study, elderly patients experienced a 5 percent fatality rate associated with diarrhea, dehydration, and subsequent complications. Severe diarrhea was seen in 40 percent. Notably, 40 percent of this study's population was between the ages of 60 and 69 years, and 20 percent was over 70 years.[5] Several other studies as well as meta-analyses suggest that adjuvant 5-FU therapy regimens for colorectal cancer are not associated with differences in efficacy or toxicity between younger and older patients, except for increased neutropenia; grade 3 diarrhea occurred in 15 percent of both younger and older patients.[6–10]

Women experience greater 5-FU toxicity than men, probably because of lower dihydropyrimidine dehydrogenase (DPD) activity. DPD is critical for the degradation of 5-FU, and severe deficiency may cause high-grade toxicity and potentially fatal side effects. In a meta-analysis examining gender and toxicity from 5-FU, women experienced 8 percent more stomatitis, 7 percent more nausea, 7 percent more vomiting, and 4 percent more diarrhea than men. Older women (greater than 60 years of age) more often experienced severe or very severe stomatitis.[11]

Capecitabine, designed for more reliable absorption from the GI tract and selective 5-FU

patient with diminished reserves (Table 29.3). As loss of fluid and electrolytes becomes severe, renal injury, metabolic acidosis, hyponatremia, hypernatremia, cardiovascular collapse, and death may occur.

More than 50 percent of patients treated with fluoropyrimidines (5-fluorouracil [5-FU]; capecitabine) and irinotecan experience diarrhea, occurring when the absorptive capacity of the colon is overwhelmed by the amount of fluid leaving the small bowel because of acutely damaged mucosa.[1,2] In the gut, the fluoropyrimidines cause mitotic arrest of epithelial crypt cells such that there are fewer mature villous enterocytes to allow normal intestinal function. Local inflammation by opportunistic organisms may stimulate secretion of fluids and electrolytes into the gut, and gram-negative enteric organisms may cross a disrupted mucosal barrier with the potential for bacteremia activation in tumor tissue, is commonly used in colorectal and breast cancer. Toxicity includes grade 3–4 diarrhea in about 10 percent of patients. Historically, patients in the United States have been relatively intolerant of the higher doses of the drug given to European patients, putatively because of the common practice of adding folic acid supplements to processed foods sold in the United States but not in Europe. Capecitabine and its metabolites are excreted by the kidneys, and its administration is contraindicated in patients whose creatinine clearance is less than 30 mL/min. Elderly patients commonly have decreased renal function caused by a progressive, age-related decline in glomerular filtration rate.[12] Creatinine level is a poor marker of renal function, particularly in the elderly, whose muscle mass is decreased. To avoid unforeseen toxicity, it is prudent to estimate the elderly individual's glomerular filtration rate. In one study of 73 older women treated with capecitabine for breast cancer, two deaths occurred from grade 4 diarrhea. The authors concluded that toxicity was increased because of relatively impaired renal function.[13] In colorectal cancer treatment, capecitabine has been compared with 5-FU in elderly patients and appears to be safe and effective. In the X-ACT (Xeloda in Adjuvant Colon Cancer) trial, capecitabine was compared to 5-FU/LV given according to the Mayo Clinic protocol (daily treatment for 5 days, repeated each month) in patients treated in the adjuvant setting for stage II and III colon cancer. Subset analysis showed that patients older than 70 years benefited as much as younger patients; rates of diarrhea were similar at 13 percent and 11 percent for 5-FU and capecitabine, respectively. Other toxicities were different: there was more neutropenia and stomatitis with 5-FU but more hand-foot syndrome with capecitabine.[14] Another study of a fixed-dose capecitabine at 2,000 mg twice daily every 2–3 weeks demonstrated greater toxicity in the elderly (median age 72), with 34 percent grade 3–4 diarrhea.[15] In practice, in the United States, many oncologists start dosing at 1,000 mg/m^2 twice daily rather than the dose specified in the package insert of 1,200 mg/m^2 twice daily and modify that dose based on tolerability. Retrospective analysis has not demonstrated a reduction in activity at this lower dose.

Irinotecan can cause both acute and delayed diarrhea. The acute diarrhea, which occurs in up to 50 percent of patients, is immediate and mediated by the cholinergic system but is gen-

erally not severe. The patient may experience other symptoms of cholinergic excess such as abdominal cramping and salivation. This occurs because of irinotecan's structural similarity to acetylcholine and can be prevented with administration of atropine. The mechanism of late irinotecan-associated diarrhea is believed to be related to the concentration of its active metabolite SN-38 in the intestinal mucosa, where it causes apoptosis. Delayed diarrhea can occur at all doses with a median time to onset of 6–11 days. Both irinotecan and SN-38 may also cause diarrhea through stimulation of pro-inflammatory cytokines and prostaglandins.[16] In one study, a higher dose, every-3-week irinotecan, was associated with less grade 3 and 4 diarrhea – 14 percent compared to 36 percent for weekly irinotecan dosing. In this analysis, age 70 and older was an independent predictor of grade 3 and 4 diarrhea (odds ratio 1.8).[17]

A prospective study of 85 patients aged 72 years and older evaluated the efficacy and safety of irinotecan and infusional 5-FU for advanced colon cancer. Eighteen percent of patients had grade 3 or 4 diarrhea, and there were two deaths.[18] Another trial of FOLFIRI (folinic acid, fluorouracil, irinotecan) in patients older than age 70 years demonstrated very similar results.[19] Irinotecan and weekly bolus 5-FU/LV (the IFL regimen[20]) produced unacceptable mortality because of enteropathy characterized by nausea, vomiting, diarrhea, cramping, dehydration, and sepsis in two large cooperative group studies, and this regimen is no longer used.[21] The median age of patients who died in the IFL-treated group was 69 years, higher than the median age of 60–63 years of patients enrolled onto other adjuvant colon cancer studies.[22,23]

Monoclonal antibodies directed against EGFR (epidermal growth factor receptor), small-molecule tyrosine kinase inhibitors, and immunomodulator drugs such as bortezomib commonly cause diarrhea (see Table 29.2). Usually, this symptom can be managed with the opiate loperamide, as described later, but in a minority of patients, such symptoms can interfere with optimal therapy and require dose reduction or discontinuation of the drug. Caution may be needed when combining these newer agents with cytotoxic chemotherapy because of overlapping toxicity. A phase I study to establish the dose-limiting toxicity and maximum-tolerated dose of erlotinib and FOLFIRI demonstrated grade 3 diarrhea and neutropenia at reduced doses and was terminated early.[24] Another phase I study demonstrated dose-limiting diarrhea with gefitinib, capecitabine, and radiation therapy in pancreatic and rectal cancer.[25] The studies included elderly patients without specific subset analysis for age.

Guidelines have been written for evaluation and management of diarrhea. Historical information should include a complete description of bowel movement frequency, duration, and stool volume and character. Close monitoring is necessary during therapy using chemotherapeutic agents known to cause diarrhea, and patients should be questioned about dizziness, orthostatic symptoms, lethargy, cramping, abdominal pain, nausea, vomiting, fever, and rectal bleeding. Symptoms should be classified as complicated or uncomplicated. Uncomplicated symptoms include grade 1 or 2 diarrhea (see Table 29.3). One algorithm for management suggests holding cytotoxic chemotherapy until symptoms resolve, dietary modification, followed by intensive administration of loperamide (4 mg initially, then 2 mg every 2 hours or 4 mg every 4 hours until the patient is free of diarrhea for 12 hours). With persistent diarrhea, stool studies to rule out enteric pathogens, such as *Clostridium difficile*, and oral antibiotics, as infection prophylaxis are recommended. Octreotide may be effective therapy in the case of loperamide failure. Deodorized tincture of opium (containing 10 mg/mL of morphine), the less concentrated camphorated tincture of opium (Paragoric, containing 0.4 mg/mL of morphine), or budesonide are may be considered if symptoms are unresolved after 48 hours. Diphenoxylate-atropine (Lomotil) is not recommended in most recent guidelines. Complicated symptoms include grade 3 or 4 diarrhea or grade 1 or 2 diarrhea and any one of the following risk factors: moderate to severe cramping, grade 2 or higher nausea and vomiting, decreased performance status, fever, sepsis, neutropenia, frank bleeding, and dehydration. Complicated diarrhea warrants hospital admission for intravenous fluids, electrolyte repletion, stool workup, antibiotics, and octreotide as vascular collapse and lethal outcomes can result from less aggressive management. Medication, history of recent travel, and dietary intake including lactose-containing products, high-osmolar supplements, and the use of so-called sugar-free products sweetened with sugar alcohols may provide additional clues regarding etiology.[26]

B. Constipation related to cancer therapy

A long-held assumption has been that the elderly are prone to constipation. A decrease in enteric neurons and changes in calcium handling may prolong transit time of waste through the colon.[27] However, when objectively studied, these so-called age-related changes in enteric physiology are not supported by substantial evidence[28] and may in fact distract the clinician from searching for a contribution by concurrent disorders, such as hypothyroidism or medications. Geriatric patients commonly use drugs such as antidepressants, anticholinergics, diuretics, iron, calcium supplements, antiemetics (particularly 5HT3 antagonists), and antacids, all of which are constipating. In addition, constipation can be the consequence of metabolic derangements such as hypercalcemia and hypokalemia, peripheral and autonomic neuropathy, spinal cord compression, and brain tumors. Other risk factors for constipation include reduced mobility, reduced fluid and food intake, dehydration, mechanical obstruction, and pain caused by problems such as fissures and hemorrhoids.

The prevalence of constipation from opioids is as high as 90 percent in cancer patients.[29] Opioids act on mu opioid receptors in the submucosal plexus of the gastrointestinal tract[30] and cause constipation by slowing transit through the gut lumen and permitting more water absorption as well as by inhibiting neurons responsible for secreting fluid into the gut. The result is dry, hard, difficult-to-pass stools that fail to distend the gut lumen. Without activation of stretch receptors, enterochromaffin cells of the gut do not release serotonin, and the bowel does not contract. This process can lead to fecal impaction, especially in older patients, for whom rectal function may already be impaired.

All opioids cause constipation, and this unfortunate side effect does not diminish with continued use. There is good evidence that compared with the water-soluble opioids morphine and oxycodone, the more lipid-soluble opioids fentanyl and buprenorphine are less likely to cause constipation but do provide equivalent analgesia.[31,32] Methadone is also thought to be less constipating. In spite of this, methadone ought to be prescribed with caution in the elderly. The half-life of methadone is over 20 hours, and its pharmacokinetics are highly variable among patients because of differences in protein binding, urinary excretion, and induction of metabolism by other drugs.[33]

Most clinicians start a prophylactic bowel program including both softeners and stimulants when prescribing narcotics, but as many as 25 percent do not.[34] Waiting to treat constipation until it is established happens all too frequently. Moreover, patients often postpone beginning a prescribed regimen until symptoms appear, at which point more aggressive intervention may become necessary.

Other constipation-inducing drugs frequently used in cancer care are those with anticholinergic properties such as tricyclic antidepressants, antihistamines, neuroleptics, and the 5HT3 antagonist antiemetics, which cause constipation in 10 percent of patients.[35]

Constipation occurs in 50 percent of patients receiving vincristine because of disruption of the microtubules within axons and interference with axonal transport. Autonomic neurotoxicity can develop, with abdominal pain, paralytic ileus, and in rare cases, megacolon.[36] In those with occult hepatic disease, metabolism of the drug may be impaired and may unexpectedly cause neurotoxicity. Most clinicians will limit the dose of vincristine to 2 mg to avoid toxicity. Oxaliplatin, despite its common toxicity of sensory neurotoxicity, is not associated with constipation. Constipation is also a common side effect of novel therapies for multiple myeloma and, increasingly, other hematologic malignancies. It is observed in 55 percent, 42 percent, and 39 percent of patients receiving thalidomide, lenalinomide, and bortezomib, respectively.[37–39]

Once the cause of constipation is identified, treatment is usually based on anecdotal experience and expert opinion. There are few evidence-based trials to guide decision making. Most would recommend adequate daily fluid intake (1.5 L or more)[40] and some physical activity, predicated on the observation that bed-bound patients are prone to constipation. On the other hand, in a large study of over 1,000 healthy adults, constipation was only weakly correlated with the level of physical activity, although some exercise was nevertheless associated with a range of other health benefits.[41] Regular physical exercise did not help chronic idiopathic constipation in healthy subjects in another observational study.[42] Constipated patients often receive recommendations about altering their diet to include more fiber with adequate fluids. One meta-analysis confirmed that dietary fiber supplementation increased stool weight and decreased transit time in both normal and constipated adults. There is a positive dose response between fiber intake, water intake, and fecal output. The recommended amount of dietary fiber is 25–30 g/d.

However, adding fiber to the diet of a cancer patient taking opioids for pain is not always an appropriate strategy, especially in those patients with severe constipation, who may experience excessive flatus and bloating because of bacterial degradation of the indigestible carbohydrate. As is true of all laxatives, fiber is contraindicated in the setting of fecal impaction or obstruction. If fiber is deemed appropriate, the best way to add it is by making small changes to the diet and establishing a routine that otherwise promotes normal bowel function and takes advantage of the gastrocolic reflex, most active after breakfast.

In terms of pharmacological treatment, laxatives are commonly prescribed, but evidence supporting their efficacy, especially in the elderly, is weak.[43] Side effects of laxatives and stool softeners include bloating, cramping, soiling, and pain, similar to symptoms caused by the constipation that is being treated. In 2005, the American College of Gastroenterology published recommendations on the management of chronic constipation; in the same year, another well-done systemic review of the efficacy and safety of traditional medical therapies for chronic constipation was published. Polyethylene glycol, sorbitol, and lactulose, all of which are hyperosmolar agents that cause water secretion into the intestine, were recommended in both publications.[44,45] The saline laxatives milk of magnesia and magnesium citrate are also hyperosmolar solutions; magnesium may interfere with absorption of certain medications and cause hypermagnesemia, potentially a problem in the elderly with renal impairment. There were insufficient data to recommend the use of stimulant laxatives such as the commonly used senna in chronic constipation. The stimulant laxatives increase intestinal motor activity but affect electrolyte balance and have worse adverse effects than other laxatives. Evidence for the effectiveness of stool softeners is limited, and they are not recommended in these recent reviews.

Methylnaltrexone, administered subcutaneously, was approved recently by the U.S. Food and Drug Administration (FDA) for refractory opioid-induced constipation. Theoretically, it antagonizes mu opioid receptors in the gastrointestinal tract but does not penetrate the central nervous system. In this way, it reverses opioid-induced gut hypomotility by blocking peripheral receptors without inhibiting the opioid's central analgesic effect. In a clinical trial of patients with advanced terminal diseases, methylnaltrexone was at least 3 times as effective as placebo in producing a bowel movement within 4 hours after the initial dose. No episodes of gut hypermotility, known as *gut withdrawal syndrome*, were observed, and there was no antagonism of analgesia. However, the drug produced a bowel movement without the help of another laxative in only half the patients, and furthermore, all patients were permitted to remain on their current laxative regimen. An oral form of the medication is available but was not tested; if effective, it would be far more convenient to administer. It has not been assessed for chronic constipation. Future studies will predict the success or failure of methylnaltrexone in cancer patients.[46]

When opiates are prescribed, it is prudent to recommend a bowel regimen to prevent constipation. Patients can be given simple titration parameters for regular bowel movements. An evaluation of underlying comorbid conditions and review of the patient's medication record should be done early. Most often, fiber supplements or osmotic laxatives such as polyethylene glycol are adequate to relieve symptoms. The patient should be educated on risks of constipation and encouraged to take a proactive approach rather than waiting for severe constipation to develop. Adequate hydration, moderate exercise, and fiber-containing diet may be effective, although there is a lack of evidence for the impact of these measures on constipation, not to mention that they may be impossible to achieve in patients who are in pain, unwell, or dying. Enemas and suppositories have their role in combination with osmotic laxatives in managing high-risk or severely obstipated patients.

C. Cancer treatment–related nausea and vomiting

In recent years, there has been considerable progress in controlling cancer treatment–related nausea and vomiting. Our understanding of the neurologic pathways initiating and controlling nausea and vomiting has expanded. There are several new, effective, and well-tolerated antiemetic drugs. As well, there is broad consensus on the likelihood and severity associated with particular chemotherapeutic drugs or multidrug regimens for causing nausea and vomiting (Table 29.4). Consequently, evidence-based guidelines on the appropriate antiemetic treatments for a given risk of emesis have also been written, although there are no recommendations specifically tailored for

Table 29.4 Emetic risk in the absence of antiemetic therapy.

High, >90%	Moderate, 30–90%	Low, 10–30%	Minimal, <10%
AC combination	Carboplatin	Asparaginase	Bleomycin
Carmustine > 250 mg/m^2	Carmustine 250 mg/m^2	Bortezomib	Busulfan
Cisplatin > 50 mg/m^2	Cisplatin < 50 mg/m^2	Capecitabine	Chlorambucil (oral)
Cyclophosphamide > 1,500 mg/m^2	Cyclophosphamide < 1,500 mg/m^2	Cetuximab	2-Chlorodeoxyadenosine
Dacarbazine	Cyclophosphamide (oral)	Cytarabine < 1 g/m^2	Fludarabine
Lomustine	Cytarabine > 1 g/m^2	Docetaxel	Hydroxyurea
Mechlorethamine	Daunorubicin	Etoposide	Methotrexate < 100 mg/m^2
Pentostatin	Doxorubicin	5-Fluorouracil < 1,000 mg/m^2	Phenylalanine mustard (oral)
Streptozocin	Cyclophosphamide (oral)	Gemcitabine	Thioguanine (oral)
Procarbazine (oral)	Epirubicin 90 mg/m^2	Methotrexate > 100 mg/m^2	Vinblastine
	Hexamethylmelamine (oral)	< 250 mg/m^2	Vincristine
	Idarubicin	Mitoxantrone	Vinorelbine
	Imatinib	Mitomycin	
	Ifosfamide	Paclitaxel	
	Irinotecan	Pemetrexed	
	Melphalan	Topotecan	
	Methotrexate 250–1,000 mg/m^2	Trastuzumab	
	Mitoxantrone > 12 mg/m^2		
	Oxaliplatin		
	Temozolomide		

Note. Adapted from Hesketh et al.[113]

Table 29.5 Antiemetic prevention based on emesis risk.

High CINV		Moderate CINV		Low CINV	
Acute	Delayed	Acute	Delayed	Acute	Delayed
5HT3RA + dexamethasone + aprepitant ± lorazepam	Dexamethasone + aprepitant ± lorazepam	Anthracycline and cyclophosphamide, or in selected patients, 5HT3RA + dexamethasone + aprepitant ± lorazepam, or other than anthracycline and cyclophosphamide, 5HT3RA + dexamethasone ± lorazepam	Aprepitant + dexamethasone ± lorazepam, dexamethasone or 5HT3RA, both ± lorazepam	Dexamethasone ± lorazepam or prochlorperazine ± lorazepam or metoclopramide ± lorazepam	

Note. CINV = chemotherapy-induced nausea and vomiting; 5HT3RA = 5HT3-receptor antagonist. From http://www.nccn.org/professionals/physician_gls/PDF/antiemesis.pdf.

the elderly (Table 29.5). The guiding principle is to prevent chemotherapy-induced nausea and vomiting (CINV) before it occurs; managing it once it is established is difficult. Second, it is critical to provide therapy for the duration of risk of CINV to avoid the phenomenon of delayed nausea. Finally, breakthrough nausea is challenging to treat and is usually best managed using a class of drugs not commonly prescribed in the prophylactic regimen. Though vomiting can be prevented in up to 90 percent of cases, nausea remains the more challenging problem and is often refractory to all therapy, still occuring in up to 50 percent of patients treated with chemotherapy despite antiemetic use.

Nausea and vomiting have been classified as acute, delayed, and anticipatory, distinctions with important implications for prevention and treatment. Factors that predict chemotherapy-related nausea and vomiting include gender, age, the chemotherapy administered, and a history of poorly controlled symptoms during prior courses of chemotherapy. Studies show that women are more susceptible than men and that younger patients are more susceptible than older patients to CINV.[47] A history of motion sickness and nausea with pregnancy predict for greater risk of CINV. Less risk of CINV has been observed in those with a history of chronic heavy alcohol consumption.[48,49]

Acute-onset nausea occurs within the first few minutes to hours after administration of chemotherapy, peaking in intensity at 6 hours and resolving by 24 hours. Delayed nausea is defined as occurring 24 hours after chemotherapy and is most often experienced with high-dose cisplatin (50 mg/m^2 or more), carboplatin (more than 300 mg/m^2), cyclophosphamide (more than 600 mg/m^2), and doxorubicin (50 mg/m^2 or more). In one study, 89 percent of patients had delayed nausea from 24 to 120 hours after receiving high-dose cisplatin, with a peak incidence occurring between 48 and 72 hours.[50] The proportion of patients experiencing delayed nausea after doxorubicin and cyclophosphamide is about 30 percent. Anticipatory nausea begins before the administration of chemotherapy and appears to be a conditioned response in patients who have developed significant nausea and vomiting during previous cycles of chemotherapy. Behavioral therapy and anxiolytics can be helpful in managing anticipatory emesis, but the best approach is prevention with an appropriate antiemetic regimen prior to the first dose of chemotherapy. Nausea related to radiation therapy occurs most often with total body irradiation, abdominal irradiation, or when the stomach or gut are in the radiation field and responds to the same drugs that control CINV, with 5HT3 receptor antagonists as arguably the most useful agents because of the high concentration of 5HT3 receptors in the gut. These antagonists may exert an anesthetic-like effect on the 5HT3 receptors.

The original work by Borison and Wang is a cornerstone for understanding the complex pathophysiology of CINV, which is still not completely defined. The emetic center in the medulla coordinates efferent respiratory, gastrointestinal, and autonomic impulses, which induce vomiting. It is stimulated by the chemotherapy trigger zone, in the area postrema at the base of the fourth ventricle, within the brain but outside the blood-brain barrier. Its location outside the blood-brain barrier permits ready exposure to chemicals, peptides, and other substances borne in the blood; furthermore, it has direct access to neurons that project to brain areas with important roles in the autonomic control of many physiological systems. For example, when exposed to chemotherapeutic drugs and other poisons, it signals the emetic center, which may be the equivalent of a number of loosely organized neuronal areas within the medulla.[51–54]

Recent investigation of neurotransmitters that act in these areas of the brain and gut has permitted the development of several very effective antiemetics. In brief, the neuroendocrine enterochromaffin cells of the stomach and gut secrete serotonin, substance-P, and neurokephalin in response to chemotherapy. In turn, these transmitters stimulate vagal and splanchnic fibers, terminating in the brain stem and activating the emetic reflex. The brain stem also has abundant neurotransmitter receptors.[55] Of the many neurotransmitters thought to be involved in CINV, serotonin (5HT3), substance-P, dopamine, and cannabinoids are among the most important.

The phenothiazine derivative prochlorperazine and metoclopromide represent two often-prescribed dopamine antagonists. As drugs used in practice for decades, they are far less costly than the newer agents but produce sedation and anticholinergic effects and are associated with extrapyramidal reactions, especially in younger individuals. In low doses, prochlorperazine is effective in preventing nausea associated with radiation therapy and in treating nausea and vomiting attributed to very low to moderately emetogenic chemotherapeutic drugs. Phenothiazines may be valuable in treating patients who experience delayed nausea.[56] Prior to the introduction of serotonin receptor antagonists, metoclopromide was considered the most effective single antiemetic agent against highly emetogenic chemotherapy such as cisplatin. It is most effective for acute vomiting when given intravenously (IV) at high doses, probably because it also competes at 5HT3 receptors at the higher doses used. As well, metoclopromide increases lower esophageal sphincter pressure and gastric emptying, contributing to the antiemetic effect.

Metoclopramide is also associated with dystonic extrapyramidal effects, more commonly observed in younger patients; diphenhydramine may be used prophylactically or therapeutically to antagonize such reactions.[57] Caution is advised when using dopamine antagonists in the elderly, who may be more sensitive to the adverse effects of the drugs, which include drowsiness, confusion, masklike facies, drooling, shuffling walk, tremor, and muscle spasm, and who may experience paradoxical restlessness and agitation.

The 5HT3 antagonists are most useful for acute and less so for delayed nausea and vomiting (Table 29.5). Adverse effects of 5HT3 antagonists are few and include constipation, headache, and a mild transaminitis. There are five serotonin antagonists, four of which are older and considered equivalent in efficacy. Comparatively, the newer agent, palonosetron, has a half-life of 40 hours or more and a greater binding affinity for the receptor. The 5HT3 antagonists have not proved to be more effective than prochlorperazine for preventing delayed nausea with the exception of palonosetron, which has not been studied in this setting.[58] The efficacy of palonosetron in preventing CINV in elderly patients was assessed in a retrospective subset analysis of two randomized phase III studies. The subset consisted of patients aged 65 years and older who received a single IV dose of palonosetron, ondansetron, or dolasetron. A greater proportion of palonosetron-treated patients were free of emesis and nausea (71 and 52%) 5 days following chemotherapy than patients treated with either ondansetron or dolasetron (51 and 38%), leading to the conclusion that palonosetron more effectively prevents CINV in the elderly[59]

The latest success in antiemetic therapy is the neurokinin-1 receptor antagonist, which selectively blocks substance-P binding at NK-1 receptors found in the central nervous system; NK-1 receptors are also found in the gastrointestinal tract. Substance-P is a tachykinin, a regulatory peptide, found to cause emesis in animals.[60] Common adverse side effects of the approved NK-1 receptor antagonist aprepitant are fatigue, hiccups, and asthenia. For highly emetogenic chemotherapy, aprepitant is indicated in combination with a serotonin-receptor antagonist and a corticosteroid for prophylaxis of acute-onset nausea and in combination with a corticosteroid for the prevention of delayed nausea and vomiting.[61] Aprepitant also reduced the occurrence of nausea and vomiting after moderately emetogenic chemotherapy. In a randomized study, patients with breast cancer treated with an anthracycline and cyclophosphamide were given either aprepitant, a serotonin-receptor antagonist, and a corticosteroid before chemotherapy, followed by aprepitant for the next 2 days, or a serotonin-receptor antagonist and a corticosteroid before chemotherapy, followed by the serotonin-receptor antagonist for the next 2 days.[62] The aprepitant-based regimen was responsible for more complete responses, defined as no vomiting and no rescue therapy throughout the acute and delayed phases of the first cycle of chemotherapy (50.8% vs. 42.5%). More patients in the aprepitant group reported minimal or no impact of CINV on daily life (63.5% vs. 55.6%).[63] Aprepitant inhibits the cytochrome P450 enzyme CYP3A4; thus attention to potential drug interactions is prudent. One such interaction involves dexamethasone, which is metabolized along the CYP3A4 pathway. Its plasma concentration doubles if aprepitant is coadministered, and guidelines suggest dose reduction of the steroid, unless it is included as part of the cancer therapy. There are many chemotherapeutic agents and drugs metabolized by CYP3A4. Although guidelines for dose adjustment do not yet exist, the potential for clinically significant drug interactions may be a concern for elderly patients who are often taking a handful of medications. Aprepitant is commonly used for cisplatin-based regimens and as standard prophylaxis for anthracycline and cyclophosphamide regimens.

Steroids are used as single agents for mild to moderate emetogenic chemotherapy and in combination with other agents for moderate- to high-risk therapy. They are effective for acute and delayed emesis.[64] The mechanism of action in this context is not fully understood but may include modulation of prostaglandin activity in the brain at the cortical level. For some, steroids may improve mood and sense of well-being. Toxicity from a short course of dexamethasone is minimal but can include insomnia, psychosis, and epigastric discomfort, among other side effects. In the elderly with diabetes, steroids can antagonize control of blood glucose.

The use of cannabinoids as antiemetics initially began with the the observation that patients who smoked marijuana during chemotherapy reported benefit. Subsequent work has shown that tetrahydrocannabinol does reduce CINV. Because of cultural taboos and a low therapeutic index at clinically useful dosages, cannabinoids are not often used clinically. Particularly in the elderly, they may produce sedation, orthostatic hypotension, ataxia, and hallucinations.

D. Oral mucositis and alimentary tract mucositis

Patients treated for head and neck cancer (HNC) experience unique side effects related to therapy concentrated on the oral cavity. Fifty percent of patients diagnosed with HNC are older than age 60 years.[65] Therapy may be aggressive if applied with curative intent and often results in long-term morbidity. Even for the most stalwart patient, the combination of surgery, radiation, and chemotherapy imposes considerable psychological and physiological demands. All patients, regardless of age, should undergo a thorough psychosocial and health assessment before therapy is begun, and the benefits of difficult treatment must be put into the context of a patient's competing comorbidities.

A dental evaluation is necessary for those who need radiotherapy to the oral cavity. Poor dental hygiene requires remediation, and carious teeth, a potential nidus for infection, should be repaired or removed.

Radiation therapy is an essential component in the management of head and neck cancer. As the concept of organ preservation has become an increasingly important goal and as concurrent chemotherapy has been shown to enhance the efficacy of radiation, its use has become more prevalent. Better treatment outcomes do come at the expense of acute side effects, such as mucositis, which many patients report as the most debilitating aspect of their treatment.[66] In one study, mucositis was observed in 100 percent and grade 3–4 mucositis in 57 percent of patients receiving radiotherapy using an altered fractionation scheme. With conventional fractionation, the incidence of mucositis was 97 percent and grade 3–4 mucositis was 34 percent (Table 29.6).[67]

Table 29.6 World Health Organization Oral Mucositis Assessment Scale.

Grade 0	No symptoms
Grade 1	Soreness and erythema; no ulceration
Grade 2	Erythema, ulcers; swallowing is possible
Grade 3	Extensive erythema, ulcers; swallowing not possible
Grade 4	Alimentation not possible

Note. From World Health Organization.[114]

Oral mucositis from radiotherapy typically peaks at 5 weeks and resolves at 8–12 weeks.[68] The influence of age on mucositis is not readily found in the literature. In one study, the adjusted risk of oral mucositis for patients who received radiation for HNC was less in the elderly; the octogenarians had the lowest risk of oral mucositis, perhaps because they received less aggressive radiotherapy.[69] In a recent retrospective study of French patients with HNC aged 80 years or more, the poor survival of patients was thought to be the result of suboptimal treatment – a failure to treat definitively to achieve durable locoregional control. The authors of the study concluded that concurrent chemoradiotherapy can be applied successfully, at least in a subset of older patients, after careful geriatric evaluation.[70]

Treatment for HNC may be interrupted or discontinued for pain or secondary infection, commonly *Candida albicans* and HSV-1.[71] Malnutrition from a poor diet may be present before treatment and will worsen, inevitably, if the patient suffers from a painful or obstructive disease affecting the upper aerodigestive tract. Most HNC patients lose weight during treatment (Table 29.7).[72] A nutritionist can be helpful in assessing the patient's nutritional needs and recommending a diet and dietary supplements. The importance of hydration and nourishment must be emphasized. One-third of patients rely temporarily on tube feeding or total parenteral nutrition (TPN) for nourishment. The need for tube feedings may be permanent if there is a significant change in architecture of the oral cavity leading to impaired swallowing and risk of aspiration or if the patient is left with a permanent tracheostomy. A feeding tube may be frustrating

Table 29.7 Factors contributing to weight loss in the head and neck cancer patient.

Dysphagia
Odynophagia
Poor dentition or poorly fitting dentures
Sialorrhea
Xerostomia
Thickened secretions
Altered taste
Altered sensation
Mucositis
Lack of supportive caregiver
Financial considerations
Gastrostomy tube feeding

or hard to manipulate, particularly in the elderly, who may lack manual dexterity. Furthermore, there are psychological and social costs associated with an inability to eat normally.[73] Eating plays an important part in social interactions, which are important in any age group and especially in the elderly. Radiation-induced trismus may interfere with communication, mastication, and oral hygiene. Secretions and saliva may pool in patients' mouths, and they may drool and need to spit often. On the other hand, xerostomia may result from long-term radiation damage to salivary glands if salivary tissue is irradiated. Permanent xerostomia may be the most prevalent late consequence of radiotherapy for HNC and a major cause of alteration in taste and consequent weight loss. Swallowing is difficult when food is not moistened properly. The preceding complications may be more pronounced in the elderly patient, who is more likely to have had swallowing dysfunction before treatment because of neural and muscular changes associated with aging such as insufficient lubrication, decreased strength of mastication, poor bolus control, and delayed swallowing.[74] There is conflicting evidence about the efficacy of amifostine in preventing xerostomia, but it has FDA approval for this indication.[75,76]

Transdermal preparations, liquid morphine, or oxycodone that can be absorbed from the oral mucosa or put easily through a gastrostomy tube are good options to treat pain from mucositis. Some of these preparations contain alcohol and sting when used. Nonalcohol preparations may be preferred. Lorazepam, which also comes as a liquid, may be helpful if the patient gags on pooled secretions. Anticholinergics such as hyoscyamine to dry secretions ought to be used cautiously in the older patient because of constipation, urinary retention, and delirium.[77] Patients learn to suck on ice chips, sip water, and use artificial saliva for hyposalivation.[78] Guidelines for effective oral hygiene include brushing with a soft brush twice daily and rinsing with bland rinses and oral moisturizers such as saline, water, and sodium bicarbonate. Mobility of the pharyngoesophageal tract ought to be maintained even if a temporary G-tube is used for sustenance; it is good practice for the patient to attempt taking small quantities of soft food or liquid to prevent pharyngeal or esophageal stenosis and an upper digestive tract that does not work. The speech pathologist is instrumental in helping diagnose problems, rehabilitating swallowing, and recommending food consistencies

Table 29.8 Chemotherapy likely to cause mucositis.

Bleomycin
Busulfan
Cytarabine
Doxorubicin
Etoposide
5-Fluorouracil
Methotrexate
Platinum coordination complexes including cisplatin and carboplatin

Note. Adapted from Peterson et al.[115]

such as a safe bolus size and other practical strategies to prevent aspiration and improve bolus transport.

Mucositis is not limited to those patients undergoing localized therapy for HNC. Systemic chemotherapy causing mucositis may begin in the oral cavity and continue along the alimentary tract (Tables 29.8 and 29.9). Diarrhea has already been discussed. The incidence of mucositis is high for particular conditioning regimens for hematopoietic stem cell transplant, even reduced-intensity or autologous regimens commonly applied in older patients, and for induction therapy for leukemia (85%).[79] Oral and esophageal mucositis can complicate multicycle chemotherapy for lymphoma (3–10%) and solid tumors such as breast cancer. Mucositis is observed in 3–9 percent of patients undergoing standard doxorubicin-based and taxane-based therapy.[80]

In GI malignancies, older age was shown to be a risk factor for mucositis in patients receiving 5-FU for colon cancer. In one study comparing raltitrexed and 5-FU according to the Mayo Clinic regimen, toxicity from stomatitis was 11 percent for those patients less than 60 years, 26 percent for those 60–69 years, and 36 percent for those over 69 years.[81] Because of this toxicity, most oncologists do not choose the Mayo Clinic regimen for 5-FU administration.

In non-small-cell lung cancer (NSCLC), survival of patients with inoperable, locally advanced disease is improved with concurrent radiation and platinum-based chemotherapy. In one study, older patients received sequential chemotherapy and daily radiotherapy, concurrent chemotherapy plus daily radiotherapy, or concurrent chemotherapy plus twice-daily radiotherapy. One-sixth of those studied were 70 years of age or older. Of those patients who received concurrent therapy, grade 3 esophagitis was significantly more common in elderly patients. However, the median survival time in the elderly patients was more favorable in patients who received concurrent therapy, and there was no difference in long-term toxicity. The authors concluded that fit elderly patients with stage III NSCLC are candidates for combined-modality therapy, acknowledging that selection bias is likely more pronounced in the elderly.[82]

Table 29.9 Updated guidelines for management of patients with oral mucositis.

Basic oral care: Regular use of soft toothbrush Assess oral cavity health and make use of dental professionals PCA with opioid in patients undergoing hematopoietic stem cell transplant	
Radiotherapy (prevention of OM): Midline radiation blocks and 3-D radiation treatment Benzydamine for moderate-dose radiation (recommendation was not unanimous)	Do not use chlorhexidine in HNC Do not use antimicrobial lozenges
Radiotherapy (treatment):	Do not use sucralfate
Standard dose chemotherapy (prevention): 30 minutes of ice chips for patients receiving bolus 5-FU or edatrexate	Do not use acyclovir
Standard-dose chemotherapy (treatment): High-dose chemotherapy with or without TBI plus HCT (prevention): Keratinocyte growth factor–1 (palifermin) 60 mg/kg/d for 3 days before conditioning and 3 days after autologous transplant Ice chips for patients receiving high-dose melphalan Low-level laser therapy before HCT if treatment center offers it	Do not use chlorhexidine Do not use pentoxifylline Do not use GM-CSF mouthwash

Note. HCT = Hematopoietic Cell Transplantation; HNC = Head and Neck Cancer; OM = oral mucositis; PCA =;Patient controlled analgesia; TBI = Total body irradiation. From Keefe et al.[80]

Acute radiation esophagitis, not to be confused with candidal esophagitis, causes thinning and, in severe cases, denudation of the epithelial mucosa. It manifests as dysphagia, odynophagia, and substernal pain and resolves with regeneration of the basal epithelium, which occurs about 3 weeks after radiation is completed.[83] Acute esophagitis is frequently managed with topical anesthetics, analgesics, and antacids. Narcotics can be used for moderate to severe pain that is not relieved by topical agents to maintain adequate hydration and calorie intake. The late effects of radiation, which may occur 3 or more months after radiotherapy, are due to chronic inflammation and fibrosis within the esophagus and may lead to altered peristalsis and stricture. The latter complication may require endoscopic dilation.

Abdominal or pelvic radiotherapy can cause enteritis in about 50 percent of patients, with cramping and diarrhea as prominent symptoms. Concurrent chemotherapy may add toxicity.[84] Late radiation effects typically manifest months to years later and are caused by an obliterative endarteritis that leads to intestinal ischemia and subsequent ulceration, bleeding, fibrosis, stricture, and obstruction. The patient may experience rapid transit though the bowel, diarrhea, malabsorption, and weight loss. Bacterial overgrowth, which may also lead to malabsorption and cause lactose intolerance, can be diagnosed by breath test; effective treatment may require cycling of antibiotics. Rifaximin, an antibiotic that is not absorbed, is a good choice, particularly in the elderly, as it minimizes the adverse effects seen with systemic antibiotics.

The large intestine is believed to be less radiosensitive than the small intestine. When acute radiation injury does involve the colon or rectum, symptoms include diarrhea, tenesmus, urgency, and bleeding. Approximately 80 percent of rectal cancers occur in the elderly.[85] Meta-analyses show that preoperative radiotherapy significantly improves local control.[86] A review examining practices for managing elderly rectal cancer patients determined that neoadjuvant regimens are much more commonly delivered to younger patients.[87] The conclusion that reasonably healthy elderly patients do not tolerate pelvic radiotherapy as well as younger patients is not well substantiated.[88,89] Two retrospective studies of rectal cancer in elderly patients aged 70 years or older suggested that the elderly can tolerate chemotherapy and radiation followed by surgery. The most common side effect was diarrhea, which

occurred in 82 percent and 49 percent of the patients in two similar studies, but with almost no grade 3–4 toxicity.[90,91] The authors cautiously note that patients with few comorbidities and better performance status had better survival. There is limited evidence for benefit associated with the use of amifostine, the free radical scavenger, to prevent acute radiation injury; it is recommended in recent practice guidelines.[92,93] It is not often used because of its cumbersome application and often intolerable side effects but may be worth considering for the high-risk patient. Sulfasalazine may also protect the patient from radiation proctitis.[94]

The most common cause of radiation injury to the rectum is treatment of prostate cancer, which generally uses higher doses of radiation compared to other pelvic malignancies and affects the anterior rectal wall. Modifications in radiation technique and dose have been employed to reduce its morbidity. Acute toxicity is treated supportively, as outlined earlier. Late complications often occur after a year or more and consist of rectal bleeding, incontinence, nocturnal bowel movements, and mucous discharge. Rarely, a patient develops ulcers, persistent incontinence, fistulas, and rectal wall breakdown requiring colostomy. Toxicity outcomes in a phase I dose-escalation study by the Radiation Therapy Oncology Group, which included elderly patients up to 87 years, were as follows: the incidence rate of rectal bleeding greater than or equal to grade 2 was 12 percent; proctitis greater than or equal to grade 2 was 7 percent; and diarrhea grade 2–3 was 3 percent. The prevalence of incontinence, ulcers, and the need for colostomy was less than 1 percent.[95] Most late complications ought to be treated supportively with sitz baths, steroid suppositories, and sucralfate enemas; surgery should be avoided, if possible, but may be a preferred solution in some patients with severe dysfunction. There is limited evidence for hyperbaric oxygen treatment and laser coagulation therapy for persistent bleeding not amenable to a conservative approach.[96,97]

E. Neutropenic enterocolitis

Neutropenic enterocolitis, also known as typhlitis, occurs primarily in immunosuppressed patients such as those with hematologic malignancies and those receiving aggressive systemic chemotherapy therapy for solid malignancies.[98,99] In the elderly, who may experience an age-related decline in bone marrow function, neutropenia sometimes occurs with chemotherapy that in general does not cause neutropenia in younger patients. Impaired defense to invasion by microorganisms because of neutropenia leads to microbial infection with enteric bacteria or fungus and necrosis of the bowel wall. The cecum is almost always involved, with symptoms mimicking appendicitis. There is usually marked diarrhea that can be bloody. Symptoms often appear about 2 weeks after cytotoxic chemotherapy, concomitant with neutropenia.[100] Stomatitis may also be present, suggesting widespread mucositis. Evaluation includes ultrasound or computerized tomography and blood and stool cultures. Treatment consists of a combination of antibiotics, antifungals, and supportive care – bowel rest, IV fluids, and possibly a trickle of enteral feeding to maintain gut integrity. Parenteral feeding may also be necessary. Neutropenic enterocolitis complicated by peritonitis, perforation, or severe bleeding may require surgery to remove necrotic or perforated bowel to prevent death. Anticholinergic, antidiarrheal, and opioid agents will aggravate ileus, but sometimes severe pain requires judicious use of opioid analgesics. Granulocyte colony-stimulating factor may be helpful if neutropenia is prolonged, but in most cases it will not speed recovery of neutrophil counts once neutropenia is established.

F. Graft-versus-host disease

Historically, allogeneic transplant has been a therapeutic approach that is less commonly offered to the elderly with diseases such as acute myeloid leukemia and myelodysplastic syndrome – although it is the best established curative therapy – because of concerns about toxicity and poor outcome. Over the last decade, with advances in therapy and supportive care, the number of elderly considered for such therapy has been growing. In our institution, fit 65-year-olds are routinely considered for transplant, and older patients are evaluated on a case-by-case basis. Graft-versus-host disease (GVHD) is a complication in 50 percent of allogeneic transplants. Earlier studies suggested that increasing age predicted its development, but current experience does not. In fact, a new study of nonmyeloablative hematopoietic stem cell transplant in older adults demonstrated no statistically significant differences in transplant-related mortality across age cohorts (40 to over 65 years of age) and no overall difference in occurrence of acute or chronic GVHD.[101–103]

The gastrointestinal tract and liver are commonly affected in both acute and chronic GVHD.

Symptoms of gastrointestinal GVHD include nausea and vomiting; severe abdominal pain and cramping; copious, watery diarrhea; malabsorption; obstruction; esophageal webbing; xerostomia; oral ulcers; dysphagia; hyperbilirubinemia; and transaminitis. Oral ulcers can be treated supportively with tacrolimus ointments and steroid rinses and dry mouth with salivary stimulants. Dilation effectively treats esophageal webbing and stricture. Pancreatic enzymes and a lactase-free diet help prevent malabsorption, a condition that can prevent important oral medications from being properly absorbed. GVHD may require long-term suppression of antigen-presenting cells and T cells, leading to absolute or functional lymphopenia and risk for infection.[104,105]

Obvious causes of acute diarrhea, which include antibiotic therapy side effects and infection by *Clostridium difficile*, among a large number of other pathogens, will not be reviewed in this chapter.

Surgery for cancer can also result in mechanical, functional, and physiological alterations to normal bowel function, leading to diarrhea by increasing transit time, causing dumping syndrome, bile salt deficiency, fat malabsorption, lactose intolerance, and bacterial overgrowth. The clinician must evaluate the elderly patient without delay and begin treating for such problems to avoid dehydration, malnutrition, and functional loss.

G. Conclusions

Supportive interventions must be expeditiously prescribed in the elderly, who are particularly susceptible to serious consequences of therapy. In the geriatric cancer population, it is often the side effects that undermine a patient's already reduced functional reserve or limit the application of effective therapy. Frequent assessment of an elderly patient's tolerance of therapy may avoid poor outcomes. As we abandon preconceptions about the ability of the elderly to endure chemotherapy, radiotherapy, and surgery based on age alone, we must learn to use the tools of supportive oncology adeptly. From a wider perspective, delivering excellent supportive care may also help conserve finite health care resources by preventing emergency visits and hospitalizations. Although there have been therapeutic breakthroughs in supportive care, particularly in antiemetic therapy, there is still much to learn in symptom management in the elderly cancer patient.

References

1. Leichman CG, Fleming TR, Muggia FM, et al. Phase II study of fluorouracil and its modulation in advanced colorectal cancer: a Southwest Oncology Group study. *J Clin Oncol*. 1995;13(6): 1303–1311.

2. Rothenberg ML, Eckardt JR, Kuhn JG, et al. Phase II trial of irinotecan in patients with progressive or rapidly recurrent colorectal cancer. *J Clin Oncol*. 1996;14(4):1128–1135.

3. Sobrero AF, Aschele C, Bertino JR. Fluorouracil in colorectal cancer – a tale of two drugs: implications for biochemical modulation. *J Clin Oncol*. 1997;15(1):368–381.

4. Mini E, Trave F, Rustum YM, et al. Enhancement of the antitumor effects of 5-fluorouracil by folinic acid. *Pharmacol Ther*. 1990;47(1):1–19.

5. Petrelli N, Douglass Jr HO, Herrera L, et al. The modulation of fluorouracil with leucovorin in metastatic colorectal carcinoma: a prospective randomized phase III trial. Gastrointestinal Tumor Study Group. *J Clin Oncol*. 1989;7(10):1419–26. Erratum, *J Clin Oncol* 1990;8(1):185.

6. Chiara S, Nobile MT, Vincenti M. Advanced colorectal cancer in the elderly: results of consecutive trials with 5 flourouracil-based chemotherapy. *Cancer Chemother Pharmacol*. 1998;42:336–340.

7. Sargent D, Goldberg, R, Jacobson S, et al. A pooled analysis of adjuvant chemotherapy for resected colon cancer in elderly patients. *New Engl J Med*. 2001;345:1091–1097.

8. Goldberg RM, Tabah-Fisch I, Bleiberg H. Pooled analysis of safety and efficacy of oxaliplatin plus fluorouracil/leucovorin administered bi-monthly in elderly patients with colorectal cancer. *J Clin Oncol*. 2006;24:4085–4091.

9. Haller DG, Catalano PJ, Macdonald JS, et al. Phase II study of fluorouracil, leucovorin and lavamisole in high-risk stage II and III colon cancer: final report of Intergroup 0089. *J Clin Oncol*. 2005;23:8671–8678.

10. Folprecht G, Cunningham D, Ross P, et al. Efficacy of 5-fluorouracil-based chemotherapy in elderly patients with metastatic colorectal cancer: a pooled analysis of clinical trials. *Ann Oncol*. 2004;15:1330–1338.

11. Sloan JA, Goldberg RM, Sargent DJ, et al. Women experience greater toxicity with fluorouracil-based chemotherapy for colorectal cancer. *J Clin Oncol*. 2002;20(6):1491–1498.

12. Balducci L, Extermann, M. Cancer chemotherapy in the older patient. *Cancer*. 1997;80(7):1317–1322.

13. Bajetta E, Procopio G, Celio L, et al. Safety and efficacy of two different doses of capecitabine in the treatment of advanced breast cancer in older women. *J Clin Oncol*. 2005;23(10):2155–2161.

14. Twelves C, Wong A, Nowacki MP. Capecitabine as adjuvant treatment for stage III colon cancer. *N Engl J Med* 2005;352(26):2692–2704.

15. Sharma R, Rivory L, Beale P, et al. A phase II study of fixed dose capecitabine and assessment of predictors of toxicity in patients with advanced metastatic colorectal cancer. *Br J Cancer*. 2006;94:964–968.

16. Sonis ST. A biological approach to mucositis. *J Support Oncol*. 2004;2(1):21–32; discussion 35–36.

17. Fuchs CS, Moore MR, Harker G, et al. Phase III comparison of two irinotecan dosing regimens in second-line therapy of metastatic colorectal cancer. *J Clin Oncol*. 2003;21(5):807–814.

18. Sastre J, Marcuello E, Masutti B, et al. Cooperative Group for the Treatment of Digestive Tumors. Irinotecan in combination with fluorouracil in a 48-hour continuous infusion as first-line chemotherapy for elderly patients with metastatic colorectal cancer: a Spanish Cooperative Group for the Treatment of Digestive Tumors study. *J Clin Oncol*. 2005;23(15):3545–3551.

19. Souglakos J, Pallis A, Kakolyris S, et al. Combination of irinotecan plus 5 fluorouracil and leucovorin (FOLFIRI regimen) as first line treatment for elderly patients with metastatic colorectal cancer: a phase II trial. *Oncology*. 2005;69:384–390.

20. Saltz LB, Cox JV, Blanke C, et al. Irinotecan plus fluorouracil and leucovorin for metastatic colorectal cancer. *Irinotecan Study Group*. *N Engl J Med*. 2000;343:905–914.

21. Rothenberg ML, Meropol NJ, Poplin EA, et al. Mortality associated with irinotecan plus bolus fluorouracil/leucovorin: summary findings of an independent panel. *J Clin Oncol*. 2001;19:3801–3807.

22. Porschen R, Bermann A, Löffler T, et al. Fluorouracil plus leucovorin as effective adjuvant chemotherapy in curatively resected stage III colon cancer: results of the trial adjCCA-01. *J Clin Oncol*. 2001;19:1787–1794.

23. Wolmark N, Rockette H, Mamounas E, et al. Clinical trial to assess the relative efficacy of fluorouracil and leucovorin, fluorouracil and levamisole, and fluorouracil, leucovorin, and levamisole in patients with Dukes' B and C carcinoma of the colon: results from National Surgical Adjuvant Breast and Bowel Project C-04. *J Clin Oncol*. 1999;17:3553–3559.

24. Messersmith WA, Laheru DA, Senzer NN, et al. Phase I trial of irinotecan, infusional 5-fluorouracil, and leucovorin (FOLFIRI) with erlotinib (OSI-774): early termination due to

increased toxicities. *Clin Cancer Res.* 2004;10(19):6522–6527.

25. Czito BG, Willett CG, Bendell JC. Increased toxicity with gefitinib, capecitabine, and radiation therapy in pancreatic and rectal cancer: phase I trial results. *J Clin Oncol.* 2006;24(4):656–662.

26. Benson III AB, Ajani JA, Catalano RB, et al. Recommended guidelines for the treatment of cancer treatment-induced diarrhea. *J Clin Oncol.* 2004;22(14):2918–2926.

27. Hanani M, Fellig Y, Udassin R, et al. Age-related changes in the morphology of the myenteric plexus of the human colon. *Auton Neurosci.* 2004;113:71–78.

28. Higgins PD, Johanson JF. Epidemiology of constipation in North America: a systemic review. *Am J Gastroenterol.* 2004;99:750–759.

29. Sykes NP. The relationship between opioid use and laxative use in terminally ill cancer patients. *Palliative Med.* 1998;12(5):375–382.

30. De Luca A, Coupar IM. Insights into opioid action in the intestinal tract. *Pharmacol Ther.* 1996;69(2):103–115.

31. Clark AJ, Ahmedzai SH, Allan LG, et al. Efficacy and safety of transdermal fentanyl and sustained-release oral morphine in patients with cancer and chronic non-cancer pain. *Curr Med Res Opin.* 2004;20(9):1419–1428.

32. Staats PS, Markowitz J, Schein J. Incidence of constipation associated with long-acting opioid therapy: a comparative study. *South Med J.* 2004;97(2):129–134.

33. Plummer JL, Gourlay GK, Cherry DA, et al. Estimation of methadone clearance: applications in the management of cancer pain. *Pain* 1988;33:313–322.

34. Goodman M, Low J, Wilkinson S. Constipation management in palliative care: a survey of practices in the United Kingdom. *J Pain Symptom Manage.* 2005;29:238–244.

35. GlaxoSmithKline. Zofran (ondansetron)–package insert. Research Triangle Park, NC; 2009.

36. Legha SS. Vincristine neurotoxicity: pathophysiology and management. *Med Toxicol.* 1986;1:421–427.

37. Millennium Pharmaceuticals Inc. Velcade (bortezomib) [package insert]. Cambridge, MA; 2007.

38. Celgene Corporation. Revlimid (lenalidomide) [package insert]. Summit, NJ; 2007.

39. Celgene Corporation. Thalomid (thalidomide) [package insert]. Summit, NJ; 2007.

40. Richmond JP, Wright ME. Review of the literature on constipation to enable development of a constipation risk assessment scale. *Clin Eff Nurs.* 2004;8:11–25.

41. Tuteja AK, Talley NJ, Joos SK, et al. Is constipation associated with decreased physical activity in normally active subjects? *Am J Gastroenterol.* 2005;100:124–129.

42. Meshkinpour H, Selod S, Movahedi H. Effects of regular exercise in management of chronic idiopathic constipation. *Dig Dis Sci.* 1998;43(11):2379–2383.

43. Jones MP, Talley NJ, Nuyts G. Lack of objective evidence of efficacy of laxatives in chronic constipation. *Dig Dis Sci.* 2002;47 2222–2230.

44. American College of Gastroenterology Chronic Constipation Task Force. An evidence-based approach to the management of chronic constipation in North America. *Am J Gastroenterol.* 2005;100(suppl 1):S1–S4.

45. Ramkumar D, Rao SS. Efficacy and safety of traditional medical therapies for chronic constipation: systematic review. *Am J Gastroenterol.* 2005;100:936–971.

46. Thomas J, Karver S, Cooney GA, et al. Methylnaltrexone for opioid-induced constipation in advanced illness. *N Engl J Med.* 2008;358(22):2332–2343.

47. Pollera CF, Giannarelli D. Prognostic factors influencing cisplatin-induced emesis: definition and validation of a predictive logistic model. *Cancer.* 1989;64:1117–1122.

48. Roila F, Tonato M, Basurto C. Protection from nausea and vomiting in cisplatin-treated patient: high dose metoclopramide combined with methylprednisolone versus metoclopramide combined with dexamethasone and diphenhydramine: a study of the Italian Oncology Group for Clinical Research. *J Clin Oncol.* 1989;7:1693–1700.

49. D'Acquisto R, Tyson LB, Gralla RJ, et al. The influence of chronic high alcohol intake on chemotherapy induced nausea and vomiting. *Proc Am Soc Clin Oncol.* 1986;5:257.

50. Kris MG, Gralla RJ, Clark RA. Incidence, course, and severity of delayed nausea and vomiting following administration of high-dose cisplatin. *J Clin Oncol.* 1985;3:1379–1384.

51. Miller AD, Bianchi AL, Bishop BP, eds. *Neural Control of the Respiratory Muscles.* Boca Raton, FL: CRC Press; 1997:239–248.

52. Andrews PL, Rudd JA. Mechanisms of acute, delayed, and anticipatory emesis induced by anticancer therapies. In: Hesketh P, ed. *Management of Nausea and Vomiting in Cancer and Cancer Treatment.* Boston: Jones and Bartlett; 2005:15–66.

53. Miller AD. Central mechanisms of vomiting. *Dig Dis Sci.* 1999;44(suppl):39S–43S.

54. Hornby PJ. Central neurocircuitry associated with emesis. *Am J Med.* 2001;111(suppl 8A):106S–112S.

55. Hesketh, P. Chemotherapy-induced nausea and vomiting. *N Engl J Med.* 2008;358(23): 2482–2494.

56. Olver IN, Wolf M, Laidlaw C, et al. A randomised double-blind study of high-dose intravenous prochlorperazine versus high-dose metoclopramide as antiemetics for cancer chemotherapy. *Eur J Cancer.* 1992;28A(11):1798–1802.

57. Kris MG, Tyson LB, Gralla RJ, et al. Extrapyramidal reactions with high-dose metoclopramide. *N Engl J Med.* 1983;309(7):433–434.

58. Hickok JT, Roscoe JA, Morrow GR, et al. 5-Hydroxytryptamine-receptor antagonists versus prochlorperazine for control of delayed nausea caused by doxorubicin: a URCC CCOP randomised controlled trial. *Lancet Oncol.* 2005;6:765–772.

59. Aapro MS, Macciocchi A, Gridelli C. Palonosetron improves prevention of chemotherapy-induced nausea and vomiting in elderly patients. *J Support Oncol.* 2005;5:369–74.

60. Carpenter DO, Briggs DB, Strominger N. Responses of neurons of canine area postrema to neurotransmitters and peptides. *Cell Mol Neurobiol.* 1983;3:113–126.

61. Emend [package insert], Whitehouse Station (NY): Merck Pharmaceuticals Corp; 2005

62. Warr DG, Hesketh PJ, Gralla RJ, et al. Efficacy and tolerability of aprepitant for the prevention of chemotherapy-induced nausea and vomiting in patients with breast cancer after moderately emetogenic chemotherapy. *J Clin Oncol.* 2005;23:2822–2830.

63. Kris MG, Hesketh PJ, Somerfield MR, et al. American Society of Clinical Oncology guideline for antiemetics in oncology: update 2006. *J Clin Oncol.* 2006;24:2932–2947. Erratum, *J Clin Oncol.* 2006;24:5341–5342.

64. Ioannidis JP, Hesketh PJ, Lau J. Contribution of dexamethasone to control of chemotherapy-induced nausea and vomiting: a meta-analysis of randomized evidence. *J Clin Oncol.* 2000;18:3409–3422.

65. Hoffman HT, Karnell LH, Funk GF. The National Cancer Data Base report on cancer of the head and neck. *Arch Otolaryngol Head Neck Surg.* 1998;124(9):951–962.

66. Bellm L, Epstein J, Rose-Ped A. Patient reports of complications of bone marrow transplantation. *Support Care Cancer.* 2000;8:33–39.

67. Trotti A, Bellm L, Epstein J. Mucositis incidence, severity and associated outcomes in patients with head and neck cancer receiving radiotherapy with or without chemotherapy: a systemic literature review. *Radiat Oncol.* 203;66:253–262.

68. Elting L, Cooksley C, Chambers M. Risk, outcome, and costs of radiation-induced oral mucositis among patients with head-and-neck malignancies. *Int J Radiat Oncol Biol Phys.* 2007;68:1110–1120.

69. Vera-Llonch M, Oster G, Hagiwara M. Oral mucositis in patients undergoing radiation treatment for head and neck carcinoma. *Cancer.* 2006;106:329–336.

70. Italiano A, Ortholan C, Dassonville O, et al. Head and neck squamous cell carcinoma in patients aged > or = 80 years: patterns of care and survival. *Cancer.* 2008;113(11):3160–3168.

71. Sonis, ST. The pathobiology of mucositis. *Nat Rev Cancer.* 2004;4:277–284.

72. Murphy B. Clinical and economic consequences of mucositis induced by chemotherapy and/or radiation therapy. *J Support Oncol.* 2007;5: 13–21.

73. Cooper JS, Pajak TF, Forastiere AA, et al. Postoperative concurrent radiotherapy and chemotherapy for high-risk squamous-cell carcinoma of the head and neck. *N Engl J Med.* 2004;350(19):1937–1944.

74. Shindler JS, Kelly JH. Swallowing disorders in the elderly. *Laryngoscope.* 2002;112(4):589–602.

75. Gosselin TK, Raj KA, Clough RW, et al. Amifostine for xerostomia – normal tissue protection at what cost? [abstract]. *Int J Radiat Oncol Biol Phys.* 2005;63(suppl 1):S128.

76. Wasserman TH, Brizel DM, Henke M, et al. Influence of intravenous amifostine on xerostomia, tumor control, and survival after radiotherapy for head-and-neck cancer: 2-year follow-up of a prospective, randomized, phase III trial. *Int J Radiat Oncol Biol Phys.* 2005;63(4):985–990.

77. Agnosti JV, Leo-Summers LS, Inouye SK. Cognitive and other adverse effects of diphenhydramine use in hospitalized older patients. *Arch Intern Med.* 2001;161(17):2091–2097.

78. Brosky ME. The role of saliva in oral health: strategies for prevention and management of xerostomia. *J Support Oncol.* 2007;5(5): 215–225.

79. Sonis ST, Oster G, Fuchs H, et al. Oral mucositis and the clinical and economic outcomes of hematopoietic stem-cell transplantation. *J Clin Oncol.* 2001;19(8):2201–2205.

80. Keefe D, Schubert M, Etling L. Updated clinical practice guidelines for the prevention and treatment of mucositis. *Cancer.* 2007;109(5):820–831.

81. Zalcberg J, Kerr D, Seymour L, et al. Haematological and non-haematological toxicity

after 5-fluorouracil and leucovorin in patients with advanced colorectal cancer is significantly associated with gender, increasing age and cycle number. Tomudex International Study Group. *Eur J Cancer*. 1998;34(12):1871–1875.

82. Langer CJ, Hsu C, Curran WJ, et al. Elderly patients with locally advanced non-small cell lung cancer benefit from combined modality therapy: secondary analysis of Radiation Therapy Oncology Group (RTOG) 94-10 [abstract]. *Proc Am Soc Clin Oncol*. 2002;21:299a.

83. O'Rourke IC, Tiver K, Bull C, et al. Swallowing performance after radiation therapy for carcinoma of the esophagus. *Cancer*. 1988;61:2022–2026.

84. Miller RC, Martenson JA, Sargent DJ, et al. Acute treatment-related diarrhea during postoperative adjuvant therapy for high-risk rectal carcinoma. *Int J Radiat Oncol Biol Phys*. 1998;41: 593–598.

85. Martijn H, Vulto JC. Should radiotherapy be avoided or delivered differently in elderly patients with rectal cancer? *Eur J Cancer*. 2007;43:2301–2306.

86. Cammà C, Giunta M, Fiorica F, et al. Preoperative radiotherapy for resectable rectal cancer: a meta-analysis. *J Am Med Assoc*. 2000;284(8):1008–1015.

87. Pignon T, Horiot JC, Bolla M, et al. Age is not a limiting factor for radical radiotherapy in pelvic malignancies. *Radiother Oncol*. 1997;42:107–120.

88. Fiorica F, Cartei F, Carau B, et al. Adjuvant radiotherapy on older and oldest elderly rectal cancer patients. *Arch Gerontol Geriatr*. 2009;49:54–59.

89. Lorchel F, Peignaux K, Créhange G, et al. Preoperative radiotherapy in elderly patients with rectal cancer. *Gastroenterol Clin Biol*. 2007;31(4):436–441.

90. Athanassiou H, Antonadou D, Coliarakis N, et al. Oncology Hellenic Group. Protective effect of amifostine during fractionated radiotherapy in patients with pelvic carcinomas: results of a randomized trial. *Int J Radiat Oncol Biol Phys*. 2003;56(4):1154–1160.

91. Kilic D, Egehan I, Ozenirler S, et al. Double-blinded, randomized, placebo-controlled study to evaluate the effectiveness of sulphasalazine in preventing acute gastrointestinal complications due to radiotherapy. *Radiother Oncol*. 2000;57:125–129.

92. Michalski JM, Winter K, Purdy JA, et al. Toxicity after three dimensional radiotherapy for prostate cancer on RTOG 9406 dose level V, *Int J Radiat Oncol Biol Phys*. 2005;62:706–713.

93. Villaviecencio RT, Rex DK, Rahmani E. Argon plasma coagulation as first line treatment for chronic proctopathy. *J Gastroenterol Hepatol*. 2004;19(10):1169–1173.

94. Dall'Era MA, Hampson NB, Hsi RA, et al. Hyperbaric oxygen therapy for radiation induced proctopathy in men treated for prostate cancer. *J Urol*. 2006;176:87–90.

95. Rolston KV, Bodey GP, Safdar A. Polymicrobial infection in patients with cancer: an underappreciated and underreported entity. *Clin Infect Dis*. 2007;45:228–233.

96. Davila ML. Neutropenic enterocolitis. *Curr Opin Gastroenterol*. 2006;22:44–47.

97. Schnoll-Sussman F, Kurtz RC. Gastrointestinal emergencies in the critically ill cancer patient. *Semin Oncol*. 2000;27:270–283.

98. Przepiorka D, Anderlini P, Saliba R, et al. Chronic graft versus host disease after allogeneic blood stem cell transplantation. *Blood*. 2001;98:1695–1700.

99. Storb R, Prentice RL, Sullivan KM, et al. Predictive factors in chronic graft-versus-host disease in patients with aplastic anemia treated by marrow transplantation from HLA-identical siblings. *Ann Intern Med*. 1983;98(4):461–466.

100. McClune B, Weisdorf DJ, DiPersio JF, et al. Non-myeloablative hematopoietic stem cell transplantation in older patients with AML and MDS: results from the Center for International Blood and Marrow Transplant Research (CIBMTR). *Blood* [abstract]. *ASH Annu Meet Abstr*. 2008;112:346.

101. McDonald GB, Shulman HM, Sullivan KM, et al. Intestinal and hepatic complications of human bone marrow transplantation. Part I. *Gastroenterology*. 1986;90(2):460–477.

102. Herrmann VM, Petruska PJ. Nutrition support in bone marrow transplant recipients. *Nutr Clin Pract*. 1993;8(1):19–27.

103. Mercadante S. Diarrhea in terminally ill patients: pathophysiology and treatment. *J Pain Symptom Manage*. 1995;10(4):298–309.

104. McDonald GB, Shulman HM, Sullivan KM, et al. Intestinal and hepatic complications of human bone marrow transplantation. Part I. *Gastroenterology*. 1986;90(2):460–477.

105. Herrmann VM, Petruska PJ. Nutrition support in bone marrow transplant recipients. *Nutr Clin Pract*. 1993;8(1):19–27.

106. Clark JW, Eder JP, Ryan D, et al. Safety and pharmacokinetics of the dual action Raf kinase and vascular endothelial growth factor receptor inhibitor, BAY 43-9006, in patients with advanced, refractory solid tumors. *Clin Cancer Res*. 2005;11(15):5472–5480.

107. Deininger MW, O'Brien SG, Ford JM, et al. Practical management of patients with chronic

myeloid leukemia receiving imatinib. *J Clin Oncol.* 2003;21(8):1637–1647.

108. Moy B, Goss PE. Lapatinib-associated toxicity and practical management recommendations. *Oncologist.* 2007;12(7):756–765.

109. Kane RC, Bross PF, Farrell AT, et al. Velcade: U.S. FDA approval for the treatment of multiple myeloma progressing on prior therapy. *Oncologist.* 2003;8(6):508–513.

110. Accessed 12/04/08: http://www.gene.com/ gene/products/information/pdf/tarceva-prescribing.pdf.

111. Hanna N, Lilenbaum R, Ansari R, et al. Phase II trial of cetuximab in patients with previously treated non-small-cell lung cancer. *J Clin Oncol.* 2006;24(33):5253–5258.

112. Van Cutsem E, Peeters M, Siena S, et al. Open-label phase III trial of panitumumab plus best supportive care compared with best supportive care alone in patients with chemotherapy-refractory metastatic colorectal cancer. *J Clin Oncol.* 2007;25(13):1658–1664.

113. Hesketh PJ, Kris MG, Grunberg SM, et al. Proposal for classifying the acute emetogenicity of cancer chemotherapy. *J Clin Oncol.* 1997;15(1): 103–109.

114. World Health Organization. *WHO Handbook for Reporting Results: Cancer Treatment.* Geneva, Switzerland: World Health Organization, 1979.

115. Peterson DE, Schubert MM. Oral toxicity. In: *The Chemotherapy Source Book.* 3rd ed. Baltimore, MD: Williams and Wilkins, 2001.

Index

419